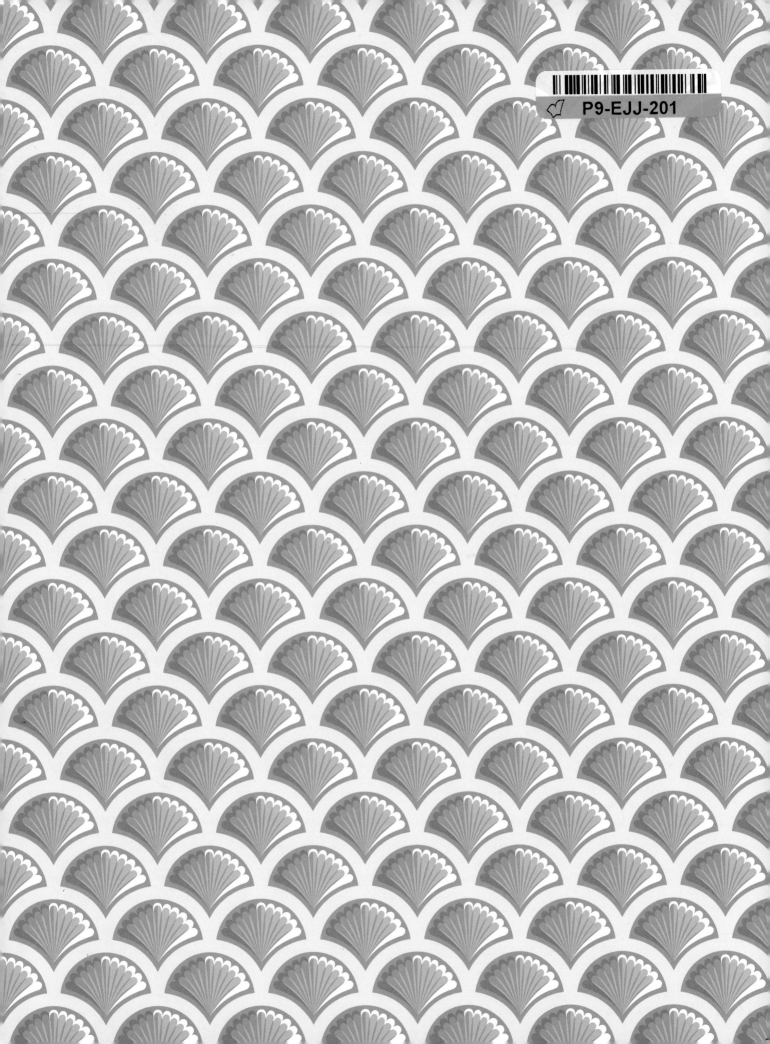

Contents

Letter of Introduction

With its founding in 1847, the American Medical Association (AMA) dedicated itself to promoting the art and science of medicine. This updated edition of the *Code of Medical Ethics (Code)* embodies this commitment in the 21st century, as the *Code* has for generations of physicians over the past 169 years. Today, as when it was first adopted, the *Code* serves two key ends in medicine: it articulates the values that ground the profession and sets out the expectations to which physicians should be held in their roles as healers, educators, scientists, and leaders in health care organizations and institutions.

In setting out the highest ideals of medical professionalism, the *Code* provides a framework for relationships of trust between patients and their physicians, regardless of specialty or geographic location, and between the profession as a whole and society.

Moreover, the *Code* provides practical guidance for physicians as they confront the challenges of day-to-day practice. Far more than a set of rules to be followed, the *Code*, through the Opinions of the AMA Council on Ethical and Judicial Affairs (Council), helps physicians think through what is at stake as they engage patients and work with colleagues to reach ethically sound decisions in complex situations.

As stewards of the *Code*, the AMA Council undertook the significant project of updating and consolidating this key professional resource to ensure that the *Code of Medical Ethics* continues to fulfill its role well into the future as the ethical touchstone for the profession of medicine. Over the course of eight years, through a rigorous process of review and consultation, the council painstakingly updated previously issued Opinions for timeliness, clarity, and consistency. The final product now features a revised chapter structure, an updated index, and a fresh new look that make guidance easier to find, easier to read, and easier to apply in day-to-day practice.

To address the challenges of 21st-century medicine, the AMA has recently launched major initiatives that span such important areas as improving outcomes for patients, transforming medical education, and nurturing sustainable, high-quality practices. Today, as part of its enduring mission, the AMA is proud to present this next generation's edition of medicine's national professional *Code of Medical Ethics*.

James L. Madara, MD
EXECUTIVE VICE PRESIDENT/ CHIEF EXECUTIVE OFFICER

Patrice A. Harris, MD
CHAIR, BOARD OF TRUSTEES

Andrew W. Gurman, MD
PRESIDENT

Foreword

The most cited 20th-century paper on medical education is Francis Peabody's 1927 "The Care of the Patient."[1] In that paper, Peabody raised two central criticisms of young doctors: that they received inadequate training on how to take care of patients and that their education was primarily in the "impersonal" hospital, so they, therefore, lacked humanity and compassion in caring for patients.

It is worth recalling that in 1847, 80 years before Peabody's article, the American Medical Association (AMA) was founded in response to a national problem of poor standards in medical and professional education. In the 1840s, the quality of medical schools was highly variable, and some schools required only 16 weeks of medical college instruction to qualify as a practicing physician. As a result, many poorly trained physicians were providing low-quality, inadequate, and "unprofessional" care to patients.

With leadership from Dr. Nathan Smith Davis, often regarded as the "father of the AMA," a national convention of medical societies meeting in New York City in May 1846 resolved to create a national organization for the medical profession. The goals of the new organization would be to develop a "uniform and elevated standard of requirements for the degree of M.D." and to adopt a single code of medical ethics to govern all physicians in the U.S.[2] The 1846 convention appointed committees to report back on these priorities at what would be the national organization's inaugural meeting in Philadelphia the following year.

Thus, in May 1847, the newly organized AMA unanimously adopted a remarkable 5000-word document by Drs. Isaac Hayes and John Bell that was essentially the first national code of medical ethics ever written, one that applied high, collective professional standards to individual practitioners across the country. The code was written for doctors by doctors and aimed to improve clinical practice and patient care by incorporating ethical and professional standards into the daily activities of physicians.

Some of the extraordinary elements of the 1847 ethics code of the AMA included:

- The medical profession was called on to treat patients with "attention, steadiness and humanity." (Chapter 1, Article 1, No. 2)
- Physicians were called upon to offer ". . . counsels, or even remonstrances . . . with politeness and a genuine love of virtue, accompanied by a sincere interest in the welfare of the person to whom they are addressed." (Chapter 1, Article I, No. 7)
- The profession could not ". . . abandon a patient because the case is deemed incurable." (Chapter 1, Article 1, No. 5)
- The profession acknowledged ". . . poverty . . . as presenting valid claims for gratuitous service." (Chapter 3, Article 1, No. 3)
- The profession accepted that "when pestilence prevails" physicians had a ". . . duty to face the danger, and to continue their labors for the alleviation of suffering, even at the jeopardy of their own lives." (Chapter 3, Article 1, No. 3)[3]

The code established guidance for both doctors and patients in their interactions and also for the reciprocal relationship between doctors and society.

The AMA *Code of Medical Ethics* "set a new moral standard in medicine not only for America but also for the world. . . . The grand moral vision inscribed in the 1847 Code of Ethics established the newly founded American Medical Association as the preeminent moral and political voice of American medicine. Throughout the rest of the nineteenth century, the AMA's Code of Ethics was the most commonly printed medical document in the English language."[4]

In fact, during the second half of the 19th century, the AMA's 1847 *Code of Medical Ethics* was viewed as the greatest achievement of the AMA.

Jumping ahead to the mid-1970s, almost 130 years after the AMA code was written, several colleagues and I developed a new field in medicine that we called clinical medical ethics. Our goal was to create a new, applied medical discipline that would improve medical care by focusing on the practice of medicine itself and by keeping at its core the patient-physician relationship. Whereas bioethics looked to philosophy, theology, and law for its ethical justifications, the foundation of clinical medical ethics is grounded squarely in medicine as a profession.

Clinical medical ethics aims to make ethics patient centered in a new way. We wanted to improve patient outcomes by strengthening the patient-physician relationship and by encouraging physicians to reach decisions that incorporate the ethical issues that arise routinely in everyday clinical practice.[5-7] In the United States, for the past 40 years, the clinical medical ethics movement has integrated ethical issues into practice, teaching, and research. This movement has defended and retained the central importance of the patient-physician relationship, a relationship that emphasizes patient autonomy, patient-centered care, and respect for the patient.

Clinical medical ethics has become so well integrated into current practice that physicians often don't realize that they are "doing" clinical ethics when they tell patients the truth, or when they obtain informed consent for a procedure, or when they make decisions based upon shared decision making, or when they work with surrogate decision makers in cases when the patient lacks capacity. These and other clinical ethical issues have become part of everyday medical practice, and many of them have become widely accepted as the standard of care.

While my colleagues and I take pride in having contributed to the development of clinical medical ethics, it is now clear to me that our work in developing clinical medical ethics was not a new invention. Rather, in the 1970s my colleagues and I were rediscovering or "reinventing" the clinical medical ethics model that had originally been created by the AMA in 1847. It was the first national medical ethics code in the world. The AMA's *Code of Medical Ethics* of 1847 was not a philosophical treatise on medicine but rather a statement about medical professionalism and ethics that focused on patients, physicians, their professional relationships, the quality of patient care, and professional standards and duties. Each of these issues, which were originally addressed in the 1847 ethics code, remains a central component of the modern clinical medical ethics movement.

In my view, Chapter 1, Article 1, of the AMA's *Code of Medical Ethics* anticipates clinical medical ethics:

> Duties of Physicians to their Patients. A physician should not only be ever ready to obey the calls of the sick, but his mind ought also to be imbued with the greatness of his mission, and of the responsibility he incurs in its discharge. . . . Physicians should therefore minister to the sick with due impressions of the importance of their office; reflecting that the ease, the health, and the lives of those committed to their charge depend on their skill, attention, and fidelity. . . . Every case committed to the charge of a Physician should be treated with attention, steadiness and humanity. . . . (Chapter 1, Article 1, Nos. 1 and 2)[3]

Each of these ideas and beliefs has been echoed and restated as part of the modern movement to develop and advance clinical medical ethics.

In an effort to meet the demands of a changing medical, scientific, and social world, the AMA's *Code of Medical Ethics* is a living document that has evolved in the 170 years since it was first written. Through its many revisions since then, major and minor, the *Code of Medical Ethics* has articulated the values and ethical standards to which members of the medical profession commit themselves. As a national standard, the *Code of Medical Ethics* addresses all physicians and physicians-in-training, regardless of location or specialty, and provides ethical guidance even when state medical societies or specialty organizations do not. It plays a vital role in enabling and strengthening medicine's ability to control its own educational, clinical, and ethical standards, a key feature of self-regulation that is essential for any professional organization.

The newly revised, modernized 2016–2017 version of the *Code of Medical Ethics* is the most extensive revision of the *Code* since 1957. In 1957, the 47 Articles of the *Code of Medical Ethics* were recast as succinct principles accompanied by annotations by the AMA's Judicial Council, the forerunners to what are now the Opinions of the Council on Ethical and Judicial Affairs (Council).

The current revisions aim to meet the needs of practicing physicians and teachers by providing guidance that is easy to find, timely, clear, and consistent. In this modernized *Code of Medical Ethics,* the Council has organized guidance around specific topics in separate chapters in a clear and orderly way. For example, the titles of five early chapters in the newly revised edition of the Opinions are:

- Patient-Physician Relationships
- Consent, Communication, and Decision Making
- Privacy, Confidentiality, and Medical Records
- Genetics and Reproductive Medicine
- Caring for Patients at the End of Life

Contrast these chapters with previous editions of the *Code of Medical Ethics*, in which material covering a given topic was often dispersed and inconvenient to locate and use. For example, in the 2014-2015 edition of the *Code of Medical Ethics*, five early chapters were:

- Opinions on Social Policy Issues
- Opinions on Interprofessional Relations
- Opinions on Hospital Relations
- Opinions on Confidentiality, Advertising, and Communications Media Relations
- Opinions on Fees and Charges

The chapter on social policy issues in the 2014-2015 edition included Opinions on a wide range of disparate topics, including mandatory parental consent to abortion; physician participation in interrogation; subject selection for clinical trials; genetic engineering; transplantation of organs from living donors; withholding or withdrawing life-sustaining treatment; the use of radio-frequency ID devices in humans; and others.

Similarly, in the 2014-2015 edition, information and opinions about the patient-physician relationship were dispersed in six separate chapters. By contrast, in the newly revised edition, all information about the patient-physician relationship is consolidated into a single chapter, Chapter 1.

I have used the AMA *Code of Medical Ethics*, particularly the Opinions of the Council, for more than 45 years. I frequently refer to the Opinions when I am struggling with an ethical decision in my clinical practice or when I am invited as a clinical ethics consultant to help patients or families reach a clinical-ethical decision. I also have used the Opinions frequently to teach medical students, residents, and fellow practitioners. Finally, in my writing and research on clinical ethics, I find the Council Opinions an excellent place to start my work because the views in the Opinions are not only clear and succinct but also supported by previous ethical analyses and legal opinions. The Opinions state clearly whether potential actions are ethical, unethical, or open to discussion and deliberation.

I must confess that in my 45 years of practice I have never read the Opinions from front to back as one might read a novel. Rather, I use the Opinions for particular problems that I encounter in my practice or as a reference source. Frequently, I find myself starting with a particular question or issue and then expanding my search to related topics.

Readers will find this updated edition of the Opinions more user friendly than ever before. First, as noted, the Opinions consolidate similar issues within a single chapter rather than scattering them throughout the volume. Second, there is a new and consistent format that is used uniformly for all Opinions. Each Opinion starts with a short statement of the key ethical values, considerations, and challenges that are raised by the specific issue. The Opinion then offers a concise description of the clinical context in which the ethical issue arises. Finally, the Opinion offers guidance for physicians, guidance that aims to be practical and concrete without being rigidly prescriptive. This newly revised edition, which required eight years to complete, makes this edition of the *Code of Medical Ethics* a far more accessible and useful resource than it has previously been for physicians, teachers, and students.

The 1847 AMA *Code of Medical Ethics* was a revolutionary document that aimed to establish a national standard for physicians' professional behavior. The 2016 update of the Opinions of the *Code of Medical Ethics* reinforces the primary focus on professional ethical standards and does so in a way that is accessible to busy practicing physicians who hope to apply clinical ethics standards to improve the care and outcome of patients.

Mark Siegler, MD
LINDY BERGMAN DISTINGUISHED SERVICE PROFESSOR OF MEDICINE AND SURGERY
EXECUTIVE DIRECTOR, BUCKSBAUM INSTITUTE FOR CLINICAL EXCELLENCE
DIRECTOR, MACLEAN CENTER FOR CLINICAL MEDICAL ETHICS
THE UNIVERSITY OF CHICAGO

References

1. Peabody FW. The care of the patient. *JAMA.* 1927;88(12):887-882.
2. American Medical Association. Proceedings of the National Medical Conventions, Held in New York, May, 1846, and in Philadelphia, May, 1847. Philadelphia, PA: TK & PG Collins; 1847:17.
3. American Medical Association. *Code of Medical Ethics of the American Medical Association.* Chicago, IL: American Medical Association; 1847.
4. Baker RB, Caplan AL, Emanuel LL, Latham SR, eds. *The American Medical Ethics Revolution: How the AMA's Code of Ethics Has Transformed Physicians' Relationships to Patients, Professionals, and Society.* Baltimore, MD: Johns Hopkins University Press; 1999: xxviii.
5. Siegler M. A legacy of Osler: teaching clinical ethics at the bedside. *JAMA.* 1978;239(10):951-956. doi:10.1001/jama.1978.03280370047023.
6. Siegler M. Clinical Ethics and Clinical Medicine. *Arch Intern Med.* 1979;139(8):914-915. doi:10.1001/archinte.1979.03630450056016.
7. Jonsen AR, Siegler M, Winslade WJ. *Clinical Ethics: A Practical Approach to Ethical Decisions in Clinical Medicine.* 8th ed. New York, NY. McGraw-Hill Education; 2015.

Council on Ethical and Judicial Affairs

2015–2016

Stephen L. Brotherton, MD
CHAIR

Ronald J. Clearfield, MD, FACR
VICE CHAIR

Dennis S. Agliano, MD, FACS

Marc Mendelsohn, MD
RESIDENT/FELLOW MEMBER

Kathryn Moseley, MD, MPH, FAAP

Alexander M. Rosenau, DO, CPE, FACEP

James E. Sabin, MD

Monique A. Spillman, MD, PhD

Kimberly A. Swartz
MEDICAL STUDENT MEMBER

The present volume reflects the efforts of numerous individuals. The Council wishes to acknowledge former members who participated in the project to modernize the *Code of Medical Ethics*:

Regina M. Benjamin, MD, MBA
CHAIR 2008-2009

Sharon P. Douglas, MD
CHAIR 2011-2012

Hilary Fairbrother, MD
RESIDENT/FELLOW MEMBER 2006-2009

Susan Dorr Goold, MD, MHSA, MA
CHAIR 2013-2014

H. Rex Greene, MD
CHAIR 2012-2013

Julia Halsey
MEDICAL STUDENT MEMBER 2010-2012

Katherine L. Harvey, MD, MPH
RESIDENT/FELLOW MEMBER 2012-2015

Mark A. Levine, MD,
CHAIR 2007-2008

Patrick W. McCormick, MD
CHAIR 2014-2015

John W. McMahon, MD*
CHAIR 2010-2011

Kavita Shah, MD
RESIDENT/FELLOW MEMBER 2009-2012
MEDICAL STUDENT MEMBER 2007-2009

Kathryn A. Skimming
MEDICAL STUDENT MEMBER 2013-2015

Dudley M. Stewart, Jr., MD*
CHAIR 2009-2010

Leon Vorobeichik
MEDICAL STUDENT MEMBER 2011-2015

* Deceased

The Council on Ethical and Judicial Affairs also wishes to acknowledge the contributions of the following individuals who served as interns with the AMA Ethics Group over the course of the project:

Kevin Abbott; Natalie Achamallah; Juan Aparicio; Ryan Bailey; Caroline Bass; Aaron Bengtson; Stephanie Bi; Sorcha Brophy; Mary Katherine Brueck; Grace Chapin; Lizz Esfeld; Joseph Gregorio; Kieran Halzhauer; Jenna Karagianis; Tobin Klusty; Jon Lee; Cassandra Leigh; Rachel Lewin; Yien Li; Allen Loup; Andreia Martinho; Courtney Matthews; Puja Parikh; Yesenia Perez; Ranola Primi; Brittany Rush; Angelique Salib; Andrew Sova; Emily Twaalfhoven; Clinton Wang; and Charley Willison.

Code *of* Medical Ethics

of the American Medical Association

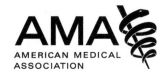

OP635516
OP632316
ISBN 978-1-62202-553-4
BP25:11/16

History

The *Code of Medical Ethics (Code)* of the American Medical Association (AMA) is rooted in an understanding of the goals of medicine as a profession, which dates back to the 5th century BCE and the Greek physician Hippocrates, to relieve suffering and promote well-being in a relationship of fidelity with the patient. As adopted by the young AMA in 1847, the *Code* drew significantly on the work of the English physician-philosopher Thomas Percival, whose 1803 code of medical ethics set standards of conduct relative to hospitals and other charities.

The *Code* is a living document that has evolved as medicine and society have changed over time. The first edition in 1847 articulated in some detail the standards of ethical conduct for physicians in relation to their patients, fellow physicians, the profession at large, and the public in three chapters, each of which also outlined the reciprocal obligations of the other parties. With minor copyediting along the way, the *Code* remained largely unchanged until 1903, when its language was updated and provisions addressing the obligations of patients and society were eliminated. At that time, the document was retitled as *Principles of Medical Ethics (Principles)*. In 1949, the *Principles* were further revised: content was reorganized and language and guidance updated to reflect the significant changes that had taken place in medical practice over the preceding decades. Debate continued, however, and six years later the chapter structure of the original document was abandoned and the *Principles* were recast in the form of a preamble and 47 separate articles.

In 1957, further revisions to the restructured *Principles* removed "superfluous wording and matters of medical etiquette" and distilled the *Principles* to a preamble and 10 statements of core values and commitments, "leaving to the [then] Judicial Council the question of interpretation of these ethical Principles (Principles of medical ethics [ed]. *JAMA*. 1957;164(13):1482.)." (Minor changes to the *Principles* were adopted in 1980 and 2001.)

The 1957 *Principles* appeared in the *Journal of the American Medical Association (JAMA)* in June 1958, accompanied by interpretive annotations. Those annotations subsequently evolved into the opinions of the Council on Ethical and Judicial Affairs (CEJA), the 1985 successor to the Judicial Council. Early annotations were offered without explanation, but since the late 1970s, CEJA reports have presented background analyses supporting the guidance set out

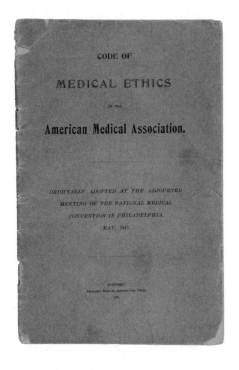

CODE OF

MEDICAL ETHICS

OF THE

American Medical Association.

ORIGINALLY ADOPTED AT THE ADJOURNED
MEETING OF THE NATIONAL MEDICAL
CONVENTION IN PHILADELPHIA.
MAY, 1847.

CHICAGO:
AMERICAN MEDICAL ASSOCIATION PRESS.

in individual opinions. Today's *Code of Medical Ethics* consists of the *Principles* and CEJA's interpretive opinions. New opinions are issued at the annual or interim meetings of the AMA House of Delegates as new CEJA reports are adopted.

By the time CEJA launched its project to comprehensively review the *Code* in 2008, opinions totaled some 220 separate statements that differed markedly in form and specificity, on topics ranging from abortion to xenotransplantation. The *Code* had become unwieldy—guidance on individual topics was hard to find; opinions varied significantly as to whether they offered general guidance or highly prescriptive statements. Some guidance was directed narrowly to dilemmas at the bedside; other guidance broadly to issues of social policy.

CEJA updated guidance that referred to outdated science or clinical practice, was overly prescriptive as a statement of ethical responsibility, or focused unduly on operational or specifically legal considerations rather than ethical responsibilities as such. In some instances, where there was significant overlap in guidance, CEJA consolidated multiple opinions on the same or closely related topics into a single, more comprehensive opinion. In other instances, CEJA extracted and recombined salient guidance scattered across two or more opinions into new, more clearly focused statements.

Throughout, CEJA's intent was to respect the accumulated wisdom represented in its constituent opinions; to ensure that guidance remains timely and useful; and to strike a balance between offering general rules for acting and providing tools for thinking about the ethical challenges physicians encounter as practicing clinicians and leaders in a rapidly changing health care environment.

American Medical Association
Principles of Medical Ethics

The nine Principles of Medical Ethics are the primary component of the *Code*. They describe the core ethical principles of the medical profession. A single Principle should not be read in isolation from others; the overall intent of the nine Principles, read together, guides physicians' behavior.

The AMA House of Delegates has the authority to establish the Principles of Medical Ethics. However, the Council on Ethical and Judicial Affairs is responsible for determining the AMA's positions on ethical issues through its interpretations of the Principles, which are expressed in the Opinions. Each Opinion identifies the Principle(s) from which the Opinion is derived.

Preamble

The medical profession has long subscribed to a body of ethical statements developed primarily for the benefit of the patient. As a member of this profession, a physician must recognize responsibility to patients first and foremost, as well as to society, to other health professionals, and to self. The following Principles adopted by the American Medical Association are not laws, but standards of conduct which define the essentials of honorable behavior for the physician.

I. A physician shall be dedicated to providing competent medical care, with compassion and respect for human dignity and rights.

II. A physician shall uphold the standards of professionalism, be honest in all professional interactions, and strive to report physicians deficient in character or competence, or engaging in fraud or deception, to appropriate entities.

III. A physician shall respect the law and also recognize a responsibility to seek changes in those requirements which are contrary to the best interests of the patient.

IV. A physician shall respect the rights of patients, colleagues, and other health professionals, and shall safeguard patient confidences and privacy within the constraints of the law.

V. A physician shall continue to study, apply, and advance scientific knowledge, maintain a commitment to medical education, make relevant information available to patients, colleagues, and the public, obtain consultation, and use the talents of other health professionals when indicated.

VI. A physician shall, in the provision of appropriate patient care, except in emergencies, be free to choose whom to serve, with whom to associate, and the environment in which to provide medical care.

VII. A physician shall recognize a responsibility to participate in activities contributing to the improvement of the community and the betterment of public health.

VIII. A physician shall, while caring for a patient, regard responsibility to the patient as paramount.

IX. A physician shall support access to medical care for all people.

Adopted June 1957; revised June 1980; revised June 2001.

Preface to the Opinions of the Council on Ethical and Judicial Affairs

Just as the AMA *Principles of Medical Ethics* are not laws, but standards of conduct, so too the Opinions in the *Code of Medical Ethics (Code)* are not laws or rules. They are guidance that identifies the essentials of ethical behavior for physicians.

Throughout the Opinions of the *Code*, the Council on Ethical and Judicial Affairs uses the words *must*, *should*, and *may* in their common understandings to distinguish different levels of ethical obligation. Use of the word *must* indicates that an action is ethically required of physicians. From the perspective of ethics and professionalism, such actions are near-absolute obligations, not matters about which physicians may use judgment or discretion. The Council uses the word *should* to indicate an action or obligation that is strongly recommended as a matter of professional ethics, but which may have some exceptions. *Should* is used to indicate what is expected of a physician in most instances, absent special circumstances or considerations. *Should* indicates that ethically there is some latitude for physician judgment and discretion. The Council uses *may* to indicate that an action is ethically permissible when qualifying conditions set out in the Opinion are met.

The Council recognizes that circumstances at times impinge on physicians' ability or opportunity to follow the guidance of the *Code* strictly as written. Recognizing when such circumstances exist and determining how best to adhere to the goals and spirit, if not the absolute letter, of guidance requires physicians to use skills of ethical discernment and reflection. Physicians are expected to have compelling reasons to deviate from guidance when, in their best judgment, they determine it is ethically appropriate or even necessary to do so.

The more stringent the ethical obligation, the stronger the justification required to deviate from it in any specific instance. Obligations indicated by *must* can be reversed or violated only in very rare circumstances, for example, when two or more core ethical values conflict in such a way that it is not possible for the physician to uphold both or all and the physician is forced to decide which value will prevail. Guidance introduced by *should* sets a general expectation for conduct, but permits more latitude for discerning alternative ways to meet the expectation. Obligations indicated by *may* call on the physician to confirm that qualifying conditions are met sufficiently to warrant taking the action addressed in guidance.

The Council also recognizes that guidance is not always equally applicable to every individual physician, depending on the nature of the physician's practice. Nonetheless, physicians are expected to be aware of guidance that may not be routinely relevant to their practice, to be sensitive to occasions when such guidance might be pertinent, and to respond in keeping with guidance when such situations occur. In this respect too, then, the *Code* relies on the reasonable exercise of judgment.

The AMA *Code* provides ethical guidance for all physicians, regardless of specialty. The AMA recognizes that other physician organizations may also have codes of ethical behavior and that physicians may, at times, have to balance guidance of other professional codes.

Preamble to the Opinions of the Council on Ethical and Judicial Affairs

Opinions of the AMA Council on Ethical and Judicial Affairs lay out the ethical responsibilities of physicians as members of the profession of medicine. In these opinions, the term "ethical" refers to matters involving moral principles, values, and practices, as well as matters of social policy involving issues of morality in the practice of medicine.

Council opinions articulate the expectations for professional conduct in the areas addressed, at times laying out specific duties and obligations. Conduct that violates these expectations or specific duties and obligations is not acceptable ethically, and is unprofessional. Violations of ethical responsibilities may justify disciplinary actions against a physician's medical society membership.

The relationship between ethics and law is complex. Ethical values and legal principles are usually closely related, but ethical responsibilities usually exceed legal duties. Conduct that is legally permissible may be ethically unacceptable. Conversely, the fact that a physician who has been charged with allegedly illegal conduct has been acquitted or exonerated in criminal or civil proceedings does not necessarily mean that the physician acted ethically.

In some cases, the law mandates conduct that is ethically unacceptable. When physicians believe a law violates ethical values or is unjust, they should work to change the law. In exceptional circumstances of unjust laws, ethical responsibilities should supersede legal duties.

1 Patient-Physician Relationships

These Opinions are offered as ethics guidance for physicians and are not intended to establish clinical practice guidelines or rules of law.

The practice of medicine is fundamentally a moral activity, the goal of which, in the words of the physician-philosopher Edmund Pellegrino, "is a right and good healing action for a particular human being."[1] At the heart of medicine lie relationships founded in a "covenant of trust" between patient and physician in which physicians commit themselves to responding to the needs and promoting the welfare of patients.[2]

Relationships between patients and physicians are inherently unequal: the fact of illness renders patients vulnerable, in greater or lesser degree, and dependent on physicians' expertise and fidelity. Yet patients bring to interactions with physicians their values, goals, and preferences as well as their needs. Patients must therefore be able to trust not only that their physicians have the knowledge and skills to provide competent care, but equally that their physicians will do so with respect for the patient as a moral agent and compassion for the patient as a human being.

A patient-physician relationship comes into being whenever a physician serves a patient's medical needs, whether both parties choose to interact or whether a patient involuntarily enters the relationship, as when a physician provides emergency care to a patient unable at the time to agree to the relationship. Although physicians have a right to choose whom they will serve, they have an ethical responsibility to exercise that right prudently and should not discriminate against patients on grounds of patients' social characteristics or disease status so long as the physician has appropriate expertise. When physicians choose not to provide certain services that conflict with their deeply held personal beliefs, they have a responsibility to be transparent with prospective patients about how they limit their practice. Once a patient-physician relationship exists, physicians have an obligation to respect patients' rights to participate in informed decision making, privacy and confidentiality, and not to be abandoned.

Opinions in the first section of this chapter provide guidance on fundamental ethical obligations in any patient-physician relationship. However, the degree of physicians' accountability for upholding specific ethical obligations and how they should meet those obligations may vary depending on the nature of the interactions they have with patients. Thus, Opinions in the second section offer guidance for a variety of different patient-physician interactions, for example, under what circumstances physicians may ethically treat family members or what considerations should prevail when physicians have competing responsibilities to different third parties.

References

1. Pellegrino ED. Toward a reconstruction of medical morality. *J Med Humanit and Bioeth.* 1987;8(1):7-18.
2. Pellegrino ED. Professionalism, profession and the virtues of the good physician. *Mt Sinai J of Med.* 2002;69(6):378-384.

Responsibilities of Physicians and Patients

Special Issues in Patient-Physician Relationships

Responsibilities of Physicians and Patients

1.1.1 Patient-Physician Relationships

The practice of medicine, and its embodiment in the clinical encounter between a patient and a physician, is fundamentally a moral activity that arises from the imperative to care for patients and to alleviate suffering. The relationship between a patient and a physician is based on trust, which gives rise to physicians' ethical responsibility to place patients' welfare above the physician's own self-interest or obligations to others, to use sound medical judgment on patients' behalf, and to advocate for their patients' welfare.

A patient-physician relationship exists when a physician serves a patient's medical needs. Generally, the relationship is entered into by mutual consent between physician and patient (or surrogate).

However, in certain circumstances a limited patient-physician relationship may be created without the patient's (or surrogate's) explicit agreement. Such circumstances include:

(a) When a physician provides emergency care or provides care at the request of the patient's treating physician. In these circumstances, the patient's (or surrogate's) agreement to the relationship is implicit.

(b) When a physician provides medically appropriate care for a prisoner under court order, in keeping with ethics guidance on court-initiated treatment.

(c) When a physician examines a patient in the context of an independent medical examination, in keeping with ethics guidance. In such situations, a limited patient-physician relationship exists.

AMA Principles of Medical Ethics: I, II, IV, VIII

Issued: 2001

Updated: 2016

Opinions on Related Matters:
1.1.7 Physician Exercise of Conscience
1.2.6 Work-Related and Independent Medical Examinations
9.1.1 Romantic or Sexual Relationships with Patients
9.1.2 Romantic or Sexual Relationships with Key Third Parties
9.7.2 Court-Initiated Medical Treatment in Criminal Cases
10.3 Peers as Patients

1.1.2 Prospective Patients

As professionals dedicated to protecting the well-being of patients, physicians have an ethical obligation to provide care in cases of medical emergency. Physicians must also uphold ethical responsibilities not to discriminate against a prospective patient on the basis of race, gender, sexual orientation or gender identity, or other personal or social characteristics that are not clinically relevant to the individual's care. Nor may physicians decline a patient based solely on the individual's infectious disease status. Physicians should not decline patients for whom they have accepted a contractual obligation to provide care.

AMA Principles of Medical Ethics: I, VI, VIII, IX

Issued: 2000

Updated: 2003, 2008, 2016

Opinions on Related Matters:
1.1.7 Physician Exercise of Conscience
1.2.1 Treating Self or Family
2.2.2 Confidential Health Care for Minors
2.3.1 Health Information Sites and Services Outside an Existing Patient-Physician Relationship
4.2.1 Assisted Reproductive Technology
8.5 Disparities in Health Care
9.6.3 Incentives to Patients for Referrals
10.3 Peers as Patients

However, physicians are not ethically required to accept all prospective patients. Physicians should be thoughtful in exercising their right to choose whom to serve.

A physician may decline to establish a patient-physician relationship with a prospective patient, or provide specific care to an existing patient, in certain limited circumstances:

(a) The patient requests care that is beyond the physician's competence or scope of practice; is known to be scientifically invalid, has no medical indication, or cannot reasonably be expected to achieve the intended clinical benefit; or is incompatible with the physician's deeply held personal, religious, or moral beliefs in keeping with ethics guidance on exercise of conscience.

(b) The physician lacks the resources needed to provide safe, competent, respectful care for the individual. Physicians may not decline to accept a patient for reasons that would constitute discrimination against a class or category of patients.

(c) Meeting the medical needs of the prospective patient could seriously compromise the physician's ability to provide the care needed by his or her other patients. The greater the prospective patient's medical need, however, the stronger is the physician's obligation to provide care, in keeping with the professional obligation to promote access to care.

(d) The individual is abusive or threatens the physician, staff, or other patients, unless the physician is legally required to provide emergency medical care. Physicians should be aware of the possibility that an underlying medical condition may contribute to this behavior.

AMA Principles of Medical Ethics: I, IV, V, VIII, IX

Issued: 1992

Updated: 2016

Opinions on Related Matters:
1.1.7 Physician Exercise of Conscience
2.1.1 Informed Consent
3.1.1 Privacy in Health Care
3.2.1 Confidentiality
5.2 Advance Directives
5.3 Withholding or Withdrawing Life-Sustaining Treatment
10.7 Ethics Committees in Health Care Institutions
10.7.1 Ethics Consultations
11.1.4 Financial Barriers to Health Care Access

1.1.3 Patient Rights

The health and well-being of patients depends on a collaborative effort between patient and physician in a mutually respectful alliance. Patients contribute to this alliance when they fulfill responsibilities they have, eg, to seek care and to be candid with their physicians.

Physicians can best contribute to a mutually respectful alliance with patients by serving as their patients' advocates and by respecting patients' rights. These include the right:

(a) To courtesy, respect, dignity, and timely, responsive attention to the patient's needs.

(b) To receive information from their physicians and to have opportunity to discuss the benefits, risks, and costs of appropriate treatment alternatives, including the risks, benefits, and costs of forgoing treatment. Patients should be able to expect that their physicians will provide guidance about what they consider the optimal course of action for the patient based on the physician's objective professional judgment.

(c) To ask questions about their health status or recommended treatment when they do not fully understand what has been described and to have their questions answered.

(d) To make decisions about the care the physician recommends and to have those decisions respected. A patient who has decision-making capacity may accept or refuse any recommended medical intervention.

(e) To have the physician and other staff respect the patient's privacy and confidentiality.

(f) To obtain copies or summaries of their medical records.

(g) To obtain a second opinion.

(h) To be advised of any conflicts of interest their physician may have in respect to their care.

(i) To continuity of care. Patients should be able to expect that their physician will cooperate in coordinating medically indicated care with other health care professionals, and that the physician will not discontinue treating them when further treatment is medically indicated without giving them sufficient notice and reasonable assistance in making alternative arrangements for care.

1.1.4 Patient Responsibilities

AMA Principles of Medical Ethics: I, IV, VI
Issued: 1994
Updated: 1998, 2000, 2001, 2016

Successful medical care requires ongoing collaboration between patients and physicians. Their partnership requires both individuals to take an active role in the healing process.

Autonomous, competent patients control the decisions that direct their health care. With that exercise of self-governance and choice comes a number of responsibilities. Patients contribute to the collaborative effort when they:

(a) Are truthful and forthcoming with their physicians and strive to express their concerns clearly. Physicians likewise should encourage patients to raise questions or concerns.

(b) Provide as complete a medical history as they can, including providing information about past illnesses, medications, hospitalizations, family history of illness, and other matters relating to present health.

(c) Cooperate with agreed-on treatment plans. Since adhering to treatment is often essential to public and individual safety, patients should disclose whether they have or have not followed the agreed-on plan and indicate when they would like to reconsider the plan.

(d) Accept care from medical students, residents, and other trainees under appropriate supervision. Participation in medical education is to the mutual benefit of patients and the health care system; nonetheless, patients' (or surrogates') refusal of care by a trainee should be respected in keeping with ethics guidance.

(e) Meet their financial responsibilities with regard to medical care or discuss financial hardships with their physicians. Patients should be aware of costs associated with using a limited resource like health care and try to use medical resources judiciously.

(f) Recognize that a healthy lifestyle can often prevent or mitigate illness and take responsibility to follow preventive measures and adopt health-enhancing behaviors.

(g) Be aware of and refrain from behavior that unreasonably places the health of others at risk. They should ask about what they can do to prevent transmission of infectious disease.

(h) Refrain from being disruptive in the clinical setting.

(i) Not knowingly initiate or participate in medical fraud.

(j) Report illegal or unethical behavior by physicians or other health care professionals to the appropriate medical societies, licensing boards, or law enforcement authorities.

AMA Principles of Medical Ethics: I, VI

Issued: 1996

Updated: 2016

Opinions on Related Matters:
1.1.7 Physician Exercise of Conscience
1.2.2 Disruptive Behavior by Patients
3.3.1 Management of Medical Records
8.5 Disparities in Health Care

1.1.5 Terminating a Patient-Physician Relationship

Physicians' fiduciary responsibility to patients entails an obligation to support continuity of care for their patients. At the beginning of a patient-physician relationship, the physician should alert the patient to any foreseeable impediments to continuity of care.

When considering withdrawing from a case, physicians must:

(a) Notify the patient (or authorized decision maker) long enough in advance to permit the patient to secure another physician.

(b) Facilitate transfer of care when appropriate.

1.1.6 Quality

As professionals dedicated to promoting the well-being of patients, physicians individually and collectively share the obligation to ensure that the care patients receive is safe, effective, patient centered, timely, efficient, and equitable.

While responsibility for quality of care does not rest solely with physicians, their role is essential. Individually and collectively, physicians should actively engage in efforts to improve the quality of health care by:

(a) Keeping current with best care practices and maintaining professional competence.

(b) Holding themselves accountable to patients, families, and fellow health care professionals for communicating effectively and coordinating care appropriately.

(c) Monitoring the quality of care they deliver as individual practitioners—eg, through personal case review and critical self-reflection, peer review, and use of other quality improvement tools.

(d) Demonstrating commitment to develop, implement, and disseminate appropriate, well-defined quality and performance improvement measures in their daily practice.

(e) Participating in educational, certification, and quality improvement activities that are well designed and consistent with the core values of the medical profession.

AMA Principles of Medical Ethics: I, V, VII, VIII

Issued: 2009

Opinions on Related Matters:
8.6 Promoting Patient Safety
11.1.1 Defining Basic Health Care
11.1.2 Physician Stewardship of Health Care Resources
11.1.4 Financial Barriers to Health Care Access

1.1.7 Physician Exercise of Conscience

Physicians are expected to uphold the ethical norms of their profession, including fidelity to patients and respect for patient self-determination. Yet physicians are not defined solely by their profession. They are moral agents in their own right and, like their patients, are informed by and committed to diverse cultural, religious, and philosophical traditions and beliefs. For some physicians, their professional calling is imbued with their foundational beliefs as persons, and at times the expectation that physicians will put patients' needs and preferences first may be in tension with the need to sustain moral integrity and continuity across both personal and professional life.

Preserving opportunity for physicians to act (or to refrain from acting) in accordance with the dictates of conscience in their professional practice is important for preserving the integrity of the medical profession, as well as the integrity of the individual physician, on which patients and the public rely. Thus,

AMA Principles of Medical Ethics: I, II, IV, VI, VIII, IX

Issued: 2015

Opinions on Related Matters:
1.1.2 Prospective Patients
1.1.5 Terminating a Patient-Physician Relationship
2.2.2 Confidential Health Care for Minors
2.2.3 Mandatory Parental Consent to Abortion
2.2.4 Treatment Decisions for Seriously Ill Newborns
4.1.2 Genetic Testing for Reproductive Decision Making
4.2.1 Assisted Reproductive Technology
4.2.7 Abortion
5.3 Withholding or Withdrawing Life-Sustaining Treatment
5.5 Medically Ineffective Interventions
5.6 Sedation to Unconsciousness in End-of-Life Care
5.7 Physician-Assisted Suicide
5.8 Euthanasia

physicians should have considerable latitude to practice in accord with well-considered, deeply held beliefs that are central to their self-identities.

Physicians' freedom to act according to conscience is not unlimited, however. Physicians are expected to provide care in emergencies, honor patients' informed decisions to refuse life-sustaining treatment, and respect basic civil liberties and not discriminate against individuals in deciding whether to enter into a professional relationship with a new patient.

In other circumstances, physicians may be able to act (or refrain from acting) in accordance with the dictates of their conscience without violating their professional obligations. Several factors impinge on the decision to act according to conscience. Physicians have stronger obligations to patients with whom they have a patient-physician relationship, especially one of long standing; when there is imminent risk of foreseeable harm to the patient or delay in access to treatment would significantly adversely affect the patient's physical or emotional well-being; and when the patient is not reasonably able to access needed treatment from another qualified physician.

In following conscience, physicians should:

(a) Thoughtfully consider whether and how significantly an action (or declining to act) will undermine the physician's personal integrity, create emotional or moral distress for the physician, or compromise the physician's ability to provide care for the individual and other patients.

(b) Before entering into a patient-physician relationship, make clear any specific interventions or services the physician cannot in good conscience provide because they are contrary to the physician's deeply held personal beliefs, focusing on interventions or services a patient might otherwise reasonably expect the practice to offer.

(c) Take care that their actions do not discriminate against or unduly burden individual patients or populations of patients and do not adversely affect patient or public trust.

(d) Be mindful of the burden their actions may place on fellow professionals.

(e) Uphold standards of informed consent and inform the patient about all relevant options for treatment, including options to which the physician morally objects.

(f) In general, physicians should refer a patient to another physician or institution to provide treatment the physician declines to offer. When a deeply held, well-considered personal belief leads a physician also to decline to refer, the physician should offer impartial guidance to patients about how to inform themselves regarding access to desired services.

(g) Continue to provide other ongoing care for the patient or formally terminate the patient-physician relationship in keeping with ethics guidance.

Special Issues in Patient-Physician Relationships

1.2.1 Treating Self or Family

Treating oneself or a member of one's own family poses several challenges for physicians, including concerns about professional objectivity, patient autonomy, and informed consent.

When the patient is an immediate family member, the physician's personal feelings may unduly influence his or her professional medical judgment. Or the physician may fail to probe sensitive areas when taking the medical history or to perform intimate parts of the physical examination. Physicians may feel obligated to provide care for family members despite feeling uncomfortable doing so. They may also be inclined to treat problems that are beyond their expertise or training.

Similarly, patients may feel uncomfortable receiving care from a family member. A patient may be reluctant to disclose sensitive information or undergo an intimate examination when the physician is an immediate family member. This discomfort may particularly be the case when the patient is a minor child, who may not feel free to refuse care from a parent.

In general, physicians should not treat themselves or members of their own families. However, it may be acceptable to do so in limited circumstances:

(a) In emergency settings or isolated settings where there is no other qualified physician available. In such situations, physicians should not hesitate to treat themselves or family members until another physician becomes available.

(b) For short-term, minor problems.

When treating self or family members, physicians have a further responsibility to:

(c) Document treatment or care provided and convey relevant information to the patient's primary care physician.

(d) Recognize that if tensions develop in the professional relationship with a family member, perhaps as a result of a negative medical outcome, such difficulties may be carried

AMA Principles of Medical Ethics: I, II, IV

Issued: 1993

Updated: 2016

Opinions on Related Matters:
1.1.6 Quality
2.1.1 Informed Consent
2.2.2 Confidential Health Care for Minors
2.2.3 Mandatory Parental Consent to Abortion
3.1.1 Privacy in Health Care
3.2.1 Confidentiality
10.3 Peers as Patients

over into the family member's personal relationship with the physician.

(e) Avoid providing sensitive or intimate care especially for a minor patient who is uncomfortable being treated by a family member.

(f) Recognize that family members may be reluctant to state their preference for another physician or decline a recommendation for fear of offending the physician.

AMA Principles of Medical Ethics: I, II, VI, IX

Issued: 2003

Updated: 2016

Opinions on Related Matters:

1.1.5 Terminating a Patient-Physician Relationship

1.2.2 Disruptive Behavior by Patients

The relationship between patients and physicians is based on trust and should serve to promote patients' well-being while respecting their dignity and rights.

Disrespectful or derogatory language or conduct on the part of either physicians or patients can undermine trust and compromise the integrity of the patient-physician relationship. It can make members of targeted groups reluctant to seek care, and create an environment that strains relationships among patients, physicians, and the health care team.

Trust can be established and maintained only when there is mutual respect. Therefore, in their interactions with patients, physicians should:

(a) Recognize that derogatory or disrespectful language or conduct can cause psychological harm to those they target.

(b) Always treat their patients with compassion and respect.

(c) Terminate the patient-physician relationship with a patient who uses derogatory language or acts in a prejudicial manner only if the patient will not modify the conduct. In such cases, the physician should arrange to transfer the patient's care.

AMA Principles of Medical Ethics: IV, V, VI

Issued: 2016

Updated: The constituent Opinions on which this guidance is based (see Concordance) were issued between 1977 and 1997, and most recently updated between 1994 and 1996.

Opinions on Related Matters:

9.6.3 Incentives to Patients for Referrals

9.6.9 Physician Self-referral

1.2.3 Consultation, Referral, and Second Opinions

Physicians' fiduciary obligation to promote patients' best interests and welfare can include consulting other physicians for advice in the care of the patient or referring patients to other professionals to provide care.

When physicians seek or provide consultation about a patient's care or refer a patient for health care services, including diagnostic laboratory services, they should:

(a) Base the decision or recommendation on the patient's medical needs, as they would for any treatment recommendation, and consult or refer the patient only to health care professionals who have appropriate knowledge and skills and are licensed to provide the services needed.

(b) Share patients' health information in keeping with ethics guidance on confidentiality.

(c) Assure the patient that he or she may seek a second opinion or choose someone else to provide a recommended consultation or service. Physicians should urge patients to familiarize themselves with any restrictions associated with their individual health plan that may bear on their decision, such as additional out-of-pocket costs to the patient for referrals or care outside a designated panel of providers.

(d) Explain clearly to the patient the rationale for the consultation, opinion, or findings and recommendations.

(e) Respect the terms of any contractual relationships they may have with health care organizations or payers that affect referrals and consultation.

Physicians may not terminate a patient-physician relationship solely because the patient seeks recommendations or care from a health care professional whom the physician has not recommended.

1.2.4 Use of Chaperones

Efforts to provide a comfortable and considerate atmosphere for the patient and the physician are part of respecting patients' dignity. These efforts may include providing appropriate gowns, private facilities for undressing, sensitive use of draping, and clearly explaining various components of the physical examination. They also include having chaperones available. Having chaperones present can also help prevent misunderstandings between patient and physician.

Physicians should:

(a) Adopt a policy that patients are free to request a chaperone and ensure that the policy is communicated to patients.

(b) Always honor a patient's request to have a chaperone.

(c) Have an authorized member of the health care team serve as a chaperone. Physicians should establish clear expectations that chaperones will uphold professional standards of privacy and confidentiality.

(d) In general, use a chaperone even when a patient's trusted companion is present.

AMA Principles of Medical Ethics: I, IV
Issued: 1998
Updated: 2016
Opinions on Related Matters:
3.1.1 Privacy in Health Care
3.2.1 Confidentiality

(e) Provide opportunity for private conversation with the patient without the chaperone present. Physicians should minimize inquiries or history taking of a sensitive nature during a chaperoned examination.

AMA Principles of Medical Ethics: I, VII

Issued: 1983

Updated: 1994, 2016

Opinions on Related Matters:
1.2.6 Work-Related and Independent Medical Examinations
3.2.3 Industry-Employed Physicians and Independent Medical Examiners

1.2.5 Sports Medicine

Many professional and amateur athletic activities, including contact sports, can put participants at risk of injury. Physicians can provide valuable help to sports participants, dancers, and others to make informed decisions about whether to initiate or continue participating in such activities.

Physicians who serve in a medical capacity at athletic, sporting, or other physically demanding events should protect the health and safety of participants.

In this capacity, physicians should:

(a) Base their judgment about an individual's participation solely on medical considerations.

(b) Not allow the desires of spectators, promoters of the event, or even the injured individual to govern a decision about whether to remove the participant from the event.

AMA Principles of Medical Ethics: I

Issued: 1997

Updated: 2016

Opinions on Related Matters:
3.2.1 Confidentiality
3.2.3 Industry-Employed Physicians and Independent Medical Examiners

1.2.6 Work-Related and Independent Medical Examinations

Physicians who are employed by businesses or insurance companies, who provide medical examinations within their realm of specialty as independent contractors, to assess individuals' health or disability face a conflict of duties. They have responsibilities both to the patient and to the employer or third party.

Such industry-employed physicians or independent medical examiners establish limited patient-physician relationships. Their relationships with patients are confined to the isolated examination; they do not monitor patients' health over time, treat them, or carry out many other duties fulfilled by physicians in the traditional fiduciary role.

In keeping with their core obligations as medical professionals, physicians who practice as industry-employed physicians or independent medical examiners should:

(a) Disclose the nature of the relationship with the employer or third party and that the physician is acting as an agent of the employer or third party before gathering health information from the patient.

(b) Explain that the physician's role in this context is to assess the patient's health or disability independently and objectively. The physician should further explain the differences between this practice and the traditional fiduciary role of a physician.

(c) Protect patients' personal health information in keeping with professional standards of confidentiality.

(d) Inform the patient about important incidental findings the physician discovers during the examination. When appropriate, the physician should suggest the patient seek care from a qualified physician and, if requested, provide reasonable assistance in securing follow-up care.

1.2.7 Use of Restraints

All individuals have a fundamental right to be free from unreasonable bodily restraint. At times, however, health conditions may result in behavior that puts patients at risk of harming themselves. In such situations, it may be ethically justifiable for physicians to order the use of chemical or physical restraint to protect the patient.

Except in emergencies, patients should be restrained only on a physician's explicit order. Patients should never be restrained punitively, for convenience, or as an alternate to reasonable staffing.

Physicians who order chemical or physical restraints should:

(a) Use best professional judgment to determine whether restraint is clinically indicated for the individual patient.

(b) Obtain the patient's informed consent to the use of restraint, or the consent of the patient's surrogate when the patient lacks decision-making capacity. Physicians should explain to the patient or surrogate:
   (i) why restraint is recommended;
   (ii) what type of restraint will be used;
   (iii) length of time for which restraint is intended to be used.

(c) Regularly review the need for restraint and document the review and resulting decision in the patient's medical record.

In certain limited situations, when a patient poses a significant danger to self or others, it may be appropriate to restrain the patient involuntarily. In such situations, the least restrictive restraint reasonable should be implemented and the restraint should be removed promptly when no longer needed.

AMA Principles of Medical Ethics: I, IV
Issued: 1992
Updated: 2016
Opinions on Related Matters:
1.2.9 Use of Remote Sensing and Monitoring Devices
2.1.1 Informed Consent

AMA Principles of Medical Ethics: I, II

Issued: 2003

Updated: 2016

Opinions on Related Matters:
2.3.6 Soliciting Charitable Contributions from Patients

1.2.8 Gifts from Patients

Patients offer gifts to a physician for many reasons. Some gifts are offered as an expression of gratitude or a reflection of the patient's cultural tradition. Accepting gifts offered for these reasons can enhance the patient-physician relationship.

Other gifts may signal psychological needs that require the physician's attention. Some patients may offer gifts or cash to secure or influence care or to secure preferential treatment. Such gifts can undermine physicians' obligation to provide services fairly to all patients; accepting them is likely to damage the patient-physician relationship.

The interaction of these factors is complex, and physicians should consider them sensitively before accepting or declining a gift.

Physicians to whom a patient offers a gift should:

(a) Be sensitive to the gift's value relative to the patient's or physician's means. Physicians should decline gifts that are disproportionately or inappropriately large, or when the physician would be uncomfortable to have colleagues know the gift had been accepted.

(b) Not allow the gift or offer of a gift to influence the patient's medical care.

(c) Decline a bequest from a patient if the physician has reason to believe accepting the gift would present an emotional or financial hardship to the patient's family.

(d) Physicians may wish to suggest that the patient or family make a charitable contribution in lieu of the bequest, in keeping with ethics guidance.

AMA Principles of Medical Ethics: I, III, V

Issued: 2007

Updated: 2016

Opinions on Related Matters:
1.2.7 Use of Restraints
2.1.1 Informed Consent

1.2.9 Use of Remote Sensing and Monitoring Devices

Sensing and monitoring devices can benefit patients by allowing physicians and other health care professionals to obtain timely information about the patient's vital signs or health status without requiring an in-person, face-to-face encounter. Implantable devices can also enable physicians to identify patients rapidly and expedite access to patients' medical records. Devices that transmit patient information wirelessly to remote receiving stations can offer convenience for both patients and physicians, enhance the efficiency and quality of care, and promote increased access to care, but also raise concerns about safety and the confidentiality of patient information.

Individually, physicians who employ remote sensing and monitoring devices in providing patient care should:

(a) Determine whether using one or more such devices is appropriate in light of individual patients' medical needs and circumstances, including patients' ability to use the chosen device appropriately.

(b) Explain how the device(s) will be used in the patient's care and what will be expected of the patient in using the technology, and disclose any limitations, risks, or medical uncertainties associated with the device(s) and data transmission.

(c) Obtain the patient's or surrogate's informed consent before implementing the device in treatment.

Collectively, physicians should:

(d) Support research into the safety, efficacy, and possible non-medical uses of remote sensing and monitoring devices, including devices intended to transmit biometric data and implantable radio frequency ID devices.

(e) Advocate for appropriate oversight of remote sensing and monitoring devices.

1.2.10 Political Action by Physicians

Like all Americans, physicians enjoy the right to advocate for change in law and policy, in the public arena, and within their institutions. Indeed, physicians have an ethical responsibility to seek change when they believe the requirements of law or policy are contrary to the best interests of patients. However, they have a responsibility to do so in ways that are not disruptive to patient care.

Physicians who participate in advocacy activities should:

(a) Ensure that the health of patients is not jeopardized and that patient care is not compromised.

(b) Avoid using disruptive means to press for reform. Strikes and other collective actions may reduce access to care, eliminate or delay needed care, and interfere with continuity of care and should not be used as a bargaining tactic. In rare circumstances, briefly limiting personal availability may be appropriate as a means of calling attention to the need for changes in patient care. Physicians should be aware that some actions may put them or their organizations at risk of violating antitrust laws or laws pertaining to medical licensure or malpractice.

(c) Avoid forming workplace alliances, such as unions, with workers who do not share physicians' primary and overriding commitment to patients.

AMA Principles of Medical Ethics: I, III, VI

Issued: 1998

Updated: 2005, 2016

Opinions on Related Matters:
11.2.2 Conflicts of Interest in Patient Care

(d) Refrain from using undue influence to pressure colleagues to participate in advocacy activities, and not punish colleagues, overtly or covertly, for deciding not to participate.

AMA Principles of Medical Ethics: V, VIII

Issued: 2014

Opinions on Related Matters:

1.2.11 Ethically Sound Innovation in Medical Practice

Innovation in medicine can range from improving an existing intervention, to introducing an innovation in one's own clinical practice for the first time, to using an existing intervention in a novel way or translating knowledge from one clinical context into another. Innovation shares features with both research and patient care, but is distinct from both.

When physicians participate in developing and disseminating innovative practices, they act in accord with professional responsibilities to advance medical knowledge, improve quality of care, and promote the well-being of individual patients and the larger community. Similarly, these responsibilities are honored when physicians enhance their own practices by expanding the range of techniques and interventions they offer to patients.

Individually, physicians who are involved in designing, developing, disseminating, or adopting innovative modalities should:

(a) Innovate on the basis of sound scientific evidence and appropriate clinical expertise.
(b) Seek input from colleagues or other medical professionals in advance or as early as possible in the course of innovation.
(c) Design innovations so as to minimize risks to individual patients and maximize the likelihood of application and benefit for populations of patients.
(d) Be sensitive to the cost implications of innovation.
(e) Be aware of influences that may drive the creation and adoption of innovative practices for reasons other than patient or public benefit.

When they offer existing innovative diagnostic or therapeutic services to individual patients, physicians must:

(f) Base recommendations on patients' medical needs.
(g) Refrain from offering such services until they have acquired appropriate knowledge and skills.
(h) Recognize that in this context informed decision making requires the physician to disclose:
    (i) how a recommended diagnostic or therapeutic service differs from the standard therapeutic approach if one exists;

    (ii) why the physician is recommending the innovative modality;

    (iii) what the known or anticipated risks, benefits, and burdens of the recommended therapy and alternatives are;

    (iv) what experience the professional community in general and the physician individually has had to date with the innovative therapy; and

    (v) what conflicts of interest the physician may have with respect to the recommended therapy.

(i) Discontinue any innovative therapies that are not benefiting the patient.

(j) Be transparent and share findings from their use of innovative therapies with peers in some manner. To promote patient safety and quality, physicians should share both immediate and delayed positive and negative outcomes.

To promote responsible innovation, the medical profession should:

(k) Require that physicians who adopt innovative treatment or diagnostic techniques into their practice have appropriate knowledge and skills.

(l) Provide meaningful professional oversight of innovation in patient care.

(m) Encourage physician-innovators to collect and share information about the resources needed to implement their innovative therapies effectively.

1.2.12 Ethical Practice in Telemedicine

Innovation in technology, including information technology, is redefining how people perceive time and distance. It is reshaping how individuals interact with and relate to others, including when, where, and how patients and physicians engage with one another.

Telehealth and telemedicine span a continuum of technologies that offer new ways to deliver care. Yet as in any mode of care, patients need to be able to trust that physicians will place patient welfare above other interests, provide competent care, provide the information patients need to make well-considered decisions about care, respect patient privacy and confidentiality, and take steps to ensure continuity of care. Although physicians' fundamental ethical responsibilities do not change, the continuum of possible patient-physician interactions in telehealth/telemedicine give rise to differing levels of accountability for physicians.

All physicians who participate in telehealth/telemedicine have an ethical responsibility to uphold fundamental fiduciary obligations by disclosing any financial or other interests the physician has in the

AMA Principles of Medical Ethics, I, IV, VI, IX

Issued: 2016

Opinions on Related Matters:
1.2.9 Use of Remote Sensing and Monitoring Devices
2.1.1 Informed Consent

telehealth/telemedicine application or service and taking steps to manage or eliminate conflicts of interests. Whenever they provide health information, including health content for websites or mobile health applications, physicians must ensure that the information they provide, or that is attributed to them, is objective and accurate.

Similarly, all physicians who participate in telehealth/telemedicine must assure themselves that telemedicine services have appropriate protocols to prevent unauthorized access and to protect the security and integrity of patient information at the patient-end of the electronic encounter, during transmission, and among all health care professionals and other personnel, who participate in the telehealth/telemedicine service, are consistent with their individual roles.

Physicians who respond to individual health queries or provide personalized health advice electronically through a telehealth service in addition should:

(a) Inform users about the limitations of the relationship and services provided.
(b) Advise site users about how to arrange for needed care when follow-up care is indicated.
(c) Encourage users who have primary care physicians to inform their primary physicians about the online health consultation, even if in-person care is not immediately needed.

Physicians, who provide clinical services through telehealth/telemedicine, must uphold the standards of professionalism expected in in-person interactions, follow appropriate ethics guidance of relevant specialty societies, and adhere to applicable law governing the practice of telemedicine. In the context of telehealth/telemedicine, they further should:

(d) Be proficient in the use of the relevant technologies and comfortable interacting with patients and/or surrogates electronically.
(e) Recognize the limitations of the relevant technologies and take appropriate steps to overcome those limitations. Physicians must ensure that they have the information they need to make well-grounded clinical recommendations when they cannot personally conduct a physical examination, such as by having another health care professional at the patient's site conduct the exam or obtain vital information through remote technologies.
(f) Be prudent in carrying out a diagnostic evaluation or prescribing medication by:
    (i)   establishing the patient's identity;
    (ii) confirming that telehealth/telemedicine services are appropriate for that patient's individual situation and medical needs;

    (iii) evaluating the indication, appropriateness and safety of any prescription in keeping with best practice guidelines and any formulary limitations that apply to the electronic interaction; and

    (iv) documenting the clinical evaluation and prescription.

(g) When the physician would otherwise be expected to obtain informed consent, tailor the informed consent process to provide information patients (or their surrogates) need about the distinctive features of telehealth/telemedicine, in addition to information about medical issues and treatment options. Patients and surrogates should have a basic understanding of how telemedicine technologies will be used in care, the limitations of those technologies, the credentials of health care professionals involved, and what will be expected of patients for using these technologies.

(h) As in any patient-physician interaction, take steps to promote continuity of care, giving consideration to how information can be preserved and accessible for future episodes of care in keeping with patients' preferences (or the decisions of their surrogates), and how follow-up care can be provided when needed. Physicians should assure themselves of how information will be conveyed to the patient's primary care physician when the patient has a primary care physician and to other physicians currently caring for the patient.

Collectively, through their professional organizations and health care institutions, physicians should:

(i) Support ongoing refinement of telehealth/telemedicine technologies, and the development and implementation of clinical and technical standards to ensure the safety and quality of care.

(j) Advocate for policies and initiatives to promote access to telehealth/telemedicine services for all patients who could benefit from receiving care electronically.

(k) Routinely monitor the telehealth/telemedicine landscape to:

    (i) identify and address adverse consequences as technologies and activities evolve; and

    (ii) identify and encourage dissemination of both positive and negative outcomes.

2 Consent, Communication, and Decision Making

These Opinions are offered as ethics guidance for physicians and are not intended to establish clinical practice guidelines or rules of law.

Patients' right to participate in decisions about their medical care, ie, to give their informed consent to treatment, is central to both professional ethics and law.[1] Patients have the right to receive information about recommendations for care to enable them to make well-considered decisions.

Informed consent means much more than the patient's signature on a document. It is a *process* that occurs when communication between a patient and a physician results in the patient's authorization or agreement to undergo a specific medical intervention. This includes information about the patient's diagnosis, the risks and benefits of treatment alternatives and the interventions the physician recommends, and who will participate in providing care.

Physicians should not withhold information from a patient in the belief that disclosure is medically contraindicated. In an emergency, when a patient is unable to participate in decisions for urgently needed care, physicians may provide care without the patient's explicit consent, but should convey relevant information once the emergency has been resolved.

When a medical condition or disorder impairs a patient's decision-making capacity, the individual may still be able to participate in some aspects of formulating a plan of care. When patients are unable to participate in decision making, surrogates may participate on their behalf, basing care decisions on the patient's own values and preferences, when those are known, or on the patient's best interests when the individual's preferences are not known.

Medical decisions for minor patients raise special issues, not least because they often involve a three-way relationship among the patient, the patient's parents or guardians, and the physicians. Minors may not have the capacity to make health care decisions on their own, and parents or guardians are responsible for doing so on their behalf. Nonetheless, physicians have a responsibility to engage minor patients in decision making at a level that is developmentally appropriate for the individual patient.

Opinions in the first section of this chapter offer guidance on fundamental issues in informed consent, while those in the second section address issues that arise in relation to medical decisions for minor patients. Opinions in the third section offer guidance for physicians when they communicate with patients through different media and on a variety of topics that may pose ethical challenges.

Reference

1. Faden RR, Beauchamp TL, King NM. *A History and Theory of Informed Consent.* New York: Oxford University Press, 1986.

Informed Consent and Shared Decision Making

2.1.1 Informed Consent

2.1.2 Decisions for Adult Patients Who Lack Capacity

2.1.3 Withholding Information from Patients

2.1.4 Use of Placebo in Clinical Practice

2.1.5 Reporting Clinical Test Results

2.1.6 Substitution of Surgeon

Decisions for Minors

2.2.1 Pediatric Decision Making

2.2.2 Confidential Health Care for Minors

2.2.3 Mandatory Parental Consent to Abortion

2.2.4 Treatment Decisions for Seriously Ill Newborns

2.2.5 Genetic Testing of Children

Communication with Patients

2.3.1 Electronic Communication with Patients

2.3.2 Professionalism in the Use of Social Media

2.3.3 Informing Families of a Patient's Death

2.3.4 Political Communications

2.3.5 Soliciting Charitable Contributions from Patients

2.3.6 Surgical Co-management

Informed Consent and Shared Decision Making

2.1.1 Informed Consent

Informed consent to medical treatment is fundamental in both ethics and law. Patients have the right to receive information and ask questions about recommended treatments so that they can make well-considered decisions about care. Successful communication in the patient-physician relationship fosters trust and supports shared decision making.

The process of informed consent occurs when communication between a patient and physician results in the patient's authorization or agreement to undergo a specific medical intervention. In seeking a patient's informed consent (or the consent of the patient's surrogate if the patient lacks decision-making capacity or declines to participate in making decisions), physicians should:

(a) Assess the patient's ability to understand relevant medical information and the implications of treatment alternatives and to make an independent, voluntary decision.

(b) Present relevant information accurately and sensitively, in keeping with the patient's preferences for receiving medical information. The physician should include information about:
  (i) the diagnosis (when known);
  (ii) the nature and purpose of recommended interventions;
  (iii) the burdens, risks, and expected benefits of all options, including forgoing treatment.

(c) Document the informed consent conversation and the patient's (or surrogate's) decision in the medical record in some manner. When the patient and surrogate has provided specific written consent, the consent form should be included in the record.

In emergencies, when a decision must be made urgently, the patient is not able to participate in decision making, and the patient's surrogate is not available, physicians may initiate treatment without prior informed consent. In such situations, the physician should inform the patient or surrogate at the earliest opportunity and obtain consent for ongoing treatment in keeping with this guidance.

AMA Principles of Medical Ethics: I, II, V, VIII

Issued: 1981

Updated: 2006, 2016

Opinions on Related Matters:
1.1.1 Patient-Physician Relationships
2.1.2 Decisions for Adult Patients Who Lack Capacity
2.1.3 Withholding Information from Patients
2.2.1 Pediatric Decision Making
2.3.7 Surgical Co-management
3.1.2 Patient Privacy and Outside Observers of the Clinical Encounter
3.1.3 Audio or Visual Recording of Patients for Education in Health Care
3.1.4 Audio or Visual Recording of Patients for Public Education
5.3 Withholding or Withdrawing Life-Sustaining Treatment
5.4 Orders Not to Attempt Resuscitation (DNAR)
5.6 Sedation to Unconsciousness in End-of-Life Care
6.1.1 Transplantation of Organs from Living Donors
6.1.2 Organ Donation after Cardiac Death
7.1.2 Informed Consent in Research
9.2.1 Medical Student Involvement in Patient Care
9.2.2 Resident and Fellow Physicians' Involvement in Patient Care
9.2.3 Performing Procedures on the Newly Deceased
9.2.5 Medical Students Practicing Clinical Skills on Fellow Students

2 Consent, Communication, and Decision Making

AMA Principles of Medical Ethics: I, III, VIII

Issued: 2001

Updated: 2004, 2016

2.1.2 Decisions for Adult Patients Who Lack Capacity

Respect for patient autonomy is central to professional ethics, and physicians should involve patients in health care decisions commensurate with the patient's decision-making capacity. Even when a medical condition or disorder impairs a patient's decision-making capacity, the patient may still be able to participate in some aspects of decision making. Physicians should engage patients whose capacity is impaired in decisions involving their own care to the greatest extent possible, including when the patient has previously designated a surrogate to make decisions on his or her behalf.

When a patient lacks decision-making capacity, the physician has an ethical responsibility to:

(a) Identify an appropriate surrogate to make decisions on the patient's behalf:

     (i)   the person the patient designated as surrogate through a durable power of attorney for health care or other mechanism;

     (ii)   a family member or other intimate associate, in keeping with applicable law and policy if the patient has not previously designated a surrogate.

(b) Recognize that the patient's surrogate is entitled to the same respect as the patient.

(c) Provide advice, guidance, and support to the surrogate.

(d) Assist the surrogate to make decisions in keeping with the standard of substituted judgment, basing decisions on:

     (i)   the patient's preferences (if any) as expressed in an advance directive or as documented in the medical record;

     (ii)   the patient's views about life and how it should be lived;

     (iii)   how the patient constructed his or her life story;

     (iv)   the patient's attitudes toward sickness, suffering, and certain medical procedures.

(e) Assist the surrogate to make decisions in keeping with the best interest standard when the patient's preferences and values are not known and cannot reasonably be inferred, such as when the patient has not previously expressed preferences or has never had decision-making capacity. Best interest decisions should be based on:

     (i)   the pain and suffering associated with the intervention;

     (ii)   the degree of and potential for benefit;

     (iii)   impairments that may result from the intervention;

     (iv)   quality of life as experienced by the patient.

(f) Consult an ethics committee or other institutional resource when:

   (i) no surrogate is available or there is ongoing disagreement about who is the appropriate surrogate;

   (ii) ongoing disagreement about a treatment decision cannot be resolved;

   (iii) the physician judges that the surrogate's decision:

      a. is clearly not what the patient would have decided when the patient's preferences are known or can be inferred;

      b. could not reasonably be judged to be in the patient's best interest;

      c. primarily serves the interests of the surrogate or other third party, rather than the patient.

2.1.3 Withholding Information from Patients

Truthful and open communication between physician and patient is essential for trust in the relationship and for respect for autonomy. Withholding pertinent medical information from patients in the belief that disclosure is medically contraindicated creates a conflict between the physician's obligations to promote patient welfare and to respect patient autonomy.

Except in emergency situations in which a patient is incapable of making an informed decision, withholding information without the patient's knowledge or consent is ethically unacceptable. When information has been withheld in such circumstances, physicians should convey that information once the emergency situation has been resolved, in keeping with relevant guidance below.

The obligation to communicate truthfully about the patient's medical condition does not mean that the physician must communicate information to the patient immediately or all at once. Information may be conveyed over time in keeping with the patient's preferences and ability to comprehend the information. Physicians should always communicate sensitively and respectfully with patients.

With respect to disclosing or withholding information, physicians should:

(a) Encourage the patient to specify preferences regarding communication of medical information, preferably before the information becomes available.

AMA Principles of Medical Ethics: I, III, V, VIII

Issued: 2006

Updated: 2016

Opinions on Related Matters:
2.1.1 Informed Consent
7.3.2 Research on Emergency Medical Interventions

(b) Honor a patient's request not to receive certain medical information or to convey the information to a designated surrogate, provided these requests appear to represent the patient's genuine wishes.

(c) Assess the amount of information the patient is capable of receiving at a given time, and tailor disclosure to meet the patient's needs and expectations in keeping with the individual's preferences.

(d) Consult with the patient's family, the physician's colleagues, or an ethics committee or other institutional resource for help in assessing the relative benefits and harms associated with delaying disclosure.

(e) Monitor the patient carefully and offer full disclosure when the patient is able to decide whether to receive the information. This should be done according to a definite plan, so that disclosure is not permanently delayed.

(f) Disclose medical errors if they have occurred in the patient's care, in keeping with ethics guidance.

AMA Principles of Medical Ethics: I, III, V, VIII

Issued: 2007

Updated: 2016

Opinions on Related Matters:
2.1.1 Informed Consent
7.3.1 Ethical Use of Placebo Controls in Research

2.1.4 Use of Placebo in Clinical Practice

A placebo is a substance provided to a patient that the physician believes has no specific pharmacological effect on the condition being treated. The use of placebo, when consistent with good medical care, is distinct from interventions that lack scientific foundation.

A placebo may still be effective if the patient knows it will be used but cannot identify it and does not know the precise timing of its use. In the clinical setting, the use of a placebo without the patient's knowledge may undermine trust, compromise the patient-physician relationship, and result in medical harm to the patient.

Physicians may use placebos for diagnosis or treatment only if they:

(a) Enlist the patient's cooperation. The physician should explain that it can be possible to achieve a better understanding of the medical condition by evaluating the effects of different medications, including the placebo.

(b) Obtain the patient's general consent to administer a placebo. The physician does not need to identify precisely when the placebo will be administered. In this way, the physician respects the patient's autonomy and fosters a trusting relationship, while the patient may still benefit from the placebo effect.

(c) Avoid giving a placebo merely to mollify a difficult patient. Giving a placebo for such reasons places the convenience of the physician above the welfare of the patient. Physicians can produce a placebo-like effect through the skillful use of reassurance and encouragement, thereby building respect and trust, promoting the patient-physician relationship, and improving health outcomes.

2.1.5 Reporting Clinical Test Results

AMA Principles of Medical Ethics: II, IV, V
Issued: 1998
Updated: 2016
Opinions on Related Matters:
1.1.6 Quality
2.1.1 Informed Consent

Patients should be able to be confident that they will receive the results of clinical tests in a timely fashion. Physicians have a corresponding obligation to be considerate of patient concerns and anxieties and ensure that patients receive test results within a reasonable time frame.

When and how clinical test results are conveyed to patients can vary considerably in different practice environments and for different clinical tests. In some instances results are conveyed by the patient's treating physician; in others, by other practice staff or directly by the laboratory or other entity.

To ensure that test results are communicated appropriately to patients, physicians should adopt, or advocate for, policies and procedures to ensure that:

(a) The patient (or surrogate decision maker if the patient lacks decision-making capacity) is informed about when he or she can reasonably expect to learn the results of clinical tests and how those results will be conveyed.

(b) The patient or surrogate is instructed what to do if he or she does not receive results in the expected time frame.

(c) Test results are conveyed sensitively, in a way that is understandable to the patient or surrogate, and the patient or surrogate receives information needed to make well-considered decisions about medical treatment and give informed consent to future treatment.

(d) Patient confidentiality is protected regardless of how clinical test results are conveyed.

(e) The ordering physician is notified before the disclosure takes place and has access to the results as they will be conveyed to the patient or surrogate, if results are to be conveyed directly to the patient or surrogate by a third party.

*AMA Principles of Medical Ethics: I, II,
IV, V*

Issued: Prior to 1977

Updated: 1994, 2016

2.1.6 Substitution of Surgeon

Patients are entitled to choose their own physicians, which includes being permitted to accept or refuse having an intervention performed by a substitute. A surgeon who allows a substitute to conduct a medical procedure on his or her patient without the patient's knowledge or consent risks compromising the trust-based relationship of patient and physician.

When one or more other appropriately trained health care professionals will participate in performing a surgical intervention, the surgeon has an ethical responsibility to:

(a) Notify the patient (or surrogate if the patient lacks decision-making capacity) that others will participate, including whether they will do so under the physician's personal supervision.

(b) Obtain the patient's or surrogate's informed consent for the intervention, in keeping with ethical and legal guidelines.

Decisions for Minors

AMA Principles of Medical Ethics: IV, VIII

Issued: 2008

Updated: 2011, 2016

2.2.1 Pediatric Decision Making

Unlike health care decisions for most adult patients, decisions for pediatric patients usually involve a three-way relationship among the minor patient, the patient's parents (or guardian), and the physician. Although children who are emancipated may consent to care on their own behalf, in general, children below the age of majority are not considered to have the capacity to make health care decisions on their own. Rather, parents or guardians are expected, and authorized, to provide or decline permission for treatment for minor patients. Nonetheless, respect and shared decision making remain important in the context of decisions for minors, and physicians have a responsibility to engage minor patients in making decisions about their own care to the greatest extent possible, including decisions about life-sustaining treatment.

Decisions for pediatric patients should be based on the child's best interest, which is determined by weighing many factors, including effectiveness of appropriate medical therapies and the needs and interests of the patient and the family as the source of support and care for the patient. When there is legitimate inability to reach consensus about what is in the best interest of the child, the wishes of the parents or guardian should generally receive preference.

For health care decisions involving minor patients, physicians should:

(a) Involve all patients in decision making at a developmentally appropriate level.

(b) Base recommendations for treatment on the likely bene-fit to the patient, taking into account the effectiveness of treatment, risks of additional suffering with and without treatment, available alternatives, and overall prognosis.

(c) For patients capable of assent, truthfully explain the medical condition, its clinical implications, and the treatment plan in a manner that takes into account the child's cognitive and emotional maturity and social circumstances.

(d) Provide a supportive environment and encourage parents to discuss their child's health status with the patient. Offer to facilitate the parent-child conversation for reluctant parents.

(e) Recognize that for certain medical conditions, such as those involving HIV/AIDS or inherited conditions, disclosing the child's health status may also reveal health information about biological relatives or disrupt existing presumptions about the child's relationships within the family.

(f) Work with parents or guardians to simplify complex treat-ment regimens whenever possible and educate them in ways to avoid behaviors that put the child or others at risk.

(g) Ensure that when decisions involve life-sustaining interven-tions, patients have opportunity to be involved in keeping with their ability to understand decisions and their desire to participate. Physicians should ensure that the patient and parents or guardian understand the patient's diagnosis, both with and without treatment. Physicians should discuss with the patient and parents or guardian the option of initiating an intervention with the intention of evaluating its clinical effectiveness after a specified amount of time to determine if it has led to improvement. Confirm that if the intervention has not achieved agreed-on goals, it may be withdrawn.

(h) Respect the decisions of the patient and parents or guardian when it is not clear whether a specific intervention promotes the patient's best interests.

(i) Seek consultation with an ethics committee or other institu-tional resource when:

(i) there is a reversible life-threatening condition and the patient (if capable) or parents or guardian refuse treat-ment the physician believes is clearly in the patient's best interest;

    (ii) there is disagreement about what the patient's best interests are. Physicians should turn to the courts to resolve disagreements only as a last resort.

(j) Provide compassionate and humane care to all pediatric patients, including patients who forgo or discontinue life-sustaining interventions.

AMA Principles of Medical Ethics: IV

Issued: 1994

Updated: 1996, 2013, 2016

Opinions on Related Matters:
3.2.1   Confidentiality

2.2.2 Confidential Health Care for Minors

Physicians who treat minors have an ethical duty to promote the developing autonomy of minor patients by involving children in making decisions about their health care to a degree commensurate with the child's abilities. A minor's decision-making capacity depends on many factors, including not only chronological age but also emotional maturity and the individual's medical experience. Physicians also have a responsibility to protect the confidentiality of minor patients, within certain limits.

In some jurisdictions, the law permits minors who are not emancipated to request and receive confidential services relating to contraception, or to pregnancy testing, prenatal care, and delivery services. Similarly, jurisdictions may permit unemancipated minors to request and receive confidential care to prevent, diagnose, or treat sexually transmitted disease, substance use disorders, or mental illness.

When an unemancipated minor requests confidential care and the law does not grant the minor decision-making authority for that care, physicians should:

(a) Inform the patient (and parent or guardian, if present) about circumstances in which the physician is obligated to inform the minor's parent or guardian, including situations when:
    (i)   involving the patient's parent or guardian is necessary to avert life- or health-threatening harm to the patient;
    (ii)   involving the patient's parent or guardian is necessary to avert serious harm to others;
    (iii) the threat to the patient's health is significant and the physician has no reason to believe that parental involvement will be detrimental to the patient's well-being.

(b) Explore the minor patient's reasons for not involving his or her parents (or guardian) and try to correct misconceptions that may be motivating the patient's reluctance to involve parents.

(c) Encourage the minor patient to involve his or her parents and offer to facilitate conversation between the patient and the parents.

(d) Inform the patient that despite the physician's respect for confidentiality the minor patient's parents/guardians may learn about the request for treatment or testing through other means (eg, insurance statements).

(e) Protect the confidentiality of information disclosed by the patient during an exam or interview or in counseling unless the patient consents to disclosure or disclosure is required to protect the interests of others, in keeping with ethics guidance and legal guidelines.

(f) Take steps to facilitate a minor patient's decision about health care services when the patient remains unwilling to involve parents or guardians, so long as the patient has appropriate decision-making capacity in the specific circumstances and the physician believes the decision is in the patient's best interest. Physicians should be aware that states provide mechanisms for unemancipated minors to receive care without parental involvement under conditions that vary from state to state.

(g) Consult experts when the patient's decision-making capacity is uncertain.

(h) Inform or refer the patient to alternative confidential services when available, if the physician is unwilling to provide services without parental involvement.

2.2.3 Mandatory Parental Consent to Abortion

AMA Principles of Medical Ethics: III, IV

Issued: 1994

Updated: 2016

Opinions on Related Matters:
2.2.1 Pediatric Decision Making
2.2.2 Confidential Health Care for Minors
3.2.1 Confidentiality

In many jurisdictions, unemancipated minors are not permitted to request or receive abortion services without their parents' (or guardian's) knowledge and consent. Physicians should ascertain the law in their state on parental involvement to ensure that their practices are consistent with their legal obligations. In many places, the issue of confidentiality for minors who seek an abortion implicates competing ethical concerns apart from the abortion issue itself.

When an unemancipated minor requests abortion services, physicians should:

(a) Strongly encourage the patient to discuss the pregnancy with her parents (or guardian).

(b) Explore the minor patient's reasons for not involving her parents (or guardian) and try to correct misconceptions that may be motivating the patient's reluctance to involve parents. If the patient is unwilling to involve her parents, encourage her to seek the advice and counsel of adults in whom she has confidence, including professional counselors, relatives, friends, teachers, or the clergy.

(c) Explain to the minor patient under what circumstances the minor's confidentiality will be abrogated, including:

    (i)   life-threatening emergency;

    (ii) when parental notification is required by applicable law.

(d) Try to ensure that the minor patient carefully considers the issues involved and makes an informed decision.

(e) Not feel or be compelled to require a minor patient to involve her parents before she decides whether to undergo an abortion.

AMA Principles of Medical Ethics: I, III, IV, V

Issued: 1994

Updated: 2016

Opinions on Related Matters:

2.2.4 Treatment Decisions for Seriously Ill Newborns

Making treatment decisions for seriously ill newborns is emotionally and ethically challenging for both parents and health care professionals. Decisions must take into account the newborn's medical needs; the interests, needs, and resources of the family; and available treatment options. Decision makers must also assess whether the choice made for the newborn will abrogate a choice the future individual would want to make for him- or herself, ie, whether the choice will undermine the child's right to an "open future." Providing information and other resources to support parents or guardians when they must make decisions about their child's care and future is a key responsibility for physicians and other health care professionals.

Decisions not to initiate care or to discontinue an intervention can be emotionally wrenching in any circumstance, but may be particularly so for a seriously ill newborn. Physicians are in a position to help parents, families, and fellow professionals understand that there is no ethical difference between withholding and withdrawing treatment—when an intervention no longer helps to achieve the goals of care or promote the quality of life desired for the patient, it is ethically appropriate to withdraw it.

To help parents formulate goals for their newborn's care and make decisions about life-sustaining treatment on their child's behalf, physicians should:

(a) Inform the parents about available therapeutic options, the nature of available interventions, and their child's expected prognosis with and without treatment.

(b) Help the parents formulate goals for care that will promote their child's best interests in light of:
   (i) the chance that the intervention will achieve the intended clinical benefit;
   (ii) the risks involved with treatment and nontreatment;
   (iii) the degree to which treatment can be expected to extend life;
   (iv) the pain and discomfort associated with the intervention;
   (v) the quality of life the child can be expected to have with and without treatment.

(c) Discuss the option of initiating an intervention with the intention of evaluating its clinical effectiveness after a given amount of time to determine whether the intervention has led to improvement. Confirm that if the intervention has not achieved agreed-on goals, it may be withdrawn. Physicians should recognize, and help parents appreciate, that it is not necessary to have prognostic certainty to withdraw life-sustaining treatment, since prognostic certainty is often unattainable and waiting may unnecessarily prolong the infant's suffering.

(d) Initiate life-sustaining and life-enhancing treatment when the child's prognosis is largely uncertain.

(e) Adhere to good clinical practice for palliative care when life-sustaining treatment is withheld or withdrawn.

(f) Provide access to counseling services or other resources to facilitate decision making and to enable parents' opportunity to talk with others who have had to make similar decisions.

(g) Seek consultation through an ethics committee or other institutional resource when disagreement about the appropriate course of action persists.

2.2.5 Genetic Testing of Children

In genetics, the ability to diagnose disease or identify predisposition to disease often precedes the ability to prevent, treat, or ameliorate the condition in question. Genetic diagnosis can carry both benefits and risks for the patient, as well as implications for others to whom the patient is biologically related. Thus, decisions to carry out genetic testing can be challenging for any patient.

AMA Principles of Medical Ethics: IV

Issued: 1996

Updated: 2016

Opinions on Related Matters:
2.2.1 Pediatric Decision Making
3.2.1 Confidentiality

Genetic testing of children implicates important concerns about the minor patient's present and future autonomy and best interests. Decisions to test must balance multiple considerations, including likely benefits, the risks of knowing genetic status (including abrogating the child's opportunity to make the choice about knowing genetic status him- or herself as an adult), features unique to the condition(s) being tested for (such as age of onset), and the availability of effective preventive, therapeutic, or palliative interventions.

With respect to genetic testing of a minor patient, including genetic testing of children being considered for adoption, physicians should:

(a) Offer diagnostic testing when the child is at risk for a condition for which effective measures to prevent, treat, or ameliorate it are available. As for any medical intervention, the physician should seek the informed consent of the minor patient's parents (or guardian) and engage the patient in decision making at a developmentally appropriate level, in keeping with ethics guidance.

(b) In general, respect the decision of the patient's parents or guardian about testing when the child is at risk for a condition with pediatric onset for which no effective measures to prevent, treat, or ameliorate the condition are available.

(c) Attempt to persuade reluctant parents or guardians to consent to testing when there are effective measures to prevent, treat, or ameliorate the condition and, in the physician's judgment, delaying testing would result in irreversible harm to the child.

(d) Regardless of the source of the testing, help the patient, parents, or guardian access appropriate counseling.

(e) Refrain from offering, providing, or recommending a genetic test:

(i) when parents or guardians request testing for a child who is at risk for a condition with adult onset for which no effective measures to prevent, treat, or ameliorate the condition are available. Physicians should inform the parents or guardian about the test and why it is not recommended. When a minor patient seeks genetic testing for such a condition, physicians should condition testing on the patient's developmental status and ability to understand the implications of testing, in keeping with ethics guidance on decisions for minor patients;

(ii) when parents or guardians request testing to determine the child's carrier status for a recessive genetic condition and there are no other health implications for the child. Physicians may provide testing when reproductive

　　　　decisions need to be made on behalf of or by a minor
　　　　patient, in keeping with ethics guidance;

(iii) for the benefit of a family member, unless testing will
　　　prevent substantial harm to the individual;

(iv) when testing will not serve the child's health interests.

(f) Seek consultation from an ethics committee or other insti-
　　tutional resource when disagreements about genetic testing
　　persist. If parents unreasonably request or refuse testing of
　　their child, the physician should take steps to change or, if
　　necessary, use legal means to override the parents' choice.

(g) Encourage parents to share genetic information with
　　the child in a manner appropriate to the child's stage of
　　development.

(h) Ensure that parents or guardians are aware of findings that
　　are not immediately relevant but will need to be shared later
　　so that the information can be conveyed to the child when it
　　becomes relevant.

Communication with Patients

2.3.1 Electronic Communication with Patients

Electronic communication, such as email or text messaging, can be
a useful tool in the practice of medicine and can facilitate communication within a patient-physician relationship. However, these
channels can raise special concerns about privacy and confidentiality, particularly when sensitive information is to be communicated.
When physicians engage in electronic communication they hold the
same ethical responsibilities to patients as they do during other clinical encounters. Any method of communication, virtual, telephonic,
or in person, should be appropriate to the patient's clinical need and
to the information being conveyed.

　　Email correspondence should not be used to establish a patient-
physician relationship. Rather, email should supplement other, more
personal encounters.

　　Physicians who choose to communicate electronically with
patients should:

(a) Uphold professional standards of confidentiality and protec-
　　tion of privacy, security, and integrity of patient information.

(b) Notify the patient of the inherent limitations of electronic
　　communication, including possible breach of privacy or con-
　　fidentiality, difficulty in validating the identity of the parties,

AMA Principles of Medical Ethics: I, IV, VI, VII

Issued: 2003

Updated: 2016

Opinions on Related Matters:
2.1.1 Informed Consent
2.3.1 Electronic Communication with Patients
3.2.1 Confidentiality

and possible delays in response. Such disclaimers do not absolve physicians of responsibility to protect the patient's interests. Patients should have the opportunity to accept or decline electronic communication before privileged information is transmitted. The patient's decision to accept or decline email communication containing privileged information should be documented in the medical record.

(c) Advise the patient of the limitations of these channels when a patient initiates electronic communication.

(d) Obtain the patient's consent to continue electronic communication when a patient initiates electronic communication.

(e) Present medical information in a manner that meets professional standards. Diagnostic or therapeutic services must conform to accepted clinical standards.

(f) Be aware of relevant laws that determine when a patient-physician relationship has been established.

AMA Principles of Medical Ethics: I, II, IV

Issued: 2011, 2016

Opinions on Related Matters:
1.2.12 Ethical Practice in Telemedicine
3.2.1 Confidentiality
9.2.1 Medical Student Involvement in Patient Care
9.2.2 Resident and Fellow Physicians' Involvement in Patient Care

2.3.2 Professionalism in the Use of Social Media

The Internet has created the ability for medical students and physicians to communicate and share information quickly and to reach millions of people easily. Participating in social networking and other similar Internet opportunities can support physicians' personal expression, enable individual physicians to have a professional presence online, foster collegiality and camaraderie within the profession, and provide opportunity to widely disseminate public health messages and other health communications. Social networks, blogs, and other forms of communication online also create new challenges to the patient-physician relationship.

Physicians and trainees have an ethical responsibility to weigh a number of considerations when maintaining a presence online:

(a) They should be cognizant of standards of patient privacy and confidentiality that must be maintained in all environments, including online, and must refrain from posting identifiable patient information online.

(b) When using the Internet for social networking, they should use privacy settings to safeguard personal information and content to the extent possible but should realize that privacy settings are not absolute and that once on the Internet, content is likely there permanently. Thus, physicians should routinely monitor their own Internet presence to ensure that the personal and professional information on their own sites and, to the extent possible, content posted about them by others is accurate and appropriate.

(c) If they interact with patients on the Internet, they must maintain appropriate boundaries of the patient-physician relationship in accordance with professional ethics guidance, just as they would in any other context.

(d) To maintain appropriate professional boundaries, they should consider separating personal and professional content online.

(e) When they see content posted by colleagues that appears unprofessional, they have a responsibility to bring that content to the attention of the individual, so that he or she can remove it or take other appropriate actions. If the behavior significantly violates professional norms and the individual does not take appropriate action to resolve the situation, the physician should report the matter to appropriate authorities.

(f) They must recognize that actions online and content posted may negatively affect their reputations among patients and colleagues, may have consequences for their medical careers (particularly for physicians-in-training and medical students), and can undermine public trust in the medical profession.

2.3.3 Informing Families of a Patient's Death

Informing a patient's family that the patient has died is a duty that is fundamental to the patient-physician relationship. When communicating this event, physicians should give foremost attention to the family's emotional needs and the integrity of the patient-physician relationship.

The following guidance applies to communicating news of a patient's death:

(a) Any physician informing a patient's family about the patient's death has a responsibility to:
  (i)   communicate this information compassionately;
  (ii) disclose the death in a timely manner.

(b) Ordinarily, the treating physician should take responsibility for informing the family. However, it may be appropriate to delegate the task to another physician if the other physician has a previous close personal relationship with the patient or family and the appropriate skill.

(c) Medical students should not be asked to inform family members of a patient's death. Medical students should be trained in communication skills relating to death and dying, and should be encouraged to accompany attending physicians when news of a patient's death is conveyed to family members.

AMA Principles of Medical Ethics: I, IV

Issued: 1992

Updated: 1994, 2016

Opinions on Related Matters:
9.2.1 Medical Student Involvement in Patient Care
9.2.2 Resident and Fellow Physicians' Involvement in Patient Care

AMA Principles of Medical Ethics: I, VII

Issued: 1999

Updated: 2016

Opinions on Related Matters:
1.2.10 Political Action by Physicians
2.3.5 Soliciting Charitable
       Contributions from Patients
3.2.1 Confidentiality

2.3.4 Political Communications

Physicians enjoy the rights and privileges of free speech shared by all Americans. It is laudable for physicians to run for political office; to lobby for political positions, parties, or candidates; and in every other way to exercise the full scope of their political rights as citizens. Physicians may exercise these rights individually or through involvement with professional societies and political action committees or other organizations.

When physicians wish to express their personal political views to a patient or a patient's family, the physician must be sensitive to the imbalance of power in the patient-physician relationship, as well as to the patient's vulnerability and desire for privacy.

Physicians must not allow differences with the patient or family about political matters to interfere with the delivery of professional care.

When expressing political views to a patient or a patient's family, physicians should:

(a) Judge both the intrusiveness of the discussion and the patient's level of comfort before initiating such a discussion.

(b) Discuss political matters only in contexts in which conversation with the patient or family about social, civic, or recreational matters is acceptable.

(c) Refrain from conversation about political matters when the patient or family is emotionally pressured by significant medical circumstances.

(d) Work toward and advocate for the reform and proper administration of laws related to health care. Physicians should stay well informed of current political questions regarding needed and proposed reforms.

(e) Stay well informed about needed or proposed policies concerning health care access and quality, medical research, and promoting public health so as to be able to advocate for patients' needs.

AMA Principles of Medical Ethics: IV, VII, VIII

Issued: 2004

Updated: 2016

Opinions on Related Matters:
1.2.8 Gifts from Patients
2.3.4 Political Communications

2.3.5 Soliciting Charitable Contributions from Patients

Charitable contributions play an important role in supporting and improving a community's health, and physicians are encouraged to participate in fundraising and other solicitation activities.

To sustain the trust that is the foundation of the patient-physician relationship and to reassure patients that their welfare is the physician's primary priority, physicians who participate in fundraising should:

(a) Assure patients that they need not contribute in order to continue receiving quality care.

(b) Refrain from directly soliciting contributions from their own patients, especially during clinical encounters.

(c) Solicit contributions by making information available, eg, in their office reception areas or by speaking at fundraising events.

(d) Protect patient privacy and confidentiality by not acknowledging that a patient is under the physician's care when approached by fundraising personnel without the prior consent of the patient.

(e) Obtain permission from the patient before releasing information for purposes of fundraising when the nature of the physician's practice could make it possible to identify the medical services provided or the patient's diagnosis.

(f) Refer patients or families who wish to make charitable contributions to appropriate information or fundraising personnel.

(g) Be sensitive to the likelihood that they may be perceived to be acting in their professional role when participating in fundraising activities as a member of the general community.

2.3.6 Surgical Co-management

Surgical co-management refers to the practice of allotting specific responsibilities of patient care to designated clinicians. Such arrangements should be made only to ensure the highest quality of care.

When engaging in this practice, physicians should:

(a) Allocate responsibilities among physicians and other clinicians according to each individual's expertise and qualifications.

(b) Work with the patient and family to designate one physician to be responsible for ensuring that care is delivered in a coordinated and appropriate manner.

(c) Participate in the provision of care by communicating with the coordinating physician and encouraging other members of the care team to do the same.

(d) Obtain patient consent for the surgical co-management arrangement of care, including disclosing significant aspects of the arrangement such as qualifications of clinicians, services each clinician will provide, and billing arrangement.

(e) Obtain informed consent for medical services in keeping with ethics guidance, including provision of all relevant medical facts.

AMA Principles of Medical Ethics: I, II, IV, V, VI

Issued: 2000

Updated: 2016

Opinions on Related Matters:
2.1.1 Informed Consent
2.1.6 Substitution of Surgeon
9.2.1 Medical Student Involvement in Patient Care
9.2.2 Resident and Fellow Physicians' Involvement in Patient Care

(f) Employ appropriate safeguards to protect patient confidentiality.

(g) Ensure that surgical co-management arrangements are in keeping with ethical and legal restrictions.

(h) Engage another caregiver based on that caregiver's skill and ability to meet the patient's needs, not in the expectation of reciprocal referrals or other self-serving reasons, in keeping with ethics guidance on consultation and referrals.

(i) Refrain from participating in unethical or illegal financial agreements, such as fee-splitting.

3 Privacy, Confidentiality, and Medical Records

These Opinions are offered as ethics guidance for physicians and are not intended to establish clinical practice guidelines or rules of law.

Respecting patients' rights to privacy and confidentiality is a core ethical obligation in medicine.[1] To receive the care they need, patients must be willing to submit to examinations that can be physically intrusive and to share highly personal and often sensitive information. When patients withhold information, eg, out of embarrassment or fear that the information may be used against them in some way, they may undermine the quality of care physicians are able to provide and compromise their own health outcomes. Patients must be able to trust that their physicians and others who participate in care will protect their dignity and safeguard the confidences they have shared.

Physicians have corresponding obligations to ensure that that trust is warranted. Thus, physicians have a responsibility to provide an environment in which intrusions on patients' physical privacy are minimized. This responsibility includes seeking patients' agreement to having third parties present during clinical encounters, especially individuals who are not part of the care team.

Physicians similarly have an obligation to protect patients' confidential information from unauthorized access. They have a responsibility to ensure that information gathered during clinical encounters, through diagnostic or treatment interventions as well as history taking and physical examinations, is appropriately recorded and is shared only with appropriate health care personnel or others to whom the patient has authorized disclosure. The obligation extends to protecting the security and integrity of medical records and to informing patients when the security of records has been breached.

Patients' right to privacy and confidentiality is not absolute, however. Patients' information may be shared without the patient's explicit authorization for purposes of health care administration and billing within the protections of state and federal law. Physicians may also have an obligation to breach confidentiality to protect other individuals or the public, eg, when the physician judges the patient to pose a risk of harm to another person or is required to report information to public health authorities.

Opinions in the first and second sections of this chapter set out physicians' fundamental ethical obligations with respect to privacy and confidentiality, and offer more specific guidance about these key obligations in different situations. Opinions in the third section provide guidance with respect to physicians' responsibilities in managing medical records.

Reference

1. Rothstein MA. Privacy and confidentiality. In Joly Y, Knoppers BM, eds. *Routledge Handbook of Medical Law and Ethics*. New York: Routledge; 2015:52-66.

Privacy

Confidentiality

Medical Records

Privacy

3.1.1 Privacy in Health Care

Protecting information gathered in association with the care of the patient is a core value in health care. However, respecting patient privacy in other forms is also fundamental, as an expression of respect for patient autonomy and a prerequisite for trust.

Patient privacy encompasses a number of aspects, including personal space (physical privacy), personal data (informational privacy), personal choices, including cultural and religious affiliations (decisional privacy), and personal relationships with family members and other intimates (associational privacy).

Physicians must seek to protect patient privacy in all settings to the greatest extent possible and should:

(a) Minimize intrusion on privacy when the patient's privacy must be balanced against other factors.

(b) Inform the patient when there has been a significant infringement on privacy of which the patient would otherwise not be aware.

(c) Be mindful that individual patients may have special concerns about privacy in any or all of these areas.

AMA Principles of Medical Ethics: I, IV

Issued: 2002

Updated: 2016

Opinions on Related Matters:
3.1.2 Patient Privacy and Outside Observers of the Clinical Encounter
3.1.3 Audio or Visual Recording of Patients for Education in Health Care
3.1.4 Audio or Visual Recording of Patients for Public Education
3.2.4 Access to Medical Records by Data Collection Companies
9.2.1 Medical Student Involvement in Patient Care
9.2.2 Resident and Fellow Physicians' Involvement in Patient Care

3.1.2 Patient Privacy and Outside Observers of the Clinical Encounter

Individuals legitimately present during patient-physician encounters include those directly involved in the patient's care, and can include other members of the health care team or employees of pharmaceutical or medical device companies when they are present to provide technical assistance, in keeping with ethics guidance.

When individuals who are not involved in providing care seek to observe patient-physician encounters, eg, for educational purposes, physicians should safeguard patient privacy by permitting such observers to be present during a clinical encounter only when:

(a) The patient has explicitly agreed to the presence of the observer(s). Outside observers should not be permitted when the patient lacks decision-making capacity, except in rare circumstances and with the consent of the patient's parent, legal guardian, or authorized decision maker.

(b) The presence of the observer will not compromise care.

AMA Principles of Medical Ethics: I, IV, VIII

Issued: 2005

Updated: 2016

Opinions on Related Matters:
3.1.1 Privacy in Health Care
3.1.3 Audio or Visual Recording of Patients for Education in Health Care
3.1.4 Audio or Visual Recording of Patients for Public Education
3.2.1 Confidentiality
3.2.4 Access to Medical Records by Data Collection Companies

(c) The observer understands and has agreed to adhere to standards of medical privacy and confidentiality.

Under no circumstances should physicians accept payment from outside observers to allow those observers to be present during a clinical encounter.

AMA Principles of Medical Ethics: I, IV, V, VIII

Issued: 2003

Updated: 2016

3.1.3 Audio or Visual Recording of Patients for Education in Health Care

Audio or visual recording of patients can be a valuable tool for educating health care professionals, but physicians must balance educational goals with patient privacy and confidentiality. The intended audience is bound by professional standards of respect for patient autonomy, privacy, and confidentiality, but physicians also have an obligation to ensure that content is accurate and complete and that the process and product of recording uphold standards of professional conduct.

To safeguard patient interests in the context of recording for purposes of educating health care professionals, physicians should:

(a) Ensure that all nonclinical personnel present during recording understand and agree to adhere to medical standards of privacy and confidentiality.

(b) Restrict participation to patients who have decision-making capacity. Recording should not be permitted when the patient lacks decision-making capacity except in rare circumstances and with the consent of the patient's parent, legal guardian, or authorized decision maker.

(c) Inform the patient (or authorized decision maker, in the rare circumstances when recording is authorized for minors or patients who lack decision-making capacity):

(i) about the purpose of recording, the intended audience(s), and the expected distribution;

(ii) about the potential benefits and harms (such as breach of privacy or confidentiality) of participating;

(iii) that participation is voluntary and that a decision not to participate (or to withdraw) will not affect the patient's care;

(iv) that the patient may withdraw consent at any time and, if so, what will be done with the recording;

(v) that use of the recording will be limited to those involved in health care education, unless the patient specifically permits use by others.

(d) Ensure that the patient has had opportunity to discuss concerns before and after recording.

(e) Obtain consent from a patient (or the authorized decision maker):

   (i)　prior to recording whenever possible; or

   (ii)　before use for educational purposes when consent could not be obtained prior to recording.

(f) Respect the decision of a patient to withdraw consent.

(g) Seek assent from the patient for participation in addition to consent by the patient's parent or guardian when participation by a minor patient is unavoidable.

(h) Be aware that the act of recording may affect patient behavior during a clinical encounter and, thereby, affect the recording's educational content and value.

(i) Be aware that the information contained in educational recordings should be held to the same protections as any other record of patient information. Recordings should be securely stored and properly destroyed, in keeping with ethics guidance for managing medical records.

(j) Be aware that recording creates a permanent record of personal patient information and may be considered part of the medical record and subject to laws governing medical records.

3.1.4 Audio or Visual Recording of Patients for Public Education

Audio or visual recording of patient care for public broadcast is one way to help educate the public about health care. However, no matter what medium is used, such recording poses challenges for protecting patient autonomy, privacy, and confidentiality. Recording cannot benefit a patient medically and may cause harm. As advocates for their patients, physicians have an obligation to protect patient interests and ensure that professional standards are upheld. Physicians also have a responsibility to ensure that information conveyed to the public is complete and accurate (including the risks, benefits, and alternatives of treatments).

Physicians involved in recording patients for public broadcast should:

(a) Participate in institutional review of requests to record patient interactions.

(b) Require that persons present for recording purposes who are not members of the health care team:

AMA Principles of Medical Ethics: I, IV, VII, VIII

Issued: 2001

Updated: 2006, 2016

Opinions on Related Matters:
3.1.1　Privacy in Health Care
3.1.2　Patient Privacy and Outside Observers of the Clinical Encounter
3.1.3　Audio or Visual Recording of Patients for Education in Health Care

(i)   minimize third-party exposure to the patient's care;

(ii) adhere to medical standards of privacy and confidentiality.

(c) Encourage recording personnel to engage medical specialty societies or other sources of independent expert review in assessing the accuracy of the product.

(d) Refuse to participate in programs that foster misperceptions or are otherwise misleading.

(e) Restrict participation to patients who have decision-making capacity. Recording should not be permitted when the patient lacks decision-making capacity except in rare circumstances and with the consent of the parent, legal guardian, or authorized decision maker.

(f) Inform a patient who is to be recorded (or authorized decision maker):

(i)   about the purpose for which patient encounters with physicians or other health care professionals will be recorded;

(ii) about the intended audience(s);

(iii) that the patient may withdraw consent at any time prior to recording and up to an agreed-on time before the completed recording is publicly broadcast, and, if so, what will be done with the recording;

(iv) that at any time the patient has the right to have recording stopped and recording personnel removed from the area;

(v)   whether the patient will be allowed to review the recording before broadcast and the degree to which the patient may edit the final product;

(vi) whether the physician was compensated for his or her participation and the terms of that compensation.

(g) Ensure that the patient has had the opportunity to address concerns before and after recording.

(h) Ensure that consent is obtained from the patient or authorized decision maker by a disinterested third party not involved with the production team to avoid potential conflict of interest.

(i) Request that recording be stopped and recording personnel removed if the physician (or other person involved in the patient's care) perceives that recording may jeopardize patient care.

(j) Ensure that the care they provide and the advice they give to patients regarding participation in recording is not influenced by potential financial gain or promotional benefit to themselves, their patients, or the health care institution.

(k) Remind patients and colleagues that recording creates a permanent record and may in some instances be considered part of the medical record.

3.1.5 Professionalism in Relationships with Media

Ensuring that the public is informed promptly and accurately about medical issues is a valuable objective. However, media requests for information about patients can pose concerns about patient privacy and confidentiality, among other issues.

Physicians who speak on health-related matters on behalf of organizations should be aware of institutional guidelines for communicating with media, where they exist.

To safeguard patient interests when working with representatives of the media, all physicians should:

(a) Obtain consent from the patient or the patient's authorized representative before releasing information.
(b) Release only information specifically authorized by the patient or patient's representative or that is part of the public record.
(c) Ensure that no statement regarding diagnosis or prognosis is made except by or on behalf of the attending physician.
(d) Refer any questions regarding criminal activities or other police matters to the proper authorities.

AMA Principles of Medical Ethics: IV

Issued: Prior to 1977

Updated: 1994, 1996, 2016

Opinions on Related Matters:
3.1.1 Privacy in Health Care
3.2.1 Confidentiality
3.2.2 Confidentiality Postmortem

Confidentiality

3.2.1 Confidentiality

Patients need to be able to trust that physicians will protect information shared in confidence. They should feel free to fully disclose sensitive personal information to enable their physician to most effectively provide needed services. Physicians in turn have an ethical obligation to preserve the confidentiality of information gathered in association with the care of the patient.

In general, patients are entitled to decide whether and to whom their personal health information is disclosed. However, specific consent is not required in all situations.

AMA Principles of Medical Ethics: III, IV, VII, VIII

Issued: 1983

Updated: 1994, 2007, 2016

Opinions on Related Matters:
2.3.2 Electronic Communication with Patients
3.1.1 Privacy in Health Care
3.2.2 Confidentiality Postmortem
3.2.4 Access to Medical Records by Data Collection Companies
3.3.2 Confidentiality and Electronic Medical Records
4.1.3 Third-Party Access to Genetic Information

When disclosing patients' personal health information, physicians should:

(a) Restrict disclosure to the minimum necessary information.
(b) Notify the patient of the disclosure, when feasible.

Physicians may disclose personal health information without the specific consent of the patient (or authorized surrogate when the patient lacks decision-making capacity):

(c) To other health care personnel for purposes of providing care or for health care operations.
(d) To appropriate authorities when disclosure is required by law.
(e) To other third parties situated to mitigate the threat when in the physician's judgment there is a reasonable probability that:
   (i) the patient will seriously harm himself or herself; or
   (ii) the patient will inflict serious physical harm on an identifiable individual or individuals.

For any other disclosures, physicians should obtain the consent of the patient (or authorized surrogate) before disclosing personal health information.

AMA Principles of Medical Ethics: IV

Issued: 2000

Updated: 2001, 2016

Opinions on Related Matters:
3.1.1 Privacy in Health Care
3.1.5 Professionalism in Relationships with Media
3.2.1 Confidentiality

3.2.2 Confidentiality Postmortem

In general, patients are entitled to the same respect for the confidentiality of their personal information after death as they were in life. Physicians have a corresponding obligation to protect patient information, including information obtained postmortem. However, the obligation to safeguard confidentiality postmortem is subject to certain exceptions that are ethically and legally justifiable because of overriding societal concerns.

Physicians may disclose autopsy results to the surrogate or other decision maker who gave consent for the procedure.

Otherwise, physicians may disclose a deceased patient's personal health information only:

(a) In accord with the patient's explicit prior consent or directive. Physicians should respect the individual's specific preferences regarding disclosure.
(b) When required by law.
(c) When in the physician's judgment disclosure will avert harm to, or benefit, identifiable individuals or the community.
(d) For purposes of medical research or education if personal identifiers have been removed.

In all circumstances, physicians should:

(e) Consider the effect disclosure is likely to have on the patient's reputation.

(f) Restrict disclosure to the minimum necessary information.

When disclosing a deceased patient's health information would result in personal gain for the physician (financial or otherwise), the physician must seek specific consent to the disclosure from the patient's authorized decision maker.

3.2.3 Industry-Employed Physicians and Independent Medical Examiners

Physicians may obtain personal information about patients outside an ongoing patient-physician relationship. For example, physicians may assess an individual's health or disability on behalf of an employer, insurer, or other third party. Or they may obtain information in providing care specifically for a work-related illness or injury. In all these situations, physicians have a responsibility to protect the confidentiality of patient information.

When conducting third-party assessments or treating work-related medical conditions, physicians may disclose information to a third party:

(a) With written or documented consent of the individual (or authorized surrogate).

(b) As required by law, including workers' compensation law where applicable.

When disclosing information to third parties, physicians should:

(c) Restrict disclosure to the minimum necessary information for the intended purpose.

(d) Ensure that individually identifying information is removed before releasing aggregate data or statistical health information about the pertinent population.

AMA Principles of Medical Ethics: IV

Issued: 1983

Updated: 1994, 1996, 1999, 2016

Opinions on Related Matters:
1.2.5 Sports Medicine
1.2.6 Work-Related and Independent Medical Examinations
3.1.1 Privacy in Health Care
3.2.1 Confidentiality
3.2.4 Access to Medical Records by Data Collection Companies
3.3.2 Confidentiality and Electronic Medical Records
11.2.2 Conflicts of Interest in Patient Care
11.2.4 Transparency in Health Care

AMA Principles of Medical Ethics: I, II, IV

Issued: 1994

Updated: 1998, 2016

Opinions on Related Matters:
3.2.1 Confidentiality
3.3.2 Confidentiality and Electronic Medical Records
3.3.3 Breach of Security in Electronic Medical Records

3.2.4 Access to Medical Records by Data Collection Companies

Information contained in patients' medical records about physicians' prescribing practices or other treatment decisions can serve many valuable purposes, such as improving quality of care. However, ethical concerns arise when access to such information is sought for marketing purposes on behalf of commercial entities that have financial interests in physicians' treatment recommendations, such as pharmaceutical or medical device companies.

Information gathered and recorded in association with the care of a patient is confidential. Patients are entitled to expect that the sensitive personal information they divulge will be used solely to enable their physician to most effectively provide needed services. Disclosing information to third parties for commercial purposes without consent undermines trust, violates principles of informed consent and confidentiality, and may harm the integrity of the patient-physician relationship.

Physicians who propose to permit third-party access to specific patient information for commercial purposes should:

(a) Only provide data that has been de-identified.
(b) Fully inform each patient whose record would be involved (or the patient's authorized surrogate when the individual lacks decision-making capacity) about the purpose(s) for which access would be granted.

Physicians who propose to permit third parties to access the patient's full medical record should:

(c) Obtain the consent of the patient (or authorized surrogate) to permit access to the patient's medical record.
(d) Prohibit access to or decline to provide information from individual medical records for which consent has not been given.
(e) Decline incentives that constitute ethically inappropriate gifts, in keeping with ethics guidance.

Medical Records

3.3.1 Management of Medical Records

Medical records serve important patient interests for present health care and future needs, as well as insurance, employment, and other purposes.

In keeping with the professional responsibility to safeguard the confidentiality of patients' personal information, physicians have an ethical obligation to manage medical records appropriately.

This obligation encompasses not only managing the records of current patients, but also retaining old records against possible future need, and providing copies or transferring records to a third party as requested by the patient or the patient's authorized representative when the physician leaves a practice, sells his or her practice, retires, or dies.

To manage medical records responsibly, physicians (or the individual responsible for the practice's medical records) should:

(a) Ensure that the practice or institution has and enforces clear policy prohibiting access to patients' medical records by unauthorized staff.

(b) Use medical considerations to determine how long to keep records, retaining information that another physician seeing the patient for the first time could reasonably be expected to need or want to know unless otherwise required by law, including:

   (i) immunization records, which should be kept indefinitely;

   (ii) records of significant health events or conditions and interventions that could be expected to have a bearing on the patient's future health care needs, such as records of chemotherapy.

(c) Make the medical record available:

   (i) as requested or authorized by the patient (or the patient's authorized representative);

   (ii) to the succeeding physician or other authorized person when the physician discontinues his or her practice (whether through departure, sale of the practice, retirement, or death);

   (iii) as otherwise required by law.

(d) Never refuse to transfer the record on request by the patient or the patient's authorized representative, for any reason.

(e) Charge a reasonable fee (if any) for the cost of transferring the record.

(f) Appropriately store records not transferred to the patient's current physician.

AMA Principles of Medical Ethics: IV, V

Issued: The constituent Opinions on which this guidance is based (see Concordance) were issued between 1977 and 1994 and most recently updated between 1994 and 2002.

Updated: 2016

Opinions on Related Matters:

3 Privacy, Confidentiality, and Medical Records

(g) Notify the patient about how to access the stored record and for how long the record will be available.

(h) Ensure that records that are to be discarded are destroyed to protect confidentiality.

AMA Principles of Medical Ethics: V

Issued: Prior to 1977

Updated: 1994, 1998, 2016

Opinions on Related Matters:
3.2.1 Confidentiality
3.2.4 Access to Medical Records by Data Collection Companies
3.3.3 Breach of Security in Electronic Medical Records

3.3.2 Confidentiality and Electronic Medical Records

Information gathered and recorded in association with the care of a patient is confidential, regardless of the form in which it is collected or stored.

Physicians who collect or store patient information electronically, whether on stand-alone systems in their own practice or through contracts with service providers, must:

(a) Choose a system that conforms to acceptable industry practices and standards with respect to:
   (i) restriction of data entry and access to authorized personnel;
   (ii) capacity to routinely monitor or audit access to records;
   (iii) measures to ensure data security and integrity;
   (iv) policies and practices to address record retrieval, data sharing, third-party access and release of information, and disposition of records (when outdated or on termination of the service relationship), in keeping with ethics guidance.
(b) Describe how the confidentiality and integrity of information is protected if the patient requests.
(c) Release patient information only in keeping with ethics guidance for confidentiality.

AMA Principles of Medical Ethics: IV, VIII

Issued: 2009

Updated: 2016

Opinions on Related Matters:
3.2.1 Confidentiality
3.2.4 Access to Medical Records by Data Collection Companies
3.3.2 Confidentiality and Electronic Medical Records

3.3.3 Breach of Security in Electronic Medical Records

When used with appropriate attention to security, electronic medical records (EMRs) promise numerous benefits for quality clinical care and health-related research. However, when a security breach occurs, patients may face physical, emotional, and dignitary harms.

Dedication to upholding trust in the patient-physician relationship, to preventing harms to patients, and to respecting patients' privacy and autonomy creates responsibilities for individual physicians, medical practices, and health care institutions when patient information is inappropriately disclosed.

The degree to which an individual physician has an ethical responsibility to address inappropriate disclosure depends in part on his or her awareness of the breach, relationship to the patient(s) affected, administrative authority with respect to the records, and authority to act on behalf of the practice or institution.

When there is reason to believe that patients' confidentiality has been compromised by a breach of the EMR, physicians should:

(a) Ensure that patients are promptly informed about the breach and potential for harm, either by disclosing directly (when the physician has administrative responsibility for the EMR), participating in efforts by the practice or health care institution to disclose, or ensuring that the practice or institution takes appropriate action to disclose.

(b) Follow all applicable state and federal laws regarding disclosure.

Physicians have a responsibility to follow ethically appropriate procedures for disclosure, which should at minimum include:

(c) Carrying out the disclosure confidentially and within a time frame that provides patients ample opportunity to take steps to minimize potential adverse consequences.

(d) Describing what information was breached; how the breach happened; what the consequences may be; what corrective actions have been taken by the physician, practice, or institution; and what steps patients themselves might take to minimize adverse consequences.

(e) Supporting responses to security breaches that place the interests of patients above those of the physician, medical practice, or institution.

(f) Providing information to patients to enable them to mitigate potential adverse consequences of inappropriate disclosure of their personal health information to the extent possible.

4 Genetics and Reproductive Medicine

These Opinions are offered as ethics guidance for physicians and are not intended to establish clinical practice guidelines or rules of law.

Ongoing developments in molecular biology and genetic technologies open new prospects for understanding health risks and for personalizing medical care to meet the unique needs and situations of individual patients. At the same time, they pose ongoing ethical challenges for patients and their families, physicians, researchers, and other stakeholders.

Issues of informed consent and privacy and confidentiality take on distinctive shapes in the context of genetic testing and information. Physicians must be skillful in presenting complex information to help patients understand what genetic testing can and cannot tell them about their current or future health status to enable patients to make well-considered decisions. Moreover, testing may return information about more than just the condition of interest, and such incidental findings may carry important but unexpected implications for patient health. Genetic information obtained about one individual also carries implications for others to whom that individual is biologically related, which raises questions about when and how a patient should disclose information to family members. Although state and federal law prohibits insurers, employers, and others from discriminating against individuals on the basis of genetic information, the possibility that third parties will use genetic information inappropriately gives special significance to concerns about protecting the privacy and confidentiality of a patient's information.

Similarly, progress in reproductive medicine continues to open new opportunities to create families for persons who are unable to have a child without medical assistance. Technologies that allow gametes to be retrieved and stored or used to create embryos on behalf of an individual or couple seeking to become parents can entangle reproductive decisions in complex webs of relationships among multiple parties whose interests may not always align. Depending on how they organize their practices, physicians will be responsible for informing gamete donors, prospective rearing parents, gestational surrogates, or all of these about potential risks and benefits of different reproductive options. Concerns about the voluntariness of participation in assisted reproduction, the possibility for conflict of interest, and obligations to provide nondirective services and to offer services fairly, without discrimination, all come into play. Assisted reproduction can also touch on deeply contested issues about the moral status of human gametes and embryos and obligations to respect the decisions prospective parents make.

Opinions in the first section offer guidance on matters involving genetics in clinical practice, while those in the second section address ethical concerns in reproductive medicine and decision making. (Opinions in Chapter 7 address related issues in the context of research.)

Genetics

Reproductive Medicine

Genetics

4.1.1 Genetic Testing and Counseling

Genetic testing can provide valuable information to support informed decision making about personal health risks and care options as well as reproductive choices. The fact that genetic information carries implications for others to whom the individual is biologically related raises ethical challenges of balancing confidentiality against the well-being of others.

Because genetic contribution to disease can be complex and highly variable, interpreting findings and helping patients understand the implications for their health and health care requires special skill and attention.

Genetic testing is most appropriate when the results of testing will have meaningful impact on the patient's care. Physicians should not encourage testing unless there is effective therapy available to prevent or ameliorate the condition tested for. Whether a genetic test is performed to help diagnose an existing health condition, to predict future health risks, or to provide information for managing a disease, it is important that the patient receive appropriate counseling.

Physicians who order genetic tests (individually or as part of a multi-test panel or large-scale sequencing) or who offer clinical genetic services should:

(a) Have appropriate knowledge and expertise to counsel patients about heritable conditions, risks for disease, and implications for health management, and to interpret findings of individual genetic tests or collaborate with other health care professionals who can provide these services, such as licensed genetic counselors.

(b) Adhere to standards of nondirective counseling and avoid imposing their personal moral values or judgment on the patient.

(c) Discuss with the patient:

   (i) what can and cannot be learned from the proposed genetic test(s) and reasons for and against testing, including the possibility of incidental findings. Physicians should ascertain whether the patient wishes to be informed about findings unrelated to the goal of testing;

   (ii) medical and psychological implications for the individual's biological relatives;

   (iii) circumstances under which the physician will expect the patient to notify biological relatives of test findings;

   (iv) that the physician will be available to assist the patient in communicating with relatives.

AMA Principles of Medical Ethics: II, IV, V, VI

Issued: The constituent Opinions on which this guidance is based (see Concordance) were issued between 1983 and 2003.

Updated: 2016

Opinions on Related Matters:
2.1.1 Informed Consent
3.2.1 Confidentiality
3.2.4 Access to Medical Records by Data Collection Companies
4.1.3 Third-Party Access to Genetic Information
4.2.1 Assisted Reproductive Technology
8.5 Disparities in Health Care

4 Genetics and Reproductive Medicine

(d) Obtain the individual's informed consent for the specific test or tests to be performed.

(e) Ensure that appropriate measures are taken to protect the confidentiality of the patient's and their biological relatives' genetic information.

AMA Principles of Medical Ethics: II, IV, V, VI

Issued: 1983

Updated: 1994, 2016

Opinions on Related Matters:

4.1.2 Genetic Testing for Reproductive Decision Making

Genetic testing can provide information to help prospective parents make informed decisions about childbearing.

Genetic testing to inform reproductive decisions was once recommended only for women or couples whose family history or medical record indicated elevated risk for a limited set of genetically mediated conditions. As procreation among individuals of diverse ancestries becomes more common and tests for more conditions become more accurate and less costly, the relevance of broad preconception, pre-implantation, or prenatal genetic screening grows stronger. Physicians may ethically provide genetic testing to inform reproductive decision making when the patient requests, but may also wish to offer broad screening to all persons who are considering having a child.

Physicians who provide reproductive health care that includes genetic testing should:

(a) Adhere to standards of nondirective counseling and avoid imposing their personal moral values or judgment on the patient.

(b) Discuss reasons for and against genetic testing and ethically inappropriate uses of genetic testing, such as to identify non-disease-related characteristics or traits.

(c) Obtain the individual's informed consent to the specific test or tests to be performed. Physicians should ascertain whether the person wishes to be informed about incidental findings.

(d) Inform the individual about any abnormal findings for the tests ordered and discuss the severity of the associated health condition, likelihood of clinical manifestation (penetrance), age at onset, and other factors relevant to a decision about childbearing.

(e) Respect an individual's decision to terminate or continue a pregnancy when testing reveals a genetic abnormality in the fetus, in accordance with applicable law.

(f) Refer the individual to another qualified physician when personal moral values prohibit the physician from providing lawful abortion services when this is a service that the person desires, in keeping with ethics guidance.

4.1.3 Third-Party Access to Genetic Information

The rapid pace of development and dissemination of genetic testing has made it possible to generate information about individuals across a wide and growing spectrum of genetic variations associated with disease risk. The prospect of access to and use of such information by third parties who have a stake in an individual's health raises ethical concerns about confidentiality and potentially inappropriate use of genetic information.

Patients who undergo genetic testing have a right to have their information kept in confidence, and a variety of state and federal laws prohibit discrimination by employers, insurers, and other third parties based on genetic information they obtain about an individual.

Physicians who provide and interpret genetic tests, or who maintain patient records that include the findings of genetic tests, have professional ethical obligations to:

(a) Maintain the confidentiality of the patient's health information, including genetic information.

(b) Release a patient's genetic information to third parties only with the patient's informed consent.

(c) Decline to participate in genetic testing at the request of third parties (eg, for purposes of establishing health care or other benefits or coverage for the individual) except when at the patient's request and with their informed consent.

AMA Principles of Medical Ethics: IV

Issued: The constituent Opinions on which this guidance is based (see Concordance) were adopted between 1991 and 1994.

Updated: 2016

Opinions on Related Matters:
1.2.6　Work-Related and Independent Medical Examinations
3.2.1　Confidentiality
3.2.4　Access to Medical Records by Data Collection Companies
7.3.7　Safeguards in the Use of DNA Databanks
8.5　Disparities in Health Care

4.1.4 Forensic Genetics

With the exception of genetic information (or material) collected under the jurisdiction of a coroner, medical examiner, or other medical legal officer, the release of genetic information from a physician's records without the patient's informed consent constitutes a breach of confidentiality. However, under limited circumstances with overriding legal and social considerations, all physicians may disclose such information to the criminal justice system.

Physicians from whom genetic information is sought for purposes of criminal justice:

(a) May ethically carry out DNA analysis on stored tissue samples or release genetic information without the consent of a living or deceased patient (or the patient's authorized surrogate) in response to a warrant or court order.

AMA Principles of Medical Ethics: III, IV

Issued: 2001

Updated: 2016

Opinions on Related Matters:
1.2.6　Work-Related and Independent Medical Examinations
2.2.1　Pediatric Decision Making
3.2.1　Confidentiality

(b) Should release only the minimum information necessary for the specific purpose.

(c) Should not be required to provide genetic information when:

    (i)   a suspect whose location is known refuses to provide a tissue sample for genetic analysis;

    (ii) a tissue sample for the suspect can be obtained from other sources (such as the body of a deceased suspect).

(d) Should decline to participate in the use of information from a genetic database created exclusively for criminal justice for any purpose other than identification.

Reproductive Medicine

AMA Principles of Medical Ethics: I, V, VII

Issued: The constituent Opinions on which this guidance is based (see Concordance) were issued between 1983 and 1998.

Updated: 2016

Opinions on Related Matters:
1.1.7 Physician Exercise of Conscience
2.2.1 Pediatric Decision Making
8.5 Disparities in Health Care

4.2.1 Assisted Reproductive Technology

Assisted reproduction offers hope to patients who want children but are unable to have a child without medical assistance. In many cases, patients who seek assistance have been repeatedly frustrated in their attempts to have a child and are psychologically very vulnerable. Patients whose health insurance does not cover assisted reproductive services may also be financially vulnerable. Candor and respect are thus essential for ethical practice.

"Assisted reproductive technology" is understood as all treatments or procedures that include the handling of human oocytes or embryos. It encompasses an increasingly complex range of interventions—such as therapeutic donor insemination, ovarian stimulation, ova and sperm retrieval, in vitro fertilization, gamete intrafallopian transfer—and may involve multiple participants.

Physicians should increase their awareness of infertility treatments and options for their patients. Physicians who offer assisted reproductive services should:

(a) Value the well-being of the patient and potential offspring as paramount.

(b) Ensure that all advertising for services and promotional materials are accurate and not misleading.

(c) Provide patients with all of the information they need to make an informed decision, including investigational techniques to be used (if any); risks, benefits, and limitations of treatment options and alternatives, for the patient and potential offspring; accurate, clinic-specific success rates; and costs.

(d) Provide patients with psychological assessment, support, and counseling or a referral to such services.

(e) Base fees on the value of the service provided. Physicians may enter into agreements with patients to refund all or a portion of fees if the patient does not conceive where such agreements are legally permitted.

(f) Not discriminate against patients who have difficult-to-treat conditions, whose infertility has multiple causes, or on the basis of race, socioeconomic status, sexual orientation, or gender identity.

(g) Participate in the development of peer-established guidelines and self-regulation.

4.2.2 Gamete Donation

Donating eggs or sperm for others to use in reproduction can enable individuals who would not otherwise be able to do so to have children. However, gamete donation also raises ethical concerns about the privacy of donors and the nature of relationships among donors and children born through use of their gametes by means of assisted reproductive technologies.

Physicians who participate in gamete retrieval and storage should:

(a) Inform prospective donors of sperm or ova:

(i)   about the clinical risks of gamete donation, including the near and long-term risks and the discomforts of ovarian hyperstimulation and egg retrieval as appropriate;

(ii)   about the need for full medical disclosure and that prospective donors will be tested for infectious disease agents and genetic disorders;

(iii) whether and how the donor will be informed if testing indicates the presence of infectious disease or genetic disorder;

(iv)   that all information collected, including test results, will be stored indefinitely;

(v)   what additional personal information will be collected about the donor;

(vi)   under what circumstances and with whom personal information, including identifying information, will be shared for clinical purposes;

(vii) how donated gametes will be stored and policies and procedures governing the use of stored gametes;

(viii) whether and how the donor will be compensated;

(ix)   the fact that state law will govern the relationship between the donor and any resulting child (or children).

AMA Principles of Medical Ethics: I, V

Issued: The constituent Opinions on which this guidance is based (see Concordance) were issued in 1993.

Updated: 2016

Opinions on Related Matters:
1.1.7 Physician Exercise of Conscience
2.1.2 Decisions for Adult Patients Who Lack Capacity
4.2.1 Assisted Reproductive Technology

4 Genetics and Reproductive Medicine

(b) Exclude prospective donors for whom testing reveals the presence of infectious disease agents.

(c) Obtain the prospective donor's consent for gamete retrieval.

(d) Discuss, document, and respect the prospective donor's preferences for how gametes may be used, including whether they may be donated for research purposes.

(e) Discuss, document, and respect the prospective donor's preferences regarding release of identifying information to any child (or children) resulting from use of the donated gametes.

(f) Adhere to good clinical practices, including ensuring that identifying information is maintained indefinitely so that:

    (i) donors can be notified in the event a child born through use of his or her gametes subsequently tests positive for infectious disease or genetic disorder that may have been transmitted by the donor;

    (ii) the number of pregnancies resulting from a single gamete donor is limited.

AMA Principles of Medical Ethics: I, V

Issued: The constituent Opinions on which this guidance is based (see Concordance) were issued in 1993.

Updated: 2016

Opinions on Related Matters:
1.1.7 Physician Exercise of Conscience
2.2.1 Pediatric Decision Making
4.2.1 Assisted Reproductive Technology

4.2.3 Therapeutic Donor Insemination

Therapeutic donor insemination using sperm from a woman's partner or a third-party donor can enable a woman or couple who might not otherwise be able to do so to fulfill the important life choice of becoming a parent (or parents).

However, the procedure also raises ethical considerations about safety for the woman and potential offspring, donor privacy, and the disposition of frozen semen, as well as the use of screening to select the sex of a resulting embryo.

Physicians who choose to provide artificial insemination should:

(a) Provide therapeutic donor insemination in a nondiscriminatory manner. Physicians should not withhold or refuse services on the basis of nonclinical considerations, such as a patient's marital status.

(b) Obtain informed consent for therapeutic donor insemination, after informing the patient (and partner, if appropriate):

    (i) about the risks, benefits, likelihood of success, and costs of the intervention;

    (ii) about the need to screen donated semen for infectious disease agents and genetic disorders when an individual proposes to donate sperm specifically for the patient's use in therapeutic donor insemination;

    (iii) about the need to address in advance what will be done with frozen sperm (if any) from a known donor in the event the donor dies;

    (iv) that state law will govern the status, obligations, and rights of the sperm donor, known or anonymous, in relation to a resulting child.

(c) When sperm is collected specifically for use by an identified patient, obtain informed consent from the prospective donor after informing the individual:

    (i) about the need to test donated semen for infectious disease agents and genetic disorders;

    (ii) whether and how the donor will be informed in the event the semen tests positive for infectious disease or genetic disorder;

    (iii) that state law will govern the status, obligations, and rights of the donor in relation to a resulting child.

(d) Counsel patients who choose to be inseminated with sperm from an anonymous donor to involve their partner (if any) in the decision.

(e) Provide sex selection of sperm only for purposes of avoiding a sex-linked inheritable disorder. Physicians should not participate in sex selection of sperm for reasons of gender preference.

4.2.4 Third-Party Reproduction

Third-party reproduction is a form of assisted reproduction in which a woman agrees to bear a child on behalf of and relinquish the child to an individual or couple who intend to rear the child. Such arrangements can promote fundamental human values by enabling individuals or couples who are otherwise unable to do so to fulfill deeply held desires to raise a child. Gestational carriers in their turn can take satisfaction in expressing altruism by helping others fulfill such desires.

    Third-party reproduction may involve therapeutic donor insemination or use of assisted reproductive technologies, such as in vitro fertilization and embryo transfer. The biological and social relationships among participants in these arrangements can form a complex matrix of roles among gestational carrier, gamete donor(s), and rearing parent(s).

    Third-party reproduction can alter social understandings of parenthood and family structure. It can also raise concerns about the voluntariness of the gestational carrier's participation and about

AMA Principles of Medical Ethics: I, II, IV

Issued: 1983

Updated: 1994, 2016

Opinions on Related Matters:
1.1.7 Physician Exercise of Conscience
2.1.2 Decisions for Adult Patients Who Lack Capacity
4.2.1 Assisted Reproductive Technology
4.2.2 Gamete Donation
4.2.3 Therapeutic Donor Insemination

4 Genetics and Reproductive Medicine

possible psychosocial harms to those involved, such as distress on the part of the gestational carrier at relinquishing the child or on the part of the child at learning of the circumstances of his or her birth. Third-party reproduction can also carry potential to depersonalize carriers, exploit economically disadvantaged women, and commodify human gametes and children. These concerns may be especially challenging when carriers or gamete donors are compensated financially for their services. Finally, third-party reproduction can raise concerns about dual loyalties or conflict of interest if a physician establishes patient-physician relationships with multiple parties to the arrangement.

Individual physicians who care for patients in the context of third-party reproduction should:

(a) Establish a patient-physician relationship with only one party (gestational carriers, gamete donor[s], or intended rearing parent[s]) to avoid situations of dual loyalty or conflict of interest.

(b) Ensure that the patient undergoes appropriate medical screening and psychological assessment.

(c) Encourage the parties to agree in advance on the terms of the agreement, including identifying possible contingencies and deciding how they will be handled.

(d) Inform the patient about the risks of third-party reproduction, including possible psychological harms to the individual(s), the resulting child, and other relationships.

(e) Satisfy themselves that the patient's decision to participate in third-party reproduction is free of coercion before agreeing to provide assisted reproductive services.

Collectively, the profession should advocate for public policy that will help ensure that the practice of third-party reproduction does not exploit disadvantaged women or commodify human gametes or children.

AMA Principles of Medical Ethics: I, III, IV, V

Issued: 1992

Updated: 1994, 2016

Opinions on Related Matters:
1.1.7 Physician Exercise of Conscience
2.1.2 Decisions for Adult Patients Who Lack Capacity
7.3.6 Research in Gene Therapy and Genetic Engineering
7.3.8 Research with Stem Cells
7.3.9 Commercial Use of Human Biological Materials

4.2.5 Storage and Use of Human Embryos

Embryos created during cycles of in vitro fertilization (IVF) that are not intended for immediate transfer are often frozen for future use. The primary goal is to minimize risk and burden by minimizing the number of cycles of ovarian stimulation and egg retrieval that an IVF patient undergoes.

While embryos are usually frozen with the expectation that they will be used for reproductive purposes by the prospective parent(s) for whom they were created, frozen embryos may also offer hope to other prospective parent(s) who would otherwise not be able to have a child. Frozen embryos also offer the prospect of advancing scientific knowledge when made available for research purposes. In all of these possible scenarios, ethical concerns arise regarding who has authority to make decisions about stored embryos and what kinds of choices they may ethically make. Decision-making authority with respect to stored embryos varies depending on the relationships between the prospective rearing parent(s) and any individual(s) who may provide gametes. At stake are individuals' interests in procreating.

When gametes are provided by the prospective rearing parent(s) or a known donor, physicians who provide clinical services that include creation and storage of embryos have an ethical responsibility to proactively discuss with the parties whether, when, and under what circumstances stored embryos may be:

(a) Used by a surviving party for purposes of reproduction in the event of the death of a partner or gamete donor.

(b) Made available to other patients for purposes of reproduction.

(c) Made available to investigators for research purposes, in keeping with ethics guidance and on the understanding that embryo(s) used for research will not subsequently be used for reproduction.

(d) Allowed to thaw and deteriorate.

(e) Otherwise disposed of.

Under no circumstances should physicians participate in the sale of stored embryos.

4.2.6 Cloning for Reproduction

Somatic cell nuclear transfer (SCNT) is the process in which the nucleus of a somatic cell of an organism is transferred into an enucleated oocyte. Cloning for reproduction, ie, the application of SCNT to create a human embryo that shares all of its nuclear genes with the donor of the human somatic cell, has been debated as having possible clinical benefit. It has been suggested that reproductive cloning might be ethically acceptable to assist individuals or couples to reproduce and to create a compatible tissue donor.

Misconceptions often surround proposals for reproductive cloning, including the mistaken notion that one's genotype determines one's individuality and using SCNT to create a human embryo would replicate a person (the donor of the somatic cell).

The possible use of SCNT in reproductive medicine also poses risks of unknown physical harms from the technology itself,

AMA Principles of Medical Ethics: V

Issued: 1999

Updated: 2003, 2016

Opinions on Related Matters:
7.3.5 Research Using Human Fetal Tissue
7.3.6 Research in Gene Therapy and Genetic Engineering
7.3.8 Research with Stem Cells

4 Genetics and Reproductive Medicine

including concerns about long-term safety, and the possibility that SCNT will be associated with genetic anomalies or have other unforeseen medical consequences. Reproductive cloning also carries the risk of psychosocial harm, including violations of privacy and autonomy and the possibility of compromising the cloned child's right to an open future by creating enormous pressures to live up to expectations based on the life of the somatic cell donor.

Reproductive cloning may have adverse effects on familial and societal relations and on the gene pool in altering reproductive patterns and the resulting genetic characteristics of a population, including posing harms to future generations if deleterious genetic mutations are introduced. Moreover, reproductive cloning has the potential to be used in a eugenic or discriminatory fashion—practices that are incompatible with the ethical norms of medicine.

In light of the physical risks of SCNT, ongoing moral debate about the status of the human embryo, and concerns about the impact of reproductive cloning on cloned children, families, and communities, reproductive cloning is not endorsed by the medical profession or by society.

Should reproductive cloning at some point be introduced into medical practice, physicians must be aware that cloning techniques must not be used without the informed consent of the somatic cell donor, the oocyte donor, and the prospective rearing parent(s), in keeping with ethics guidance for assisted reproduction.

Further, any child produced by reproductive cloning would be entitled to the same rights, freedoms, and protections as every other individual in society, irrespective of the fact that the child's nuclear genes derive from a single individual.

As professionals dedicated to protecting the well-being of patients, physicians should not participate in using SCNT to produce children. Because SCNT technology is not limited to any single country, physicians should help establish international guidelines governing its uses before experimentally proven techniques are introduced into clinical practice.

AMA Principles of Medical Ethics: III, IV

Issued: Prior to 1977

Opinions on Related Matters:
1.1.7　Physician Exercise of Conscience
2.1.2　Decisions for Adult Patients Who Lack Capacity
4.1.2　Genetic Testing for Reproductive Decision Making

4.2.7 Abortion

The *Principles of Medical Ethics* of the AMA do not prohibit a physician from performing an abortion in accordance with good medical practice and under circumstances that do not violate the law.

5 Caring for Patients at the End of Life

These Opinions are offered as ethics guidance for physicians and are not intended to establish clinical practice guidelines or rules of law.

Caring for patients at the end of life is a privilege that draws deeply on physicians' profession-defining commitment to alleviate suffering. Medicine's advancing power to intervene to delay death has proven double-edged, however, tempting physicians, patients, and families to pursue aggressive care that may not always be in the patient's interest. Interventions intended to prolong life can all too easily come to have the unsought effect of only prolonging death.

Physicians and other health care professionals are challenged to help patients and families identify what matters most to them when cure is not possible and to negotiate difficult decisions about what trade-off to accept between quality of life and length of life, what interventions to accept, and when to refuse efforts to sustain life. Through the process of advance care planning, physicians can help patients and families express their values and preferences, define goals for the patient's care, and, ideally, identify who will make decisions on the patient's behalf when he or she can no longer do so. Encouraging patients to set out their values, goals for care, and treatment preferences in oral or written advance directives helps to ensure that their wishes will guide the recommendations and actions of the health care team and thus to promote respect for patient autonomy and self-determination.

Respect for patients' right to refuse life-sustaining interventions is central to ethical practice in end-of-life care, and physicians thus have an obligation not to allow their personal beliefs and values to override the decision of a patient who has decision-making capacity. Physicians have a similar responsibility to respect the decisions made by patients' authorized surrogates. This does not mean, however, that physicians are ethically required to offer or to provide on request interventions that, in their best professional judgment, cannot reasonably be expected to yield the intended clinical benefit or achieve agreed-on goals for care. Rather they have a responsibility to preserve the integrity of medical judgment, to address patients' or surrogates' fears and clarify misunderstandings, and to resolve disagreements about care, at the bedside when possible or through consultation with an ethics committee or similar resource when necessary. In all cases, physicians are expected to uphold their obligation to provide compassionate care and not to abandon a patient.

Although their commitment of fidelity to patients is foremost, physicians have further responsibilities to uphold the fundamental values of medicine and therefore not to take actions that are contrary to the role of healer with which they are entrusted.

5.1 Advance Care Planning

The process of advance care planning is widely recognized as a way to support patient self-determination, facilitate decision making, and promote better care at the end of life. Although often thought of primarily for terminally ill patients or those with chronic medical conditions, advance care planning is valuable for everyone, regardless of age or current health status. Planning in advance for decisions about care in the event of a life-threatening illness or injury gives individuals the opportunity to reflect on and express the values they want to have govern their care, to articulate the factors that are important to them for quality of life, and to make clear any preferences they have with respect to specific interventions. Importantly, these discussions also give individuals the opportunity to identify who they would want to make decisions for them should they not have decision-making capacity.

Proactively discussing with patients what they would or would not want if recovery from illness or injury is improbable also gives physicians opportunity to address patients' concerns and expectations and clarify misunderstandings individuals may have about specific medical conditions or interventions. Encouraging patients to share their views with their families or other intimates and record them in advance directives, and to name a surrogate decision maker, helps to ensure that patients' own values, goals, and preferences will inform care decisions even when they cannot speak for themselves.

Physicians must recognize, however, that patients and families approach decision making in many different ways, informed by culture, faith traditions, and life experience, and should be sensitive to each patient's individual situations and preferences when broaching discussion of planning for care at the end of life.

Physicians should routinely engage their patients in advance care planning in keeping with the following guidance:

(a) Regularly encourage all patients, regardless of age or health status, to:
   (i) think about their values and perspectives on quality of life and articulate what goals they would have for care if they faced a life-threatening illness or injury, including any preferences they may have about specific medical interventions (such as pain management, medically administered nutrition and hydration, mechanical ventilation, use of antibiotics, dialysis, or cardiopulmonary resuscitation);

AMA Principles of Medical Ethics: I, IV

Issued: 2011

Updated: 2016

Opinions on Related Matters:
1.1.1 Patient-Physician Relationships
2.1.1 Informed Consent
2.1.2 Decisions for Adult Patients Who Lack Capacity
5.3 Withholding or Withdrawing Life-Sustaining Treatment
2.2.2 Confidential Health Care for Minors

5 Caring for Patients at the End of Life

(ii) identify someone they would want to have make decisions on their behalf if they did not have decision-making capacity;

(iii) make their views known to their designated surrogate and to (other) family members or intimates.

(b) Be prepared to answer questions about advance care planning, to help patients formulate their views, and to help them articulate their preferences for care (including their wishes regarding time-limited trials of interventions and surrogate decision maker). Physicians should also be prepared to refer patients to additional resources for further information and guidance if appropriate.

(c) Explain how advance directives, as written articulations of patients' preferences, are used as tools to help guide treatment decisions in collaboration with patients themselves when they have decision-making capacity, or with surrogates when they do not, and explain the surrogate's responsibilities in decision making. Involve the patient's surrogate in this conversation whenever possible.

(d) Incorporate notes from the advance care planning discussion into the medical record. Patient values, preferences for treatment, and designation of surrogate decision maker should be included in the notes to be used as guidance when the patient is unable to express his or her own decisions. If the patient has an advance directive document or written designation of proxy, include a copy (or note the existence of the directive) in the medical record and encourage the patient to give a copy to his or her surrogate and others to help ensure it will be available when needed.

(e) Periodically review with the patient his or her goals, preferences, and chosen decision maker, which often change over time or with changes in health status. Update the patient's medical records accordingly when preferences have changed to ensure that these continue to reflect the individual's current wishes. If applicable, assist the patient with updating his or her advance directive or designation of proxy forms. Involve the patient's surrogate in these reviews whenever possible.

5.2 Advance Directives

Respect for autonomy and fidelity to the patient are widely acknowledged as core values in the professional ethics of medicine. For patients who lack decision-making capacity, these values are fulfilled through third-party decision making and the use of advance directives. Advance directives also support continuity of care for patients when they transition across care settings, physicians, or health care teams.

Advance directives, whether oral or written, advisory or a formal statutory document, are tools that give patients of all ages and health status the opportunity to express their values, goals for care, and treatment preferences to guide future decisions about health care. Advance directives also allow patients to identify whom they want to make decisions on their behalf when they cannot do so themselves. They enable physicians and surrogates to make good-faith efforts to respect the patient's goals and implement the patient's preferences when the patient does not have decision-making capacity.

An advance directive never takes precedence over the contemporaneous wishes of a patient who has decision-making capacity.

In emergency situations when a patient is not able to participate in treatment decisions and there is no surrogate or advance directive available to guide decisions, physicians should provide medically appropriate interventions when urgently needed to meet the patient's immediate clinical needs. Interventions may be withdrawn at a later time in keeping with the patient's preferences when they become known and in accordance with ethics guidance for withdrawing treatment.

Before initiating or continuing treatment, including, but not limited to, life-sustaining interventions, the physician should:

(a) Assess the patient's decision-making capacity in the current clinical circumstances.

(b) Ascertain whether the patient has an advance directive and, if so, whether it accurately reflects his or her current values and preferences. Determine whether the patient's current clinical circumstances meet relevant thresholds set out in the directive.

(c) Ascertain whether the patient has named a health care proxy (eg, orally or through a formal legal document). If the patient has not, ask who the patient would want to have make decisions should he or she become unable to do so.

(d) Document the conversation, including the patient's goals for care, and specific preferences regarding interventions and surrogate decision maker, in the medical record; incorporate any written directives (as available) into the medical record to ensure they are accessible to the health care team.

AMA Principles of Medical Ethics: I, IV

Issued: 1998

Updated: 2016

Opinions on Related Matters:
1.1.1 Patient-Physician Relationships
2.1.2 Decisions for Adult Patients Who Lack Capacity
5.1 Advance Care Planning
5.3 Withholding or Withdrawing Life-Sustaining Treatment
5.4 Orders Not to Attempt Resuscitation (DNAR)
5.6 Sedation to Unconsciousness in End-of-Life Care

5 Caring for Patients at the End of Life

(e) When treatment decisions must be made by the patient's surrogate, help the surrogate understand how to carry out the patient's wishes in keeping with the advance directive (when available), including whether the directive applies in the patient's current clinical circumstances and what medically appropriate interventions are available to achieve the patient's goals for care. When conflicts arise between the advance directive and the wishes of the patient's surrogate, the attending physician should seek assistance from an ethics committee or other appropriate institutional resource.

(f) When a patient who lacks decision-making capacity has no advance directive and there is no surrogate available and willing to make treatment decisions on the patient's behalf, or no surrogate can be identified, the attending physician should seek assistance from an ethics committee or other appropriate resource in ascertaining the patient's best interest.

(g) Document physician orders to implement treatment decisions in the medical record, including both orders for specific, ongoing interventions (eg, palliative interventions) and orders to forgo specific interventions (eg, orders not to attempt resuscitation, not to intubate, not to provide antibiotics or dialysis).

AMA Principles of Medical Ethics: I, III, IV, V

Issued: The constituent Opinions on which this guidance is based (see Concordance) were issued in 1984.

Updated: 2016

Opinions on Related Matters:

5.3 Withholding or Withdrawing Life-Sustaining Treatment

Decisions to withhold or withdraw life-sustaining interventions can be ethically and emotionally challenging to all involved. However, a patient who has decision-making capacity appropriate to the decision at hand has the right to decline any medical intervention or ask that an intervention be stopped, even when that decision is expected to lead to his or her death and regardless of whether the individual is terminally ill. When a patient lacks appropriate capacity, the patient's surrogate may decline an intervention or ask that an intervention be stopped in keeping with ethics guidance for surrogate decision making.

While there may be an emotional difference between not initiating an intervention at all and discontinuing it later in the course of care, there is no ethical difference between withholding and withdrawing treatment. When an intervention no longer helps to achieve the patient's goals for care or desired quality of life, it is ethically appropriate for physicians to withdraw it.

Physicians should elicit patient goals of care and preferences regarding life-sustaining interventions early in the course of care, including the patient's surrogate in that discussion whenever possible. When facing decisions about withholding or withdrawing life-sustaining treatment, the physician should:

(a) Review with the patient the individual's advance directive, if there is one. Otherwise, elicit the patient's values, goals for care, and treatment preferences. Include the patient's surrogate in the conversation if possible, even when the patient retains decision-making capacity.

(b) Document the patient's preferences and identify the patient's surrogate in the medical record and ensure that the record includes the patient's written advance directive or durable power of attorney for health care (DPAHC), where applicable.

(c) Support the decision-making process by providing all relevant medical information to the patient and/or surrogate.

(d) Discuss with the patient and/or surrogate the option of initiating an intervention with the intention of evaluating its clinical effectiveness after a given amount of time to determine if it has led to improvement. Confirm that if the intervention has not achieved agreed-on goals, it may be withdrawn.

(e) Reassure the patient and/or surrogate that all other medically appropriate care will be provided, including aggressive palliative care and appropriate symptom management if that is what the patient wishes.

(f) Explain that the surrogate should make decisions to withhold or withdraw life-sustaining interventions when the patient lacks decision-making capacity and there is a surrogate available and willing to make decisions on the patient's behalf, in keeping with ethics guidance for substituted judgment or best interests as appropriate.

(g) Seek consultation through an ethics committee or other appropriate resource in keeping with ethics guidance when:

(i) the patient or surrogate and the health care team cannot reach agreement about a decision to withhold or withdraw life-sustaining treatment;

(ii) there is no surrogate available and willing to make decisions on behalf of a patient who does not have decision-making capacity or no surrogate can be identified;

(iii) in the physician's best professional judgment a decision by the patient's surrogate clearly violates the patient's previously expressed values, goals for care, or treatment preferences, or is not in the patient's medical interest.

(h) Ensure that relevant standards for good clinical practice and palliative care are followed when implementing any decision to withdraw a life-sustaining intervention.

AMA Principles of Medical Ethics: I, IV, VIII

Issued: 1992

Updated: 1994, 2005, 2016

5.4 Orders Not to Attempt Resuscitation (DNAR)

The ethical obligation to respect patient autonomy and self-determination requires that the physician respect decisions to refuse care, even when such decisions will result in the patient's death. Whether a patient declines or accepts medically appropriate resuscitative interventions, physicians should not permit their personal value judgments to obstruct implementation of the patient's decision.

Orders not to attempt resuscitation (DNAR orders) direct the health care team to withhold resuscitative measures in accord with a patient's wishes. DNAR orders can be appropriate for any patient medically at risk of cardiopulmonary arrest, regardless of the patient's age or whether the patient is terminally ill. DNAR orders apply in any care setting, in or out of hospital, within the constraints of applicable law.

In the event a patient suffers a cardiopulmonary arrest when there is no DNAR order in the medical record, resuscitation should be attempted if it is medically appropriate. If it is found after the "code" is initiated that the patient would not have wanted resuscitation, the physician should order that resuscitative efforts be stopped.

Physicians should address the potential need for resuscitation early in the patient's course of care, while the patient has decision-making capacity, and should encourage the patient to include his or her chosen surrogate in the conversation. Before entering a DNAR order in the medical record, the physician should:

(a) Candidly describe the procedures involved in resuscitation, the likelihood of medical benefit in the patient's clinical circumstances, and the likelihood of achieving the patient's desired goals for care or quality of life to address any misconceptions the patient may have about probable outcomes of resuscitation.

(b) Ascertain the patient's wishes with respect to resuscitation—directly from the patient when the individual has decision-making capacity, or from the surrogate when the patient lacks capacity. If the patient has an advance directive, the physician should review the directive with the patient and confirm that the preferences set out in the directive about resuscitation are current and valid. The DNAR order should be tailored to reflect the particular patient's preferences and clinical circumstances.

(c) Reinforce with the patient, loved ones, and the health care team that DNAR orders apply only to resuscitative interventions as they relate to the patient's goals for care. Other medically appropriate interventions, such as antibiotics, dialysis, or appropriate symptom management, will be provided or withheld in accordance with the patient's wishes.

(d) Revisit and revise decisions about resuscitation—with appropriate documentation in the medical record—as the patient's clinical circumstances change. Confirm whether the patient wants the DNAR order to remain in effect when obtaining consent for surgical or other interventions that carry a known risk for cardiopulmonary arrest and adhere to those wishes.

(e) Document in the medical record the patient's clinical status, prognosis, current decision-making capacity, and preferences with respect to resuscitation, as well as the physician's medical judgment about the appropriateness of resuscitation.

When the patient cannot express preferences regarding resuscitation or does not have decision-making capacity and has not previously indicated his or her preferences, the physician has an ethical responsibility to:

(f) Candidly and compassionately discuss these issues with the patient's authorized surrogate and document the surrogate's decision in the medical record.

(g) Revisit with the surrogate decisions about resuscitation as the patient's clinical circumstances change, revising the decision as needed and updating the medical record accordingly.

(h) Seek consultation with an ethics committee or other appropriate institutional resource if disagreement about a DNAR order that cannot be resolved at the bedside.

When the patient's preferences cannot be determined and the individual has no surrogate, the physician should consult with an ethics committee or other appropriate institutional resource before entering an order not to attempt resuscitation.

AMA Principles of Medical Ethics: I, IV, V

Issued: The constituent Opinions on which this guidance is based (see Concordance) were issued in 1994 and 1997.

Updated: 2016

5.5 Medically Ineffective Interventions

At times patients (or their surrogates) request interventions that the physician judges not to be medically appropriate. Such requests are particularly challenging when the patient is terminally ill or suffers from an acute condition with an uncertain prognosis and therapeutic options range from aggressive, potentially burdensome life-extending intervention to comfort measures only. Requests for interventions that are not medically appropriate challenge the physician to balance obligations to respect patient autonomy and not to abandon the patient with obligations to be compassionate, yet candid, and to preserve the integrity of medical judgment.

Physicians should only recommend and provide interventions that are medically appropriate—ie, scientifically grounded—and that reflect the physician's considered medical judgment about the risks and likely benefits of available options in light of the patient's goals for care. Physicians are not required to offer or to provide interventions that, in their best medical judgment, cannot reasonably be expected to yield the intended clinical benefit or achieve agreed-on goals for care. Respecting patient autonomy does not mean that patients should receive specific interventions simply because they (or their surrogates) request them.

Many health care institutions have promoted policies regarding so-called "futile" care. However, physicians must remember that it is not possible to offer a single, universal definition of futility. The meaning of the term "futile" depends on the values and goals of a particular patient in specific clinical circumstances.

As clinicians, when a patient (or surrogate on behalf of a patient who lacks decision-making capacity) requests care that the physician or other members of the health care team judge not to be medically appropriate, physicians should:

(a) Discuss with the patient the individual's goals for care, including desired quality of life, and seek to clarify misunderstandings. Include the patient's surrogate in the conversation if possible, even when the patient retains decision-making capacity.

(b) Reassure the patient (and/or surrogate) that medically appropriate interventions, including appropriate symptom management, will be provided unless the patient declines particular interventions (or the surrogate does so on behalf of a patient who lacks capacity).

(c) Negotiate a mutually agreed-on plan of care consistent with the patient's goals and with sound clinical judgment.

(d) Seek assistance from an ethics committee or other appropriate institutional resource if the patient (or surrogate) continues to request care that the physician judges not to be medically appropriate, respecting the patient's right to appeal when review does not support the request.

(e) Seek to transfer care to another physician or another institution willing to provide the desired care in the rare event that disagreement cannot be resolved through available mechanisms, in keeping with ethics guidance. If transfer is not possible, the physician is under no ethical obligation to offer the intervention.

As leaders within their institutions, physicians should encourage the development of institutional policy that:

(f) Acknowledges the need to make context-sensitive judgments about care for individual patients.

(g) Supports physicians in exercising their best professional judgment.

(h) Takes into account community and institutional standards for care.

(i) Uses scientifically sound measures of function or outcome.

(j) Ensures consistency and due process in the event of disagreement over whether an intervention should be provided.

5.6 Sedation to Unconsciousness in End-of-Life Care

The duty to relieve pain and suffering is central to the physician's role as healer and is an obligation physicians have to their patients. When a terminally ill patient experiences severe pain or other distressing clinical symptoms that do not respond to aggressive, symptom-specific palliation, it can be appropriate to offer sedation to unconsciousness as an intervention of last resort.

Sedation to unconsciousness must never be used to intentionally cause a patient's death.

When considering whether to offer palliative sedation to unconsciousness, physicians should:

(a) Restrict palliative sedation to unconsciousness to patients in the final stages of terminal illness.

(b) Consult with a multi-disciplinary team (if available), including an expert in the field of palliative care, to ensure that symptom-specific treatments have been sufficiently employed and that palliative sedation to unconsciousness is now the most appropriate course of treatment.

(c) Document the rationale for all symptom management interventions in the medical record.

AMA Principles of Medical Ethics: I, VII

Issued: 2008

Updated: 2016

Opinions on Related Matters:
1.1.1 Patient-Physician Relationships
2.1.1 Informed Consent
2.1.2 Decisions for Adult Patients Who Lack Capacity
5.7 Physician-Assisted Suicide
5.8 Euthanasia
10.7 Ethics Committees in Health Care Institutions
10.7.1 Ethics Consultations

(d) Obtain the informed consent of the patient (or authorized surrogate when the patient lacks decision-making capacity).

(e) Discuss with the patient (or surrogate) the plan of care relative to:

   (i)   degree and length of sedation;

   (ii) specific expectations for continuing, withdrawing, or withholding future life-sustaining treatments.

(f) Monitor care once palliative sedation to unconsciousness is initiated.

Physicians may offer palliative sedation to unconsciousness to address refractory clinical symptoms, not to respond to existential suffering arising from such issues as death anxiety, isolation, or loss of control. Existential suffering should be addressed through appropriate social, psychological, or spiritual support.

AMA Principles of Medical Ethics: I, IV

Issued: 1994

Opinions on Related Matters:
1.1.1 Patient-Physician Relationships
1.1.7 Physician Exercise of Conscience
2.1.1 Informed Consent
2.1.2 Decisions for Adult Patients Who Lack Capacity
5.6   Sedation to Unconsciousness in End-of-Life Care
5.8   Euthanasia

5.7 Physician-Assisted Suicide

Physician-assisted suicide occurs when a physician facilitates a patient's death by providing the necessary means and/or information to enable the patient to perform the life-ending act (eg, the physician provides sleeping pills and information about the lethal dose, while aware that the patient may commit suicide).

It is understandable, though tragic, that some patients in extreme duress—such as those suffering from a terminal, painful, debilitating illness—may come to decide that death is preferable to life. However, permitting physicians to engage in assisted suicide would ultimately cause more harm than good.

Physician-assisted suicide is fundamentally incompatible with the physician's role as healer, would be difficult or impossible to control, and would pose serious societal risks.

Instead of engaging in assisted suicide, physicians must aggressively respond to the needs of patients at the end of life. Physicians:

(a) Should not abandon a patient once it is determined that cure is impossible.

(b) Must respect patient autonomy.

(c) Must provide good communication and emotional support.

(d) Must provide appropriate comfort care and adequate pain control.

5.8 Euthanasia

Euthanasia is the administration of a lethal agent by another person to a patient for the purpose of relieving the patient's intolerable and incurable suffering.

It is understandable, though tragic, that some patients in extreme duress—such as those suffering from a terminal, painful, debilitating illness—may come to decide that death is preferable to life.

However, permitting physicians to engage in euthanasia would ultimately cause more harm than good.

Euthanasia is fundamentally incompatible with the physician's role as healer, would be difficult or impossible to control, and would pose serious societal risks. Euthanasia could readily be extended to incompetent patients and other vulnerable populations.

The involvement of physicians in euthanasia heightens the significance of its ethical prohibition. The physician who performs euthanasia assumes unique responsibility for the act of ending the patient's life. Instead of engaging in euthanasia, physicians must aggressively respond to the needs of patients at the end of life. Physicians:

(a) Should not abandon a patient once it is determined that a cure is impossible.
(b) Must respect patient autonomy.
(c) Must provide good communication and emotional support.
(d) Must provide appropriate comfort care and adequate pain control.

AMA Principles of Medical Ethics: I, IV

Issued: 1994

Opinions on Related Matters:
1.1.1 Patient-Physician Relationships
1.1.7 Physician Exercise of Conscience
2.1.1 Informed Consent
2.1.2 Decisions for Adult Patients Who Lack Capacity
5.6 Sedation to Unconsciousness in End-of-Life Care
5.7 Physician-Assisted Suicide

5 Caring for Patients at the End of Life

6 Organ Procurement and Transplantation

*These Opinions are offered as ethics guidance for physicians and are not
intended to establish clinical practice guidelines or rules of law.*

Transplantation offers a last hope for patients whose organs are failing. However, the chronic shortage of organs and tissues available for transplant under the model of voluntary, affirmative, altruistic donation that prevails in the United States has resulted in a variety of proposals intended to increase the supply of transplantable organs and tissues.

Different proposals seek to balance the rights and welfare of prospective donors with the benefits of increasing the supply of organs and tissues in different ways. Some focus on alternative models for informed consent, for example, mandated choice, in which individuals are required to express their preferences regarding donation at the time of performing a state-regulated task like getting a driver's license, or presumed consent, in which individuals are presumed to be willing to donate organs when they die unless they explicitly refuse to donate. Others suggest using financial or other incentives to increase donation rates. Still others look to identify new protocols for procuring organs beyond traditional cadaveric donation, for example, donation from living donors or donation after cardiac death.

Other approaches to alleviating the ongoing shortage of transplantable organs and tissues focus on allowing organ donors to designate recipients (directed donation), on redefining criteria for who may become a donor to allow organs to be donated by individuals who previously would not have been eligible, and on improving the efficiency of organ retrieval and transplantation.[1,2] Under these approaches, concerns about risks and outcomes for organ and tissue recipients come to the fore.

Ensuring that consent is voluntary and sufficiently informed is a central concern in organ donation and transplantation. Situations of living donation in particular can raise concerns that donors may experience coercion, for example, through emotional ties to the patient in need of transplant or financial inducement, especially when donors are socioeconomically disadvantaged.

Conflict of interest is also of concern. Physicians' fiduciary obligation to promote the interests and welfare of their patients argues strongly that organ procurement and organ transplant teams should not overlap.

Fairness in the allocation of organs and tissues is likewise a key ethical consideration in the context of organ transplantation. Except in situations of directed donation, about the ethical propriety of which there is ongoing debate, ethically sound criteria for allocating organs and tissues include likelihood of benefit, urgency of need, and quality of life. Organs should not be allocated on the basis of non-medical considerations.

Finally, situations of living donation that involve multiple parties and complex chains of donor-recipient exchanges may raise special concerns about protecting the privacy and confidentiality of both donors and recipients.

Opinions in the first section provide guidance for physicians on ethical concerns in organ donation and procurement, while those in the second section set out fundamental conditions for ethically sound transplantation practice. The third section provides guidance in the unique situation of transplantation of organs and tissues from nonhuman sources.

References

1. CST/CNTRP increased risk donor working group. Guidance on the use of increased infectious risk donors for organ transplantation. *Transplantation.* 2014;98(4):365-369.
2. Tector AJ, Mangus RS, Chestovich P, et al. Use of extended criteria livers decreases wait time for liver transplantation without adversely impacting posttransplant survival. *Ann Surg.* 2006;244(3):439-450.

Organ Procurement

6.1.1 Transplantation of Organs from Living Donors

Donation of nonvital organs and tissue from living donors can increase the supply of organs available for transplantation, to the benefit of patients with end-stage organ failure. Enabling individuals to donate nonvital organs is in keeping with the goals of treating illness and relieving suffering so long as the benefits to both donor and recipient outweigh the risks to both.

Living donors expose themselves to harm to benefit others; novel variants of living organ donation call for special safeguards for both donors and recipients.

Physicians who participate in donation of nonvital organs and tissues by a living individual should:

(a) Ensure that the prospective donor is assigned an advocacy team, including a physician, dedicated to protecting the donor's well-being.

(b) Avoid conflicts of interest by ensuring that the health care team treating the prospective donor is as independent as possible from the health care team treating the prospective transplant recipient.

(c) Carefully evaluate prospective donors to identify serious risks to the individual's life or health, including psychosocial factors that would disqualify the individual from donating; address the individual's specific needs; and explore the individual's motivations to donate.

(d) Secure agreement from all parties to the prospective donation in advance so that, should the donor withdraw, his or her reasons for doing so will be kept confidential.

(e) Determine that the prospective living donor has decision-making capacity and adequately understands the implications of donating a nonvital organ, and that the decision to donate is voluntary.

(f) In general, decline proposed living organ donations from unemancipated minors or legally incompetent adults, who are not able to understand the implications of a living donation or give voluntary consent to donation.

(g) In exceptional circumstances, enable donation of a nonvital organ or tissue from a minor who has substantial decision-making capacity when:

  (i) the minor agrees to the donation;

  (ii) the minor's legal guardians consent to the donation;

AMA Principles of Medical Ethics: I, V, VII, VIII

Issued: 2005

Updated: 2011, 2015

Opinions on Related Matters:
2.1.1 Informed Consent
2.1.2 Decisions for Adult Patients Who Lack Capacity
6.1.2 Organ Donation after Cardiac Death
6.1.6 Anencephalic Newborns as Organ Donors

(iii) the intended recipient is someone to whom the minor
has an emotional connection.

(h) Seek advice from another adult trusted by the prospective
minor donor when circumstances warrant, or from an independent body such as an ethics committee, pastoral service,
or other institutional resource.

(i) Inform the prospective donor:

(i) about the donation procedure and possible risks and
complications for the donor;

(ii) about the possible risks and complications for the transplant recipient;

(iii) about the nature of the commitment the donor is making
and the implications for other parties;

(iv) that the prospective donor may withdraw at any time
before undergoing the intervention to remove the organ
or collect tissue, whether the context is paired, domino,
or chain donation;

(v) that if the donor withdraws, the health care team will
report simply that the individual was not a suitable candidate for donation.

(j) Obtain the prospective donor's separate consent for donation
and for the specific intervention(s) to remove the organ or
collect tissue.

(k) Ensure that living donors do not receive payment of any kind
for any of their solid organs. Donors should be compensated
fairly for the expenses of travel, lodging, meals, lost wages,
and medical care associated with the donation only.

(l) Permit living donors to designate a recipient, whether related
to the donor or not.

(m) Decline to facilitate a living donation to a known recipient
if the transplantation cannot reasonably be expected to yield
the intended clinical benefit or achieve agreed-on goals for
the intended recipient.

(n) Permit living donors to designate a stranger as the intended
recipient if doing so produces a net gain in the organ pool
without unreasonably disadvantaging others on the waiting
list. Variations on donation to a stranger include:

(i) prospective donors who respond to public solicitations
for organs or who wish to participate in a paired donation ("organ swap," as when donor-recipient pairs Y
and Z with incompatible blood types are recombined to
make compatible pairs: donor Y with recipient Z and
donor Z with recipient Y);

(ii) domino paired donation;

(iii) nonsimultaneous extended altruistic donation ("chain
donation").

(o) When the living donor does not designate a recipient, allocate organs according to the algorithm that governs the distribution of deceased donor organs.

(p) Protect the privacy and confidentiality of donors and recipients, which may be difficult in novel donation arrangements that involve many patients and in which donation-transplant cycles may be extended over time (as in domino or chain donation).

(q) Monitor prospective donors and recipients in proposed nontraditional donation arrangements for signs of psychological distress during screening and after the transplant is complete.

(r) Support the development and maintenance of a national database of living donor outcomes to support better understanding of associated harms and benefits and enhance the safety of living donation.

6.1.2 Organ Donation after Cardiac Death

Increasing the supply of organs available for transplant serves the interests of patients and the public and is in keeping with physicians' ethical obligation to contribute to the health of the public and to support access to medical care. Physicians should support innovative approaches to increasing the supply of organs for transplantation, but must balance this obligation with their duty to protect the interests of their individual patients.

Organ donation after cardiac death is one approach being undertaken to make greater numbers of transplantable organs available. In what is known as "controlled" donation after cardiac death, a patient who has decided to forgo life-sustaining treatment (or the patient's authorized surrogate when the patient lacks decision-making capacity) may be offered the opportunity to discontinue life support under conditions that would permit the patient to become an organ donor by allowing organs to be removed promptly after death is pronounced. Organ retrieval under this protocol thus differs from usual procedures for cadaveric donation when the patient has died as a result of catastrophic illness or injury.

Donation after cardiac death raises a number of special ethical concerns, including how and when death is declared, potential conflicts of interest for physicians in managing the withdrawal of life support for a patient whose organs are to be retrieved for transplantation, and the use of a surrogate decision maker.

In light of these concerns, physicians who participate in retrieving organs under a protocol of donation after cardiac death should observe the following safeguards:

AMA Principles of Medical Ethics: I, III, V

Issued: 1996

Updated: 2005, 2016

Opinions on Related Matters:
2.1.1 Informed Consent
2.1.2 Decisions for Adult Patients Who Lack Capacity
5.3 Withholding or Withdrawing Life-Sustaining Treatment
6.1.1 Transplantation of Organs from Living Donors

(a) Promote the development of and adhere to clinical criteria for identifying prospective donors whose organs are reasonably likely to be suitable for transplantation.

(b) Promote the development of and adhere to clear and specific institutional policies governing donation after cardiac death.

(c) Avoid actual or perceived conflicts of interest by:

   (i) ensuring that the health care professionals who provide care at the end of life are distinct from those who will participate in retrieving organs for transplant;

   (ii) ensuring that no member of the transplant team has any role in the decision to withdraw treatment or the pronouncement of death.

(d) Ensure that the decision to withdraw life-sustaining treatment is made prior to and independent of any offer of opportunity to donate organs (unless organ donation is spontaneously broached by the patient or surrogate).

(e) Obtain informed consent for organ donation from the patient (or surrogate), including consent specifically to the use of interventions intended not to benefit the patient but to preserve organs in order to improve the opportunity for successful transplantation.

(f) Ensure that relevant standards for good clinical practice and palliative care are followed when implementing the decision to withdraw a life-sustaining intervention.

AMA Principles of Medical Ethics: I, III, V, VII, VIII, IX

Issued: 2002

Updated: 2016

Opinions on Related Matters:

6.1.3 Studying Financial Incentives for Cadaveric Organ Donation

Physicians' ethical obligations to contribute to the health of the public and to support access to medical care extend to participating in efforts to increase the supply of organs for transplantation. However, offering financial incentives for donation raises ethical concerns about potential coercion, the voluntariness of decisions to donate, and possible adverse consequences, including reducing the rate of altruistic organ donation and unduly encouraging perception of the human body as a source of profit.

These concerns merit further study to determine whether, overall, the benefits of financial incentives for organ donation outweigh their potential harms. It would be appropriate to carry out pilot studies among limited populations to investigate the effects of such financial incentives for the purpose of examining and possibly revising current policies in the light of scientific evidence.

Physicians who develop or participate in pilot studies of financial incentives to increase donation of cadaveric organs should ensure that the study:

(a) Is strictly limited to circumstances of voluntary cadaveric donation with an explicit prohibition of the selling of organs.

(b) Is scientifically well designed and clearly defines measurable outcomes and time frames in a written protocol.

(c) Has been developed in consultation with the population among whom it is to be carried out.

(d) Has been reviewed and approved by an appropriate oversight body, such as an institutional review board, and is carried out in keeping with guidelines for ethical research.

(e) Offers incentives of only modest value and at the lowest level that can reasonably be expected to increase organ donation.

6.1.4 Presumed Consent and Mandated Choice for Organs from Deceased Donors

AMA Principles of Medical Ethics: I, III, V

Issued: 2005

Updated: 2016

Opinions on Related Matters:
2.1.1 Informed Consent
6.1.2 Organ Donation after Cardiac Death
6.1.3 Studying Financial Incentives for Cadaveric Organ Donation
6.2.2 Directed Donation of Organs for Transplantation

Organ transplantation offers hope for patients suffering end-stage organ failure. However, the supply of organs for transplantation is inadequate to meet the clinical need. Proposals to increase donation have included studying possible financial incentives for donation and changing the approach to consent for cadaveric donation through "presumed consent" and "mandated choice."

Both presumed consent and mandated choice models contrast with the prevailing traditional model of voluntary consent to donation, in which prospective donors indicate their preferences, but the models raise distinct ethical concerns. Under presumed consent, deceased individuals are presumed to be organ donors unless they have indicated their refusal to donate. Donations under presumed consent would be ethically appropriate only if it could be determined that individuals were aware of the presumption that they were willing to donate organs and if effective and easily accessible mechanisms for documenting and honoring refusals to donate had been established. Physicians could proceed with organ procurement based on presumed consent only after verifying that there was no documented prior refusal and that the family was not aware of any objection to donation by the deceased.

Under mandated choice, individuals are required to express their preferences regarding donation at the time they execute a state-regulated task. Donations under mandated choice would be ethically appropriate only if an individual's choice was made on the basis of a meaningful exchange of information about organ donation in keeping with the principles of informed consent. Physicians could proceed with organ procurement based on mandated choice only after verifying that the individual's consent to donate was documented.

These models merit further study to determine whether either or both can be implemented in a way that meets fundamental ethical criteria for informed consent and provides clear evidence that their benefits outweigh ethical concerns.

Physicians who propose to develop or participate in pilot studies of presumed consent or mandated choice should ensure that the study adheres to the following guidance:

(a) Is scientifically well designed and defines clear, measurable outcomes in a written protocol.

(b) Has been developed in consultation with the population among whom it is to be carried out.

(c) Has been reviewed and approved by an appropriate oversight body and is carried out in keeping with guidelines for ethical research.

Unless there are data that suggest a positive effect on donation, neither presumed consent nor mandated choice for cadaveric organ donation should be widely implemented.

AMA Principles of Medical Ethics: I, V

Issued: 2008

Updated: 2016

Opinions on Related Matters:
2.1.1 Informed Consent
11.2.2 Conflicts of Interest in Patient Care

6.1.5 Umbilical Cord Blood Banking

Transplants of umbilical cord blood have been recommended or performed to treat a variety of conditions. Cord blood is also a potential source of stem and progenitor cells with possible therapeutic applications. Nonetheless, collection and storage of cord blood raise ethical concerns with regard to patient safety, autonomy, and potential for conflict of interest. In addition, storage of umbilical cord blood in private as opposed to public banks can raise concerns about access to cord blood for transplantation.

Physicians who provide obstetrical care should be prepared to inform pregnant women of the various options regarding cord blood donation or storage and the potential uses of donated samples.

Physicians who participate in collecting umbilical cord blood for storage should:

(a) Ensure that collection procedures do not interfere with standard delivery practices or the safety of a newborn or the mother.

(b) Obtain informed consent for the collection of umbilical cord blood stem cells before the onset of labor whenever feasible.

Physicians should disclose their ties to cord blood banks, public or private, as part of the informed consent process.

(c) Decline financial or other inducements for providing samples to cord blood banks.

(d) Encourage women who wish to donate umbilical cord blood to donate to a public bank, if one is available, when there is low risk of predisposition to a condition for which umbilical cord blood cells are therapeutically indicated:

  (i) in view of the cost of private banking and limited likelihood of use;

  (ii) to help increase availability of stem cells for transplantation.

(e) Discuss the option of private banking of umbilical cord blood when there is a family predisposition to a condition for which umbilical cord stem cells are therapeutically indicated.

(f) Continue to monitor ongoing research into the safety and effectiveness of various methods of cord blood collection and use.

6.1.6 Anencephalic Newborns as Organ Donors

Permitting parents of an anencephalic newborn to donate their child's organs has been proposed as a way to increase the organ supply for pediatric transplantation.

However, organ donation in these circumstances also raises concerns, particularly about the accuracy of diagnosis and the potential implications for other vulnerable individuals who lack decision-making capacity and are not able to participate in decisions to donate their organs, although anencephalic newborns are thought to be unique among other brain-damaged beings because they lack past consciousness and have no potential for future consciousness.

In the context of prospective organ donation from an anencephalic newborn, physicians may ethically:

(a) Provide ventilator assistance and other medical therapies that are necessary to sustain organ perfusion and viability until such time as a determination of death can be made in accordance with accepted medical standards.

(b) Retrieve and transplant the organs of an anencephalic newborn only after such determination of death, and in accordance with ethics guidance for transplantation and for medical decisions for minors.

AMA Principles of Medical Ethics: I, III, V

Issued: 1992

Updated: 1994, 1996, 2016

Opinions on Related Matters:
2.1.2 Decisions for Adult Patients Who Lack Capacity
2.2.1 Pediatric Decision Making
2.2.4 Treatment Decisions for Seriously Ill Newborns

Organ Transplantation

AMA Principles of Medical Ethics: I, III, V

Issued: Prior to 1977

Updated: 1994, 2016

Opinions on Related Matters:
2.1.1   Informed Consent
6.1.1   Transplantation of Organs from Living Donors
6.1.2   Organ Donation after Cardiac Death

6.2.1 Guidance for Organ Transplantation from Deceased Donors

Transplantation offers hope to patients with organ failure. As in all patient-physician relationships, the physician's primary concern must be the well-being of the patient. However, organ transplantation is also unique in that it involves two patients, donor and recipient, both of whose interests must be protected. Concern for the patient should always take precedence over advancing scientific knowledge.

Physicians who participate in transplantation of organs from deceased donors should:

(a) Avoid actual or perceived conflicts of interest by ensuring that:

    (i) to the greatest extent possible the health care professionals who provide care at the end of life are not directly involved in retrieving or transplanting organs from the deceased donor. Physicians should encourage health care institutions to distinguish the roles of health care professionals who solicit or coordinate organ transplantation from those who provide care at the time of death;

    (ii) no member of the transplant team has any role in the decision to withdraw treatment or the pronouncement of death.

(b) Ensure that death is determined by a physician not associated with the transplant team and in accordance with accepted clinical and ethical standards.

(c) Ensure that transplant procedures are undertaken only by physicians who have the requisite medical knowledge and expertise and are carried out in adequately equipped medical facilities.

(d) Ensure that the prospective recipient (or the recipient's authorized surrogate if the individual lacks decision-making capacity) is fully informed about the procedure and has given voluntary consent in keeping with ethics guidance.

(e) Except in situations of directed donation, ensure that organs for transplantation are allocated to recipients on the basis of ethically sound criteria, including but not limited to likelihood of benefit, urgency of need, change in quality of life, duration of benefit, and, in certain cases, amount of resources required for successful treatment.

(f) Ensure that organs for transplantation are treated as a national, rather than a local or regional, resource.

(g) Refrain from placing transplant candidates on the waiting lists of multiple local transplant centers, but rather place candidates on a single waiting list for each type of organ.

6.2.2 Directed Donation of Organs for Transplantation

Efforts to increase the supply of organs available for transplant can serve the interests of individual patients and the public and are in keeping with physicians' obligations to promote the welfare of their patients and to support access to care. Although public solicitations for directed donation—ie, for donation to a specific patient—may benefit individual patients, such solicitations have the potential to adversely affect the equitable distribution of organs among patients in need, the efficacy of the transplant system, and trust in the overall system.

Donation of needed organs to specified recipients has long been permitted in organ transplantation. However, solicitation of organs from potential donors who have no pre-existing relationship with the intended recipient remains controversial. Directed donation policies that produce a net gain of organs for transplantation and do not unreasonably disadvantage other transplant candidates are ethically acceptable.

Physicians who participate in soliciting directed donation of organs for transplantation on behalf of their patients should:

(a) Support ongoing collection of empirical data to monitor the effects of solicitation of directed donations on the availability of organs for transplantation.

(b) Support the development of evidence-based policies for solicitation of directed donation.

(c) Ensure that solicitations do not include potentially coercive inducements. Donors should receive no payment beyond reimbursement for travel, lodging, lost wages, and the medical care associated with donation.

(d) Ensure that prospective donors are fully evaluated for medical and psychosocial suitability by health care professionals who are not part of the transplant team, regardless of any relationship, or lack of relationship, between prospective donor and transplant candidate.

(e) Refuse to participate in any transplant that he or she believes to be ethically improper and respect the decisions of other health care professionals should they choose not to participate on ethical or moral grounds.

AMA Principles of Medical Ethics: VII, VIII, IX

Issued: 2006

Updated: 2016

Opinions on Related Matters:
2.1.1 Informed Consent
6.1.1 Transplantation of Organs from Living Donors
6.1.2 Organ Donation after Cardiac Death

Special Issues in Organ Procurement and Transplantation

AMA Principles of Medical Ethics: IV, VII

Issued: 2001

Updated: 2016

Opinions on Related Matters:
2.1.1 Informed Consent
7.1.1 Physician Involvement in Research

6.3.1 Xenotransplantation

Physicians have an obligation to participate in efforts to increase the supply of organs available for transplantation. In fulfilling that obligation, they must also be mindful of their obligations to protect the interests of patients and the welfare of the public. Xenotransplantation, ie, using organs or tissues from nonhuman animal species for transplantation into human patients, is a possible novel means of addressing the shortage of transplantable organs that can pose distinctive ethical challenges with respect to patient safety and public health.

Some forms of transplantation, implantation, or infusion into a human recipient of organs or tissues from a nonhuman animal source have a significant history in clinical practice—for example the use of porcine heart valves. Other proposed procedures are more controversial and are restricted to research protocols.

Physicians who choose to participate in clinical research that involves transplantation of organs or tissues from nonhuman sources should:

(a) Encourage education and public discussion of xenotransplantation in light of the unique risks such procedures pose to individual patients and the public.

(b) Ensure that research in which they participate is well designed and adheres to institutional review board requirements, applicable national guidelines, and ethical standards for research with human participants.

(c) Ensure that research in which they participate is adequately funded to assure lifelong surveillance of xenotransplant recipients and treatment of medical complications related to transplantation.

(d) Ensure that recruitment is restricted to patients with serious or life-threatening conditions for whom no adequately safe and effective alternative therapies are available unless there is documented, very high assurance of safety.

(e) Ensure that if participation by individuals who lack decision-making capacity is contemplated, appropriate measures are taken to safeguard their interests. In exceptional circumstances, minors with substantial decision-making capacity may, with the informed consent of their legal guardians, be considered as recipients in xenotransplantation. When an unemancipated minor proposes to participate

in xenotransplantation, it may be appropriate to seek advice
from another adult trusted by the minor or to seek consultation with an independent body, such as an ethics committee,
pastoral service, or other counseling resource.

(f) Ensure that participants are informed about and consent to
the unique risks and burdens posed by xenotransplantation,
including:

(i)   novel infectious diseases (zoonoses);

(ii) potential psychological concerns arising from receiving
an organ or tissue from a nonhuman animal;

(iii) the need for lifelong surveillance and ongoing clinical
and laboratory monitoring, with archiving of biological
samples, when appropriate;

(iv) the need to inform intimate contacts of potential risk to
their health;

(v)   the need for an autopsy when appropriate.

(g) Ensure that high standards of care and humane treatment of
all animals used in research are upheld.

7 Research and Innovation

These Opinions are offered as ethics guidance for physicians and are not intended to establish clinical practice guidelines or rules of law.

Ethically sound research with human participants rests on three fundamental principles: respect for persons, beneficence, and justice.[1] Before a study ever enrolls participants, it must meet conditions of value and scientific validity. That is, a study must, first, be designed to evaluate an intervention that could improve health or test a hypothesis that can generate important knowledge, and, second, be methodologically rigorous.[2] The study's potential benefits should be proportionate to the risks imposed on participants, and the study should be designed and conducted in a way that minimizes those risks and protects the privacy and confidentiality of participants. Physician-investigators and other study personnel further have an obligation to preserve the integrity of the scientific enterprise.

In the context of research with human participants, ethical practice requires a robust process of informed consent that not only discloses risks, but also provides information to help a prospective participant understand the nature of the study and the differences between participating in research and receiving clinical care, and that the individual may not benefit personally from participating.

The principle of justice requires that participants be selected fairly and, in particular, that vulnerable or disadvantaged populations not be exploited for the benefit of others—a concern that is heightened in studies carried out internationally. Finally, to close the circle of value, study results must be disseminated to appropriate audiences.

Opinions in the first section of this chapter lay out general guidance relevant to all research with human participants, including issues of consent, study design, conflicts of interest, and research misconduct. The second section provides guidance with respect to the obligation to share results, while the third section offers guidance on special topics in clinical research.

References

1. National Commission for the Protection of Human Subjects of Biomedical and Behavioral Research. *The Belmont Report: Ethical Principles and Guidelines for the Protection of Human Subjects of Research.* Washington, DC: National Commission; 1979. www.fda.gov/ohrms /dockets/ac/05/briefing/2005-4178b_09_02_Belmont%20Report.pdf. Accessed April 18, 2016.
2. Emanuel EJ, Wendler D, Grady C. What makes clinical research ethical? *JAMA.* 2000(283):2701-2711.

7 Research and
Innovation

Physician Involvement in Research

7.1.1 Physician Involvement in Research

Biomedical and health research is intended to contribute to the advancement of knowledge and the welfare of society and future patients, rather than to the specific benefit of the individuals who participate as research subjects.

However, research involving human participants should be conducted in a manner that minimizes risks and avoids unnecessary suffering. Because research depends on the willingness of participants to accept risk, they must be able to make informed decisions about whether to participate or continue in a given protocol.

Physician-researchers share their responsibility for the ethical conduct of research with the institution that carries out research. Institutions have an obligation to oversee the design, conduct, and dissemination of research to ensure that scientific, ethical, and legal standards are upheld. Institutional review boards (IRBs) as well as individual investigators should ensure that each participant has been appropriately informed and has given voluntary consent.

Physicians who are involved in any role in research with human participants have an ethical obligation to ensure that participants' interests are protected and to safeguard participants' welfare, safety, and comfort.

To fulfill these obligations, individually, physicians who are involved in research should:

(a) Participate only in those studies for which they have relevant expertise.

(b) Ensure that voluntary consent has been obtained from each participant or from the participant's legally authorized representative if the participant lacks the capacity to consent, in keeping with ethics guidance. This requires that:

   (i) prospective participants receive the information they need to make well-considered decisions, including informing them about the nature of the research and potential harms involved;

   (ii) physicians make all reasonable efforts to ensure that participants understand the research is not intended to benefit them individually;

   (iii) physicians also make clear that the individual may refuse to participate or may withdraw from the protocol at any time.

(c) Assure themselves that the research protocol is scientifically sound and meets ethical guidelines for research with human

AMA Principles of Medical Ethics: I, II, III, V

Issued: The constituent Opinions on which this guidance is based (see Concordance) were issued between 1977 and 2001.

Updated: 2016

Opinions on Related Matters:
1.1.1 Patient-Physician Relationships
1.2.11 Ethically Sound Innovation in Medical Practice
2.1.1 Informed Consent
2.1.2 Decisions for Adult Patients Who Lack Capacity
3.2.1 Confidentiality
4.1.3 Third-Party Access to Genetic Information
6.3.1 Xenotransplantation
11.2.2 Conflicts of Interest in Patient Care

7 Research and Innovation

participants. Informed consent can never be invoked to justify an unethical study design.

(d) Demonstrate the same care and concern for the well-being of research participants that they would for patients to whom they provide clinical care in a therapeutic relationship. Physician-researchers should advocate for access to experimental interventions that have proven effectiveness for patients.

(e) Be mindful of conflicts of interest and assure themselves that appropriate safeguards are in place to protect the integrity of the research and the welfare of human participants.

(f) Adhere to rigorous scientific and ethical standards in conducting, supervising, and disseminating results of the research.

AMA Principles of Medical Ethics: I, III, V

Issued: The constituent Opinions on which this guidance is based (see Concordance) were issued between 1977 and 1997.

Updated: 2016

7.1.2 Informed Consent in Research

Informed consent is an essential safeguard in research. The obligation to obtain informed consent arises out of respect for persons and a desire to respect the autonomy of the individual deciding whether to volunteer to participate in biomedical or health research. For these reasons, no person may be used as a subject in research against his or her will.

Physicians must ensure that the participant (or legally authorized representative) has given voluntary, informed consent before enrolling a prospective participant in a research protocol. With certain exceptions, to be valid, informed consent requires that the individual have the capacity to provide consent and have sufficient understanding of the subject matter involved to form a decision. The individual's consent must also be voluntary.

A valid consent process includes:

(a) Ascertaining that the individual has decision-making capacity.

(b) Reviewing the process and any materials to ensure that they are understandable to the study population.

(c) Disclosing:
    (i)   the nature of the experimental drug(s), device(s), or procedure(s) to be used in the research;
    (ii) any conflicts of interest relating to the research, in keeping with ethics guidance;
    (iii) any known risks or foreseeable hazards, including pain or discomfort that the participant might experience;
    (iv) the likelihood of therapeutic or other direct benefit for the participant;

(v) that there are alternative courses of action open to the participant, including choosing standard or no treatment instead of participating in the study;

(vi) the nature of the research plan and implications for the participant;

(vii) the differences between the physician's responsibilities as a researcher and as the patient's treating physician.

(d) Answering questions the prospective participant has.

(e) Refraining from persuading the individual to enroll.

(f) Avoiding encouraging unrealistic expectations.

(g) Documenting the individual's voluntary consent to participate.

Participation in research by minors or other individuals who lack decision-making capacity is permissible in limited circumstances when:

(h) Consent is given by the individual's legally authorized representative, under circumstances in which informed and prudent adults would reasonably be expected to volunteer themselves or their children in research.

(i) The participant gives his or her assent to participation, where possible. Physicians should respect the refusal of an individual who lacks decision-making capacity.

(j) There is potential for the individual to benefit from the study.

In certain situations, with special safeguards in keeping with ethics guidance, the obligation to obtain informed consent may be waived in research on emergency interventions.

7.1.3 Study Design and Sampling

To be ethically justifiable, biomedical and health research that involves human subjects must uphold fundamental principles of respect for persons, beneficence, and justice. These principles apply not only to the conduct of research, but equally to the selection of research topics and study design.

Well-designed, ethically sound research aligns with the goals of medicine, addresses questions relevant to the population among whom the study will be carried out, balances the potential for benefit against the potential for harm, employs study designs that will yield scientifically valid and significant data, and generates useful knowledge. For example, research to develop biological or chemical weapons is antithetical to the goals of the medical profession, whereas research to develop defenses against such weapons can be ethically justifiable.

AMA Principles of Medical Ethics: I, II, III, V, VII

Issued: The constituent Opinions on which this guidance is based (see Concordance) were issued between 1977 and 2004.

Updated: 2016

Opinions on Related Matters:
8.5 Disparities in Health Care

Physicians who engage in biomedical or health research with human participants thus have an ethical obligation to ensure that any study with which they are involved:

(a) Is consistent with the goals and fundamental values of the medical profession.

(b) Addresses research question(s) that will contribute meaningfully to medical knowledge and practice.

(c) Is scientifically well designed to yield valid data to answer the research question(s), including using appropriate population and sampling controls, clear and appropriate inclusion/exclusion criteria, a statistically sound plan for data collection and analysis, appropriate controls, and, when applicable, criteria for discontinuing the study (stopping rules).

(d) Minimizes risks to participants, including risks associated with recruitment and data collection activities, without compromising scientific integrity.

(e) Provides mechanisms to safeguard confidentiality.

(f) Does not disproportionately recruit participants from historically disadvantaged populations or populations whose ability to provide fully voluntary consent is compromised. Participants who otherwise meet inclusion/exclusion criteria should be recruited without regard to race, ethnicity, gender, or economic status.

(g) Recruits participants who lack the capacity to give informed consent only when the study stands to benefit that class of participants and participants with capacity would not yield valid results. In this event, assent should be sought from the participant and consent should be obtained from the prospective participant's legally authorized representative, in keeping with ethics guidance.

(h) Has been reviewed and approved by appropriate oversight bodies.

AMA Principles of Medical Ethics: II, IV, V

Issued: The constituent Opinions on which this guidance is based (see Concordance) were issued between 1992 and 2001.

Updated: 2016

Opinions on Related Matters:
7.3.9 Commercial Use of Human Biological Materials
11.2.2 Conflicts of Interest in Patient Care

7.1.4 Conflicts of Interest in Research

Increasing numbers of physicians, both within and outside academic health centers, are becoming involved in partnerships with industry to conduct biomedical and health research. As they do so, physicians must be mindful of the conflicts such engagement poses to the integrity of the research and the welfare of human participants. In addition to financial conflicts of interest created by incentives to conduct trials and recruit subjects, physicians must be sensitive to the differing roles of clinician and investigator, which may require them to balance dual commitments to participants and science. This conflict of commitment is particularly acute when a physician-investigator has treated or continues to treat a patient who is eligible to enroll as a participant in a clinical trial the physician is conducting.

Minimizing and mitigating conflicts of interest in clinical research is imperative if the medical community is to justify and maintain trust in the medical research community.

Physicians who engage in research should:

(a) Decline financial compensation that awards in excess of the physician's research efforts and does not reflect fair market value. Physicians should not accept payment solely for referring patients to research studies.

(b) Ensure that the research protocol includes provision for funding participants' medical care in the event of complications associated with the research. A physician should not double-bill a third-party payer for additional expenses related to conducting the trial if he or she has already received funds from a sponsor for those expenses.

(c) As part of the informed consent process, disclose to prospective participants the nature and source of funding and financial incentives offered to the investigators. This disclosure should be included in any written consent materials.

(d) Avoid engaging in any research where there is an understanding that limitations can be placed on the presentation or publication of results by the research sponsor.

(e) Refrain from knowingly participating in a financial relationship with a commercial entity with whom they have a research relationship until the research relationship ends and the research results have been published or otherwise disseminated to the public.

(f) Disclose material ties to companies whose products they are investigating or other ties that create real or perceived conflicts of interest to:
  (i) institutions where the research will be carried out;
  (ii) organizations that are funding the research;
  (iii) any journal or publication where the research results are being submitted.

(g) Physicians who have leadership roles in institutions that conduct biomedical and health research as well as the entities that fund research with human participants should promote the development of guidelines on conflicts of interest that clarify physician-investigators' responsibilities.

AMA Principles of Medical Ethics: I, III, V

Issued: Prior to 1977

Updated: 1994, 1998, 2016

Opinions on Related Matters:
9.4.2 Reporting Incompetent or
Unethical Behavior by Colleagues

7.1.5 Misconduct in Research

Biomedical and health research is intended to advance medical knowledge to benefit future patients. To achieve those goals, physicians who are involved in such research maintain the highest standards of professionalism and scientific integrity.

Physicians with oversight responsibilities in biomedical or health research have a responsibility to ensure that allegations of scientific misconduct are addressed promptly and fairly. They should ensure that procedures to resolve such allegations:

(a) Do not damage science.

(b) Resolve charges expeditiously.

(c) Treat all parties fairly and justly. Review procedures should be sensitive to parties' reputations and vulnerabilities.

(d) Maintain the integrity of the process. Real or perceived conflicts of interest must be avoided.

(e) Maintain accurate and thorough documentation throughout the process.

(f) Maintain the highest degree of confidentiality.

(g) Take appropriate action to discharge responsibilities to all individuals involved, as well as to the public, research sponsors, the scientific literature, and the scientific community.

Disseminating Research Results

AMA Principles of Medical Ethics: I, II, III, V, VII

Issued: The constituent Opinions on which this guidance is based (see Concordance) were issued between 1977 and 2004.

Updated: 2016

Opinions on Related Matters:
3.1.5 Professionalism in Relationships with Media
8.8 Required Reporting of Adverse Events

7.2.1 Principles for Disseminating Research Results

Physicians have an ethical responsibility to learn from and contribute to the total store of scientific knowledge. When they engage in biomedical or health research, physicians have obligations as scientists, which include disseminating research findings. Prompt presentation to scientific peers and publication of research findings are foundational to good medical care and promote enhanced patient care, early evaluation of clinical innovations, and rapid dissemination of improved techniques.

To fulfill their ethical responsibilities with respect to sharing research findings for the ultimate benefit of patients, physicians should:

(a) Advocate for timely and transparent dissemination of research data and findings. Physicians should not intentionally withhold information for reasons of personal gain.

(b) Report the results of research accurately, including subsequent negative findings. This is particularly important where the findings do not support the research hypothesis.

(c) Maintain a commitment to peer review.

(d) Disclose sponsorship and conflicts of interest relating to the research, in keeping with ethics guidance.

(e) Be responsible in their release of research results to the media, ensuring that any information the researcher provides is prompt and accurate and that informed consent to the release of information has been obtained from research participants (or participants' legally authorized representative when the participant lacks decision-making capacity) prior to releasing any identifiable information.

In rare circumstances, the potential for misuse of research results could affect the decision about when and whether to disseminate research findings. Physician-researchers should assess foreseeable ramifications of their research in an effort to balance the promise of benefit against potential harms from corrupt application. Only under rare circumstances should findings be withheld, and then only to the extent required to reasonably protect against misuse.

7.2.2 Release of Data from Unethical Experiments

AMA Principles of Medical Ethics: II, V, VII
Issued: 1998
Updated: 2016

Research that violates the fundamental principle of respect for persons and basic standards of human dignity, such as Nazi experiments during World War II or from the US Public Health Service Tuskegee Syphilis Study, is unethical and of questionable scientific value. Data obtained from such cruel and inhumane experiments should virtually never be published. If data from unethical experiments can be replaced by data from ethically sound research and achieve the same ends, then such must be done. In the rare instances when ethically tainted data have been validated by rigorous scientific analysis and are the only data of such nature available, and human lives would certainly be lost without the knowledge obtained from the data, it may be permissible to use or publish findings from unethical experiments.

Physicians who engage with data from unethical experiments as authors, peer reviewers, or editors of medical publications should:

(a) Disclose that the data derive from studies that do not meet contemporary standards for the ethical conduct of research.

(b) Clearly describe and acknowledge the unethical nature of the experiment(s) from which the data are derived.

(c) Provide ethically compelling reasons for which the data are being released or cited, such as the need to save human lives when no other relevant data are available.

(d) Pay respect to those who were the victims of the unethical experimentation.

AMA Principles of Medical Ethics: V, VII

Issued: The constituent Opinions on which this guidance is based (see Concordance) were issued between 1977 and 1998.

Updated: 2016

Opinions on Related Matters:
7.1.4 Conflicts of Interest in Research
7.3.9 Commercial Use of Human Biological Materials
11.2.2 Conflicts of Interest in Patient Care

7.2.3 Patents and Dissemination of Research Products

A patent grants the holder the right, for a limited time, to prevent others from commercializing his or her inventions. By requiring full disclosure of the invention, and thus enabling another trained in the art to replicate it, the patent system protects the holder's discovery, yet also fosters information sharing. Patenting is also thought to encourage private investment into research.

With respect to genetic research, patenting raises unique questions. Arguments have been made that the patenting of human genetic material sets a troubling precedent for the ownership or commodification of human life. However, DNA sequences are not tantamount to human life, and it is unclear where and whether qualities uniquely human are found in genetic material. Moreover, while genetic research holds great potential for developing new medical therapies, it remains unclear what role patenting will play in ensuring such development.

Physicians who develop medical innovations may ethically patent their discoveries or products but should uphold the following guidance:

(a) Not use patents (or other means, such as trade secrets or confidentiality agreements) to limit the availability of medical innovations. Patent protection should not hinder the goal of achieving better medical treatments and technologies.

(b) Not allow patents to languish. Physicians who hold patents should negotiate and structure licensing agreements in such a way as to encourage the development of better medical technology.

(c) For patents on genetic materials, recognize that:
   (i) patents on processes, eg, to isolate and purify gene sequences, are ethically preferable to patents on the substances themselves;
   (ii) patents on purified proteins (substance patents) are ethically preferable to patents on genes or DNA sequences.

Descriptions for (substance) patents on proteins, genes, or genetic sequences should be carefully constructed to ensure that the patent holder does not limit the use of a naturally occurring form of the substance in question.

Special Issues in Research

7.3.1 Ethical Use of Placebo Controls in Research

A fundamental requirement of biomedical and health research is that it must provide scientifically valid data. In some research, this can best be achieved by comparing an intervention against a control to identify the effects of the intervention. Used appropriately, a placebo control can provide valuable data, particularly when there is no accepted therapy for the condition under study.

The existence of an accepted therapy does not necessarily preclude use of placebo controls, but because use of a placebo deprives participants in the control arm of access to accepted therapy for some period of time, it requires thoughtful ethical justification. In general, the use of a placebo control will more easily be justified as the severity and number of negative side effects of standard therapy increase.

To ensure that the interests of human participants are protected, physician-researchers and those who serve on oversight bodies should give careful attention to issues of methodological rigor, informed consent, characteristics of the medical condition under study, and safety and monitoring, in keeping with the following guidance:

(a) Evaluate each study protocol to determine whether a placebo control is scientifically necessary or an alternative study design using a different type of control would be sufficient for the purposes of the research. Placebo controls are ethically justifiable when no other research design will yield the requisite data.

(b) Assess the use of placebo controls in relation to the characteristics of the condition under study in keeping with the following considerations:

(i) Studies that involve conditions likely to cause death or irreversible damage cannot ethically employ placebo controls if an alternative therapy would prevent or slow the progression of illness;

(ii) Studies that involve illnesses characterized by severe or painful symptoms require a thorough exploration of alternatives to the use of a placebo control;

AMA Principles of Medical Ethics: I, V

Issued: The constituent Opinions on which this guidance is based (see Concordance) were issued between 1997 and 2000.

Updated: 2016

Opinions on Related Matters:
2.1.1 Informed Consent
2.1.2 Decisions for Adult Patients Who Lack Capacity
2.1.4 Use of Placebo in Clinical Practice
7.1.2 Informed Consent in Research

(iii) In general, the more severe the consequences or symptoms of the illness under study, the more difficult it will be to justify the use of a placebo control when alternative therapy exists. Consequently, there will almost certainly be conditions for which placebo controls cannot ethically be justified.

(c) Design studies to minimize the amount of time participants are on placebo without compromising the scientific integrity of the study or the value of study data.

(d) Pay particular attention to the informed consent process when enrolling participants in research that uses a placebo control. In addition to general guidance for informed consent in research, physician-researchers (or other health care professionals) who obtain informed consent from prospective subjects should:

(i)   describe the differences among the research arms, emphasizing the essential intervention(s) that will or will not be performed in each;

(ii) be sensitive to the possible need for additional safeguards in the consent process, such as having a neutral third party obtain consent or using a consent monitor to oversee the consent process.

(e) Ensure that interim data analysis and monitoring are in place to allow researchers to terminate a study because of either positive or negative results, thus protecting participants from remaining on placebo longer than needed to ensure the scientific integrity of the study.

(f) Avoid using surgical placebo controls—ie, a control arm in which participants undergo surgical procedures that have the appearance of therapeutic interventions but during which the essential therapeutic maneuver is not performed—when there is a standard treatment that is efficacious and acceptable to the patient and forgoing standard treatment would result in significant injury. In these situations, physician-researchers must offer standard treatment as part of the study design. Use of surgical placebo controls may be justified when:

(i)   an existing, accepted surgical procedure is being tested for efficacy. Use of a placebo control is not justified to test the effectiveness of an innovative surgical technique that represents only a minor modification of an existing, accepted surgical procedure;

(ii) a new surgical procedure is developed with the prospect of treating a condition for which there is no known surgical therapy. In such cases, the use of placebo must be evaluated in light of whether the current standard of care includes a nonsurgical treatment and the risks, benefits, and side effects of that treatment;

(iii) the standard (nonsurgical) treatment is not efficacious or not acceptable to the patient;

(iv) additional safeguards are in place in the informed consent process.

7.3.2 Research on Emergency Medical Interventions

Emergency medicine often applies standard interventions that have not been scientifically evaluated for safety and effectiveness in the context of emergency care and may render unsatisfactory outcomes. However, in life-threatening situations, patients may not be able to give informed consent and a surrogate decision maker may not be readily available, making it challenging to carry out ethically sound research. Soliciting input from the community before a research protocol is approved can help address some concerns, but not all.

Given the insufficiency of standard treatment alternatives, it can be appropriate, in certain situations and with special safeguards, to provide experimental treatment without a participant's informed consent.

To protect the rights and welfare of participants in research on emergency medical interventions, physician-researchers must adhere to the following criteria:

(a) The experimental intervention has a realistic probability of providing benefit equal to or greater than standard care.

(b) The risks associated with the research are reasonable in light of the critical nature of the medical condition and the risks associated with standard treatment.

(c) Study participants are randomized fairly.

(d) The trial is overseen by an independent data and safety monitoring board.

(e) The prospective participant lacks the capacity to give informed consent at the time he or she must be enrolled due to the emergency situation and requirements of the research protocol, and it would not have been feasible to obtain prospective informed consent because the life-threatening emergency situation could not have been anticipated.

(f) The window of opportunity to administer the experimental intervention is so narrow as to make it unfeasible to obtain consent from the prospective participant's surrogate or other legally authorized representative.

AMA Principles of Medical Ethics: I, V

Issued: 1997

Updated: 2016

Opinions on Related Matters:
2.1.1 Informed Consent
7.1.2 Informed Consent in Research

(g) Participants, or their representatives, are informed as soon as possible that the individual has been enrolled in the research and asked to give consent to further participation.

(h) The representative of a patient who dies while participating in the research must be informed that the individual was involved in an experimental protocol.

(i) Study results will be publicly disclosed.

AMA Principles of Medical Ethics: I, IV, VII, VIII, IX

Issued: 2001

Updated: 2016

Opinions on Related Matters:
2.1.1 Informed Consent
7.1.2 Informed Consent in Research
7.1.3 Study Design and Sampling
8.5 Disparities in Health Care

7.3.3 International Research

Biomedical and health research in international settings often raises special ethical questions, particularly when research is carried out in resource-poor settings by sponsors or researchers from resource-rich countries. Physicians engaged in international research may encounter differing cultural traditions, economic conditions, health care systems, and ethical or regulatory standards and traditions than in the US.

While fundamental requirements to ensure scientifically sound research and to protect the welfare, safety, and comfort of human participants apply in any research setting, physicians who are involved in international research may need to address special concerns about selection of research topic and study design, informed consent, and the impact of the research on the participating community.

In addition to following general ethical guidelines for biomedical and health research, physicians who are involved in international research have obligations to:

Study design

(a) Ensure that the research responds to a medical need in the region in which it is undertaken.

(b) Ensure that the research does not exploit the populations and communities from which participants will be drawn.

(c) Be sensitive to special considerations in assessing the risks and benefits of the research in the particular setting and employ a research design that minimizes risks to the participant population by:

    (i) ascertaining that there is genuine uncertainty within the clinical community about the comparative merits of the experimental intervention and the intervention that will be offered as a control for the population to be enrolled;

    (ii) obtaining relevant input from representatives of the host community and from the research population;

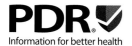
Visit PDR.net/Updates to view full new and updated drug labeling.

LABELING UPDATES

KEY			
■ **Boxed Warning**	▲ Other Warnings*	● Updates to Indications/Dosage	◆ Other Updates†
	*Warnings & Precautions; Adverse Reactions; Drug Interactions; and Contraindications		†Other labeling changes; added to PDR database

		◆	**Arranon** (nelarabine)
▲		◆	**Depakote ER** (divalproex sodium)
▲		◆	**Duopa** (carbidopa/levodopa)
▲		◆	**Gleevec** (imatinib mesylate)
▲		◆	**Kaletra** (lopinavir/ritonavir)
▲		◆	**Norvir** (ritonavir)
▲		◆	**Sprycel** (dasatinib)
▲		◆	**Tarka** (trandolapril/verapamil hydrochloride)

▲		◆	**Tasigna** (nilotinib)
		◆	**Trilipix** (fenofibric acid)
▲		◆	**Trintellix** (vortioxetine)
	●	◆	**Vascepa** (icosapent ethyl)
▲	●	◆	**Zofran** (ondansetron, ondansetron hydrochloride) ODT Orally Disintegrating Tablets, Oral Solution, and Tablets
		◆	**Zykadia** (ceritinib)

To have full prescribing information faxed or mailed to you, call 1-800-261-2313.

(iii) considering the harm that is likely to result for the host community or research population if the research is not carried out.

(d) In some instances, a three-armed protocol that offers the standard of care in the US, an intervention that meets a level of care that can be attained in and sustained by the host community, and a placebo may offer the most ethically desirable means for evaluating the safety and efficacy of an intervention in a given population.

Informed consent

(e) Ensure that a suitable process for informed consent is in place. If consent is to be meaningful, physicians (or other health professionals) who obtain consent must communicate with sensitivity to local customs. Notwithstanding, they should always ensure that individual participants are informed and that their voluntary consent is sought.

Impact on the host community

(f) Foster research with the potential for lasting benefits to the host community, especially when the research is carried out among populations that are severely deficient in health care resources. This can be achieved by:

(i) facilitating development of a health care infrastructure that will be of use during and after the research period itself;

(ii) encouraging sponsors to provide interventions that have been demonstrated to be beneficial to all study participants after the study concludes.

7.3.4 Maternal-Fetal Research

Maternal-fetal research, ie, research intended to benefit pregnant women and/or their fetuses, must balance the health and safety of the woman who participates and the well-being of the fetus with the desire to develop new and innovative therapies. One challenge in such research is that pregnant women may face external pressure or expectations to enroll from partners, family members, or others that may compromise their ability to make a fully voluntary decision about whether to participate.

Physicians engaged in maternal-fetal research should demonstrate the same care and concern for the pregnant woman and fetus that they would in providing clinical care.

AMA Principles of Medical Ethics: I, III, V

Issued: 1980

Updated: 1994, 2016

Opinions on Related Matters:
2.1.1 Informed Consent
7.1.2 Informed Consent in Research

In addition to adhering to general guidelines for the ethical conduct of research and applicable law, physicians who are involved in maternal-fetal research should:

(a) Base studies on scientifically sound clinical research with animals and nongravid human participants that has been carried out prior to conducting maternal-fetal research whenever possible.

(b) Enroll a pregnant woman in maternal-fetal research only when there is no simpler, safer intervention available to promote the well-being of the woman or fetus.

(c) Obtain the informed, voluntary consent of the pregnant woman.

(d) Minimize risks to the fetus to the greatest extent possible, especially when the intervention under study is intended primarily to benefit the pregnant woman.

AMA Principles of Medical Ethics: I, III, IV, V

Issued: The constituent Opinions on which this guidance is based (see Concordance) were issued between 1980 and 1992.

Updated: 2016

7.3.5 Research Using Human Fetal Tissue

Research with human fetal tissue has led to the development of a number of important research and medical advances, such as the development of polio vaccine. Fetal tissue has also been used to study the mechanism of viral infections and to diagnose viral infections and inherited diseases, as well as to develop transplant therapies for a variety of conditions, eg, parkinsonism.

However, the use of fetal tissue for research purposes also raises a number of ethical considerations, including the degree to which a woman's decision to have an abortion might be influenced by the opportunity to donate fetal tissue. Concerns have also been raised about potential conflict of interest when there is possible financial benefit to those who are involved in the retrieval, storage, testing, preparation, and delivery of fetal tissues.

To protect the interests of pregnant women, as well as the integrity of science, physicians who are involved in research that uses human fetal tissue should:

(a) Abstain from offering money in exchange for fetal tissue.

(b) In all instances, obtain the woman's voluntary, informed consent in keeping with ethics guidance, including when using fetal tissue from a spontaneous abortion for purposes of research or transplantation. Informed consent includes a disclosure of the nature of the research including the purpose of using fetal tissue, as well as informing the woman of a right to refuse to participate.

(c) Ensure that when fetal tissue from an induced abortion is used for research purposes:

   (i) the woman's decision to terminate the pregnancy is made prior to and independent of any discussion of using the fetal tissue for research purposes;

   (ii) decisions regarding the technique used to induce abortion and the timing of the abortion in relation to the gestational age of the fetus are based on concern for the safety of the pregnant woman.

(d) Ensure that when fetal tissue is to be used for transplantation in research or clinical care:

   (i) the donor does not designate the recipient of the tissue;

   (ii) both the donor and the recipient of the tissue give voluntary, informed consent.

(e) Ensure that health care personnel involved in the termination of a pregnancy do not benefit from their participation in the termination, or from use of the fetal tissue for transplantation.

7.3.6 Research in Gene Therapy and Genetic Engineering

Gene therapy involves the replacement or modification of a genetic variant to restore or enhance cellular function or to improve the response to nongenetic therapies. Genetic engineering involves the use of recombinant DNA techniques to introduce new characteristics or traits. In medicine, the goal of gene therapy and genetic engineering is to alleviate human suffering and disease. As with all therapies, this goal should be pursued only within the ethical traditions of the profession, which gives primacy to the welfare of the patient.

In general, genetic manipulation should be reserved for therapeutic purposes. Efforts to enhance "desirable" characteristics or to "improve" complex human traits are contrary to the ethical tradition of medicine. Because of the potential for abuse, genetic manipulation of nondisease traits or the eugenic development of offspring may never be justifiable.

Moreover, genetic manipulation can carry risks to both the individuals into whom modified genetic material is introduced and future generations. Somatic cell gene therapy targets nongerm cells and thus does not carry risk to future generations. Germ-line therapy, in which a genetic modification is introduced into the genome of human gametes or their precursors, is intended to result in the expression of the modified gene in the recipient's offspring

AMA Principles of Medical Ethics: I, V, VII

Issued: The constituent Opinions on which this guidance is based (see Concordance) were issued between 1980 and 1988.

Updated: 2016

Opinions on Related Matters:
2.1.1 Informed Consent
3.2.1 Confidentiality
4.1.3 Third-Party Access to Genetic Information
7.1.2 Informed Consent in Research
7.3.7 Safeguards in the Use of DNA Databanks

and subsequent generations. Germ-line therapy thus may be associated with increased risk and the possibility of unpredictable and irreversible results that adversely affect the welfare of subsequent generations.

Thus, in addition to fundamental ethical requirements for the appropriate conduct of research with human participants, research in gene therapy or genetic engineering must put in place additional safeguards to vigorously protect the safety and well-being of participants and future generations.

Physicians should not engage in research involving gene therapy or genetic engineering with human participants unless the following conditions are met:

(a) Experience with animal studies is sufficient to assure that the experimental intervention will be safe and effective and its results predictable.

(b) No other suitable, effective therapies are available.

(c) Gene therapy is restricted to somatic cell interventions, in light of the far-reaching implications of germ-line interventions.

(d) Evaluation of the effectiveness of the intervention includes determination of the natural history of the disease or condition under study and follow-up examination of the participants' descendants.

(e) The research minimizes risks to participants, including those from any viral vectors used.

(f) Special attention is paid to the informed consent process to ensure that the prospective participant (or legally authorized representative) is fully informed about the distinctive risks of the research, including use of viral vectors to deliver the modified genetic material, possible implications for the participant's descendants, and the need for follow-up assessments.

Physicians should be aware that gene therapy or genetic engineering interventions may require additional scientific and ethical review, and regulatory oversight, before they are introduced into clinical practice.

7.3.7 Safeguards in the Use of DNA Databanks

AMA Principles of Medical Ethics: I, IV, V, VII

Issued: 2002

Updated: 2016

Opinions on Related Matters:
2.1.1 Informed Consent
3.2.1 Confidentiality
4.1.1 Genetic Testing and Counseling
4.1.3 Third-Party Access to Genetic Information
7.1.2 Informed Consent in Research

DNA databanks facilitate population-based research into the genetic components of complex diseases. These databanks derive their power from integrating genetic and clinical data, as well as data on health, lifestyle, and environment about large samples of individuals. However, the use of DNA databanks in genomic research also raises the possibility of harm to individual participants, their families, and even populations.

Breach of confidentiality of information contained in DNA databanks may result in discrimination or stigmatization and may carry implications for important personal choices, such as reproductive choices. Human participants who contribute to research involving DNA databanks have a right to be informed about the nature and scope of the research and to make decisions about how their information may be used.

In addition to having adequate training to be able to discuss genomic research and related ethical issues with patients or prospective research participants, physician-researchers who are involved in genomic research using DNA databanks should:

Research involving individuals

(a) Obtain informed consent from participants in genomic research, in keeping with ethics guidance. In addition, physicians should put special emphasis in the consent process on disclosing:

   (i) the specific privacy standards to which the study will adhere, including whether the information or biological sample will be encrypted and remain identifiable to the researcher or will be completely de-identified;

   (ii) whether participants whose data will be encrypted rather than de-identified can expect to be contacted in the future about findings or be invited to participate in additional research, either related to the current protocol or for other research purposes;

   (iii) whether researchers or participants stand to gain financially from research findings, and any conflicts of interest researchers may have in regard to the research, in keeping with ethics guidance;

   (iv) when, if ever, archived information or samples will be discarded;

   (v) participants' freedom to refuse use of their biological materials without penalty.

Research involving identifiable communities

(b) When research is to be conducted within a defined subset of the general population, physicians should:

(i)   consult with the community in advance to design a study that is sensitive to community concerns and that will minimize harm for the community, as well as for individual participants. Physicians should not carry out a study when there is substantial opposition to the research within the community of interest;

(ii) protect confidentiality by encrypting any demographic or identifying information that is not required for the study's purpose.

AMA Principles of Medical Ethics: V

Issued: 2011

Opinions on Related Matters:
2.1.1 Informed Consent
4.2.5 Storage and Use of Human Embryos
4.2.6 Cloning for Reproduction
7.1.2 Informed Consent in Research

7.3.8 Research with Stem Cells

Human stem cells are widely seen as offering a source of potential treatment for a range of diseases and are thus the subject of much research. Clinical studies have validated the use of adult stem cells in a limited number of therapies, but have yet to confirm the utility of embryonic stem cells.

Physicians who conduct research using stem cells obtained from any source (established tissue, umbilical cord blood, or embryos) must, at a minimum:

(a) Adhere to institutional review board (IRB) requirements.

(b) Ensure that the research is carried out with appropriate oversight and monitoring.

(c) Ensure that the research is carried out with appropriate informed consent. In addition to disclosure of research risks and potential benefits, at minimum, the consent disclosure should address:

(i)   for a donor of cells to be used in stem cell research:
   a. the process by which stem cells will be obtained;
   b. what specifically will be done with the stem cells;
   c. whether an immortal cell line will result;
   d. the primary and anticipated secondary uses of donated embryos and/or derived stem cells, including potential commercial uses.

(ii) for a recipient of stem cells in clinical research:
   a. the types of tissue from which the stem cells derive (eg, established tissue, umbilical cord blood, or embryos);
   b. unique risks posed by investigational stem cell products (when applicable), such as tumorigenesis,

immunological reactions, unpredictable behavior of cells, and unknown long-term health effects.

The professional community as well as the public remains divided about the use of embryonic stem cells for either research or therapeutic purposes. The conflict regarding research with embryonic stem cells centers on the moral status of embryos, a question that divides ethical opinion and that cannot be resolved by medical science. Regardless whether they are obtained from embryos donated by individuals or couples undergoing in vitro fertilization, or from cloned embryos created by somatic cell nuclear transfer (SCNT), use of embryonic stem cells currently requires the destruction of the human embryo from which the stem cells derive.

The pluralism of moral visions that underlies this debate must be respected. Participation in research involving embryonic stem cells requires respect for embryos, research participants, donors, and recipients. Embryonic stem cell research does not violate the ethical standards of the profession. Every physician remains free to decide whether to participate in stem cell research or to use its products. Physicians should continue to be guided by their commitment to the welfare of patients and the advancement of medical science.

Physicians who conduct research using embryonic stem cells should be able to justify greater risks for subjects, and the greater respect due embryos than stem cells from other sources, based on expectations that the research offers substantial promise of contributing significantly to scientific or therapeutic knowledge.

7.3.9 Commercial Use of Human Biological Materials

Research using human tissues has resulted in numerous commercially available products for use in both research and treatment. The development of these products raises questions about who holds property rights in human biological materials, how to distribute profits derived from human tissues equitably, and what constitutes appropriately informed consent when patients donate biological materials to research that may ultimately result in one or more commercial products.

Physicians involved in research with human biological materials should:

(a) Disclose potential commercial applications to the tissue donor before a profit is realized on products developed from biological materials.

AMA Principles of Medical Ethics: II, V

Issued: 1994

Updated: 2016

Opinions on Related Matters:
2.1.1 Informed Consent
4.2.2 Gamete Donation
4.2.5 Storage and Use of Human Embryos
7.1.2 Informed Consent in Research
7.1.4 Conflicts of Interest in Research
7.3.7 Safeguards in the Use of DNA Databanks
11.2.2 Conflicts of Interest in Patient Care

(b) Obtain informed consent to use biological materials in research from the tissue donor. Human biological materials and their products may not be used for commercial purposes without the consent of the tissue donor.

(c) Share profits from the commercial use of human biological materials with the tissue donor in accordance with lawful contractual agreements.

Physicians must make diagnostic and treatment recommendations in keeping with standards of good medical practice. They must not allow the commercial potential of the patient's tissue to influence professional judgment.

8 Physicians and the Health of the Community

These Opinions are offered as ethics guidance for physicians and are not intended to establish clinical practice guidelines or rules of law.

Physicians' primary ethical obligation is to individual patients, but they also have a well-recognized responsibility to protect and promote public health. To fulfill these dual responsibilities, physicians must balance the rights and welfare of individuals with the needs and safety of the community.

What considerations come into play and how physicians should weigh different considerations in striking that balance may vary with context. In some contexts, patients' own interests may align with those of the public, as when the safety of both the individual and others is best served by persuading patients not to drive when their ability to do so safely is compromised by a medical or mental health condition. In the limit case, it will still be in the patient's interest when a physician is required to report the individual to appropriate authorities in a position to revoke the patient's driving privileges.

In other contexts, the interests of the individual and the public diverge. In the context of highly transmissible infectious disease, for example, physicians' responsibility to protect the community may outweigh individual liberty and informed consent, justifying the use of isolation or quarantine for individuals to prevent the spread of disease. In general, when civil liberties are abrogated in the interests of the public good, physicians have an obligation to advocate for and impose the least restrictive means that will achieve the public health goal. Similarly, physicians' obligation to protect the privacy and confidentiality of individual patients may yield to the need for surveillance and mandatory reporting. At the same time, physicians retain the obligation to disclose the minimum information necessary for the public health purpose.

Physicians may also be expected to take on new obligations in discharging their responsibility to protect the health of the community, notably the duty to treat even in the face of personal risk. Physicians likewise have an obligation to adopt preventive measures and accept limitations on their own practice when they are themselves at risk of transmitting disease, an obligation that stems in part from the need to protect the workforce.

Finally, in meeting the needs of individual patients, physicians have a responsibility to the community to promote access to care and to address disparities in health outcomes across populations of patients when those outcomes are not directly attributable to patients' medical needs or preferences.

8.1 Routine Universal Screening for HIV

Physicians' primary ethical obligation is to their individual patients. However, physicians also have a long-recognized responsibility to participate in activities to protect and promote the health of the public. Routine universal screening of adult patients for HIV helps promote the welfare of individual patients, avoid injury to third parties, and protect public health.

Medical and social advances have enhanced the benefits of knowing one's HIV status and at the same time have minimized the need for specific written informed consent prior to HIV testing. Nonetheless, the ethical tenets of respect for autonomy and informed consent require that physicians continue to seek patients' informed consent, including informed refusal of HIV testing.

To protect the welfare and interests of individual patients and fulfill their public health obligations in the context of HIV, physicians should:

(a) Support routine, universal screening of adult patients for HIV with opt-out provisions.

(b) Make efforts to persuade reluctant patients to be screened, including explaining potential benefits to the patient and to the patient's close contacts.

(c) Continue to uphold respect for autonomy by respecting a patient's informed decision to opt out.

(d) Test patients without prior consent only in limited cases in which the harms to individual autonomy are offset by significant benefits to known third parties, such as testing to protect occupationally exposed health care professionals or patients.

(e) Work to ensure that patients who are identified as HIV positive receive appropriate follow-up care and counseling.

(f) Attempt to persuade patients who are identified as HIV positive to cease endangering others.

(g) Be aware of and adhere to state and local guidelines regarding public health reporting and disclosure of HIV status when a patient who is identified as HIV positive poses significant risk of infecting an identifiable third party. The doctor may, if permitted, notify the endangered third party without revealing the identity of the source person.

(h) Safeguard the confidentiality of patient information to the greatest extent possible when required to report HIV status.

AMA Principles of Medical Ethics: I, VI, VII

Issued: 2008

Updated: 2010, 2016

Opinions on Related Matters:
1.1.1 Patient-Physician Relationships
1.1.2 Prospective Patients
1.1.3 Patient Rights
2.1.1 Informed Consent

AMA Principles of Medical Ethics: I, III, IV, VII

Issued: 2000

Updated: 2016

Opinions on Related Matters:

8.2 Impaired Drivers and Their Physicians

A variety of medical conditions can impair an individual's ability to operate a motor vehicle safely, whether a personal car or boat or a commercial vehicle, such as a bus, train, plane, or commercial vessel. Those who operate a vehicle when impaired by a medical condition pose threats to both public safety and their own well-being. Physicians have unique opportunities to assess the impact of physical and mental conditions on patients' ability to drive safely and have a responsibility to do so in light of their professional obligation to protect public health and safety. In deciding whether or how to intervene when a patient's medical condition may impair driving, physicians must balance dual responsibilities to promote the welfare and confidentiality of the individual patient and to protect public safety.

Not all physicians are in a position to evaluate the extent or effect of a medical condition on a patient's ability to drive, particularly physicians who treat patients only on a short-term basis. Nor do all physicians necessarily have appropriate training to identify and evaluate physical or mental conditions in relation to the ability to drive. In such situations, it may be advisable to refer a potentially at-risk patient for assessment.

To serve the interests of their patients and the public, within their areas of expertise physicians should:

(a) Assess at-risk patients individually for medical conditions that might adversely affect driving ability, using best professional judgment and keeping in mind that not all physical or mental impairments create an obligation to intervene.

(b) Tactfully but candidly discuss driving risks with the patient and, when appropriate, the family when a medical condition may adversely affect the patient's ability to drive safely. Help the patient (and family) formulate a plan to reduce risks, including options for treatment or therapy if available, changes in driving behavior, or other adjustments.

(c) Recognize that safety standards for those who operate commercial transportation are subject to governmental medical standards and may differ from standards for private licenses.

(d) Be aware of applicable state requirements for reporting to the licensing authority those patients whose impairments may compromise their ability to operate a motor vehicle safely.

(e) Prior to reporting, explain to the patient (and family, as appropriate) that the physician may have an obligation to report a medically at-risk driver:

(i)   when the physician identifies a medical condition clearly related to the ability to drive;

(ii) when continuing to drive poses a clear risk to public safety or the patient's own well-being and the patient ignores the physician's advice to discontinue driving;

(iii) when required by law.

(f) Inform the patient that the determination of inability to drive safely will be made by other authorities, not the physician.

(g) Disclose only the minimum necessary information when reporting a medically at-risk driver, in keeping with ethics guidance on respect for patient privacy and confidentiality.

8.3 Physicians' Responsibilities in Disaster Response and Preparedness

Whether at the national, regional, or local level, responses to disasters require extensive involvement from physicians individually and collectively. Because of their commitment to care for the sick and injured, individual physicians have an obligation to provide urgent medical care during disasters. This obligation holds even in the face of greater than usual risks to physicians' own safety, health, or life.

However, the physician workforce is not an unlimited resource. Therefore, when providing care in a disaster with its inherent dangers, physicians also have an obligation to evaluate the risks of providing care to individual patients versus the need to be available to provide care in the future.

With respect to disaster, whether natural or manmade, individual physicians should:

(a) Take appropriate advance measures, including acquiring and maintaining appropriate knowledge and skills to ensure they are able to provide medical services when needed.

Collectively, physicians should:

(b) Provide medical expertise and work with others to develop public health policies that:
   (i) are designed to improve the effectiveness and availability of medical services during a disaster;
   (ii) are based on sound science;
   (iii) are based on respect for patients.

(c) Advocate for and participate in ethically sound research to inform policy decisions.

AMA Principles of Medical Ethics: V, VI, VII, VIII

Issued: 2004

Updated: 2016

Opinions on Related Matters:
8.4   Ethical Use of Quarantine and Isolation

AMA Principles of Medical Ethics: I, III, VI, VII, VIII

Issued: 2006

Updated: 2016

Opinions on Related Matters:
8.3 Physicians' Responsibilities in Disaster Response and Preparedness

8.4 Ethical Use of Quarantine and Isolation

Although physicians' primary ethical obligation is to their individual patients, they also have a long-recognized public health responsibility. In the context of infectious disease, this may include the use of quarantine and isolation to reduce the transmission of disease and protect the health of the public. In such situations, physicians have a further responsibility to protect their own health to ensure that they remain able to provide care. These responsibilities potentially conflict with patients' rights of self-determination and with physicians' duty to advocate for the best interests of individual patients and to provide care in emergencies.

With respect to the use of quarantine and isolation as public health interventions in situations of epidemic disease, individual physicians should:

(a) Participate in implementing scientifically and ethically sound quarantine and isolation measures in keeping with the duty to provide care in epidemics.

(b) Educate patients and the public about the nature of the public health threat, potential harm to others, and benefits of quarantine and isolation.

(c) Encourage patients to adhere voluntarily to quarantine and isolation.

(d) Support mandatory quarantine and isolation when a patient fails to adhere voluntarily.

(e) Inform patients about and comply with mandatory public health reporting requirements.

(f) Take appropriate protective and preventive measures to minimize transmission of infectious disease from physician to patient, including accepting immunization for vaccine-preventable disease, in keeping with ethics guidance.

(g) Seek medical evaluation and treatment if they suspect themselves to be infected, including adhering to mandated public health measures.

The medical profession, in collaboration with public health colleagues and civil authorities, has an ethical responsibility to:

(h) Ensure that quarantine measures are ethically and scientifically sound:

    (i) use the least restrictive means available to control disease in the community while protecting individual rights;

    (ii) without bias against any class or category of patients.

(i) Advocate for the highest possible level of confidentiality when personal health information is transmitted in the context of public health reporting.

(j) Advocate for access to public health services to ensure timely detection of risks and implementation of public health interventions, including quarantine and isolation.

(k) Advocate for protective and preventive measures for physicians and others caring for patients with communicable disease.

(l) Develop educational materials and programs about quarantine and isolation as public health interventions for patients and the public.

8.5 Disparities in Health Care

Stereotypes, prejudice, or bias based on gender expectations and other arbitrary evaluations of any individual can manifest in a variety of subtle ways. Differences in treatment that are not directly related to differences in individual patients' clinical needs or preferences constitute inappropriate variations in health care. Such variations may contribute to health outcomes that are considerably worse in members of some populations than those of members of majority populations.

This represents a significant challenge for physicians, who ethically are called on to provide the same quality of care to all patients without regard to medically irrelevant personal characteristics.

To fulfill this professional obligation in their individual practices, physicians should:

(a) Provide care that meets patient needs and respects patient preferences.

(b) Avoid stereotyping patients.

(c) Examine their own practices to ensure that inappropriate considerations about race, gender identity, sexual orientation, sociodemographic factors, or other nonclinical factors do not affect clinical judgment.

(d) Work to eliminate biased behavior toward patients by other health care professionals and staff who come into contact with patients.

(e) Encourage shared decision making.

(f) Cultivate effective communication and trust by seeking to better understand factors that can influence patients' health care decisions, such as cultural traditions, health beliefs and health literacy, language or other barriers to communication, and fears or misperceptions about the health care system.

The medical profession has an ethical responsibility to:

(g) Help increase awareness of health care disparities.

(h) Strive to increase the diversity of the physician workforce as a step toward reducing health care disparities.

AMA Principles of Medical Ethics: I, IV, VII, VIII, IX

Issued: The constituent Opinions on which this guidance is based (see Concordance) were issued in 1992.

Updated: 2016

Opinions on Related Matters:
1.1.2 Prospective Patients
1.1.7 Physician Exercise of Conscience
4.2.1 Assisted Reproductive Technology

8 Physicians and the Health of the Community

(i) Support research that examines health care disparities, including research on the unique health needs of all genders, ethnic groups, and medically disadvantaged populations, and the development of quality measures and resources to help reduce disparities.

AMA Principles of Medical Ethics: I, II, III, IV, VIII

Issued: The constituent Opinions on which this guidance is based (see Concordance) were issued between 1981 and 2003.

Updated: 2016

Opinions on Related Matters:
1.1.6 Quality
2.1.3 Withholding Information from Patients

8.6 Promoting Patient Safety

In the context of health care, an error is an unintended act or omission or a flawed system or plan that harms or has the potential to harm a patient. Patients have a right to know their past and present medical status, including conditions that may have resulted from medical error. Open communication is fundamental to the trust that underlies the patient-physician relationship, and physicians have an obligation to deal honestly with patients at all times, in addition to their obligation to promote patient welfare and safety. Concern regarding legal liability should not affect the physician's honesty with the patient.

Even when new information regarding the medical error will not alter the patient's medical treatment or therapeutic options, individual physicians who have been involved in a (possible) medical error should:

(a) Disclose the occurrence of the error, explain the nature of the (potential) harm, and provide the information needed to enable the patient to make informed decisions about future medical care.

(b) Acknowledge the error and express professional and compassionate concern toward patients who have been harmed in the context of health care.

(c) Explain efforts that are being taken to prevent similar occurrences in the future.

(d) Provide for continuity of care to patients who have been harmed during the course of care, including facilitating transfer of care when a patient has lost trust in the physician.

Physicians who have discerned that another health care professional (may have) erred in caring for a patient should:

(e) Encourage the individual to disclose.

(f) Report impaired or incompetent colleagues, in keeping with ethics guidance.

As professionals uniquely positioned to have a comprehensive view of the care patients receive, physicians must strive to ensure patient safety and should play a central role in identifying, reducing, and preventing medical errors. Both as individuals and collectively as a profession, physicians should:

(g) Support a positive culture of patient safety, including compassion for peers who have been involved in a medical error.

(h) Enhance patient safety by studying the circumstances surrounding medical error. A legally protected review process is essential for reducing health care errors and preventing patient harm.

(i) Establish and participate fully in effective, confidential, protected mechanisms for reporting medical errors.

(j) Participate in developing means for objective review and analysis of medical errors.

(k) Ensure that investigation of root causes and analysis of error leads to measures to prevent future occurrences and that these measures are conveyed to relevant stakeholders.

8.7 Routine Universal Immunization of Physicians

As professionals committed to promoting the welfare of individual patients and the health of the public and to safeguarding their own and their colleagues' well-being, physicians have an ethical responsibility to take appropriate measures to prevent the spread of infectious disease in health care settings. Conscientious participation in routine infection control practices, such as hand washing and respiratory precautions, is a basic expectation of the profession. In some situations, however, routine infection control is not sufficient to protect the interests of patients, the public, and fellow health care workers.

In the context of a highly transmissible disease that poses significant medical risk for vulnerable patients or colleagues or threatens the availability of the health care workforce, particularly a disease that has potential to become epidemic or pandemic, and for which there is an available, safe, and effective vaccine, physicians should:

(a) Accept immunization absent a recognized medical, religious, or philosophic reason to not be immunized.

(b) Accept a decision of the medical staff leadership or health care institution, or other appropriate authority, to adjust practice activities if not immunized (eg, wear masks or refrain from direct patient care). It may be appropriate in some circumstances to inform patients about immunization status.

AMA Principles of Medical Ethics: I, II

Issued: 2011

Opinions on Related Matters:
8.3 Physicians' Responsibilities in Disaster Response and Preparedness
8.4 Ethical Use of Quarantine and Isolation
8.6 Promoting Patient Safety

8 Physicians and the Health of the Community

AMA Principles of Medical Ethics: I, V, VII

Issued: 1993

Updated: 1994, 2016

Opinions on Related Matters:
8.6   Promoting Patient Safety

8.8 Required Reporting of Adverse Events

Physicians' professional commitment to advance scientific knowledge and make relevant information available to patients, colleagues, and the public carries with it the responsibility to report suspected adverse events resulting from the use of a drug or medical device.

Mandated pre- and post-marketing studies provide basic safeguards for public health, but are inherently limited in their ability to detect rare or unexpected consequences of use of a drug or medical device. Thus, spontaneous reports of adverse events, especially rare or delayed effects or effects in vulnerable populations, are irreplaceable as a source of information about the safety of drugs and devices. As the professionals who prescribe and monitor the use of drugs and medical devices, physicians are best positioned to observe and communicate about adverse events.

Cases in which there is clearly a causal relationship between use of a drug or device and an adverse event, especially a serious event, will be rare. Physicians need not be certain that there is such an event, or even that there is a reasonable likelihood of a causal relationship, to suspect that an adverse event has occurred. A physician who suspects that an adverse reaction to a drug or medical device has occurred has an ethical responsibility to:

(a) Communicate that information to the professional community through established reporting mechanisms.

(b) Promptly report serious adverse events requiring hospitalization, death, or medical or surgical intervention to the appropriate regulatory agency.

AMA Principles of Medical Ethics: VII

Issued: 2008

Updated: 2016

Opinions on Related Matters:
1.1.1   Patient-Physician Relationships
2.1.1   Informed Consent

8.9 Expedited Partner Therapy

Expedited partner therapy seeks to increase the rate of treatment for partners of patients with sexually transmitted infections through patient-delivered therapy without the partner receiving a medical evaluation or professional prevention counseling.

Although expedited partner therapy has been demonstrated to be effective at reducing the burden of certain diseases, such as gonorrhea and chlamydia, it also has ethical implications. Expedited partner therapy potentially abrogates the standard informed consent process, compromises continuity of care for patients' partners, encroaches upon the privacy of patients and their partners, increases the possibility of harm by a medical or allergic reaction, leaves other diseases or complications undiagnosed, and may violate state practice laws.

Before initiating expedited partner therapy, physicians should:

(a) Determine the legal status of expedited partner therapy in the jurisdiction in which they practice.

(b) Seek guidance from public health officials.

(c) Engage in open discussions with patients to ascertain partners' ability to access medical services.

(d) Initiate expedited partner therapy only when the physician reasonably believes that a patient's partner(s) will be unwilling or unable to seek treatment within the context of a traditional patient-physician relationship.

When initiating expedited partner therapy, physicians should:

(e) Instruct patients regarding expedited partner therapy and the medications involved.

(f) Answer any questions the patient has.

(g) Provide to patients educational materials to share with their partners that:

(i) encourage the partner to consult a physician as a preferred alternative to expedited partner therapy;

(ii) disclose the risk of potential adverse drug reactions;

(iii) disclose the possibility of dangerous interactions between the medication delivered by the patient and other medications the partner may be taking;

(iv) disclose that the partner may be affected by other sexually transmitted diseases that may be left untreated by the medication delivered by the patient.

(h) Make reasonable efforts to refer the patient's partner(s) to appropriate health care professionals.

8.10 Preventing, Identifying, and Treating Violence and Abuse

AMA Principles of Medical Ethics: I, III
Issued: 2008
Updated: 2016
Opinions on Related Matters:
1.1.1 Patient-Physician Relationships

All patients may be at risk for interpersonal violence and abuse, which may adversely affect their health or ability to adhere to medical recommendations. In light of their obligation to promote the well-being of patients, physicians have an ethical obligation to take appropriate action to avert the harms caused by violence and abuse.

To protect patients' well-being, physicians individually should:

(a) Become familiar with:

(i) how to detect violence or abuse, including cultural variations in response to abuse;

(ii) community and health resources available to abused or vulnerable persons;

(iii) public health measures that are effective in preventing violence and abuse;

(iv) legal requirements for reporting violence or abuse.

(b) Consider abuse as a possible factor in the presentation of medical complaints.

(c) Routinely inquire about physical, sexual, and psychological abuse as part of the medical history.

(d) Not allow diagnosis or treatment to be influenced by misconceptions about abuse, including beliefs that abuse is rare, does not occur in "normal" families, is a private matter best resolved without outside interference, or is caused by victims' own actions.

(e) Treat the immediate symptoms and sequelae of violence and abuse and provide ongoing care for patients to address long-term consequences that may arise from being exposed to violence and abuse.

(f) Discuss any suspicion of abuse sensitively with the patient, whether or not reporting is legally mandated, and direct the patient to appropriate community resources.

(g) Report suspected violence and abuse in keeping with applicable requirements. Before doing so, physicians should:

(i) inform patients about requirements to report;

(ii) obtain the patient's informed consent when reporting is not required by law. Exceptions can be made if a physician reasonably believes that a patient's refusal to authorize reporting is coerced and therefore does not constitute a valid informed treatment decision.

(h) Protect patient privacy when reporting by disclosing only the minimum necessary information.

Collectively, physicians should:

(i) Advocate for comprehensive training in matters pertaining to violence and abuse across the continuum of professional education.

(j) Provide leadership in raising awareness about the need to assess and identify signs of abuse, including advocating for guidelines and policies to reduce the volume of unidentified cases and help ensure that all patients are appropriately assessed.

(k) Advocate for mechanisms to direct physicians to community or private resources that might be available to aid their patients.

(l) Support research in the prevention of violence and abuse, and collaborate with public health and community organizations to reduce violence and abuse.

(m) Advocate for change in mandatory reporting laws if evidence indicates that such reporting is not in the best interests of patients.

8.11 Health Promotion and Preventive Care

AMA Principles of Medical Ethics: V, VII

Issued: 2014

Opinions on Related Matters:
1.1.1 Patient-Physician Relationships
1.1.6 Quality

Medicine and public health share an ethical foundation stemming from the essential and direct role that health plays in human flourishing. While a physician's role tends to focus on diagnosing and treating illness once it occurs, physicians also have a professional commitment to prevent disease and promote health and well-being for their patients and the community.

The clinical encounter provides an opportunity for the physician to engage the patient in the process of health promotion. Effective elements of this process may include educating and motivating patients regarding healthy lifestyle, helping patients by assessing their needs, preferences, and readiness for change, and recommending appropriate preventive care measures. Implementing effective health promotion practices is consistent with physicians' duties to patients and also with their responsibilities as stewards of health care resources.

While primary care physicians are typically the patient's main source for health promotion and disease prevention, specialists can play an important role, particularly when the specialist has a close or long-standing relationship with the patient or when recommended action is particularly relevant for the condition that the specialist is treating. Additionally, while all physicians must balance a commitment to individual patients with the health of the public, physicians who work solely or primarily in a public health capacity should uphold accepted standards of medical professionalism by implementing policies that appropriately balance individual liberties with the social goals of public health policies.

Health promotion should be a collaborative, patient-centered process that promotes trust and recognizes patients' self-directed roles and responsibilities in maintaining health. In keeping with their professional commitment to the health of patients and the public, physicians should:

(a) Keep current with preventive care guidelines that apply to their patients and ensure that the interventions they recommend are well supported by the best available evidence.

(b) Educate patients about relevant modifiable risk factors.

(c) Recommend and encourage patients to have appropriate vaccinations and screenings.

(d) Encourage an open dialogue regarding circumstances that may make it difficult to manage chronic conditions or maintain a healthy lifestyle, such as transportation, work and home environments, and social support systems.

(e) Collaborate with the patient to develop recommendations that are most likely to be effective.

(f) When appropriate, delegate health promotion activities to other professionals or other resources available in the community who can help counsel and educate patients.

(g) Consider the health of the community when treating their own patients, and identify and notify public health authorities if and when they notice patterns in patient health that may indicate a health risk for others.

(h) Recognize that modeling health behaviors can help patients make changes in their own lives.

Collectively, physicians should:

(i) Promote training in health promotion and disease prevention during medical school residency and in continuing medical education.

(j) Advocate for healthier schools, workplaces, and communities.

(k) Create or promote healthier work and training environments for physicians.

(l) Advocate for community resources designed to promote health and provide access to preventive services.

(m) Support research to improve the evidence for disease prevention and health promotion.

9 Professional Self-regulation

These Opinions are offered as ethics guidance for physicians and are not intended to establish clinical practice guidelines or rules of law.

Medicine is founded in a "covenant of trust" between patient and physician. Patients must be able to trust that their physicians will acquire and maintain the knowledge, skills, and values that are central to the healing profession. In exchange for medicine's promise to be trustworthy, society grants the profession considerable authority to set the ethical and professional standards of practice and the privilege to self-regulate.[1,2]

As a self-regulating profession, medicine accepts responsibility for articulating and holding its members and members in training to core ethical values in their interactions with patients, the public, one another, and the organizations and institutions in which they practice.

The duty of self-regulation thus ranges widely over the many settings and relationships in which physicians engage professionally. As clinical practitioners, physicians promise to respect patients and patients' intimates and to avoid exploiting the power differential inherent in patient-physician relationships. They likewise commit themselves to lifelong learning in the service of their patients. As educators, physicians promise to instill the ethical precepts of the profession and to be fair and respectful in their conduct toward trainees. As custodians of professional values and conduct, they promise to identify lapses in their own behavior or that of colleagues and to address fairly and compassionately conduct that puts patients, the reputation of the profession, or public trust at risk.

Opinions in the first section of this chapter address the need to maintain ethical boundaries in relationships with patients and colleagues. Those in the second section provide guidance on salient issues in education and training across the professional life span.

Opinions in the third section offer guidance with respect to physicians whose ability to practice safely and ethically are compromised, while the fourth section addresses responsibilities for disciplining incompetent or unethical behavior, including questions of due process.

Guidance regarding physicians' relationships with health care organizations and institutions is offered in Opinions in the fifth section, and about physicians' interactions with manufacturers of health care products in the sixth section, along with issues of physician self-promotion.

Finally, Opinions in the seventh section articulate physicians' ethical responsibilities in relation to government agencies, especially with respect to activities in which physicians may be expected to serve the interests of the state in conflict with their primary commitment of fidelity to patients.

References

1. Wynia MK, Papadakis MA, Sullivan WM, Hafferty FW. More than a list of values and desired behaviors: a foundational understanding of medical professionalism. *Acad Med.* 2014;89(5):712-714.

2. Cruess SR, Cruess RL. The medical profession and self-regulation: a current challenge. *Virtual Mentor* 2005;7(4).

Sexual Boundaries

9.1.1 Romantic or Sexual Relationships with Patients

Romantic or sexual interactions between physicians and patients that occur concurrently with the patient-physician relationship are unethical. Such interactions detract from the goals of the patient-physician relationship and may exploit the vulnerability of the patient, compromise the physician's ability to make objective judgments about the patient's health care, and ultimately be detrimental to the patient's well-being.

A physician must terminate the patient-physician relationship before initiating a dating, romantic, or sexual relationship with a patient.

Likewise, sexual or romantic relationships between a physician and a former patient may be unduly influenced by the previous physician-patient relationship. Sexual or romantic relationships with former patients are unethical if the physician uses or exploits trust, knowledge, emotions, or influence derived from the previous professional relationship, or if a romantic relationship would otherwise foreseeably harm the individual.

In keeping with a physician's ethical obligations to avoid inappropriate behavior, a physician who has reason to believe that nonsexual, nonclinical contact with a patient may be perceived as or may lead to romantic or sexual contact should avoid such contact.

AMA Principles of Medical Ethics: I, II, IV

Issued: 1989

Updated: 1992, 2016

Opinions on Related Matters:
1.1.1 Patient-Physician Relationships
1.1.2 Prospective Patients
2.1.1 Informed Consent

9.1.2 Romantic or Sexual Relationships with Key Third Parties

Patients are often accompanied by third parties who play an integral role in the patient-physician relationship, including, but not limited to, spouses or partners, parents, guardians, or surrogates. Sexual or romantic interactions between physicians and third parties such as these may detract from the goals of the patient-physician relationship, exploit the vulnerability of the third party, compromise the physician's ability to make objective judgments about the patient's health care, and ultimately be detrimental to the patient's well-being.

Third parties may be deeply involved in the clinical encounter and in medical decision making. The physician interacts and communicates with these individuals and often is in a position to offer them information, advice, and emotional support. The more

AMA Principles of Medical Ethics: I, II

Issued: 1998

Updated: 2016

Opinions on Related Matters:
1.1.1 Patient-Physician Relationships
1.1.2 Prospective Patients
2.1.1 Informed Consent
2.1.2 Decisions for Adult Patients Who Lack Capacity

deeply involved the individual is in the clinical encounter and in medical decision making, the stronger the argument against sexual or romantic contact between the physician and a key third party. Physicians should avoid sexual or romantic relations with any individual whose decisions directly affect the health and welfare of the patient.

For these reasons, physicians should refrain from sexual or romantic interactions with key third parties when the interaction would exploit trust, knowledge, influence, or emotions derived from a professional relationship with the third party or could compromise the patient's care.

Before initiating a relationship with a key third party, physicians should take into account:

(a) The nature of the patient's medical problem and the likely effect of a relationship on patient care.
(b) The length of the professional relationship.
(c) The degree of the third party's emotional dependence on the physician.
(d) The importance of the clinical encounter to the third party and the patient.
(e) Whether the patient-physician relationship can be terminated in keeping with ethics guidance and what implications doing so would have for the patient.

AMA Principles of Medical Ethics: II, IV, VII

Issued: 1992

Updated: 1994, 2016

Opinions on Related Matters:
9.2.4 Disputes between Medical Supervisors and Trainees
9.4.2 Reporting Incompetent or Unethical Behavior by Colleagues
9.5.4 Civil Rights and Medical Professionals
9.5.5 Gender Discrimination in Medicine

9.1.3 Sexual Harassment in the Practice of Medicine

Sexual harassment can be defined as unwelcome sexual advances, requests for sexual favors, and other verbal or physical conduct of a sexual nature.

Sexual harassment in the practice of medicine is unethical. Sexual harassment exploits inequalities in status and power; abuses the rights and trust of those who are subjected to such conduct; interferes with an individual's work performance, and may influence or be perceived as influencing professional advancement in a manner unrelated to clinical or academic performance, harm professional working relationships, and create an intimidating or hostile work environment; and is likely to jeopardize patient care. Sexual relationships between medical supervisors and trainees are not acceptable, even if consensual. The supervisory role should be eliminated if the parties wish to pursue their relationship.

Physicians should promote and adhere to strict sexual harassment policies in medical workplaces. Physicians who participate in grievance committees should be broadly representative with respect to gender identity or sexual orientation, profession, and employment status; have the power to enforce harassment policies; and be accessible to the persons they are meant to serve.

Physician Education and Training

9.2.1 Medical Student Involvement in Patient Care

Having contact with patients is essential for training medical students, and both patients and the public benefit from the integrated care that is provided by health care teams that include medical students. However, the obligation to develop the next generation of physicians must be balanced against patients' freedom to choose from whom they receive treatment.

All physicians share an obligation to ensure that patients are aware that medical students may participate in their care and have the opportunity to decline care from students. Attending physicians may be best suited to fulfill this obligation. Before involving medical students in a patient's care, physicians should:

(a) Convey to the patient the benefits of having medical students participate in their care.

(b) Inform the patients about the identity and training status of individuals involved in care. Students, their supervisors, and all health care professionals should avoid confusing terms and properly identify themselves to patients.

(c) Inform the patient that trainees will participate before a procedure is undertaken when the patient will be temporarily incapacitated.

(d) Discuss student involvement in care with the patient's surrogate when the patient lacks decision-making capacity.

(e) Confirm that the patient is willing to permit medical students to participate in care.

AMA Principles of Medical Ethics: V, VII

Issued: 2001

Updated: 2016

Opinions on Related Matters:
1.1.1 Patient-Physician Relationships
2.1.1 Informed Consent

9 Professional
Self-regulation

AMA Principles of Medical Ethics: I, II, V, VIII

Issued: 2005

Updated: 2016

Opinions on Related Matters:
1.1.1   Patient-Physician Relationships
2.1.1   Informed Consent

9.2.2 Resident and Fellow Physicians' Involvement in Patient Care

Residents and fellows have dual roles as trainees and caregivers. Residents and fellows share responsibility with physicians involved in their training to facilitate educational and patient care goals.

Residents and fellows are physicians first and foremost and should always regard the interests of patients as paramount. When they are involved in patient care, residents and fellows should:

(a) Interact honestly with patients, including clearly identifying themselves as members of a team that is supervised by the attending physician and clarifying the role they will play in patient care. They should notify the attending physician if a patient refuses care from a resident or fellow.

(b) Participate fully in established mechanisms in their training programs and hospital systems for reporting and analyzing errors. They should cooperate with attending physicians in communicating errors to patients.

(c) Monitor their own health and level of alertness so that these factors do not compromise their ability to care for patients safely. Residents and fellows should recognize that providing patient care beyond time permitted by their programs (eg, "moonlighting" or other activities that interfere with adequate rest during off hours) might be harmful to themselves and patients.

Physicians involved in training residents and fellows should:

(d) Take steps to help ensure that training programs are structured to be conducive to the learning process as well as to promoting the patient's welfare and dignity.

(e) Address patient refusal of care from a resident or fellow. If, after discussion, a patient does not want to participate in training, the physician may exclude residents or fellows from the patient's care. If appropriate, the physician may transfer the patient's care to another physician or nonteaching service or another health care facility.

(f) Provide residents and fellows with appropriate faculty supervision and availability of faculty consultants, and with graduated responsibility relative to level of training and expertise.

(g) Observe pertinent regulations and seek consultation with appropriate institutional resources, such as an ethics committee, to resolve educational or patient care conflicts that arise in the course of training. All parties involved in such conflicts must continue to regard patient welfare as the first priority. Conflict resolution should not be punitive, but should aim at assisting residents and fellows to complete their training successfully.

9.2.3 Performing Procedures on the Newly Deceased

Medical training sometimes involves practicing procedures on newly deceased patients, in particular, critical medical skills for which adequate educational alternatives are not available. Such training must balance protecting the interests of newly deceased patients, their families, society, and the profession with the need to educate health care providers.

Physicians should work to develop clear institutional policies for performing procedures on newly deceased patients for training purposes. Before medical trainees practice any procedure on a newly deceased patient, the supervising physician has an ethical responsibility to ensure that:

(a) The interests of all parties are respected and the risks and benefits of permitting the procedure have been carefully considered, including:
  (i) the rights of deceased patients and their families;
  (ii) benefits to trainees and society;
  (iii) risks to trainees, staff, the institution, and the profession.
(b) The procedure is carried out:
  (i) as part of an appropriately structured training sequence;
  (ii) in a manner and an environment that is respectful of the values of all involved parties.
(c) Permitting trainees to perform the procedure is in keeping with the previously expressed preferences of the deceased individual regarding handling of the body or procedures performed after death.
(d) Permission for a trainee to perform the procedure is obtained from the decedent's family if the individual's preferences are not known. Procedures should never be performed for training purposes if the decedent's wishes are not known and permission is not available from an appropriate surrogate.
(e) The procedure is entered in the medical record.

AMA Principles of Medical Ethics: I, V

Issued: 2001

Updated: 2016

Opinions on Related Matters:
2.1.1 Informed Consent
2.3.4 Informing Families of a Patient's Death
3.2.1 Confidentiality

9 Professional
Self-regulation

AMA Principles of Medical Ethics: II, III, VII

Issued: 1994

Updated: 2016

Opinions on Related Matters:
9.4.1 Peer Review and Due Process
9.5.4 Civil Rights and Medical Professionals
9.5.5 Gender Discrimination in Medicine

9.2.4 Disputes between Medical Supervisors and Trainees

The relationship between medical students, resident physicians or fellows, and their supervisors is a major determinant of the quality of medical education. When conflicts arise, it is essential to ensure that disputes are resolved fairly.

Retaliatory or punitive actions against those who raise complaints are unethical and are a legitimate cause for filing a grievance with the appropriate institutional committee.

Physicians who are involved in training or supervising medical students, residents, and fellows should ensure that institutional policies and procedures are in place to:

(a) Protect complainants' confidentiality whenever possible, so long as protecting confidentiality does not hinder the subject's ability to respond to the complaint.

(b) Carefully monitor employment and evaluation files to prevent possible tampering.

(c) Permit resident physicians and fellows to access their employment files and copy the contents, within the provisions of applicable law.

(d) Support medical students, residents, and fellows in fulfilling their responsibility to:

   (i) withdraw from care ordered by a supervisor when the trainee believes the order reflects serious errors in clinical or ethical judgment, or physician impairment, that could pose a risk of imminent harm to the patient or others, provided withdrawing does not itself threaten the patient's immediate welfare;

   (ii) communicate concerns to the physician issuing the orders and, if necessary, to the persons or institutional programs responsible for mediating such disputes, which may involve third parties.

AMA Principles of Medical Ethics: IV, V

Issued: 2000

Updated: 2016

Opinions on Related Matters:
2.1.1 Informed Consent
3.2.1 Confidentiality
10.3 Peers as Patients

9.2.5 Medical Students Practicing Clinical Skills on Fellow Students

Medical students often learn basic clinical skills by practicing on classmates, patients, or trained instructors. Unlike patients in the clinical setting, students who volunteer to act as "patients" are not seeking to benefit medically from the procedures being performed on them. Their goal is to benefit from educational instruction, yet their right to make decisions about their own bodies remains.

To protect medical students' privacy, autonomy, and sense of propriety in the context of practicing clinical skills on fellow students, instructors should:

(a) Explain to students how the clinical skills will be performed, making certain that students are not placed in situations that violate their privacy or sense of propriety.

(b) Discuss the confidentiality, consequences, and appropriate management of a diagnostic finding.

(c) Ask students to specifically consent to clinical skills being performed by fellow students. The stringency of standards for ensuring explicit, noncoerced informed consent increases as the invasiveness and intimacy of the procedure increase.

(d) Allow students the choice of whether to participate prior to entering the classroom.

(e) Never require that students provide a reason for their unwillingness to participate.

(f) Never penalize students for refusing to participate. Instructors must refrain from evaluating students' overall performance based on their willingness to volunteer as "patients."

9.2.6 Continuing Medical Education

Physicians should strive to further their medical education throughout their careers, to ensure that they serve patients to the best of their abilities and live up to professional standards of excellence.

Participating in certified continuing medical education (CME) activities is critical to fulfilling this professional commitment to lifelong learning. As attendees of CME activities, physicians should:

(a) Select activities that are of high quality and are appropriate for the physician's educational needs.

(b) Choose activities that are carried out in keeping with ethics guidance and applicable professional standards.

(c) Claim only the credit commensurate with the extent of participation in the CME activity.

(d) Decline any subsidy offered by a commercial entity other than the physician's employer to compensate the physician for time spent or expenses of participating in a CME activity.

AMA Principles of Medical Ethics: I, V

Issued: 1993

Updated: 2013

Opinions on Related Matters:
9.2.7 Financial Relationships with Industry in Continuing Medical Education
11.2.2 Conflicts of Interest in Patient Care

9 Professional
Self-regulation

AMA Principles of Medical Ethics: I, V

Issued: 2011

9.2.7 Financial Relationships with Industry in Continuing Medical Education

In an environment of rapidly changing information and emerging technology, physicians must maintain the knowledge, skills, and values central to a healing profession. They must protect the independence and commitment to fidelity and service that define the medical profession.

Financial or in-kind support from pharmaceutical, biotechnology, or medical device companies that have a direct interest in physicians' recommendations creates conditions in which external interests could influence the availability or content of continuing medical education (CME). Financial relationships between such sources and individual physicians who organize CME, teach in CME, or have other roles in continuing professional education can carry similar potential to influence CME in undesired ways.

CME that is independent of funding or in-kind support from sources that have financial interests in physicians' recommendations promotes confidence in the independence and integrity of professional education, as does CME in which organizers, teachers, and others involved in educating physicians do not have financial relationships with industry that could influence their participation. When possible, CME should be provided without such support or the participation of individuals who have financial interests in the educational subject matter.

In some circumstances, support from industry or participation by individuals who have financial interests in the subject matter may be needed to enable access to appropriate, high-quality CME. In these circumstances, physician-learners should be confident that vigorous efforts will be made to maintain the independence and integrity of educational activities.

Individually and collectively physicians must ensure that the profession independently defines the goals of physician education, determines educational needs, and sets its own priorities for CME. Physicians who attend CME activities should expect that, in addition to complying with all applicable professional standards for accreditation and certification, their colleagues who organize, teach, or have other roles in CME will:

(a) Be transparent about financial relationships that could potentially influence educational activities.

(b) Provide the information physician-learners need to make critical judgments about an educational activity, including:

    (i)   the source(s) and nature of commercial support for the activity;

(ii) the source(s) and nature of any individual financial relationships with industry related to the subject matter of the activity;

(iii) what steps have been taken to mitigate the potential influence of financial relationships.

(c) Protect the independence of educational activities by:

(i) ensuring independent, prospective assessment of educational needs and priorities;

(ii) adhering to a transparent process for prospectively determining when industry support is needed;

(iii) giving preference in selecting faculty or content developers to similarly qualified experts who do not have financial interests in the educational subject matter;

(iv) ensuring a transparent process for making decisions about participation by physicians who may have a financial interest in the educational subject matter;

(v) permitting individuals who have a substantial financial interest in the educational subject matter to participate in CME only when their participation is central to the success of the educational activity; the activity meets a demonstrated need in the professional community; and the source, nature, and magnitude of the individual's specific financial interest is disclosed;

(vi) taking steps to mitigate potential influence commensurate with the nature of the financial interest(s) at issue, such as prospective peer review.

Physician Wellness

9.3.1 Physician Health and Wellness

When physician health or wellness is compromised, so may be the safety and effectiveness of the medical care provided. To preserve the quality of their performance, physicians have a responsibility to maintain their health and wellness, broadly construed as preventing or treating acute or chronic diseases, including mental illness, disabilities, and occupational stress.

To fulfill this responsibility individually, physicians should:

(a) Maintain their health and wellness by:

(i) following healthy lifestyle habits;

(ii) ensuring that they have a personal physician whose objectivity is not compromised.

AMA Principles of Medical Ethics: I, II, IV

Issued: The constituent Opinions on which this guidance is based (see Concordance) were issued in 1986 and 2004.

Updated: 2016

Opinions on Related Matters:
9.3.2 Physician Responsibilities to Impaired Colleagues

(b) Take appropriate action when their health or wellness is compromised, including:

   (i) engaging in honest assessment of their ability to continue practicing safely;

   (ii) taking measures to mitigate the problem;

   (iii) taking appropriate measures to protect patients, including measures to minimize the risk of transmitting infectious disease commensurate with the seriousness of the disease;

   (iv) seeking appropriate help as needed, including help in addressing substance abuse. Physicians should not practice if their ability to do so safely is impaired by use of a controlled substance, alcohol, or other chemical agent or by a health condition.

Collectively, physicians have an obligation to ensure that colleagues are able to provide safe and effective care, which includes promoting health and wellness among physicians.

AMA Principles of Medical Ethics: II

Issued: The constituent Opinions on which this guidance is based (see Concordance) were issued in 1992 and 2004.

Updated: 2016

Opinions on Related Matters:
9.3.1 Physician Health and Wellness

9.3.2 Physician Responsibilities to Impaired Colleagues

Physical or mental health conditions that interfere with a physician's ability to engage safely in professional activities can put patients at risk, compromise professional relationships, and undermine trust in medicine. While protecting patients' well-being must always be the primary consideration, physicians who are impaired are deserving of thoughtful, compassionate care.

To protect patient interests and ensure that their colleagues receive appropriate care and assistance, individually physicians have an ethical obligation to:

(a) Intervene in a timely manner to ensure that impaired colleagues cease practicing and receive appropriate assistance from a physician health program.

(b) Report impaired colleagues in keeping with ethics guidance and applicable law.

(c) Assist recovered colleagues when they resume patient care.

Collectively, physicians have an obligation to ensure that their colleagues are able to provide safe and effective care. This obligation is discharged by:

(d) Promoting health and wellness among physicians.

(e) Establishing mechanisms to assure that impaired physicians promptly cease practice.

(f) Supporting peers in identifying physicians in need of help.

(g) Establishing or supporting physician health programs that provide a supportive environment to maintain and restore health and wellness.

Peer Review and Disciplinary Action

9.4.1 Peer Review and Due Process

Physicians have mutual obligations to hold one another to the ethical standards of their profession. Peer review, by the ethics committees of medical societies, hospital credentials and utilization committees, or other bodies, has long been established by organized medicine to scrutinize professional conduct. Peer review is recognized and accepted as a means of promoting professionalism and maintaining trust. The peer review process is intended to balance physicians' right to exercise medical judgment freely with the obligation to do so wisely and temperately.

Fairness is essential in all disciplinary or other hearings where the reputation, professional status, or livelihood of the physician or medical student may be adversely affected.

Individually, physicians and medical students who are involved in reviewing the conduct of fellow professionals, medical students, residents, or fellows should:

(a) Always adhere to principles of a fair and objective hearing, including:
(i) a listing of specific charges;
(ii) adequate notice of the right of a hearing;
(iii) the opportunity to be present and to rebut the evidence;
(iv) the opportunity to present a defense.

(b) Ensure that the reviewing body includes a significant number of persons at a similar level of training.

(c) Disclose relevant conflicts of interest and, when appropriate, recuse themselves from a hearing.

Collectively, through the medical societies and institutions with which they are affiliated, physicians should ensure that such bodies provide procedural safeguards for due process in their constitutions and bylaws or policies.

AMA Principles of Medical Ethics: II, III, VII

Issued: The constituent Opinions on which this guidance is based (see Concordance) were issued prior to 1977.

Updated: 1994, 2016

Opinions on Related Matters:
9.4.2 Reporting Incompetent or Unethical Behavior by Colleagues
9.4.3 Discipline and Medicine

AMA Principles of Medical Ethics: II

Issued: The constituent Opinions on which this guidance is based (see Concordance) were issued between 1977 and 1992.

Updated: 2016

Opinions on Related Matters:
9.4.1   Peer Review and Due Process
9.4.3   Discipline and Medicine

9.4.2 Reporting Incompetent or Unethical Behavior by Colleagues

Medicine has a long tradition of self-regulation, based on physicians' enduring commitment to safeguard the welfare of patients and the trust of the public. The obligation to report incompetent or unethical conduct that may put patients at risk is recognized in both the ethical standards of the profession and in law, and physicians should be able to report such conduct without fear or loss of favor.

Reporting a colleague who is incompetent or who engages in unethical behavior is intended not only to protect patients, but also to help ensure that colleagues receive appropriate assistance from a physician health program or other service to be able to practice safely and ethically. Physicians must not submit false or malicious reports.

Physicians who become aware of or strongly suspect that conduct threatens patient welfare or otherwise appears to violate ethical or legal standards should:

    (a) Report the conduct to appropriate clinical authorities in the first instance so that the possible impact on patient welfare can be assessed and remedial action taken. This should include notifying the peer review body of the hospital, or the local or state medical society when the physician of concern does not have hospital privileges.

    (b) Report directly to the state licensing board when the conduct in question poses an immediate threat to the health and safety of patients or violates state licensing provisions.

    (c) Report to a higher authority if the conduct continues unchanged despite initial reporting.

    (d) Protect the privacy of any patients who may be involved to the greatest extent possible, consistent with due process.

    (e) Report the suspected violation to appropriate authorities.

Physicians who receive reports of alleged incompetent or unethical conduct should:

    (f) Evaluate the reported information critically and objectively.

    (g) Hold the matter in confidence until it is resolved.

    (h) Ensure that identified deficiencies are remedied or reported to other appropriate authorities for action.

    (i) Notify the reporting physician when appropriate action has been taken, except in cases of anonymous reporting.

9.4.3 Discipline and Medicine

Incompetence, corruption, dishonesty, or unethical conduct on the part of members of the medical profession is reprehensible. In addition to posing a real or potential threat to patients, such conduct undermines the public's confidence in the profession. The obligation to address misconduct falls on both individual physicians and the profession as a whole.

The goal of disciplinary review is both to protect patients and to help ensure that colleagues receive appropriate assistance from a physician health program or other service to enable them to practice safely and ethically. Disciplinary review must not be undertaken falsely or maliciously.

Individually, physicians should report colleagues whose behavior is incompetent or unethical, in keeping with ethics guidance.

Collectively, medical societies have a civic and professional obligation to:

(a) Report to the appropriate governmental body or state board of medical examiners credible evidence that may come to their attention involving the alleged criminal conduct of any physician relating to the practice of medicine.

(b) Initiate disciplinary action whenever a physician is alleged to have engaged in misconduct whenever there is credible evidence tending to establish unethical conduct, regardless of the outcome of any civil or criminal proceedings relating to the alleged misconduct.

(c) Impose a penalty, up to and including expulsion from membership, on a physician who violates ethical standards.

AMA Principles of Medical Ethics: II, III, VII
Issued: Prior to 1977
Updated: 1994, 2016
Opinions on Related Matters:
9.4.1 Peer Review and Due Process
9.4.2 Reporting Incompetent or Unethical Behavior by Colleagues

9.4.4 Physicians with Disruptive Behavior

The importance of respect among all health professionals as a means of ensuring good patient care is foundational to ethics. Physicians have a responsibility to address situations in which individual physicians behave disruptively, ie, speak or act in ways that may negatively affect patient care, including conduct that interferes with the individual's ability to work with other members of the health care team, or that of others to work with the physician.

Disruptive behavior is different from criticism offered in good faith with the aim of improving patient care and from collective action on the part of physicians. Physicians must not submit false or malicious reports of disruptive behavior.

Physicians who have leadership roles in a health care institution must be sensitive to the unintended effects institutional structures,

AMA Principles of Medical Ethics: I, II, VIII
Issued: 2000
Updated: 2016
Opinions on Related Matters:
9.3.2 Physician Responsibilities to Impaired Colleagues
9.5.4 Civil Rights and Medical Professionals
11.2.1 Professionalism in Health Care Systems

9 Professional Self-regulation

policies, and practices may have on patient care and professional staff.

As members of the medical staff, physicians should develop and adopt policies or bylaw provisions that:

(a) Establish a body authorized to receive, review, and act on reports of disruptive behavior, such as a medical staff wellness committee. Members must be required to disclose relevant conflicts of interest and to recuse themselves from a hearing when they have a conflict.

(b) Establish procedural safeguards that protect due process.

(c) Clearly state principal objectives in terms that ensure high standards of patient care, and promote a professional practice and work environment.

(d) Clearly describe the behaviors or types of behavior that will prompt intervention.

(e) Provide a channel for reporting and appropriately recording instances of disruptive behavior. A single incident may not warrant action, but individual reports may help identify a pattern that requires intervention.

(f) Establish a process to review or verify reports of disruptive behavior.

(g) Establish a process to notify a physician that his or her behavior has been reported as disruptive, and provide opportunity for the physician to respond to the report.

(h) Provide for monitoring and assessing whether a physician's disruptive conduct improves after intervention.

(i) Provide for evaluative and corrective actions that are commensurate with the behavior, such as self-correction and structured rehabilitation. Suspending the individual's responsibilities or privileges should be a mechanism of final resort.

(j) Identify who will be involved in the various stages of the process, from reviewing reports to notifying physicians and monitoring conduct after intervention.

(k) Provide clear guidance for protecting confidentiality.

(l) Ensure that individuals who report instances of disruptive behavior are appropriately protected.

Physician Involvement in Health Care Institutions

9.5.1 Organized Medical Staff

The organized medical staff performs essential hospital functions even though it may often consist primarily of independent practicing physicians who are not hospital employees. The core responsibilities of the organized medical staff are the promotion of patient safety and the quality of care.

Members of the organized medical staff may choose to act as a group for the purpose of communicating and dealing with the governing board and others with respect to matters that concern the interest of the organized medical staff and its members. This is ethical so long as there is no adverse effect on patient safety and the quality of care.

AMA Principles of Medical Ethics: IV, VI

Issued: 1983

Updated: 1994, 2004, 2016

Opinions on Related Matters:
9.5.2 Staff Privileges
9.5.3 Accreditation
9.5.4 Civil Rights and Medical Professionals
9.5.5 Gender Discrimination in Medicine

9.5.2 Staff Privileges

The purpose of medical staff privileging is to improve the quality and efficiency of patient care in the hospital.

Physicians who are involved in granting, denying, or terminating hospital privileges have an ethical responsibility to be guided by concern for the welfare and best interests of patients. They should:

(a) Base privilege decisions on:
   (i) the candidate's training, experience, and demonstrated competence;
   (ii) the availability of facilities;
   (iii) the overall medical needs of the community, the hospital, and especially patients.

(b) Avoid basing privilege decisions on:
   (i) numbers of patients the candidate has admitted to the facility;
   (ii) economic or insurance status of patients admitted by the candidate;
   (iii) personal friendships, antagonisms, jurisdictional disputes, or fear of competition.

AMA Principles of Medical Ethics: IV, VI, VII

Issued: 1983

Updated: 1994, 2016

Opinions on Related Matters:
9.5.1 Organized Medical Staff
9.5.3 Accreditation
9.5.4 Civil Rights and Medical Professionals
9.5.5 Gender Discrimination in Medicine
11.2.1 Professionalism in Health Care Systems

AMA Principles of Medical Ethics: II, IV, VII

Issued: 1982

Updated: 2016

Opinions on Related Matters:
11.2.1 Professionalism in Health Care Systems
11.2.2 Conflicts of Interest in Patient Care

9.5.3 Accreditation

Physicians who engage in activities that involve the accreditation, approval, or certification of institutions, facilities, and programs that provide patient care or medical education or certify the attainment of specialized professional competence have the ethical responsibility to develop and apply standards that are:

(a) Relevant, fair, reasonable, and nondiscriminatory.
(b) Focused on the quality of patient care achieved.

They must avoid adopting or using standards as a means of minimizing competition solely for economic gain.

AMA Principles of Medical Ethics: IV

Issued: Prior to 1977

Updated: 1994, 2008, 2016

Opinions on Related Matters:
9.4.1 Peer Review and Due Process
9.5.5 Gender Discrimination in Medicine

9.5.4 Civil Rights and Medical Professionals

Opportunities in medical society activities or membership, medical education and training, employment and remuneration, academic medicine, and all other aspects of professional endeavors must not be denied to any physician or medical trainee because of race, color, religion, creed, ethnic affiliation, national origin, gender or gender identity, sexual orientation, age, family status, or disability or for any other reason unrelated to character, competence, ethics, professional status, or professional activities.

AMA Principles of Medical Ethics: II, VII

Issued: 1994

Updated: 2016

Opinions on Related Matters:
9.5.1 Organized Medical Staff
9.5.2 Staff Privileges
9.5.4 Civil Rights and Medical Professionals

9.5.5 Gender Discrimination in Medicine

Inequality of professional status in medicine among individuals based on gender can compromise patient care, undermine trust, and damage the working environment. Physician leaders in medical schools and medical institutions should advocate for increased leadership in medicine among individuals of underrepresented genders and equitable compensation for all physicians.

Collectively, physicians should actively advocate for and develop family-friendly policies that:

(a) Promote fairness in the workplace, including providing for:
  (i) retraining or other programs that facilitate re-entry by physicians who take time away from their careers to have a family;
  (ii) on-site child care services for dependent children;
  (iii) job security for physicians who are temporarily not in practice due to pregnancy or family obligations.
(b) Promote fairness in academic medical settings by:

(i) ensuring that tenure decisions make allowance for family obligations by giving faculty members longer to achieve standards for promotion and tenure;

(ii) establishing more reasonable guidelines regarding the quantity and timing of published material needed for promotion or tenure that emphasize quality over quantity and encourage the pursuit of careers based on individual talent rather than tenure standards that undervalue teaching ability and overvalue research;

(iii) fairly distributing teaching, clinical, research, and administrative responsibilities, and access to tenure tracks;

(iv) structuring the mentoring process through a fair and visible system.

(c) Take steps to mitigate gender bias in research and publication.

Physician Promotion and Marketing Practices

9.6.1 Advertising and Publicity

There are no restrictions on advertising by physicians except those that can be specifically justified to protect the public from deceptive practices. A physician may publicize himself or herself as a physician through any commercial publicity or other form of public communication (including any newspaper, magazine, telephone directory, radio, television, direct mail, or other advertising) provided that the communication shall not be misleading because of the omission of necessary material information, shall not contain any false or misleading statement, and shall not otherwise operate to deceive.

Because the public can sometimes be deceived by the use of medical terms or illustrations that are difficult to understand, physicians should design the form of communication to communicate the information contained therein to the public in a readily comprehensible manner. Aggressive, high-pressure advertising and publicity should be avoided if they create unjustified medical expectations or are accompanied by deceptive claims. The key issue, however, is whether advertising or publicity, regardless of format or content, is true and not materially misleading.

The communication may include (1) the educational background of the physician, (2) the basis on which fees are determined (including charges for specific services), (3) available credit or other methods of payment, and (4) any other nondeceptive information.

AMA Principles of Medical Ethics: II

Issued: Issued in 1996 in response to federal regulatory action.

Nothing in this opinion is intended to discourage or to limit advertising and representations that are not false or deceptive within the meaning of Section 5 of the Federal Trade Commission Act. At the same time, however, physicians are advised that certain types of communications have a significant potential for deception and should therefore receive special attention. For example, testimonials of patients as to the physician's skill or the quality of the physician's professional services tend to be deceptive when they do not reflect the results that patients with conditions comparable to the testimoniant's condition generally receive.

Objective claims regarding experience, competence, and the quality of physicians and the services they provide may be made only if they are factually supportable. Similarly, generalized statements of satisfaction with a physician's services may be made if they are representative of the experiences of that physician's patients.

Because physicians have an ethical obligation to share medical advances, it is unlikely that a physician will have a truly exclusive or unique skill or remedy. Claims that imply such a skill or remedy therefore can be deceptive. Statements that a physician has an exclusive or unique skill or remedy in a particular geographic area, if true, however, are permissible. Similarly, a statement that a physician has cured or successfully treated a large number of cases involving a particular serious ailment is deceptive if it implies a certainty of result and creates unjustified and misleading expectations in prospective patients.

Consistent with federal regulatory standards that apply to commercial advertising, a physician who is considering the placement of an advertisement or publicity release, whether in print, radio, or television, should determine in advance that the communication or message is explicitly and implicitly truthful and not misleading. These standards require the advertiser to have a reasonable basis for claims before they are used in advertising. The reasonable basis must be established by those facts known to the advertiser, and those that a reasonable, prudent advertiser should have discovered. Inclusion of the physician's name in advertising may help to assure that these guidelines are being met.

9.6.2 Gifts to Physicians from Industry

Relationships among physicians and professional medical organizations and pharmaceutical, biotechnology, and medical device companies help drive innovation in patient care and contribute to the economic well-being of the community to the ultimate benefit of patients and the public. However, an increasingly urgent challenge for both medicine and industry is to devise ways to preserve strong, productive collaborations at the same time that they take clear, effective action to prevent relationships that damage public trust and tarnish the reputation of both parties.

Gifts to physicians from industry create conditions that carry the risk of subtly biasing—or being perceived to bias—professional judgment in the care of patients.

To preserve the trust that is fundamental to the patient-physician relationship and public confidence in the profession, physicians should:

(a) Decline cash gifts in any amount from an entity that has a direct interest in physicians' treatment recommendations.

(b) Decline any gifts for which reciprocity is expected or implied.

(c) Accept an in-kind gift for the physician's practice only when the gift:
    (i) will directly benefit patients, including patient education;
    (ii) is of minimal value.

(d) Academic institutions and residency and fellowship programs may accept special funding on behalf of trainees to support medical students', residents', and fellows' participation in professional meetings, including educational meetings, provided that:
    (i) the program identifies recipients based on independent institutional criteria;
    (ii) funds are distributed to recipients without specific attribution to sponsors.

AMA Principles of Medical Ethics: II

Issued: 1993

Updated: 2014

Opinions on Related Matters:
1.1.1 Patient-Physician Relationships
1.2.8 Gifts from Patients
7.1.4 Conflicts of Interest in Research
9.2.6 Continuing Medical Education
9.2.7 Financial Relationships with Industry in Continuing Medical Education
11.2.2 Conflicts of Interest in Patient Care

9 Professional Self-regulation

AMA Principles of Medical Ethics: I, II, VIII

Issued: 2004

Updated: 2016

Opinions on Related Matters:
11.2.2 Conflicts of Interest in Patient Care

9.6.3 Incentives to Patients for Referrals

Endorsement by current patients can be a strong incentive to direct new patients to a medical practice, and physicians often rely on word of mouth as a source of referrals. However, to be ethically appropriate, word-of-mouth referrals must be voluntary on the part of current patients and should reflect honestly on the practice.

Physicians must not offer financial incentives or other valuable incentives to current patients in exchange for recruitment of other patients. Such incentives can distort the information patients provide and skew the expectations of prospective patients, thus compromising the trust that is the foundation of patient-physician relationships.

AMA Principles of Medical Ethics: II

Issued: 1999

Updated: 2016

Opinions on Related Matters:
9.6.5 Sale of Non-Health-Related Goods
11.2.2 Conflicts of Interest in Patient Care

9.6.4 Sale of Health-Related Products

The sale of health-related products by physicians can offer convenience for patients, but can also pose ethical challenges. "Health-related products" are any products other than prescription items that, according to the manufacturer or distributor, benefit health. "Selling" refers to dispensing items from the physician's office or website in exchange for money or endorsing a product that the patient may order or purchase elsewhere that results in remuneration for the physician.

Physician sale of health-related products raises ethical concerns about financial conflict of interest, risks placing undue pressure on the patient, and threatens to erode patient trust, undermine the primary obligation of physicians to serve the interests of their patients before their own, and demean the profession of medicine.

Physicians who choose to sell health-related products from their offices or through their office website or other online venues have ethical obligations to:

(a) Offer only products whose claims of benefit are based on peer-reviewed literature or other sources of scientific review of efficacy that are unbiased, sound, systematic, and reliable. Physicians should not offer products whose claims of benefit lack scientific validity.

(b) Address conflict of interest and possible exploitation of patients by:

    (i) fully disclosing the nature of their financial interest in the sale of the product(s), either in person or through written notification, and informing patients of the availability of the product or other equivalent products elsewhere;

(ii) limiting sales to products that serve immediate and pressing needs of their patients (eg, to avoid requiring a patient on crutches to travel to a local pharmacy to purchase the product). Distributing products free of charge or at cost makes products readily available and helps to eliminate the elements of personal gain and financial conflict of interest that may interfere or appear to interfere with the physician's independent medical judgment.

(c) Provide information about the risks, benefits, and limits of scientific knowledge regarding the products in language that is understandable to patients.

(d) Avoid exclusive distributorship arrangements that make the products available only through physician offices. Physicians should encourage manufacturers to make products widely accessible to patients.

9.6.5 Sale of Non-Health-Related Goods

Unlike the sale of health-related products, sale of non-health-related products by physicians through their offices or websites, even at cost, does not offer health benefits to patients. The sale of non-health-related goods by physicians presents a conflict of interest and threatens to erode the primary obligation of physicians to serve the interests of their patients before their own. Furthermore, this activity risks placing undue pressure on the patient and demeaning the practice of medicine.

However, such sales can be acceptable under the following limited conditions:

(a) The goods in question are low-cost.
(b) The physician takes no share in profit from their sale.
(c) The sale is:
  (i) for the benefit of community organizations;
  (ii) conducted in a dignified manner;
  (iii) conducted in such a way as to assure that patients are not pressured into making purchases;
  (iv) not a regular part of the physician's business.

AMA Principles of Medical Ethics: I, II

Issued: 1998

Updated: 2016

Opinions on Related Matters:
9.6.4 Sale of Health-Related Products
11.2.2 Conflicts of Interest in Patient Care

9 Professional Self-regulation

AMA Principles of Medical Ethics: II, III, IV, V

Issued: 2002

Updated: 2016

Opinions on Related Matters:
1.1.1 Patient-Physician Relationships
2.1.1 Informed Consent
11.2.2 Conflicts of Interest in Patient Care

9.6.6 Prescribing and Dispensing Drugs and Devices

In keeping with physicians' ethical responsibility to hold the patient's interests as paramount, in their role as prescribers and dispensers of drugs and devices, physicians should:

(a) Prescribe drugs, devices, and other treatments based solely on medical considerations, patient need, and reasonable expectations of effectiveness for the particular patient.

(b) Dispense drugs in their office practices only if such dispensing primarily benefits the patient.

(c) Avoid direct or indirect influence of financial interests on prescribing decisions by:

　(i) declining any kind of payment or compensation from a drug company or device manufacturer for prescribing its products, including offers of indemnification;

　(ii) respecting the patient's freedom to choose where to fill prescriptions. In general, physicians should not refer patients to a pharmacy the physician owns or operates.

AMA Principles of Medical Ethics: II, III

Issued: 1999

Updated: 2016

Opinions on Related Matters:
1.1.1 Patient-Physician Relationships
2.1.1 Informed Consent
9.6.8 Direct-to-Consumer Diagnostic Imaging Tests
11.2.2 Conflicts of Interest in Patient Care

9.6.7 Direct-to-Consumer Advertisement of Prescription Drugs

Direct-to-consumer advertising may raise awareness about diseases and treatment and may help inform patients about the availability of new diagnostic tests, drugs, treatments, and devices. However, direct-to-consumer advertising also carries the risk of creating unrealistic expectations for patients and conflicts of interest for physicians, adversely affecting patients' health and safety, and compromising patient-physician relationships.

In the context of direct-to-consumer advertising of prescription drugs, physicians individually should:

(a) Remain objective about advertised tests, drugs, treatments, and devices, avoiding bias for or against advertised products.

(b) Engage in dialogue with patients who request tests, drugs, treatments, or devices they have seen advertised to:

　(i) assess and enhance the patient's understanding of the test, drug, or device;

　(ii) educate patients about why an advertised test, drug, or device may not be suitable for them, including providing cost-effectiveness information about different options.

(c) Resist commercially induced pressure to prescribe tests, drugs, or devices that may not be indicated.

(d) Obtain informed consent before prescribing an advertised test, drug, or device, in keeping with professional standards.

(e) Deny requests for an inappropriate test, drug, or device.

(f) Consider reporting to the sponsoring manufacturer or appropriate authorities direct-to-consumer advertising that:

　(i)　promotes false expectations;

　(ii)　does not enhance consumer education;

　(iii)　conveys unclear, inaccurate, or misleading health education messages;

　(iv)　fails to refer patients to their physicians for additional information;

　(v)　does not identify the target population at risk;

　(vi)　encourages consumer self-diagnosis and treatment.

Collectively, physicians should:

(g) Encourage and engage in studies that examine the impact of direct-to-consumer advertising on patient health and medical care.

(h) Whenever possible, assist authorities to enforce existing law by reporting advertisements that do not:

　(i)　provide a fair and balanced discussion of the use of the drug product for the disease, disorder, or condition;

　(ii)　clearly explain warnings, precautions, and potential adverse reactions associated with the drug product;

　(iii)　present summary information in language that can be understood by the consumer;

　(iv)　comply with applicable regulations;

　(v)　provide collateral materials to educate both physicians and consumers.

9.6.8 Direct-to-Consumer Diagnostic Imaging Tests

Diagnostic imaging tests are sometimes marketed directly to consumers before they have been scientifically validated. This can help consumers prevent disease and promote health, but may also expose patients to risk without benefit, create conflicts of interests for physicians, and be abused for profits.

Individually, physicians who offer diagnostic imaging services that have not been scientifically validated and for which a patient has not been referred by another physician have an ethical obligation to:

(a) Perform a requested diagnostic imaging test only when, in the physician's judgment, the possible benefits of the service outweigh its risks.

AMA Principles of Medical Ethics: I, II, V, VIII

Issued: 2005

Updated: 2016

Opinions on Related Matters:
1.1.1 Patient-Physician Relationships
2.1.1 Informed Consent
9.6.7 Direct-to-Consumer Advertisement of Prescription Drugs
11.2.2 Conflicts of Interest in Patient Care

9 Professional Self-regulation

(b) Recognize that in agreeing to perform diagnostic imaging on request, the physician:
   (i) establishes a patient-physician relationship, with all the ethical and professional obligations such relationship entails;
   (ii) assumes responsibility for relevant clinical evaluation, including pre- and post-test counseling about the test, its results, and indicated follow-up. Physicians may choose to refer the patient for post-test counseling to an appropriate physician who accepts the patient.
(c) Obtain the patient's informed consent. In addition to the usual elements of informed consent, the physician should disclose:
   (i) that the diagnostic imaging test has not been validated scientifically;
   (ii) the inaccuracies inherent in the proposed test;
   (iii) the possibility of inconclusive results;
   (iv) the likelihood of false positive and false negative results;
   (v) circumstances that may require further assessments and additional cost.
(d) Ensure that the patient's interests are primary and place patient welfare above physician interests when the physician has a financial interest in the imaging facility.
(e) Ensure that any advertisements for the services are truthful and not misleading or deceptive, in keeping with ethics guidance and applicable law.

Collectively, physicians should:

(f) Advocate for the conduct of appropriate trials aimed at determining the predictive power of diagnostic imaging tests and their sensitivity and specificity for target populations.
(g) Develop suitable guidelines for specific diagnostic imaging tests when adequate scientific data become available.

AMA Principles of Medical Ethics: II, III, VIII

Issued: 2009

Opinions on Related Matters:
1.1.1 Patient-Physician Relationships
1.2.3 Consultation, Referral, and Second Opinions
2.1.1 Informed Consent
11.2.2 Conflicts of Interest in Patient Care

9.6.9 Physician Self-referral

Business arrangements among physicians in the health care marketplace have the potential to benefit patients by enhancing quality of care and access to health care services. However, these arrangements can also be ethically challenging when they create opportunities for self-referral in which patients' medical interests can be in tension with physicians' financial interests. Such arrangements can undermine a robust commitment to professionalism in medicine as well as trust in the profession.

In general, physicians should not refer patients to a health care facility that is outside their office practice and at which they do not directly provide care or services when they have a financial interest in that facility. Physicians who enter into legally permissible contractual relationships—including acquisition of ownership or investment interests in health facilities, products, or equipment; or contracts for service in group practices—are expected to uphold their responsibilities to patients first.

When physicians enter into arrangements that provide opportunities for self-referral, they must:

(a) Ensure that referrals are based on objective, medically relevant criteria.

(b) Ensure that the arrangement:

    (i)   is structured to enhance access to appropriate, high-quality health care services or products;

    (ii) within the constraints of applicable law:

        a. does not require physician-owners/investors to make referrals to the entity or otherwise generate revenues as a condition of participation;

        b. does not prohibit physician-owners/investors from participating in or referring patients to competing facilities or services; and

        c. adheres to fair business practices vis-à-vis the medical professional community—eg, by ensuring that the arrangement does not prohibit investment by nonreferring physicians.

(c) Take steps to mitigate conflicts of interest, including:

    (i)   ensuring that financial benefit is not dependent on the physician-owner or investor's volume of referrals for services or sales of products;

    (ii) establishing mechanisms for utilization review to monitor referral practices;

    (iii) identifying or if possible making alternate arrangements for care of the patient when conflicts cannot be appropriately managed or mitigated.

(d) Disclose their financial interest in the facility, product, or equipment to patients; inform them of available alternatives for referral; and assure them that their ongoing care is not conditioned on accepting the recommended referral.

9 Professional
Self-regulation

Physician Interactions with Government Agencies

AMA Principles of Medical Ethics: II, IV, V, VII

Issued: 2004

Updated: 2016

Opinions on Related Matters:
11.2.2 Conflicts of Interest in Patient Care

9.7.1 Medical Testimony

Medical evidence is critical in a variety of legal and administrative proceedings. As citizens and as professionals with specialized knowledge and experience, physicians have an obligation to assist in the administration of justice.

Whenever physicians serve as witnesses, they must:

(a) Accurately represent their qualifications.

(b) Testify honestly.

(c) Not allow their testimony to be influenced by financial compensation. Physicians must not accept compensation that is contingent on the outcome of litigation.

Physicians who testify as fact witnesses in legal claims involving a patient they have treated must hold the patient's medical interests paramount by:

(d) Protecting the confidentiality of the patient's health information, unless the physician is authorized or legally compelled to disclose the information.

(e) Delivering honest testimony. This requires that they engage in continuous self-examination to ensure that their testimony represents the facts of the case.

(f) Declining to testify if the matters could adversely affect their patients' medical interests unless the patient consents or unless ordered to do so by legally constituted authority.

(g) Considering transferring the care of the patient to another physician if the legal proceedings result in placing the patient and the physician in adversarial positions.

Physicians who testify as expert witnesses must:

(h) Testify only in areas in which they have appropriate training and recent, substantive experience and knowledge.

(i) Evaluate cases objectively and provide an independent opinion.

(j) Ensure that their testimony:

(i) reflects current scientific thought and standards of care that have gained acceptance among peers in the relevant field;

(ii) appropriately characterizes the theory on which testimony is based if the theory is not widely accepted in the profession;

(iii) considers standards that prevailed at the time the event under review occurred when testifying about a standard of care.

Organized medicine, including state and specialty societies and medical licensing boards, has a responsibility to maintain high standards for medical witnesses by assessing claims of false or misleading testimony and issuing disciplinary sanctions as appropriate.

9.7.2 Court-Initiated Medical Treatment in Criminal Cases

Court-initiated medical treatments raise important questions as to the rights of prisoners, the powers of judges, and the ethical obligations of physicians. Although convicted criminals have fewer rights and protections than other citizens, being convicted of a crime does not deprive an offender of all protections under the law. Court-ordered medical treatments raise the question whether professional ethics permits physicians to cooperate in administering and overseeing such treatment. Physicians have civic duties, but medical ethics do not require a physician to carry out civic duties that contradict fundamental principles of medical ethics, such as the duty to avoid doing harm.

In limited circumstances physicians can ethically participate in court-initiated medical treatments. Individual physicians who provide care under court order should:

(a) Participate only if the procedure being mandated is therapeutically efficacious and is therefore undoubtedly not a form of punishment or solely a mechanism of social control.

(b) Treat patients based on sound medical diagnoses, not court-defined behaviors. While a court has the authority to identify criminal behavior, a court does not have the ability to make a medical diagnosis or to determine the type of treatment that will be administered. When the treatment involves inpatient therapy, surgical intervention, or pharmacological treatment, the physician's diagnosis must be confirmed by an independent physician or a panel of physicians not responsible to the state. A second opinion is not necessary in cases of court-ordered counseling or referrals for psychiatric evaluations.

(c) Decline to provide treatment that is not scientifically validated and consistent with nationally accepted guidelines for clinical practice.

(d) Be able to conclude, in good conscience and to the best of his or her professional judgment, that to the extent possible

AMA Principles of Medical Ethics: I, III

Issued: 1998

Updated: 2016

Opinions on Related Matters:
1.1.1 Patient-Physician Relationships
2.1.1 Informed Consent
3.2.1 Confidentiality

the patient voluntarily gave his or her informed consent, recognizing that an element of coercion is inevitably present. When treatment involves inpatient therapy, surgical intervention, or pharmacological treatment, an independent physician or a panel of physicians not responsible to the state should confirm that voluntary consent was given.

AMA Principles of Medical Ethics: I

Issued: 1980

Updated: 1996, 1999, 2000, 2016

Opinions on Related Matters:
1.1.1 Patient-Physician Relationships
2.1.1 Informed Consent
3.2.1 Confidentiality
6.2.1 Guidance for Organ Transplantation from Deceased Donors
9.7.5 Torture

9.7.3 Capital Punishment

Debate over capital punishment has occurred for centuries and remains a volatile social, political, and legal issue. An individual's opinion on capital punishment is the personal moral decision of the individual. However, as a member of a profession dedicated to preserving life when there is hope of doing so, a physician must not participate in a legally authorized execution.

Physician participation in execution is defined as actions that fall into one or more of the following categories:

(a) Would directly cause the death of the condemned.
(b) Would assist, supervise, or contribute to the ability of another individual to directly cause the death of the condemned.
(c) Could automatically cause an execution to be carried out on a condemned prisoner.

These include, but are not limited to:

(d) Determining a prisoner's competence to be executed. A physician's medical opinion should be merely one aspect of the information taken into account by a legal decision maker, such as a judge or hearing officer.
(e) Treating a condemned prisoner who has been declared incompetent to be executed for the purpose of restoring competence, unless a commutation order is issued before treatment begins. The task of re-evaluating the prisoner should be performed by an independent medical examiner.
(f) Prescribing or administering tranquilizers and other psychotropic agents and medications that are part of the execution procedure.
(g) Monitoring vital signs on site or remotely (including monitoring electrocardiograms).
(h) Attending or observing an execution as a physician.
(i) Rendering of technical advice regarding execution.

And, when the method of execution is lethal injection:

(j) Selecting injection sites.

(k) Starting intravenous lines as a port for a lethal injection device.

(l) Prescribing, preparing, administering, or supervising injection drugs or their doses or types.

(m) Inspecting, testing, or maintaining lethal injection devices.

(n) Consulting with or supervising lethal injection personnel.

The following actions do not constitute physician participation in execution:

(o) Testifying as to the prisoner's medical history and diagnoses or mental state as they relate to competence to stand trial, testifying as to relevant medical evidence during trial, testifying as to medical aspects of aggravating or mitigating circumstances during the penalty phase of a capital case, or testifying as to medical diagnoses as they relate to the legal assessment of competence for execution.

(p) Certifying death, provided that the condemned has been declared dead by another person.

(q) Witnessing an execution in a totally nonprofessional capacity.

(r) Witnessing an execution at the specific voluntary request of the condemned person, provided that the physician observes the execution in a nonprofessional capacity.

(s) Relieving the acute suffering of a condemned person while awaiting execution, including providing tranquilizers at the specific voluntary request of the condemned person to help relieve pain or anxiety in anticipation of the execution.

(t) Providing medical intervention to mitigate suffering when an incompetent prisoner is undergoing extreme suffering as a result of psychosis or any other illness.

No physician should be compelled to participate in the process of establishing a prisoner's competence or be involved with treatment of an incompetent, condemned prisoner if such activity is contrary to the physician's personal beliefs. Under those circumstances, physicians should be permitted to transfer care of the prisoner to another physician.

Organ donation by condemned prisoners is permissible only if:

(u) The decision to donate was made before the prisoner's conviction.

(v) The donated tissue is harvested after the prisoner has been pronounced dead and the body removed from the death chamber.

(w) Physicians do not provide advice on modifying the method of execution for any individual to facilitate donation.

AMA Principles of Medical Ethics: I, III, VII, VIII

Issued: 2006

Updated: 2016

Opinions on Related Matters:
1.1.1 Patient-Physician Relationships
9.7.5 Torture

9.7.4 Physician Participation in Interrogation

Interrogation is defined as questioning related to law enforcement or to military and national security intelligence gathering, designed to prevent harm or danger to individuals, the public, or national security. Interrogations of criminal suspects, prisoners of war, or any other individuals who are being held involuntarily ("detainees") are distinct from questioning used by physicians to assess an individual's physical or mental condition. To be appropriate, interrogations must avoid the use of coercion—ie, threatening or causing harm through physical injury or mental suffering.

Physicians who engage in any activity that relies on their medical knowledge and skills must continue to uphold principles of medical ethics. Questions about the propriety of physician participation in interrogations and in the development of interrogation strategies may be addressed by balancing obligations to individuals with obligations to protect third parties and the public. The further removed the physician is from direct involvement with a detainee, the more justifiable is a role serving the public interest.

Applying this general approach, physician involvement with interrogations during law enforcement or intelligence gathering should be guided by the following:

(a) Physicians may perform physical and mental assessments of detainees to determine the need for and to provide medical care. When so doing, physicians must disclose to the detainee the extent to which others have access to information included in medical records. Treatment must never be conditional on a patient's participation in an interrogation.

(b) Physicians must neither conduct nor directly participate in an interrogation, because a role as physician-interrogator undermines the physician's role as healer and thereby erodes trust in the individual physician-interrogator and in the medical profession.

(c) Physicians must not monitor interrogations with the intention of intervening in the process, because this constitutes direct participation in interrogation.

(d) Physicians may participate in developing effective interrogation strategies for general training purposes. These strategies must not threaten or cause physical injury or mental suffering and must be humane and respect the rights of individuals.

When physicians have reason to believe that interrogations are coercive, they must report their observations to the appropriate authorities. If authorities are aware of coercive interrogations but have not intervened, physicians are ethically obligated to report the offenses to independent authorities that have the power to investigate or adjudicate such allegations.

9.7.5 Torture

Torture refers to the deliberate, systematic, or wanton administration of cruel, inhumane, and degrading treatments or punishments during imprisonment or detainment. Physicians must oppose and must not participate in torture for any reason. Participation in torture includes, but is not limited to, providing or withholding any services, substances, or knowledge to facilitate the practice of torture. Physicians must not be present when torture is used or threatened.

Physicians may treat prisoners or detainees if doing so is in the prisoner's or detainee's best interest, but physicians should not treat individuals to verify their health so that torture can begin or continue.

Physicians who treat torture victims should not be persecuted.

Physicians should help provide support for victims of torture and, whenever possible, strive to change situations in which torture is practiced or the potential for torture is great.

AMA Principles of Medical Ethics: I, III

Issued: 1999

Opinions on Related Matters:
1.1.1 Patient-Physician Relationships
2.1.1 Informed Consent
9.7.4 Physician Participation in Interrogation

9 Professional Self-regulation

10 Interprofessional Relationships

*These Opinions are offered as ethics guidance for physicians and are not
intended to establish clinical practice guidelines or rules of law.*

Physicians interact with other health care professionals and with health care
organizations and institutions in a variety of ways—as peers and professional colleagues,
as administrators and supervisors, as members of ethics committees or as ethics
consultants, as educators and mentors, and as patients themselves. Yet physicians still
have a fundamental responsibility to act professionally toward other physicians and
medical staff.

In light of their shared professional commitments and responsibilities, physicians'
relationships with nurses, medical staff, and allied health professionals should be
based on mutual respect and trust. Physicians should also treat each other with similar
respect and trust. And if a physician is asked to provide care for a fellow physician, the
treating physician must recognize that providing medical care for a peer can pose unique
challenges for objectivity, open exchange of information, privacy and confidentiality,
and informed consent.

Throughout their formal education and their practice of medicine, physicians profess
and are therefore held to standards of medical ethics and professionalism. Complying
with these standards enables physicians to earn the trust of their patients and the public.
These ethical obligations are not suspended when a physician assumes a position that
does not directly involve patient care; rather, they are binding on physicians in nonclinical
roles to the extent that physicians rely on medical training, experience, or perspective to
carry out those roles. When physicians make decisions in nonclinical roles, they should
strive to protect the health of individuals and communities.

When physicians assume leadership roles in their health care facilities, they frequently
find themselves in the position of having to account for not only the best interests
of individual patients, but also the best interests of others, including populations of
patients and the medical staff. Adhering to professional medical standards in this context
includes placing the interests of patients above other considerations, such as personal
interests (eg, financial incentives) or employer business interests (eg, profit). Professional
medical standards also demand the use of fair and just criteria when making care-related
determinations.

Finally, when physicians provide ethics consultations or serve on ethics committees,
they have a primary responsibility to support informed, deliberative decision making and
to promote respect for the values, needs, and interests of all participants.

10 Interprofessional
Relationships

10.1 Ethics Guidance for Physicians in Nonclinical Roles

Physicians earn and maintain the trust of their patients and the public by upholding norms of fidelity to patients, on which the physician's professional identity rests.

Even when they fulfill roles that do not involve directly providing care for patients in clinical settings, physicians are seen by patients and the public, as well as their colleagues and coworkers, as professionals who have committed themselves to the values and norms of medicine. Whatever roles they may play in the system of health care delivery, when physicians use the knowledge and values they gained through medical training and practice in roles that affect the care and well-being of individual patients or groups of patients, they are functioning within the sphere of their profession.

When physicians take on obligations that compete with their fiduciary obligations to patients, those fiduciary obligations may ethically be tempered by the following considerations:

(a) The impact of the nonclinical role on the health of individuals and communities.

(b) The degree to which they are perceived to be acting as representatives of the medical profession.

(c) The extent to which they rely on their medical training or expertise to fulfill the nonclinical role.

AMA Principles of Medical Ethics: I, VII

Issued: 1994

Updated: 1998, 2007, 2016

Opinions on Related Matters:
1.1.1 Patient-Physician Relationships
10.1.1 Ethical Obligations of Medical Directors

10.1.1 Ethical Obligations of Medical Directors

Physicians' core professional obligations include acting in and advocating for patients' best interests. When they take on roles that require them to use their medical knowledge on behalf of third parties, physicians must uphold these core obligations.

When physicians accept the role of medical director and must make benefit coverage determinations on behalf of health plans or other third parties or determinations about individuals' fitness to engage in an activity or need for medical care, they should:

(a) Use their professional expertise to help craft plan guidelines to ensure that all enrollees receive fair, equal consideration.

(b) Review plan policies and guidelines to ensure that decision-making mechanisms:
(i) are objective, flexible, and consistent;
(ii) rest on appropriate criteria for allocating medical resources in keeping with ethics guidance.

AMA Principles of Medical Ethics: I, III, VII

Issued: 1999

Updated: 2016

Opinions on Related Matters:
1.1.1 Patient-Physician Relationships
10.1 Ethics Guidance for Physicians in Nonclinical Roles

10 Interprofessional Relationships

(c) Apply plan policies and guidance evenhandedly to all patients.

(d) Encourage third-party payers to provide needed medical services to all plan enrollees and to promote access to services by the community at large.

(e) Put patient interests over personal interests (financial or other) created by the nonclinical role.

AMA Principles of Medical Ethics: II, VI, VIII

Issued: 2009

Updated: 2016

Opinions on Related Matters:
1.1.1 Patient-Physician Relationships
10.4 Nurses
10.5 Allied Health Professionals

10.2 Physician Employment by a Nonphysician Supervisee

Physicians' relationships with midlevel practitioners must be based on mutual respect and trust as well as their shared commitment to patient well-being. Health care professionals recognize that clinical tasks should be shared and delegated in keeping with each practitioner's training, expertise, and scope of practice. Given their comprehensive training and broad scope of practice, physicians have a professional responsibility for the quality of overall care that patients receive, even when aspects of that care are delivered by nonphysician clinicians.

Accepting employment to supervise a nonphysician employer's clinical practice can create ethical dilemmas for physicians. If maintaining an employment relationship with a midlevel practitioner contributes significantly to the physician's livelihood, the personal and financial influence that employer status confers creates an inherent conflict for a physician who is simultaneously an employee and a clinical supervisor of his or her employer.

Physicians who are simultaneously employees and clinical supervisors of nonphysician practitioners must:

(a) Give precedence to their ethical obligation to act in the patient's best interest.

(b) Exercise independent professional judgment, even if that puts the physician at odds with the employer-supervisee.

AMA Principles of Medical Ethics: VI

Issued: 2008

Updated: 2016

Opinions on Related Matters:
1.1.1 Patient-Physician Relationships

10.3 Peers as Patients

The opportunity to care for a fellow physician or physician-in-training is a privilege and may represent a gratifying experience and serve as a show of respect or competence. However, physicians must recognize that providing medical care for a fellow professional can pose special challenges for objectivity, open exchange of information, privacy and confidentiality, and informed consent.

In emergencies or isolated rural settings when options for care by other physicians are limited or where no other qualified physician is available, physicians should not hesitate to treat colleagues.

Physicians must make the same fundamental ethical commitments when treating peers as when treating any other patient. Physicians who provide medical care to a colleague should:

(a) Exercise objective professional judgment and make unbiased treatment recommendations despite the personal or professional relationship they may have with the patient.

(b) Be sensitive to the potential psychological discomfort of the physician-patient, especially when eliciting sensitive information or conducting an intimate examination.

(c) Respect the physical and informational privacy of physician-patients. Discuss how to respond to inquiries from colleagues about the physician-patient's medical care. Recognize that special measures may be needed to ensure privacy.

(d) Provide information to enable the physician-patient to make voluntary, well-informed decisions about care. The treating physician should not assume that the physician-patient is knowledgeable about his or her medical condition.

Physicians-in-training and medical students (when they provide care as part of their supervised training) face unique challenges when asked to provide or participate in care for peers, given the circumstances of their roles in residency programs and medical schools. Except in emergency situations or when other care is not available, physicians-in-training should not be required to provide medical care for fellow trainees, faculty members, or attending physicians if they are reluctant to do so.

10.4 Nurses

Like physicians, nurses hold a primary ethical obligation to promote patients' well-being. Nurses' training, expertise, and scope of practice complement physicians' professional commitments and expertise.

While physicians have overall responsibility for the quality of care that patients receive, good nursing practice requires that nurses voice their concerns when, in the nurse's professional judgment, a physician order is in error or is contrary to good medical practice.

In light of their shared professional commitments, physicians' relationships with nurses should be based on mutual respect and trust. As leaders of the health care team, physicians should:

AMA Principles of Medical Ethics: IV, V

Issued: 1983

Updated: 1994, 2016

Opinions on Related Matters:
10.2 Physician Employment by a Nonphysician Supervisee
10.5 Allied Health Professionals

10 Interprofessional Relationships

(a) Listen respectfully and take seriously the concerns a nurse raises about the physician's order and explain the order to the nurse and modify if appropriate.

(b) Recognize nurses' professional responsibility not to follow orders that are contrary to good medical practice.

(c) Acknowledge that in an emergency situation when the physician is not immediately available, to protect the patient's health, nurses may have a professional obligation to take prompt action contrary to the physician's order.

(d) Seek assistance from the ethics committee or other institutional resource to resolve disagreement in nonemergent situations when disagreement about patient care persists.

AMA Principles of Medical Ethics: I, V, VII

Issued: 1997

Updated: 2016

Opinions on Related Matters:
10.2 Physician Employment by a Nonphysician Supervisee
10.4 Nurses

10.5 Allied Health Professionals

Physicians often practice in concert with optometrists, nurse anesthetists, nurse midwives, and other allied health professionals. Although physicians have overall responsibility for the quality of care that patients receive, allied health professionals have training and expertise that complements physicians'. With physicians, allied health professionals share a common commitment to patient well-being.

In light of this shared commitment, physicians' relationships with allied health professionals should be based on mutual respect and trust. It is ethically appropriate for physicians to:

(a) Help support high-quality education that is complementary to medical training, including by teaching in recognized schools for allied health professionals.

(b) Work in consultation with or employ appropriately trained and credentialed allied health professionals.

(c) Delegate provision of medical services to an appropriately trained and credentialed allied health professional within the individual's scope of practice.

10.6 Industry Representatives in Clinical Settings

Representatives of medical device manufacturers can play an important role in patient safety and quality of care by providing information about the proper use of their companies' devices or equipment and by offering technical assistance to physicians. However, allowing industry representatives to be present in clinical settings while care is being given also raises concerns. Their presence can pose challenges for patient autonomy, privacy, and confidentiality as well as safety and professionalism in caregiving.

Physicians have a responsibility to protect patient interests and thus have a corresponding obligation to exercise good professional judgment in inviting industry representatives into the clinical setting. Physicians should recognize that in this setting appropriately trained industry representatives function as consultants. Participation by industry representatives should not be allowed to substitute for training physicians to use devices and equipment safely themselves.

Physicians who invite industry representatives into the clinical setting should ensure that:

(a) The representative's participation will improve the safety and effectiveness of patient care.

(b) The representative's qualifications to provide the desired assistance have been appropriately screened.

(c) The patient is aware that an industry representative will facilitate care, has been informed about the scope and nature of the representative's role in care, and has agreed to the representative's participation.

(d) The representative understands and is committed to upholding medical standards of respect for patient privacy and confidentiality.

(e) The representative has agreed to abide by the policies of the health care institution governing his or her presence and clinical activities.

(f) The representative does not exceed the bounds of his or her training, is adequately supervised, and does not engage in the practice of medicine.

AMA Principles of Medical Ethics: I, IV, V

Issued: 2007

Updated: 2016

Opinions on Related Matters:
2.1.1 Informed Consent
3.1.1 Privacy in Health Care
3.1.2 Patient Privacy and Outside Observers of the Clinical Encounter
3.1.4 Audio or Visual Recording of Patients for Public Education
3.2.1 Confidentiality

10 Interprofessional Relationships

AMA Principles of Medical Ethics: II, IV, VII

Issued: 1994

Updated: 2016

10.7 Ethics Committees in Health Care Institutions

In making decisions about health care, patients, families, and physicians and other health care professionals often face difficult, potentially life-changing situations. Such situations can raise ethically challenging questions about what would be the most appropriate or preferred course of action. Ethics committees, or similar institutional mechanisms, offer assistance in addressing ethical issues that arise in patient care and facilitate sound decision making that respects participants' values, concerns, and interests.

In addition to facilitating decision making in individual cases (as a committee or through the activities of individual members functioning as ethics consultants), many ethics committees assist in ethics-related educational programming and policy development within their institutions.

To be effective in providing the intended support and guidance in any of these capacities, ethics committees should:

(a) Serve as advisors and educators rather than decision makers. Patients, physicians and other health care professionals, health care administrators, and other stakeholders should not be required to accept committee recommendations. Nonetheless, physicians and other institutional stakeholders should explain their reasoning when they choose not to follow the committee's recommendations in an individual case.

(b) Respect the rights and privacy of all participants and the privacy of committee deliberations, and take appropriate steps to protect the confidentiality of information disclosed during the discussions.

(c) Ensure that all stakeholders have timely access to the committee's services for facilitating decision making in nonemergent situations and as feasible for urgent consultations.

(d) Be structured, staffed, and supported appropriately to meet the needs of the institution and its patient population. Committee membership should represent diverse perspectives, expertise, and experience, including one or more community representatives.

(e) Adopt and adhere to policies and procedures governing the committee and, where appropriate, the activities of individual members as ethics consultants, in keeping with medical staff bylaws. This includes standards for resolving competing responsibilities and for documenting committee recommendations in the patient's medical record when facilitating decision making in individual cases.

(f) Draw on the resources of appropriate professional organizations, including guidance from national specialty societies, to inform committee recommendations.

Ethics committees that serve faith-based or other mission-driven heath care institutions have a dual responsibility to:

(g) uphold the principles to which the institution is committed;

(h) to make clear to patients, physicians, and other stakeholders that the institution's defining principles will inform the committee's recommendations.

10.7.1 Ethics Consultations

The goal of ethics consultation is to support informed, deliberative decision making on the part of patients, families, physicians, and the health care team. By helping to clarify ethical issues and values, facilitating discussion, and providing expertise and educational resources, ethics consultants promote respect for the values, needs, and interests of all participants, especially when there is disagreement or uncertainty about treatment decisions.

Whether they serve independently or through an institutional ethics committee or similar mechanism, physicians who provide ethics consultation services should:

(a) Seek to balance the concerns of all stakeholders, focusing on protecting the patient's needs and values.

(b) Serve as advisors and educators rather than decision makers. Patients, physicians and other members of the care team, health care administrators, and other stakeholders should not be required to accept the consultant's recommendations. Nonetheless, physicians and other institutional stakeholders should explain their reasoning when they choose not to follow the consultant's recommendations in an individual case.

(c) Inform the patient when an ethics consultation has been requested (if the request was not made by the patient or family) and seek the patient's agreement to participate. Ethics consultants should respect the decision of a patient or family not to participate, whether that decision is indicated formally through explicit refusal or informally by not taking part in discussions.

(d) Respect the rights and privacy of all participants, and ensure that appropriate steps are taken to protect the confidentiality of information disclosed in the consultation.

AMA Principles of Medical Ethics: IV, V

Issued: 1998

Updated: 2016

Opinions on Related Matters:
1.1.1 Patient-Physician Relationships
1.1.7 Physician Exercise of Conscience
2.1.1 Informed Consent
2.1.2 Decisions for Adult Patients Who Lack Capacity
2.2.1 Pediatric Decision Making
4.2.1 Assisted Reproductive Technology
5.3 Withholding or Withdrawing Life-Sustaining Treatment
5.4 Orders Not to Attempt Resuscitation (DNAR)
5.6 Sedation to Unconsciousness in End-of-Life Care
6.1.1 Transplantation of Organs from Living Donors
10.7 Ethics Committees in Health Care Institutions
10.7.1 Ethics Consultations

(e) Have appropriate expertise or training—eg, familiarity with the relevant professional literature, training in clinical or philosophical ethics, or competence in conflict resolution—and relevant experience to fulfill their role effectively.

(f) Adopt and adhere to policies and procedures governing ethics consultation activities in keeping with medical staff bylaws, including accountability and standards for documenting the consultation in the patient's medical record.

(g) Ensure that all stakeholders have timely access to consultation services in nonemergent situations and as feasible for urgent consultations.

11 Financing and Delivery of Health Care

*These Opinions are offered as ethics guidance for physicians and are not
intended to establish clinical practice guidelines or rules of law.*

Relationships between individual patients and their physicians remain at the heart of
medicine, but those relationships are embedded in an increasingly complex system of
health care institutions and payers. As health care has become more complex and costlier,
new challenges have emerged for physicians. Today's physicians must often navigate
competing responsibilities to multiple parties as they strive to provide safe, high-quality
care for their patients.

Payment models and incentive mechanisms intended to contain costs and improve
quality may create conflicts of interest that work against the goal of providing care that is
responsive to the unique needs, values, and preferences of individual patients. Changing
arrangements for delivering health care can affect patients' choices about where
and from whom to receive care and physicians' relationships with both patients and
professional colleagues, while tools designed to influence physicians' decision making
can impinge on professional judgment and undermine physicians' ability to advocate for
their patients.

In their roles as practicing clinicians, physicians are in a unique position to understand
and try to mitigate the impact of these changes on individual patients. As leaders in
health care organizations, they are in a position to address the dilemmas posed by
the evolving policies and practices of health care organizations and institutions. As a
profession, physicians collectively are in a position to help shape the societal policies that
create the conditions under which patients at large receive health care.

Coupled with medicine's core commitment of fidelity and service to patients, these
opportunities define ethical responsibilities to promote access to care for individuals and
for populations of patients; to help shape fair, transparent policies for allocating health
care resources at the institutional and societal level; to be prudent stewards of the shared
societal resources with which they are entrusted; and to promote and sustain standards
of professionalism.

Opinions in the first section of this chapter provide guidance on aspects of physicians'
ethical responsibilities to address questions of access to care, individually and collectively,
while those in the second section offer guidance on the ethical responsibilities of
physicians in health care organizations. Opinions in the third section address ethical
issues in the context of particular questions about fees for medical and nonmedical
services.

Access to Health Care

Health Care Organizations and Physician Practice

Fees and Charges

Access to Health Care

11.1.1 Defining Basic Health Care

Health care is a fundamental human good because it affects our opportunity to pursue life goals, reduces our pain and suffering, helps prevent premature loss of life, and provides information needed to plan for our lives. Society has an obligation to make access to an adequate level of care available to all its members, regardless of ability to pay.

Physicians regularly confront the effects of lack of access to adequate care and have a corresponding responsibility to contribute their expertise to societal decisions about what health care services should be included in a minimum package of care for all.

Individually and collectively as a profession, physicians should advocate for fair, informed decision making about basic health care that:

(a) Is transparent.

(b) Strives to include input from all stakeholders, including the public, throughout the process.

(c) Protects the most vulnerable patients and populations, with special attention to historically disadvantaged groups.

(d) Considers best available scientific data about the efficacy and safety of health care services.

(e) Seeks to improve health outcomes to the greatest extent possible, in keeping with principles of wise stewardship.

(f) Monitors for variations in care that cannot be explained on medical grounds to ensure that the defined threshold of basic care does not have discriminatory impact.

(g) Provides for ongoing review and adjustment in consideration of innovation in medical science and practice to ensure continued, broad public support for the defined threshold of basic care.

AMA Principles of Medical Ethics: VII

Issued: 1994

Updated: 2016

Opinions on Related Matters:
1.1.6 Quality
8.5 Disparities in Health Care

11.1.2 Physician Stewardship of Health Care Resources

Physicians' primary ethical obligation is to promote the well-being of individual patients. Physicians also have a long-recognized obligation to patients in general to promote public health and access to care. This obligation requires physicians to be prudent stewards of the shared societal resources with which they are entrusted. Managing health care resources responsibly for the benefit of all

AMA Principles of Medical Ethics: I, V, VII, VIII, IX

Issued: 2012

Opinions on Related Matters:
1.1.6 Quality
2.1.1 Informed Consent
8.5 Disparities in Health Care
11.1.4 Financial Barriers to Health Care Access

patients is compatible with physicians' primary obligation to serve the interests of individual patients.

To fulfill their obligation to be prudent stewards of health care resources, physicians should:

(a) Base recommendations and decisions on patients' medical needs.

(b) Use scientifically grounded evidence to inform professional decisions when available.

(c) Help patients articulate their health care goals, and help patients and their families form realistic expectations about whether a particular intervention is likely to achieve those goals.

(d) Endorse recommendations that offer reasonable likelihood of achieving the patient's health care goals.

(e) Choose the course of action that requires fewer resources when alternative courses of action offer similar likelihood and degree of anticipated benefit compared to anticipated harm for the individual patient but require different levels of resources.

(f) Be transparent about alternatives, including disclosing when resource constraints play a role in decision making.

(g) Participate in efforts to resolve persistent disagreement about whether a costly intervention is worthwhile, which may include consulting other physicians, an ethics committee, or other appropriate resource.

Physicians are in a unique position to affect health care spending. But individual physicians alone cannot and should not be expected to address the systemic challenges of wisely managing health care resources. Medicine as a profession must create conditions for practice that make it feasible for individual physicians to be prudent stewards by:

(h) Encouraging health care administrators and organizations to make cost data transparent (including cost accounting methodologies) so that physicians can exercise well-informed stewardship.

(i) Ensuring that physicians have the training they need to be informed about health care costs and how their decisions affect overall health care spending.

(j) Advocating for policy changes, such as medical liability reform, that promote professional judgment and address systemic barriers that impede responsible stewardship.

11.1.3 Allocating Limited Health Care Resources

Physicians' primary ethical obligation is to promote the well-being of their patients. Policies for allocating scarce health care resources can impede their ability to fulfill that obligation, whether those policies address situations of chronically limited resources, such as ICU (intensive care unit) beds, medications, or solid organs for transplantation, or "triage" situations in times of scarcity, such as access to ventilators during an influenza pandemic.

As professionals dedicated to protecting the interests of their patients, physicians thus have a responsibility to contribute their expertise to developing allocation policies that are fair and safeguard the welfare of patients.

Individually and collectively through the profession, physicians should advocate for policies and procedures that allocate scarce health care resources fairly among patients, in keeping with the following criteria:

(a) Base allocation policies on criteria relating to medical need, including urgency of need, likelihood and anticipated duration of benefit, and change in quality of life. In limited circumstances, it may be appropriate to take into consideration the amount of resources required for successful treatment. It is not appropriate to base allocation policies on social worth, perceived obstacles to treatment, patient contribution to illness, past use of resources, or other non-medical characteristics.

(b) Give first priority to those patients for whom treatment will avoid premature death or extremely poor outcomes, then to patients who will experience the greatest change in quality of life, when there are very substantial differences among patients who need access to the scarce resource(s).

(c) Use an objective, flexible, transparent mechanism to determine which patients will receive the resource(s) when there are not substantial differences among patients who need access to the scarce resource(s).

(d) Explain the applicable allocation policies or procedures to patients who are denied access to the scarce resource(s) and to the public.

AMA Principles of Medical Ethics: I, VII

Issued: 1981

Updated: 1994, 2016

Opinions on Related Matters:
1.1.6 Quality
6.2.1 Guidance for Organ Transplantation from Deceased Donors
11.1.1 Defining Basic Health Care
11.1.2 Physician Stewardship of Health Care Resources
11.2.1 Professionalism in Health Care Systems
11.2.4 Transparency in Health Care

AMA Principles of Medical Ethics: I, II, VI, VII, IX

Issued: 2009

Opinions on Related Matters:
1.1.1 Patient-Physician Relationships
1.1.6 Quality
8.5 Disparities in Health Care
11.1.2 Physician Stewardship of Health
Care Resources

11.1.4 Financial Barriers to Health Care Access

Health care is a fundamental human good because it affects our opportunity to pursue life goals, reduces our pain and suffering, helps prevent premature loss of life, and provides information needed to plan for our lives. As professionals, physicians individually and collectively have an ethical responsibility to ensure that all persons have access to needed care regardless of their economic means.

In view of this obligation, individual physicians should:

(a) take steps to promote access to care for individual patients, such as providing pro bono care in their office or through freestanding facilities or government programs that provide health care for the poor, or, when permissible, waiving insurance copayments in individual cases of hardship. Physicians in the poorest communities should be able to turn for assistance to colleagues in more prosperous communities.

(b) individual physicians should help patients obtain needed care through public or charitable programs when patients cannot do so themselves.

Physicians, individually and collectively through their professional organizations and institutions should:

(c) participate in the political process as advocates for patients (or support those who do) so as to diminish financial obstacles to access health care.

The medical profession must:

(d) work to ensure that societal decisions about the distribution of health resources safeguard the interests of all patients and promote access to health services.

All stakeholders in health care, including physicians, health facilities, health insurers, professional medical societies, and public policy makers must work together to ensure sufficient access to appropriate health care for all people.

Health Care Organizations and Physician Practice

11.2.1 Professionalism in Health Care Systems

Containing costs, promoting high-quality care for all patients, and sustaining physician professionalism are important goals. Models for financing and organizing the delivery of health care services often aim to promote patient safety and to improve quality and efficiency. However, they can also pose ethical challenges for physicians that could undermine the trust essential to patient-physician relationships.

Payment models and financial incentives can create conflicts of interest among patients, health care organizations, and physicians. They can encourage undertreatment and overtreatment, as well as dictate goals that are not individualized for the particular patient.

Structures that influence where and by whom care is delivered—such as accountable care organizations, group practices, health maintenance organizations, and other entities that may emerge in the future—can affect patients' choices, the patient-physician relationship, and physicians' relationships with fellow health care professionals.

Formularies, clinical practice guidelines, and other tools intended to influence decision making may impinge on physicians' exercise of professional judgment and ability to advocate effectively for their patients, depending on how they are designed and implemented.

Physicians in leadership positions within health care organizations should ensure that practices for financing and organizing the delivery of care:

(a) Are transparent.
(b) Reflect input from key stakeholders, including physicians and patients.
(c) Recognize that over-reliance on financial incentives may undermine physician professionalism.
(d) Ensure ethically acceptable incentives that:
   (i) are designed in keeping with sound principles and solid scientific evidence. Financial incentives should be based on appropriate comparison groups and cost data and adjusted to reflect complexity, case mix, and other factors that affect physician practice profiles. Practice guidelines, formularies, and other tools should be based on best available evidence and developed in keeping with ethics guidance;

AMA Principles of Medical Ethics: I, II, III, V

Issued: 2014

Opinions on Related Matters:
1.1.6 Quality
8.5 Disparities in Health Care
11.1.3 Allocating Limited Health Care Resources
11.2.2 Conflicts of Interest in Patient Care
11.2.3 Contracts to Deliver Health Care Services
11.2.4 Transparency in Health Care

    (ii) are implemented fairly and do not disadvantage identifiable populations of patients or physicians or exacerbate health care disparities;

    (iii) are implemented in conjunction with the infrastructure and resources needed to support high-value care and physician professionalism;

    (iv) mitigate possible conflicts between physicians' financial interests and patient interests by minimizing the financial impact of patient care decisions and the overall financial risk for individual physicians.

(e) Encourage, rather than discourage, physicians (and others) to:

    (i)   provide care for patients with difficult-to-manage medical conditions;

    (ii) practice at their full capacity, but not beyond.

(f) Recognize physicians' primary obligation to their patients by enabling physicians to respond to the unique needs of individual patients and providing avenues for meaningful appeal and advocacy on behalf of patients.

(g) Are routinely monitored to:

    (i)   identify and address adverse consequences;

    (ii) identify and encourage dissemination of positive outcomes.

All physicians should:

(h) Hold physician-leaders accountable to meeting conditions for professionalism in health care systems.

(i) Advocate for changes in health care payment and delivery models to promote access to high-quality care for all patients.

AMA Principles of Medical Ethics: II

Issued: The constituent Opinions on which this guidance is based (see Concordance) were issued in 1986.

Updated: 2016

Opinions on Related Matters:
1.1.1 Patient-Physician Relationships
2.1.1 Informed Consent
7.1.4 Conflicts of Interest in Research
9.6.9 Physician Self-referral
11.2.1 Professionalism in Health Care Systems

11.2.2 Conflicts of Interest in Patient Care

The primary objective of the medical profession is to render service to humanity; reward or financial gain is a subordinate consideration. Under no circumstances may physicians place their own financial interests above the welfare of their patients.

Treatment or hospitalization that is willfully excessive or inadequate constitutes unethical practice. Physicians should not provide wasteful and unnecessary treatment that may cause needless expense solely for the physician's financial benefit or for the benefit of a hospital or other health care organization with which the physician is affiliated.

Where the economic interests of the hospital, health care organization, or other entity are in conflict with patient welfare, patient welfare takes priority.

11.2.3 Contracts to Deliver Health Care Services

Physicians have a fundamental ethical obligation to put the welfare of patients ahead of other considerations, including personal financial interests. This obligation requires them to consider carefully the terms and conditions of contracts to deliver health care services before entering into such contracts to ensure that those contracts do not create untenable conflicts of interests.

Ongoing evolution in the health care system continues to bring changes to medicine, including changes in reimbursement mechanisms, models for health care delivery, restrictions on referral and use of services, clinical practice guidelines, and limitations on benefits packages. While these changes are intended to enhance quality, efficiency, and safety in health care, they can also put at risk physicians' ability to uphold professional ethical standards of informed consent and fidelity to patients and can impede physicians' freedom to exercise independent professional judgment and tailor care to meet the needs of individual patients.

As physicians enter into various differently structured contracts to deliver health care services—with group practices, hospitals, health plans, or other entities—they should be mindful that while many arrangements have the potential to promote desired improvements in care, some arrangements also have the potential to impede patients' interests.

When contracting to provide health care services, physicians should:

(a) Carefully review the terms of proposed contracts or have a representative do so on their behalf to assure themselves that the arrangement:

  (i) minimizes conflict of interest with respect to proposed reimbursement mechanisms, financial or performance incentives, restrictions on care, or other mechanisms intended to influence physicians' treatment recommendations or direct what care patients receive, in keeping with ethics guidance;

  (ii) does not compromise the physician's own financial well-being or ability to provide high-quality care through unrealistic expectations regarding utilization of services or terms that expose the physician to excessive financial risk;

  (iii) allows the physician to appropriately exercise professional judgment;

  (iv) includes a mechanism to address grievances and supports advocacy on behalf of individual patients;

  (v) permits disclosure to patients.

AMA Principles of Medical Ethics: I, II, III, V, VI, VIII, IX

Issued: The constituent Opinions on which this guidance is based (see Concordance) were issued between 1996 and 1998.

Updated: 2016

Opinions on Related Matters:
1.1.1 Patient-Physician Relationships
1.1.6 Quality
11.2.1 Professionalism in Health Care Systems
11.2.4 Transparency in Health Care

(b) Negotiate modification or removal of any terms that unduly compromise physicians' ability to uphold ethical standards.

AMA Principles of Medical Ethics: III, IV, VI, VII

Issued: 2014

Opinions on Related Matters:
9.5.2 Staff Privileges
9.6.9 Physician Self-referral
11.2.1 Professionalism in Health Care Systems

11.2.3.1 Restrictive Covenants

Competition among physicians is ethically justifiable when it is based on such factors as quality of services, skill, experience, conveniences offered to patients, fees, or credit terms.

Covenants not to compete restrict competition, can disrupt continuity of care, and may limit access to care.

Physicians should not enter into covenants that:

(a) Unreasonably restrict the right of a physician to practice medicine for a specified period of time or in a specified geographic area on termination of a contractual relationship; and

(b) Do not make reasonable accommodation for patients' choice of physician.

Physicians in training should not be asked to sign covenants not to compete as a condition of entry into any residency or fellowship program.

AMA Principles of Medical Ethics: I, II, III, V, VI

Issued: The constituent Opinions on which this guidance is based (see Concordance) were issued between 1986 and 1996.

Updated: 2016

Opinions on Related Matters:
1.1.1 Patient-Physician Relationships
2.1.1 Informed Consent
11.2.1 Professionalism in Health Care Systems
11.2.2 Conflicts of Interest in Patient Care
11.2.3 Contracts to Deliver Health Care Services

11.2.4 Transparency in Health Care

Respect for patients' autonomy is a cornerstone of medical ethics. Patients must rely on their physicians to provide information that patients would reasonably want to know to make informed, well-considered decisions about their health care. Thus, physicians have an obligation to inform patients about all appropriate treatment options, the risks and benefits of alternatives, and other information that may be pertinent, including the existence of payment models, financial incentives, and formularies, guidelines, or other tools that influence treatment recommendations and care. Restrictions on disclosure can impede communication between patient and physician and undermine trust, patient choice, and quality of care.

Although health plans and other entities may have primary responsibility to inform patient-members about plan provisions that will affect the availability of care, physicians share in this responsibility.

Individually, physicians should:

(a) Disclose any financial and other factors that could affect the patient's care.

(b) Disclose relevant treatment alternatives, including those that may not be covered under the patient's health plan.

(c) Encourage patients to be aware of the provisions of their health plan.

Collectively, physicians should advocate that health plans with which they contract disclose to patient-members:

(d) Plan provisions that limit care, such as formularies or constraints on referrals.

(e) Plan provisions for obtaining desired care that would otherwise not be provided, such as provision for off-formulary prescribing.

(f) Plan relationships with pharmacy benefit management organizations and other commercial entities that have an interest in physicians' treatment recommendations.

11.2.5 Retainer Practices

Physicians are free to enter into contracts to provide special non-medical services and amenities with individual patients who are willing and able to pay additional costs out of pocket for such services. While such retainer contracts are one among many diverse models for delivering and paying for health care, they can also raise ethical concerns about access, quality, and continuity of care.

Regardless of the model within which they practice, physicians must uphold their primary professional obligation of fidelity and their responsibility to treat all patients with courtesy and respect for patients' rights and dignity, and ensure that all patients in the physician's practice receive the same quality of medical care, regardless of contractual arrangements for special, nonmedical services and amenities.

Physicians who enter into retainer contracts with patients must:

(a) Present the terms of the retainer arrangement clearly to patients, including implications for the patient's current health care insurance, if known, and take care not to imply that more or better medical services will be provided under a retainer contract.

(b) Ensure that patient decisions to accept retainer contracts are voluntary and that patients are free to opt out of entering into a retainer agreement.

(c) Facilitate transfer of care for any patient who chooses not to participate in a retainer practice. If it is not feasible to transfer a patient's care to another local physician, the physician should continue to provide care under the terms of the patient's existing health care insurance until other appropriate arrangements for ongoing care can be made.

AMA Principles of Medical Ethics: I, II, VI, VIII, IX

Issued: 2003

Updated: 2016

Opinions on Related Matters:
1.1.1 Patient-Physician Relationships
8.5 Disparities in Health Care
11.1.4 Financial Barriers to Health Care Access
11.2.1 Professionalism in Health Care Systems
11.2.4 Transparency in Health Care

(d) Ensure that treatment recommendations for all patients are based on scientific evidence, relevant professional guidelines, sound professional judgment, and prudent stewardship.

(e) Uphold standards of honesty and transparency in billing and clearly distinguish charges for special services or amenities provided under a retainer contract from medical services reimbursable by the patient's health care insurance or third-party payer.

(f) Uphold professional obligations to promote access to health care and to provide care to those in need regardless of ability to pay, in keeping with ethics guidance.

Fees and Charges

AMA Principles of Medical Ethics: II, VI

Issued: The constituent Opinions on which this guidance is based (see Concordance) were issued between 1977 and 1984.

Updated: 2016

Opinions on Related Matters:
11.3.2 Fees for Nonclinical and Administrative Services

11.3.1 Fees for Medical Services

Physicians are expected to conduct themselves as honest, responsible professionals. They should be knowledgeable about and conform to relevant laws and should adhere to professional ethical standards and sound business practice. Physicians should not recommend, provide, or charge for unnecessary medical services. Nor should they make intentional misrepresentations to increase the level of payment they receive or to secure noncovered health benefits for their patients.

With regard to fees for medical services, physicians should:

(a) Charge reasonable fees based on the:
  (i)   kind of service(s);
  (ii) difficulty or uniqueness of the service(s) performed;
  (iii) time required to perform the service(s);
  (iv) skill required to perform the service(s);
  (v)   experience of the physician;
  (vi) quality of the physician's performance.

(b) Charge only for the service(s) that are personally rendered or for services performed under the physician's direct personal observation, direction, or supervision. If possible, when services are provided by more than one physician, each physician should submit his or her own bill to the patient and be compensated separately. When physicians have professional colleagues assist in the performance of a service, the physician may pay a reasonable amount for such assistance and recoup that amount through fees charged to the patient, provided the patient is notified in advance of the financial arrangement.

(c) Itemize separately charges for diagnostic, laboratory, or clinical services provided by other health care professionals and indicate who provided the service when fees for others' services cannot be billed directly to the patient, in addition to charges for the physician's own professional services.

(d) Not charge excessive fees, contingent fees, or fees solely to facilitate hospital admission. Physicians must not charge a markup or commission, or profit on services rendered by other health care professionals.

(e) Extend professional courtesy at their discretion, recognizing that it is not an ethical requirement and is prohibited in many jurisdictions.

11.3.2 Fees for Nonclinical and Administrative Services

Physicians individually and collectively should promote access to care for individual patients, in part through being prudent stewards of resources. Thus, physicians have a responsibility to balance patients' needs and expectations with responsible business practices.

With respect to fees for nonclinical or administrative services provided in conjunction with patient care, physicians should:

(a) Clearly notify patients in advance of fees charged by the practice (if any) for nonclinical or administrative services.

(b) Base fees (if any) on reasonable costs to the practice for:
   (i) providing special documentation on patient request for such purposes as insurance reimbursement to the patient, certification of immunization or fitness, or similar nonclinical services;
   (ii) missed appointments or appointments not cancelled in advance in keeping with the published policy of the practice;
   (iii) acquisition or processing charges in relation to diagnostic, laboratory, or clinical services, copies of medical records, or similar nonclinical services.

AMA Principles of Medical Ethics: II, VI

Issued: The constituent Opinions on which this guidance is based (see Concordance) were issued prior to 1977.

Updated: 2016

Opinions on Related Matters:
11.3.1 Fees for Medical Services

11.3.3 Interest and Finance Charges

Financial obstacles to medical care can directly affect patients' well-being and may diminish physicians' ability to use their knowledge and skills on patients' behalf. Physicians should not be expected to risk the viability of their practices or compromise

AMA Principles of Medical Ethics: II, VI, IX

Issued: Prior to 1977
Updated: 1994, 2016

quality of care by routinely providing care without compensation. Patients should make reasonable efforts to meet their financial responsibilities or to discuss financial hardships with their physicians.

To preserve patients' dignity and help sustain the patient-physician relationship, physicians should be candid about financial matters and:

(a) Clearly notify patients in advance about policy and practice with respect to delinquent accounts, including under what circumstances:
  (i)   payment will be requested at the time of service;
  (ii) interest or finance charges may be levied;
  (iii) a past due account will be sent to a collection agency.
(b) Ensure that no bills are sent to collection without the physician's knowledge.
(c) Use discretion and compassion in hardship cases, in keeping with ethics guidance regarding financial barriers to health care access.

AMA Principles of Medical Ethics: II

Issued: The constituent Opinions on which this guidance is based (see Concordance) were issued between 1977 and 1997.

Updated: 2016

Opinions on Related Matters:
9.6.9 Physician Self-referral

11.3.4 Fee Splitting

Patients must be able to trust that their physicians will be honest with them and will make treatment recommendations, including referrals, based on medical need, the skill of other health care professionals or facilities to whom the patient is referred, and the quality of products or services provided.

Payment by or to a physician or health care institution solely for referral of a patient is fee splitting and is unethical.

Physicians may not accept:

(a) Any payment of any kind, from any source, for referring a patient other than distributions of a health care organization's revenues as permitted by law.
(b) Any payment of any kind, from any source, for prescribing a specific drug, product, or service.
(c) Payment for services relating to the care of a patient from any health care facility or organization to which the physician has referred the patient.
(d) Payment referring a patient to a research study.

Physicians in a capitated primary care practice may not refer patients based on whether the referring physician has negotiated a discount for specialty services.

Guide to the Use of Annotations

The *Code of Medical Ethics* (*Code*) of the American Medical Association, consisting of the Principles of Medical Ethics and Opinions of the Council on Ethical and Judicial Affairs (CEJA) that interpret them, is an important source of guidance for responsible professional conduct. Together, the Principles and Opinions have served as the primary statement of the values to which physicians commit themselves as members of the medical profession.

The impact of the *Code* has been significant. Attorneys, judges, and scholars in medical ethics have looked to the Principles and Opinions for legal advocacy and decision making in health care. These Annotations are designed to provide a research and reference tool for practitioners, scholars, jurists, and others. Annotations summarize all reported court decisions and selected state attorney general opinions that make substantive reference to Principles or Opinions, as well as selected articles from the medical, legal, and ethics literature.

Each case annotation offers a synopsis of facts and legal issues, then focuses on the court's reference to the Principle(s) or Opinion(s) and the role it played in the decision. Where necessary, each case annotation includes a cross-reference to the relevant provision(s) of the version of the Principles and Opinions as they appeared in the 2014-2015 edition of the *Code. Note that the Annotations have not been updated for this edition of the Code.*

Journal annotations provide a general summary of the subject article and indicate which specific Principle(s) or Opinion(s) the article references, with appropriate cross-reference to the Principle or Opinion as it appeared in the 2014-2015 edition of the *Code*. Each journal annotation indicates whether the article *refers to* the Principle or Opinion in a general way; specifically *cites* the Principle or Opinion; or directly *quotes* the language of the Principle or Opinion.

To facilitate efficient use of this resource, both case and journal annotations identify the specific page(s) where the Principle(s) or Opinion(s) are discussed. An Index of Cases and an Index of Articles are also provided to enhance the usefulness of this compendium.

The Principles and Opinions have a long and evolving history. Over time, some Principles and Opinions have been substantially amended or eliminated. Moreover, in 2008, CEJA launched an ambitious project to review each of the more than 200 individual Opinions included in the *Code* at that time. Over the course of nearly 8 years, with input from the member organizations represented in the AMA House of Delegates and other stakeholders, CEJA updated the Opinions to ensure that guidance remains relevant and consistent. CEJA reorganized the Opinions into more intuitive, topically based chapters and recast the guidance of each individual Opinion into a uniform format to make guidance easy to find and use. Annotations for each constituent opinion are presented here in sequence. Users are advised to carefully review the particular case or article under consideration with respect to the user's specific interest. A Concordance maps the updated Opinions in the present volume to their predecessors in the 2014-2015 edition of the *Code*.

CEJA thanks the individuals who supervised preparation of these Annotations under contract to the AMA, along with the students and staff who ably provided research, editing, and other assistance to the project:

Kelly Armstrong, PhD
SOUTHERN ILLINOIS UNIVERSITY
SCHOOL OF MEDICINE
DEPARTMENTS OF MEDICAL HUMANITIES AND
INTERNAL MEDICINE

W. Eugene Basanta, JD, LLM
SOUTHERN ILLINOIS UNIVERSITY
SCHOOL OF LAW
CENTER FOR HEALTH LAW AND POLICY

Frank G. Houdek, JD, MLS
ASSOCIATE DEAN
SOUTHERN ILLINOIS UNIVERSITY
SCHOOL OF LAW

Connie Poole, AMLS
SOUTHERN ILLINOIS UNIVERSITY
SCHOOL OF MEDICINE
DEPARTMENT OF INFORMATION AND
COMMUNICATION SCIENCES

Annotations

Principles of Medical Ethics

Preamble

Haw. 1995 After physician was convicted of attempted first-degree sexual abuse and kidnapping, the civil court affirmed the Board of Medical Examiner's decision to suspend him from practicing medicine for one year. In challenging Board's action, physician argued, among other things, that convictions were not related to his qualifications, functions, or duties as a physician. The court disagreed with all of physician's points of error on appeal. In considering physician's claim that convictions were not related to his duties as a physician, the court referred to the Preamble as reflecting a duty to the public generally. *Loui v. Board of Medical Examiners, 78 Haw. 21, 889 P.2d 705, 714.*

Ind. 1991 Plaintiff sued physician for injuries caused by physician's patient as the result of medication administered by the physician. Weighing (1) the relationship between the parties, (2) the reasonable foreseeability of harm to the injured party, and (3) public policy, the court held that a physician generally owes no duty to unknown third parties who may be injured by the physician's treatment of a patient. Concurring opinion quoted the Preamble, which mandates that a physician "recognize responsibility . . . to society," arguing that there is no absolute immunity to third-party suits. *Webb v. Jarvis, 575 N.E.2d 992, 998.*

N.J. 1979 In wrongful death action against a psychiatrist whose patient murdered plaintiff's decedent, the court concluded, in accord with Principle 9 (1957) [now Principle IV], that a psychiatrist may owe a duty to warn potential victims of possible danger from psychiatrist's patient despite the general emphasis on confidentiality. The court also noted the Preamble and Principles 1 and 3 (1957) [now revised Preamble, Principle I, and Opinion 5.05] in discussing the psychiatrist-patient relationship. *McIntosh v. Milano, 168 N.J. Super. 466, 403 A.2d 500, 510, 512-13.*

Journal 2011 Discusses the development of lethal autonomous robots, as well as issues raised by this new military technology. Concludes discussion on the advancement and acceptance of lethal autonomous robots is needed on the national and international levels in order to successfully manage advancements in robotic technology. Cites Preamble and Principles I and VI. Allenby, Arkin, Barrett, Borenstein, Gaudet, Kittrie, Lin, Lucas, Marchant, O'Meara, & Silberman, *International Governance of Autonomous Military Robots, 12 Colum. Sci. & Tech. L. Rev. 272, 291 (2011).*

Journal 2010 Analyzes factors contributing to the emergence of medical repatriation and evaluates whether this practice comports with current legal and ethical standards. Proposes changes to federal regulations that govern hospitals and clarifications to medical ethical standards. Quotes the Preamble and Principles I, II, III, IV, V, VI, VII, VIII, and IX. Zoellner, *Medical Repatriation: Examining the Legal and Ethical Implications of an Emerging Practice, 32 Wash. U. J. L. & Pol'y 515, 530-532 (2010).*

Journal 2009 Examines the ethical guidelines regarding physicians' participation in interrogations and statutory approaches aimed at eliminating such physician involvement. Concludes that to maintain the integrity of the medical profession, physician involvement in interrogations must be precluded by legislative action. Quotes Preamble and Opinions 2.067 and 2.068. Cites Opinions 2.06 and 2.068. Bahnassi, *Keeping Doctors Out of the Interrogation Room: A New Ethical Obligation That Requires the Backing of the Law, 19 Health Matrix 447, 449-51, 461, 464, 465-67, 469-70, 474-75 (2009).*

Journal 2009 Explores the Supreme Court's *Baze v. Rees* decision and the three-drug protocol for lethal injection. Discusses the necessity of judicial intervention to improve lethal injection protocols. Concludes courts should carefully consider their approach to challenges to lethal injection as an opportunity to prevent violation of Eighth Amendment rights. Quotes Preamble and Opinion 1.02. Cites Opinion 2.06. Berger, *Lethal Injection and the Problem of Constitutional Remedies*, 27 Yale L. & Pol'y Rev. 259, 319, 320 (2009).

Journal 2009 Discusses the essential role of professionals in the community and the conflicting moral obligations facing professionals. Concludes the legal profession's insistence that priority be given exclusively to the client's interests prevents it from successfully addressing ethical problems. Cites Preamble and Principle VII. Greenstein, *Against Professionalism*, 22 Geo. J. Legal Ethics 327, 349 (2009).

Journal 2009 Explores the nature of the physician-patient relationship and the impact of increased availability of medical information on patient autonomy and physician responsibility to exercise independent judgment. Concludes physicians must treat patients in accordance with their fiduciary obligation to use their own judgment when confronted with a patient demanding unnecessary medical services. Quotes Preamble, Principles I and VIII, and Opinions 2.035, 8.03, and 10.015. Hafemeister, *The Fiduciary Obligation of Physicians to "Just Say No" If an "Informed" Patient Demands Services That Are Not Medically Indicated*, 39 Seton Hall L. Rev. 335, 372, 373, 374 (2009).

Journal 2009 Discusses the right of health care professionals to refuse to provide health care services to lesbian, gay, or bisexual (LGB) individuals, because of moral or religious objections, and its impact on access to health care services, including assisted reproduction and elder health care services, for such patients. Concludes physicians should adhere to professional ethical standards to promote LGB patients' autonomy and equal access to care. Quotes Preamble. Cites Opinion 10.05. Reibman, *The Patient Wanted the Doctor to Treat Her in the Closet, but the Janitor Wouldn't Open the Door: Healthcare Provider Rights of Refusal Versus LGB Rights to Reproductive and Elder Healthcare*, 28 Temp. J. Sci. Tech. & Envtl. L. 65, 90-91 (2009).

Journal 2009 Discusses the tension between duties of confidentiality and to protect third parties owed by mental health professionals to their patients and the public. Analyzes current Illinois law regarding these duties. Argues because Illinois law causes confusion regarding a professional's duty to disclose, inappropriately restricts the protected class, and leads to unnecessary breaches of confidentiality, clarification is necessary. Quotes Preamble and Opinion 5.05. Wood, *Protective Privilege versus Public Peril: How Illinois Has Failed to Balance Patient Confidentiality With the Mental Health Professional's Duty to Protect the Public*, 29 N. Ill. U. L. Rev. 571, 581, 598 (2009).

Journal 2008 Discusses issues arising from the increase in retail clinics and their impact on patients. Concludes the growth of retail clinics should be established on the same principles as traditional clinics to maximize their benefits to patients and to the health care community. Quotes Preamble. Hsu, *Legal Issues Concerning Retail Clinics*, 20 Health Law 13, 22 (June 2008).

Journal 2008 Examines the ethical reasons why physicians choose to provide treatment in disaster situations, even at great risk to themselves. Concludes that individual values play a substantial role in such decision making. Quotes Preamble, Opinion 9.131, and Ch. III, Art. 1, Sec. 1 (1847) [now Opinions 2.25 and 9.067]. Iserson, Heine, Larkin, Moskop, Baruch, & Aswegan, *Fight or Flight: The Ethics of Emergency Physician Disaster Response*, 51 Annals of Emergency Med. 345, 346-47 (2008).

Journal 2007 Compares the role of conscience clauses in various professions. Concludes that conscience clauses in the area of health care must not impede access to care. Quotes Preamble and Principles V, VI, and VIII. Chudoba, *Conscience in America: The Slippery Slope of Mixing Morality With Medicine*, 36 Sw. U. L. Rev. 85, 86, 103, 104, 105 (2007).

Journal 2007 Addresses physician liability for an extramarital affair with a patient's spouse. Concludes that such an affair should be regarded as a breach of a fiduciary duty. Quotes Preamble, Principles I, II, and VIII, and Opinions 8.145, 9.04, 9.123, and 10.015. Demaine, *"Playing Doctor" With the Patient's Spouse: Alternative Conceptions of Health Professional Liability*, 14 Va. J. Soc. Pol'y & L. 308, 325, 330-31, 331-32 (2007).

Journal 2007 Compares laws of client abandonment with those of patient abandonment by physicians. Concludes that physicians should be required to show good cause to justify abandonment. Quotes Ch. II, Art. I, Sec. 5 (1903) [now Preamble]. References Opinion 8.115. LeBlanc, *Abandoning Patients and Clients: Where Medicine Can Learn From Law*, 1 Charleston L. Rev. 237, 237-38, 256 (2007).

Journal 2007 Analyzes scientific, ethical, and legal issues raised in the exhumation and genetic analysis of historical figures. Concludes that biohistorical review boards should be created to generate guidelines for such research. Quotes Preamble and Opinion 2.08. Cites Opinions 2.079, 2.105, 5.05, 5.051, 5.075, 8.03, 8.031, 9.095, and 9.10. Paradise & Andrews, *Tales From the Crypt: Scientific, Ethical, and Legal Considerations for Biohistorical Analysis of Deceased Historical Figures*, 26 Temp. J. Sci. Tech. & Envtl. L. 223, 287-88 (2007).

Journal 2007 Examines how the subject of medical ethics is taught in US medical schools. Concludes that ethics should be broadly integrated into the curriculum throughout medical school. Quotes Preamble. Rooksby, *Ethics Education in Medical Schools: Problems, Practices, and Possibilities*, 10 Quinnipiac Health L. J. 181, 205 (2007).

Journal 2006 Examines the legal and public health issues raised by increased rates of hepatitis C in prison populations. Concludes that reform is needed to provide adequate health care to prisoners and that courts have the power to require such care under the Eighth Amendment. Quotes Preamble, Principles VII, VIII, and IX, and Opinion 10.015. Brunsden, *Hepatitis C in Prisons: Evolving Toward Decency Through Adequate Medical Care and Public Health Reform, 54 UCLA L. Rev. 465, 500 (2006).*

Journal 2006 Considers the interaction of laws, rules, and guidelines in the area of health law. Suggests that the legislature should revise current laws to reflect local variability in practice. Quotes Preamble and Principles VII and IX. Heimer, *Responsibility in Health Care: Spanning the Boundary Between Law and Medicine, 41 Wake Forest L. Rev. 465, 498 (2006).*

Journal 2006 Examines a mental health professional's competing duties of confidentiality and reporting a patient's threats of violence. Suggests new legislation should clarify duty to report a threat. Quotes Preamble and Principles III, IV, and VIII. Cites Opinion 5.05. Mossman, *Critique of Pure Risk Assessment or, Kant Meets Tarasoff, 75 U. Cin. L. Rev. 523, 579 (2006).*

Journal 2006 Addresses the problem of disruptive dialysis patients. Concludes that the dialysis care system must change to prevent dismissal of these patients. Quotes Preamble. Smetanka, *Who Will Protect the "Disruptive" Dialysis Patient? 32 Am. J. L. & Med. 53, 89 (2006).*

Journal 2004 Discusses the "no-harm" doctrine as a long-held legal and moral principle. Concludes that this doctrine protects personal liberties and shields citizens from harmful religious or secular action. Quotes Preamble. Hamilton, *Religious Institutions, the No-Harm Doctrine, and the Public Good, 2004 B.Y.U. L. Rev. 1099, 1175, 1176 (2004).*

Journal 2004 Analyzes various issues relating to the role of mental health professionals in capital punishment in light of Albert Bandura's model of "mechanisms of moral disengagement." Concludes that facilitating participation of mental health professionals in executions creates conflicts with the humanistic norms of the profession. Quotes Preamble and Opinions 1.01, 1.02, 2.06, 2.067, 2.20, 2.21, 2.211, and 8.14. Judges, *The Role of Mental Health Professionals in Capital Punishment: An Exercise in Moral Disengagement, 41 Hous. L. Rev. 515, 562, 568, 569, 570, 571-72, 581, 586, 588, 598 (2004).*

Journal 2003 Examines policy options for integration of traditional and modern medicine. Concludes that solid cross-sectoral linkages between different traditions can stabilize an integrated health care system. Quotes Preamble and Principle V. Holliday, *Traditional Medicines in Modern Societies: An Exploration of Integrationist Options Through East Asian Experience, 28 J. Med. & Phil. 373, 387 (2003).*

Journal 2003 Considers conflicts of interest and potential liability that a team physician faces when treating an injured athlete. Concludes that an athlete's health should be the team physician's primary concern in making treatment decisions. References Principles I and II. Landis, *The Team Physician: An Analysis of the Causes of Action, Conflicts, Defenses and Improvements, 1 DePaul J. Sports L. & Contemp. Probs. 139, 144 (2003).*

Journal 2002 Explores the implications of withholding medical treatment when abortion results in a live birth. Concludes that, in these situations, abortive parents and physicians should not solely decide the child's best interest. Quotes Preamble, Principles I and III, and Opinions 2.035, 2.20, and 2.215. Casagrande, *Children Not Meant to Be: Protecting the Interests of the Child When Abortion Results in Live Birth, 6 Quinnipiac Health L. J. 19, 44, 45, 47-48 (2002).*

Journal 2002 Considers the dilemma of informed consent in the context of prescribing psychotropic medication to patients with mental illness and mental retardation. Recognizes the need for substituted decision-making in certain situations. Concludes that legislation would help address this issue. Quotes Preamble, Principles I, III, IV, VIII, and IX, and Opinion 8.08. O'Sullivan & Borcherding, *Informed Consent for Medication in Persons With Mental Retardation and Mental Illness, 12 Health Matrix 63, 75, 86, 87, 88 (2002).*

Journal 2002 Discusses legal and medical policies that protect confidentiality in the physician-patient relationship. Concludes that reducing the current level of privacy protection would jeopardize health care. Quotes Preamble and Opinions 2.136, 5.05, and 10.01. References Principles VIII and IX. Sciarrino, *Ferguson v. City of Charleston: "The Doctor Will See You Now, Be Sure to Bring Your Privacy Rights in With You!" 12 Temp. Pol. & Civ. Rts. L. Rev. 197, 213, 215, 220, 221, 222 (2002).*

Journal 2000 Examines the increased prominence of medical ethics in light of various changes in medicine and society. Concludes with observations regarding how "preventive ethics" can enhance patient care. Quotes Preamble. Nandi, *Ethical Aspects of Clinical Practice, 135 Arch. Surg. 22, 23 (2000).*

Journal 2000 Examines current laws prohibiting discrimination in the context of access to health care, placing emphasis on people with HIV/AIDS. Considers the implications of *Bragdon v. Abbott*. Concludes that everyone should be entitled to health care in the absence of an acceptable justification for its denial. Quotes Preamble, Principle VI, and Opinion 9.131. Shepherd, *HIV, the ADA, and the Duty to Treat, 37 Hous. L. Rev. 1055, 1061, 1083-84 (2000).*

Journal 1999 Asserts that patient autonomy is closely linked to patient-physician discourse. Proposes a constitutional framework for evaluating how governmental regulations may interfere with such discourse. Concludes by emphasizing the importance of protecting the quality of physician-patient discourse. Quotes Preamble and Opinion 8.03. Gatter, *Protecting Patient-Doctor Discourse: Informed Consent and Deliberative Autonomy, 78 Or. L. Rev. 941, 956 (1999).*

Journal 1998 Argues that the doctrine of informed consent should not be abandoned. Explains why informed consent is needed. Suggests that even if physicians cannot determine patients' best interests, they can determine patients' reasonable interests. Quotes Preamble. White & Zimbelman, *Abandoning Informed Consent: An Idea Whose Time Has Not Yet Come*, 23 J. Med. Phil. 477, 496 (1998).

Journal 1997 Examines noncompetition clauses in the medical field. Reviews policy concerns and historical and common-law analyses of agreements not to compete. Posits that the more commercialized the medical profession becomes, the more noncompetition clauses infringe upon the physician-patient relationship and patients' rights. Quotes Opinions 9.02 and 9.06. Cites Preamble and Opinion 6.11. Comment, *Noncompetition Clauses in Physician Employment Contracts in Oregon*, 76 Or. L. Rev. 195, 204-06 (1997).

Journal 1997 Considers principles of confidentiality in the physician-patient relationship. Notes the current trend emphasizing public reporting obligations of physicians to protect members of society. Emphasizes need for balance between patient rights and societal interests. Quotes Principle IV and Opinion 5.05. References Preamble. Jozefowicz, *The Case Against Having Professional Privilege in the Physician-Patient Relationship*, 16 Med. & L. 385, 386-87, 391 (1997).

Journal 1997 Discusses the need for balance between business ethics and medical ethics in the context of managed care. Explores two models for integrating ethics and managed care. Proposes the adoption of a collective responsibility model to improve quality of care. Quotes Principles I, II, III, IV, and V. Cites Preamble. References Opinion 8.13. Regan, *Regulating the Business of Medicine: Models for Integrating Ethics and Managed Care*, 30 Colum. J. L. & Soc. Probs. 635, 651, 656, 657 (1997).

Journal 1996 Considers the impact of gag clauses on the physician-patient relationship. Undertakes an extensive legal, ethical, and policy analysis. Concludes that gag clauses are violative of legal and ethical principles. Quotes Principles II, V, and VI, and Fundamental Elements (1). Cites Preamble. Martin & Bjerknes, *The Legal and Ethical Implications of Gag Clauses in Physician Contracts*, XXII Am. J. Law & Med. 433, 465-66 (1996).

Journal 1996 Considers prearraignment forensic evaluations. Notes the prohibition against use of such evaluations. Examines underlying ethical precepts. Observes that

principles of beneficence are misapplied to forensic psychiatry in this context. Advocates a new ethical framework. Quotes Preamble. References Principle IV and Opinion 5.05. Ornish, Mills, & Ornish, *Prearraignment Forensic Evaluations: Toward a New Policy*, 24 Bull. Am. Acad. Psychiatry Law 453, 454, 469 (1996).

Journal 1995 Examines the metaphor of physicians as fiduciaries. Considers how the law holds physicians accountable in this regard. Quotes Preamble. Cites Opinion 8.03 (1986) [now Opinion 8.032]. Rodwin, *Strains in the Fiduciary Metaphor: Divided Physician Loyalties and Obligations in a Changing Health Care System*, XXI Am. J. Law & Med. 241, 246, 250 (1995).

Journal 1994 Reviews the evolution of the physician-patient relationship, with attention to patient autonomy. Examines the changing health care delivery environment. Quotes Preamble, Principles I, II, III, IV, V, and VI, Fundamental Elements (1) and (2), and Opinions 1.02 and 8.07 (1981) [now Opinion 8.08]. Cites Opinion 1.01. Szczygiel, *Beyond Informed Consent*, 21 Ohio N. U. L. Rev. 171, 217, 218, 220, 225, 226, 256 (1994).

Journal 1993 Discusses ethical issues that may arise in the context of caring for the critically ill. Emphasizes the need for organization of patient care when multiple providers are involved. Quotes Preamble. Bruening, Andrew, & Smith, *Concurrent Care: An Ethical Issue for Family Physicians*, 36 J. Fam. Practice 606, 607 (1993).

Journal 1991 Examines the informed consent doctrine and how it was broadened in *Moore v. Regents of the University of California*. Concludes that, in California, under Moore, a physician must disclose to patients any economic or research interest he or she might have in the patient's medical treatment. Quotes Preamble. Guise, *Expansion of the Scope of Disclosure Required Under the Informed Consent Doctrine: Moore v. The Regents of the University of California*, 28 San Diego L. Rev. 455, 462 (1991).

Journal 1990 Discusses the moral dilemma in deciding whether to withdraw artificial nutrition and hydration from a patient and the appropriate role of the judiciary. Concludes that judicial decisions do not represent the moral viewpoint of society and that moral pronouncements should not be made in the courtroom. Quotes Preamble, Principles I, II, III, IV, V, VI, and VII, and Opinion 2.20. Peccarelli, *A Moral Dilemma: The Role of Judicial Intervention in Withholding or Withdrawing Nutrition and Hydration*, 23 John Marshall L. Rev. 537, 539, 540, 541 (1990).

Principle I

10th Cir. 2001 Plaintiffs, former employees of a public medical center, brought suit against medical director under 42 USC § 1983, based upon medical director's racially and sexually harassing actions and statements. The district court awarded compensatory and punitive damages against the

medical director. Affirming the award of damages, the court quoted Principles I and IV and concluded that the medical director's behavior impacted not only plaintiffs, but the overall public health. *Nieto v. Kapoor*, 268 F.3d 1208, 1223 n. 12.

D. Kan. 1995 Plaintiff, an occupational medicine physician, alleged that defendant, medical group, wrongfully discharged him in violation of public policy and in breach of the implied covenant of good faith and fair dealing. Defendant complained that plaintiff consistently granted excess time off to patients. Even though defendant warned plaintiff that he would be terminated if he continued this practice, plaintiff refused to comply stating that he was ethically obligated to serve the best interests of his patients. Plaintiff claimed that to place the defendant's interests above his legal and ethical duties to his patients would violate public policy as set out by statute and the Principles of Medical Ethics, with apparent reference to Principle I. Since plaintiff failed to show that defendant's practice caused harm to patients or deviated from accepted standards, the court disregarded plaintiff's public policy exception to the employment-at-will doctrine and granted defendant's motion for summary judgment. *Aiken v. Business & Indus. Health Group, 886 F. Supp. 1565, 1571.*

N.J. 1979 In wrongful death action against a psychiatrist whose patient murdered plaintiff's decedent, the court concluded, in accord with Principle 9 (1957) [now Principle IV], that a psychiatrist may owe a duty to warn potential victims of possible danger from psychiatrist's patient despite the general emphasis on confidentiality. The court also noted the Preamble and Principles 1 and 3 (1957) [now revised Preamble, Principle I, and Opinion 5.05] in discussing the psychiatrist-patient relationship. *McIntosh v. Milano, 168 N.J. Super. 466, 403 A.2d 500, 510, 512-13.*

Ohio 2009 Physician appealed from a judgment affirming an order of the State Medical Board that permanently revoked appellant's certificate to practice medicine. The Board found that appellant's sexual contact with patients violated Ohio statutes governing physician conduct and the Code of Ethics of the AMA, citing Principles I, II, IV, and VIII. The Court of Appeals held that Ohio state law allows the Board to revoke a physician's certificate if it finds that the person violated any provision of the Code of Ethics of the AMA. *D'Souza v. State Med. Bd. of Ohio, 2009 WL 5108774, 6.*

Ohio 2000 Hospital sought court order permitting administration of antipsychotic medication to an involuntarily committed mentally ill patient without consent. The court said that forced medication is permitted in certain instances, including where medical personnel determine that patients present an imminent risk of harm to themselves or others. Quoting Principle I, the court found that placing such authority in a physician's hands is appropriate. Because the treating physician testified the patient did not pose a risk, the court ruled forced medication could not be required on this basis. *Steele v. Hamilton County Cmty. Mental Health Bd., 90 Ohio St. 3d 176, 736 N.E.2d 10, 18.*

Ohio 1991 State medical board revoked license of physician who had consensual sexual relations with his patient. The court upheld the board's ruling that this violated Principles I, II, and IV. Dissenting judge, citing AMA Council on Ethical and Judicial Affairs, Sexual Misconduct in the Practice of Medicine, 266 *JAMA* 2741 [now Opinion 8.14], argued that until 1991, the AMA did not clearly deem sexual contact with a patient unethical. *Pons v. Ohio State Medical Bd., 66 Ohio St. 3d 619, 623, 625, 614 N.E.2d 748, 752, 753.*

Ohio App. 2005 The Ohio State Medical Board permanently revoked the license of the appellant, a psychiatrist, for having inappropriate physical and sexual contact with a female patient. The trial court affirmed the Board's ruling, and the appellant appealed. The Board claimed that the appellant's relationship with his patient violated the AMA's Code of Medical Ethics, citing Principles I, II, and IV. The appellate court affirmed, stating that permanent revocation of the appellant's license was not excessive and was not a violation of due process as the Board may revoke the appellant's license if treatment did not meet minimal standards of care and violated any provision of the AMA's Code of Medical Ethics. *Schechter v. Ohio State Med. Bd., 2005 WL 1869733, 9.*

Ohio App. 1999 Physician appealed trial court's affirmation of state medical board's decision to suspend his medical license because the physician engaged in sexual relationships with mothers of his pediatric patients. On appeal the physician claimed that he was denied due process because physicians were not adequately notified that having sexual relations with parents of pediatric patients was unethical. The physician also claimed that the board had not presented adequate evidence that AMA Principles I and IV extend to the parents of pediatric patients. The court quoted Principles I and IV, and stated that medical experts who testified were of the opinion that having sexual relationships with parents of pediatric patients constituted ethical violations. *Gladieux v. Ohio State Medical Board, 1999 WL 770959, *2, *4.*

Journal 2011 Discusses the development of lethal autonomous robots, as well as issues raised by this new military technology. Concludes discussion on the advancement and acceptance of lethal autonomous robots is needed on the national and international levels in order to successfully manage advancements in robotic technology. Cites Preamble and Principles I and VI. Allenby, Arkin, Barrett, Borenstein, Gaudet, Kittrie, Lin, Lucas, Marchant, O'Meara, & Silberman, *International Governance of Autonomous Military Robots, 12 Colum. Sci. & Tech. L. Rev. 272, 291 (2011).*

Journal 2011 Discusses compassion in the medical field and a proposed change to New Zealand law creating a patient's right to be treated with compassion. Concludes in order to eliminate the need for compassion legislation, physicians should have more education on suffering and patient values, and regulators should inform health care providers about what constitutes inappropriate behavior by setting standards of conduct. Quotes Principle I. Paterson, *Can We Mandate Compassion? 41 Hastings Center Rep. 20, 21 (Mar.-Apr. 2011).*

Journal 2011 Argues that regulation of physicians' off-label use of prescription medications is necessary to prevent harm to both the patient and to society via unnecessary increases in health care spending. Concludes the state should intervene in the physician-patient relationship when physicians prescribe medicine off-label that is not justified by high-quality evidence of safety and efficacy. Quotes Principles I and V. Rosoff & Coleman, *The Case for Legal Regulation of Physicians' Off-Label Prescribing*, 86 Notre Dame L. Rev. 649, 675 (2011).

Journal 2010 Argues the medicalization of the concepts of "health" and "harm" has led to a simplistic use of evidence to answer complicated ethical questions, such as the permissibility of the reduction of twins to a singleton. Concludes empirical evidence cannot be a substitute for ethical deliberation. References Principle I. McClimans, *Elective Twin Reductions: Evidence and Ethics*, 24 Bioethics 295, 297 (2010).

Journal 2010 Analyzes factors contributing to the emergence of medical repatriation and evaluates whether this practice comports with current legal and ethical standards. Proposes changes to federal regulations that govern hospitals and clarifications to medical ethical standards. Quotes the Preamble and Principles I, II, III, IV, V, VI, VII, VIII, and IX. Zoellner, *Medical Repatriation: Examining the Legal and Ethical Implications of an Emerging Practice*, 32 Wash. U. J. L. & Pol'y 515, 530-532 (2010).

Journal 2009 Explores emerging issues in conflict management systems design (CMSD). Concludes as the practice of CMSD in the organizational context continues to expand, practitioners should openly discuss the emerging issues of the field. References Principles I, II, V, and VIII. Costantino, *Second Generation Organizational Conflict Management Systems Design: A Practitioner's Perspective on Emerging Issues*, 14 Harv. Negot. L. Rev. 81, 95 (2009).

Journal 2009 Discusses tobacco use in psychiatric institutions and its impact on the health and behavior of patients. Concludes legislative action should be taken to remove tobacco from psychiatric institutions to provide patients with the health and safety benefits of smoke-free facilities. Quotes Principles I and III. Hackett, *Smoke-Free State Psychiatric Facility Grounds: Is Legislation Necessary and Appropriate to Remove Tobacco From These Treatment Settings?* 53 N. Y. L. Sch. L. Rev. 99, 122-23 (2009).

Journal 2009 Discusses whether patients have a right to pain management. Concludes that no physician duty is established by law or ethics to provide pain management outside the traditional physician-patient relationship. Cites Principles I, II, IV, and VIII. Hall & Boswell, *Ethics, Law, and Pain Management as a Patient Right*, 12 Pain Physician 499, 500 (2009).

Journal 2009 Examines the advent of a consumerist model of providing health care services to patients. Concludes that patients as consumers cannot, by themselves, achieve the desired policy goals of containing health care costs and optimizing care quality because the demands on patients and health care providers are too numerous. Cites Principle I. Hall & Schneider, *When Patients Say No (To Save Money): An Essay on the Tectonics of Health Law*, 41 Conn. L. Rev. 743, 770 (2009).

Journal 2009 Explores the nature of the physician-patient relationship and the impact of increased availability of medical information on patient autonomy and physician responsibility to exercise independent judgment. Concludes physicians must treat patients in accordance with their fiduciary obligation to use their own judgment when confronted with a patient demanding unnecessary medical services. Quotes Preamble, Principles I and VIII, and Opinions 2.035, 8.03, and 10.015. Hafemeister, *The Fiduciary Obligation of Physicians to "Just Say No" if an "Informed" Patient Demands Services That Are Not Medically Indicated*, 39 Seton Hall L. Rev. 335, 372, 373, 374 (2009).

Journal 2008 Explores the legal, ethical, and policy implications of concierge medicine. Argues physicians engaged in concierge care must strive to meet ethical and legal standards, and take care to communicate clearly with patients about services and fees. Quotes Opinion 8.055. Cites Principles II and VI and Opinion 8.055. Portman & Romanow, *Concierge Medicine: Legal Issues, Ethical Dilemmas, and Policy Challenges*, 1 J. Health & Life Sci. L. 1, 4, 28-29 (2008).

Journal 2008 Examines the development of bioethics and environmental ethics, as well as laws promoting the role of bioethicists in decision making. Concludes environmental ethicists must convince legislatures of the role of environmental ethics in order to have a greater impact on decision making. Quotes Principles I, II, III, IV, V, VI, VII, VIII, and IX. Robertson, *Seeking a Seat at the Table: Has Law Left Environmental Ethics Behind as It Embraces Bioethics?* 32 Wm. & Mary Envtl. L. & Pol'y Rev. 273, 307 (2008).

Journal 2008 Explores the fiduciary relationship between physicians and patients, professional and ethical obligations of both physicians and lawyers, and the implications for conflict resolution in health care. Concludes physicians must put patient interests above their own and lawyers must work to discern clients' best interests and support client welfare. Quotes Principle VIII and Opinions 8.12 and 10.015. Cites Principles I and II and Opinions 10.01 and 10.015. Scott, *Doctors as Advocates, Lawyers as Healers*, 29 Hamline J. Pub. L. Pol'y, 331, 340-41, 347, 371 (2008).

Journal 2007 Addresses physician liability for an extramarital affair with a patient's spouse. Concludes that such an affair should be regarded as a breach of a fiduciary duty. Quotes Preamble, Principles I, II, and VIII, and Opinions 8.145, 9.04, 9.123, and 10.015. Demaine, *"Playing Doctor" With the Patient's Spouse: Alternative Conceptions of Health Professional Liability*, 14 Va. J. Soc. Pol'y & L. 308, 325, 330-31, 331-32 (2007).

Journal 2007 Discusses the evolution of informed consent doctrine. Concludes that, in context of research, informed consent exceptions should be substantially narrowed. Quotes Ch. I, Art. I, Sec. 4 (May 1847) [now Opinion 8.082], and Ch. I, Art. I, Sec. 1 (May 1847) [now Principles I and VIII]. References Opinions 2.08 and 8.08. Grimm, *Informed Consent for All! No Exceptions*, 37 N. M. L. Rev. 39, 39, 61 (2007).

Journal 2007 Highlights inconsistencies in applying judicial deference to medical ethics. Concludes that courts should afford greater deference to established medical ethics standards. Quotes Principle I and Opinion 2.06 and Ch. II, Art. I, Sec. 3 (May 1847) [now Opinion 5.02]. Cites Opinions 4.01 and 7.05. Lerman, *Second Opinion: Inconsistent Deference to Medical Ethics in Death Penalty Jurisprudence*, 95 Geo. L. J. 1941, 1945, 1974-75, 1976, 1977 (2007).

Journal 2007 Argues that issuance of apologies from physicians who commit medical errors will diminish the number of malpractice suits brought. Concludes that patients desire apologies in the case of medical errors and are less likely to sue when they are given. Cites Principles I, II, III, and IV and Opinion 8.12. Tabler, *Should Physicians Apologize for Medical Errors?* 19 Health Lawyer 23, 25 (Jan. 2007).

Journal 2006 Examines ethical dilemmas physicians may face as providers of pay-for-performance medical care. Concludes that this strategy offers a benefit to patients as long as physicians uphold stringent ethical standards and work together to ensure optimum patient care. Cites Principles I, V, VIII, and IX and Opinions 2.035, 2.095, 6.01, 8.021, 8.03, 8.0501, 8.053, 8.054, and 8.121. Bostick, Sade, & McMahon, *Report of the Council on Ethical and Judicial Affairs: Physician Pay-For-Performance Programs*, 3 Ind. Health L. Rev. 429, 430, 431, 432-33, 434, 435, 436 (2006).

Journal 2006 Explores conscience clause legislation relating to the dispensing of oral contraceptives. Concludes that such legislation must balance the interests of the patient and the health care provider. Cites Principles I, II, III, IV, V, VI, VII, VIII, and IX. Collins, *Conscience Clauses and Oral Contraceptives: Conscientious Objection or Calculated Obstruction?* 15 Ann. Health L. 37, 54 (2006).

Journal 2006 Discusses mentally incompetent inmates and capital punishment. Proposes that, to be permissible, involuntary medication of death-row inmates must represent the best medically appropriate treatment. Quotes Principles I, III, and VIII and Opinion 2.06. Gabos, *The Perils of Singleton v. Norris: Ethics and Beyond*, 32 Am. J. L. & Med. 117, 118, 125-26, 127 (2006).

Journal 2005 Considers the legal and ethical implications of tracking dementia patients with global positioning system (GPS) technology. Concludes that GPS tracking may infringe on fundamental rights of privacy, autonomy, and human dignity and that the only justification for tracking is to prevent harm to the individual being tracked. References Principle I. Eltis, *Predicating Dignity on Autonomy? The Need for Further Inquiry Into the Ethics of Tagging and Tracking Dementia Patients With GPS Technology*, 13 Elder L. J. 387, 403 (2005).

Journal 2005 Examines issues surrounding tort reform proposals. Concludes that more can be done to correct the current tort system before moving toward a "one size fits all" approach. Quotes Principles I, II, III, IV, V, VI, VII, VIII, and IX. Messerly & Warwick, *Nowhere to Turn: A Glance at the Facts Behind the Supposed Need for Tort "Reform,"* 28 Hamline L. Rev. 489, 506 (2005).

Journal 2003 Considers the legal, medical, and ethical issues of physician-patient confidentiality in disclosure of paternity. Concludes that a balancing test should be applied to making determinations regarding disclosure of paternity. Quotes Principles I, IV, and V and Opinions 1.02, 5.055, and 10.01. Cites Principle II and Opinion 5.05. Richards & Wolf, *Medical Confidentiality and Disclosure of Paternity*, 48 S. D. L. Rev. 409, 411, 412, 413 (2003).

Journal 2002 Explores the implications of withholding medical treatment when abortion results in a live birth. Concludes that, in these situations, abortive parents and physicians should not solely decide the child's best interest. Quotes Preamble, Principles I and III, and Opinions 2.035, 2.20, and 2.215. Casagrande, *Children Not Meant to Be: Protecting the Interests of the Child When Abortion Results in Live Birth*, 6 Quinnipiac Health L. J. 19, 44, 45, 47-48 (2002).

Journal 2002 Analyzes the expanded use of the Civil False Claims Act in prosecuting health care fraud. Concludes that, in enforcing the law, government must balance its promises to beneficiaries, health care providers, and the public. Quotes Principles I, II, and IV. Krause, *"Promises to Keep": Health Care Providers and the Civil False Claims Act*, 23 Cardozo L. Rev. 1363, 1365 (2002).

Journal 2002 Considers the dilemma of informed consent in the context of prescribing psychotropic medication to patients with mental illness and mental retardation. Recognizes the need for substituted decision-making in certain situations. Concludes that legislation would help address this issue. Quotes Preamble, Principles I, III, IV, VIII, and IX, and Opinion 8.08. O'Sullivan & Borcherding, *Informed Consent for Medication in Persons With Mental Retardation and Mental Illness*, 12 Health Matrix 63, 75, 86, 87, 88 (2002).

Journal 2002 Examines the origin and dynamics of the scope-of-practice laws governing health care providers. Concludes that the current system is not working and offers recommendations for change. Quotes Principles I and II. Safriet, *Closing the Gap Between Can and May in Health-Care Providers' Scopes of Practice: A Primer for Policymakers*, 19 Yale J. on Reg. 301, 311 (2002).

Journal 2001 Discusses the physician unionization debate with emphasis on the perspective of physicians. Concludes that physicians' arguments against managed care articulate a moral claim in favor of collective bargaining rights. Quotes

Principle I. Fine, *Exploitation of the Elite: A Case for Physician Unionization*, 45 St. Louis L. J. 207, 207 (2001).

Journal 2000 Examines the AMA Code of Ethics. Explores historical developments. Concludes that professional ethical principles meaningfully affect the conduct of physicians and make a difference to the patients and the public they serve. Cites Principle I. Baker & Emanuel, *The Efficacy of Professional Ethics: The AMA Code of Ethics in Historical and Current Perspective*, 30 Hastings Center Rep. S13, S14 (July/Aug. 2000).

Journal 2000 Considers the rules governing expert testimony. Explores professional ethical standards affecting expert witnesses and concludes that codes of ethics have not succeeded in eliminating biased expert testimony. Recommends creation of an organization to assist courts in obtaining reliable expert witness testimony. Quotes Principle III and Opinion 6.01. Cites Principles I, II, and V and Opinions 1.02 and 9.07. Murphy, *Expert Witnesses at Trial: Where Are the Ethics?* 14 Geo. J. Legal Ethics 217, 231-32 (2000).

Journal 1999 Analyzes the federal rules of evidence from a feminist perspective. Proposes a new "apology" evidence rule to serve as an exception to the general rule that statements by party opponents are admissible during trial. Suggests that physicians who commit medical errors may ease patients' anger by apologizing. The new evidence rule would permit physicians to be more forthcoming in this regard. Quotes Principles I and II. Orenstein, *Apology Excepted: Incorporating a Feminist Analysis Into Evidence Policy Where You Would Least Expect It*, 28 S.W. U. L. Rev. 221, 264 (1999).

Journal 1998 Explores the impact of managed care on the health care system. Discusses legal and ethical conflicts that have arisen and emphasizes the need to balance the interests of patients with the integrity of the system. Quotes Principle I. Field, *New Ethical Relationships Under Health Care's New Structure: The Need for a New Paradigm*, 43 Vill. L. Rev. 467, 468 (1998).

Journal 1998 Discusses managed care and the expansion of physicians' duties under such programs. Focuses on the current legal standard of care for physicians. Proposes that physicians who are mandated by managed care organizations to provide services performed by specialists be held to the same standard of care as other physicians who are required to deliver those services. Quotes Principle I. Friedland, *Managed Care and the Expanding Scope of Primary Care Physicians' Duties: A Proposal to Redefine Explicitly the Standard of Care*, 26 J. Law Med. & Ethics 100, 104 (1998).

Journal 1998 Examines the US Supreme Court's decision in *Zinermon v. Burch* in relation to other Supreme Court decisions regarding the role of the courts in mental health treatment determinations. Argues that the government must strike a balance between the duty to care for the mentally ill and the duty to respect individual liberty. Provides

approaches legislatures could adopt regarding mental health issues. References Principles I and III. Nidich, *Zinermon v. Burch and Voluntary Admissions to Public Hospitals: A Common Sense Proposal for Compromise*, 25 N. Ky. L. Rev. 699, 710 (1998).

Journal 1997 Discusses the practice of physician deselection by managed care organizations. Suggests that deselection harms the physician-patient relationship and creates a conflict of interest. Argues that solutions to deselection should consider effects on the patient rather than on the physician. Quotes Principle III. Cites Principle I and Opinions 8.05 and 8.13. Liner, *Physician Deselection: The Dynamics of a New Threat to the Physician-Patient Relationship*, 23 Am. J. Law & Med. 511, 513, 527 (1997).

Journal 1997 Discusses the need for balance between business ethics and medical ethics in the context of managed care. Explores two models for integrating ethics and managed care. Proposes the adoption of a collective responsibility model to improve quality of care. Quotes Principles I, II, III, IV, and V. Cites Preamble. References Opinion 8.13. Regan, *Regulating the Business of Medicine: Models for Integrating Ethics and Managed Care*, 30 Colum. J. L. & Soc. Probs. 635, 651, 656, 657 (1997).

Journal 1996 Discusses the trend toward conserving resources expended on health care by withholding services absent a showing of necessity. Claims that the high standard of care physicians owe patients is jeopardized by medical treatment decisions based on coverage concerns. Concludes that the legal structure regarding health care plans should be changed. Quotes Preamble, Principles I, II, III, IV, V, VI, and VII, and Opinion 2.03. Hirshfeld & Thomason, *Medical Necessity Determinations: The Need for a New Legal Structure*, 6 Health Matrix 3, 8-9 (1996).

Journal 1995 Examines the rights of health care professionals to refuse to participate in patient care on the basis of conscientious objection. Suggests steps that health care facilities may take when dealing with health care professionals who object to participating in patient care. Quotes Principles I and VI and Opinions 1.02, 2.035, and 9.055. Dellinger & Vickery, *When Staff Object to Participating in Care*, 28 J. Health & Hospital Law 269, 272, 276 (1995).

Journal 1994 Considers whether an exception should be made to physician-patient confidentiality that would allow a physician to reveal parental medical history to a child. Concludes that such an exception would not completely erode physician-patient confidentiality. Quotes Principle IV, Fundamental Elements (4), and Opinion 5.05. Cites Principle I and Fundamental Elements (1). Friedland, *Physician-Patient Confidentiality: Time to Re-examine a Venerable Concept in Light of Contemporary Society and Advances in Medicine*, 15 J. Legal Med. 249, 257, 264, 276 (1994).

Journal 1994 Argues that physician aid-in-dying should be protected by the US Constitution and that patients should have a federal cause of action to challenge prohibitive state statutes. Considers how such a cause of action might affect public policy. Quotes Principles I and III. References Opinion 2.06. Note, *Toward a More Perfect Union: A Federal Cause of Action for Physician Aid-in-Dying, 27 U. Mich. J. L. Ref. 521, 538 (1994).*

Journal 1994 Reviews the evolution of the physician-patient relationship, with attention to patient autonomy. Examines the changing health care delivery environment. Quotes Preamble, Principles I, II, III, IV, V, and VI, Fundamental Elements (1) and (2), and Opinions 1.02 and 8.07 (1981) [now Opinion 8.08]. Cites Opinion 1.01. Szczygiel, *Beyond Informed Consent, 21 Ohio N. U. L. Rev. 171, 217, 218, 220, 225, 226, 256 (1994).*

Journal 1993 Discusses physicians' duty to disclose to patients medical treatment alternatives that are not readily available. Proposes that based on the historical development and legal requirements of the informed consent doctrine, physicians should be required to inform patients of non–readily available alternatives or face liability for breach of such obligation. Quotes Principles I, II, III, IV, and V and Opinion 8.08. Note, *Informed Choice: Physicians' Duty to Disclose Nonreadily Available Alternatives, 43 Case W. Res. L. Rev. 491, 491, 498-99, 508, 509 (1993).*

Journal 1990 Discusses the moral dilemma in deciding whether to withdraw artificial nutrition and hydration from a patient and the appropriate role of the judiciary. Concludes that judicial decisions do not represent the moral viewpoint of society and that moral pronouncements should not be made in the courtroom. Quotes Preamble, Principles I, II, III, IV, V, VI, and VII, and Opinion 2.20. Peccarelli, *A Moral Dilemma: The Role of Judicial Intervention in Withholding or Withdrawing Nutrition and Hydration, 23 John Marshall L. Rev. 537, 539, 540, 541 (1990).*

Journal 1986 Observes that the AMA policy on capital punishment expressly forbids psychiatrists from making determinations of competency for execution. Compares the psychiatrist's determination of competency for execution to the behavior of Nazi physicians, and condemns as inherently dishonest any therapy not grounded in the patient's best interests. References Principle I and Opinion 2.06. Sargent, *Treating the Condemned to Death, 16 Hastings Center Rep. 5, 5 (Dec. 1986).*

Principle II

E.D. Mo. 2007 Defendant-physician's husband, also a physician, suffered brain damage during surgery, yet continued to practice medicine. Following a patient death, plaintiff brought a wrongful death action against the physician and a separate action against his wife for negligent failure to report her husband's impairment. The court found that the wife, although a physician, had no duty to warn of her husband's "dangerous propensities." Plaintiff cited Principle II's ethical requirement to report a fellow physician's deficiencies in competence. However, the court noted that the defendant was not a member of the AMA and that Missouri law does not impose such a duty. *Phelps v. DeMello, 2007 WL 1063567, 3.*

Cal. App. 2004 Trial court sustained a demur to the appellants' first amended complaint. The appellate court quoted Principles II and V in concluding the coroner's practice of hiring a pathologist who had a close working relationship with a company which treats individuals whose death the pathologist may be required to investigate was a questionable policy due to the pathologist's wide discretion. The appellate court, however, affirmed the trial court's decision that appellants had not stated any viable claims. *Miller v. Rupf, 2004 WL 2092015, 11 n. 9.*

Cal. App. 1956 Physician-petitioner sought mandamus against local medical association whose bylaws provided for the expulsion of any member who violated the Principles. Petitioner had been expelled under the provision for alleged violation of Principles Ch. III, Art IV, Sec. 4 (1947) [now Opinions 9.04 and 9.07] for making disparaging statements regarding another physician in a report used in judicial proceedings. In holding that application of the provision to petitioner was contrary to public policy, the court noted that the physician's statements had been made at the request of a civil litigant and enjoyed a statutory testimonial privilege. Further, the court found that the AMA's right to formulate ethical principles did not extend to defining the duties of witnesses. Expulsion was also based on petitioner's critical comments about other physicians overheard by their patients in violation of Principles Ch. III, Art. IV, Sec. 1 (1947) [now Principle II and Opinion 9.04]. The court found application of this Principle under the circumstances reasonable and not contrary to public policy. *Bernstein v. Alameda-Contra Costa Medical Ass'n, 139 Cal. App. 2d 241, 293 P.2d 862, 863, 863 nn.1, 2, 865 nn.4, 6, 866, 866 n.8, 867.*

Fla. App. 1995 The court considered the issue of the effect of § 455.241(2) of the Florida Statutes on right of defense in a medical malpractice action to engage in ex parte communications with plaintiff's nonparty treating physician. The court held that a 1988 amendment to § 455.241(2) negated the applicability of the statute to medical malpractice cases. The dissent, citing *Petrillo v. Syntex Laboratories, Inc.,* 148 Ill. App. 3d 581, 499 N.E.2d 952 (1986), quoted Principles II and IV and Opinions 5.05, 5.06, and 5.08 as strong public policy support for its position that ex parte communications should be barred altogether. *Castillo-Plaza v. Green, 655 So. 2d 197, 206 n.4.*

Ill. App. 1986 Defense attorney in product liability suit was held in contempt of court for conducting ex parte discussions with plaintiff-patient's treating physician without patient's consent and contrary to authorized methods of discovery.

The court held that the strong public policy favoring physician-patient confidentiality articulated in Principles II and IV and Opinions 5.05, 5.06, 5.07, and 5.08 justified a rule against such ex parte discussions. Further, the court held that the public has the right to rely on physicians to faithfully execute their ethical obligations. *Petrillo v. Syntex Laboratories, Inc., 148 Ill. App. 3d 581, 499 N.E.2d 952, 957, 958, 959.*

Ky. App. 1978 Plaintiff-physician attempted to enjoin defendant medical society from expelling him for actions contrary to a variety of Principles, the most relevant to his alleged unethical behavior being Principle 4 (1957) [now Principles II and III]. After reviewing the procedures followed by the medical society in considering the evidence pertaining to the charges, the court affirmed judgment dismissing the action, concluding that plaintiff was not deprived of due process. *Kirk v. Jefferson County Medical Soc'y, 577 S.W.2d 419, 421.*

Md. App. 2007 The Maryland State Board of Physicians suspended the medical license of physician-appellant upon finding he lied to a peer review committee and left an anesthetized patient unattended. The circuit court affirmed suspension and the physician appealed. Quoting Principle II to support finding a breach of the physician's duty of honesty, the court ruled there was a reasonable factual and legal basis for the Board's decision. *Cornfeld v. State Board of Physicians, 174 Md. App. 456, 921 A.2d 893, 906-07.*

Md. App. 1993 State Board of Physician Quality Assurance received a complaint that psychiatrist was having a romantic relationship with a former patient. When, as part of its investigation, the Board subpoenaed psychiatrist's records, patient raised the constitutional right to privacy. The court held that the state's interest in investigating possible disciplinary action against psychiatrist outweighed patient's constitutional right to privacy. The court cited Principle II as a potential basis to justify the Board's investigation of possible unprofessional conduct by physician. *Dr. K. v. State Board of Physician Quality Assur., 98 Md. App. 103, 632 A.2d 453, 456, cert. denied, 334 Md. 18, 637 A.2d 1191 (1994), and cert. denied, 115 S. Ct. 75, 130 L. Ed. 29 (1994).*

Mass. 1955 Plaintiff-physician was charged under state licensing statute by defendant-board with conspiracy and fee-splitting. Both parties sought a declaratory judgment as to whether the defendant-board had jurisdiction to determine plaintiff's guilt or innocence. In holding that the board was qualified to determine if plaintiff's actions constituted gross misconduct under the statute, the court referred to Principles Ch. I, Secs. 1 and 6 (1947) [now Principle II and Opinion 6.02], delineating, in part, limitations on payment for medical services. These provisions, the court said, reflected the medical profession's understanding of its peculiar obligations. *Forziati v. Board of Registration in Medicine, 333 Mass. 125, 128 N.E.2d 789, 791.*

Mich. App. 2007 Plaintiff-physician had privileges at defendant-hospital. After a decline in referrals, plaintiff

sued the hospital and two physicians for tortious interference with a business relationship and civil conspiracy. Plaintiff attempted to establish illegitimate business practices on the part of defendants by showing that a defendant-physician was not qualified to handle the cases referred to him. With apparent reference to Principle II, plaintiff claimed that this defendant improperly held himself out to have expertise in the field of gynecologic oncology. The court found the honesty requirement in Principle II to be too vague to support any of the claims brought by the plaintiff and affirmed summary judgment for defendants. *Boike v. McLaren Health Care Corp., 2007 WL 1932029, 4.*

Mich. App. 1968 Physician was properly dismissed from hospital staff for violating Principle 4 (1957) [now Principle II and Opinion 9.11] when on numerous occasions physician vilified other physicians, swore and screamed in the hospital, and quarreled with staff and hospital visitors. *Anderson v. Board of Trustees of Caro Community Hosp., 10 Mich. App. 348, 159 N.W.2d 347, 348-50.*

Minn. 1970 Defendant-physician appealed order to answer interrogatories, claiming that a medical malpractice plaintiff is prohibited from compelling expert testimony from a defendant to prove a charge of malpractice without calling other medical witnesses. In holding that a defendant could be compelled to provide expert medical opinion in response to interrogatories, the court quoted Principle 1 (1957) [now Principle II and Opinion 8.12] for the proposition that physicians owe a duty of disclosure to their patients. *Anderson v. Florence, 288 Minn. 351, 181 N.W.2d 873, 880, 880 n.7.*

N.Y. Sup. 1965 Physician sued publishing company to bar insertion of advertisement for baby and child care products in physician's book, seeking declaration that book contract was void to the extent that it allowed inclusion of such an advertisement. Physician asserted that the advertisement was contrary to public policy, citing Opinions and Reports of the Judicial Council Sec. 5, Para. 29 (1965) [now Opinion 5.02], which stated that a doctor should not lend his name to any product. In rejecting the physician's claim, the court was willing to give careful consideration to the Association's view but concluded that it did not, in itself, constitute an expression of public policy. *Spock v. Pocket Books, Inc., 48 Misc. 2d 812, 266 N.Y.S.2d 77, 79.*

Ohio 2009 Physician appealed from a judgment affirming an order of the state medical board that permanently revoked appellant's certificate to practice medicine. The board found that appellant's sexual contact with patients violated Ohio statutes governing physician conduct and the code of ethics of the AMA, citing Principles I, II, IV, and VIII. The Court of Appeals held that Ohio state law allows the board to revoke a physician's certificate if it finds that the person violated any provision of the code of ethics of the AMA. *D'Souza v. State Med. Bd. of Ohio, 2009 WL 5108774, 6.*

Ohio 1991 State medical board revoked license of physician who had consensual sexual relations with his patient. The court upheld the board's ruling that this violated Principles I,

II, and IV. Dissenting judge, citing AMA Council on Ethical and Judicial Affairs, Sexual Misconduct in the Practice of Medicine, 266 *JAMA* 2741 [now Opinion 8.14], argued that until 1991, the AMA did not clearly deem sexual contact with a patient unethical. *Pons v. Ohio State Medical Bd., 66 Ohio St. 3d 619, 623, 625, 614 N.E.2d 748, 752, 753.*

Ohio 1980 A physician, charged with violating the state medical licensing statute by distributing controlled substances without a proper license and writing prescriptions for narcotics in the name of one person when they were intended for another, challenged the state medical board's decision to suspend his license and place him on two years' probation. Under the statute, a physician could be disciplined for various activities including violation of any provision of a code of ethics of a national professional organization such as the AMA. The board found in part that the physician's actions violated Principles 4 and 7 (1957) [now Principles II and III and Opinions 8.06 and 9.04]. The trial court reversed, holding that the board had insufficient evidence for its decision, and the court of appeals affirmed. On appeal, the supreme court held that expert testimony was not required at a hearing before a medical licensing board because they were experts and could determine for themselves whether the Principles had been violated. *Arlen v. State, 61 Ohio St. 2d 168, 399 N.E.2d 1251, 1252, 1253-54.*

Ohio App. 2005 The Ohio State Medical Board permanently revoked the license of the appellant, a psychiatrist, for having inappropriate physical and sexual contact with a female patient. The trial court affirmed the board's ruling, and the appellant appealed. The board claimed that the appellant's relationship with his patient violated the AMA's Code of Medical Ethics, citing Principles I, II, and IV. The appellate court affirmed, stating that permanent revocation of the appellant's license was not excessive and was not a violation of due process as the board may revoke the appellant's license if treatment did not meet minimal standards of care and violated any provision of the AMA's Code of Medical Ethics. *Schechter v. Ohio State Med. Bd., 2005 WL 1869733, 9.*

Journal 2010 Analyzes factors contributing to the emergence of medical repatriation and evaluates whether this practice comports with current legal and ethical standards. Proposes changes to federal regulations that govern hospitals and clarifications to medical ethical standards. Quotes the Preamble and Principles I, II, III, IV, V, VI, VII, VIII, and IX. Zoellner, *Medical Repatriation: Examining the Legal and Ethical Implications of an Emerging Practice, 32 Wash. U. J. L. & Pol'y 515, 530-532 (2010).*

Journal 2009 Explores emerging issues in conflict management systems design (CMSD). Concludes as the practice of CMSD in the organizational context continues to expand, practitioners should openly discuss the emerging issues of the field. References Principles I, II, V, and VIII. Costantino, *Second Generation Organizational Conflict Management Systems Design: A Practitioner's Perspective on Emerging Issues, 14 Harv. Negot. L. Rev. 81, 95 (2009).*

Journal 2009 Discusses the interaction between statutes and case law governing the medical field and the core principles of medical professionalism. Concludes the legal framework of medical professionalism does not encompass all the elements required of a medical professional. Quotes Principles II, III, IV, V, VI, VII, and VIII. Fichter, *The Law of Doctoring: A Study of the Codification of Medical Professionalism, 19 Health Matrix 317, 338, 339, 340, 343, 351 (2009).*

Journal 2009 Discusses whether patients have a right to pain management. Concludes that no physician duty is established by law or ethics to provide pain management outside the traditional physician-patient relationship. Cites Principles I, II, IV, and VIII. Hall & Boswell, *Ethics, Law, and Pain Management as a Patient Right, 12 Pain Physician 499, 500 (2009).*

Journal 2008 Discusses procedural guidelines for treating HIV-positive patients seeking cosmetic surgery for lipodystrophy syndrome. Concludes that this patient group is increasing in number, and that physicians could risk violating legal and ethical rules by refusing to provide treatment. Quotes Principle II and Opinion 9.131. Davison, Reisman, Pellegrino, Larson, Dermody, & Hutchison, *Perioperative Guidelines for Elective Surgery in the Human Immunodeficiency Virus–Positive Patient, 121 Plastic and Reconstructive Surgery 1831, 1838 (2008).*

Journal 2008 Explores the legal, ethical, and policy implications of concierge medicine. Argues physicians engaged in concierge care must strive to meet ethical and legal standards, and take care to communicate clearly with patients about services and fees. Quotes Opinion 8.055. Cites Principles II and VI and Opinion 8.055. Portman & Romanow, *Concierge Medicine: Legal Issues, Ethical Dilemmas, and Policy Challenges, 1 J. Health & Life Sci. L. 1, 4, 28-29 (2008).*

Journal 2008 Examines the development of bioethics and environmental ethics, as well as laws promoting the role of bioethicists in decision making. Concludes environmental ethicists must convince legislatures of the role of environmental ethics in order to have a greater impact on decision making. Quotes Principles I, II, III, IV, V, VI, VII, VIII, and IX. Robertson, *Seeking a Seat at the Table: Has Law Left Environmental Ethics Behind as It Embraces Bioethics? 32 Wm. & Mary Envtl. L. & Pol'y Rev. 273, 307 (2008).*

Journal 2008 Explores the fiduciary relationship between physicians and patients, professional and ethical obligations of both physicians and lawyers, and the implications for conflict resolution in health care. Concludes physicians must put patient interests above their own and lawyers must work to discern clients' best interests and support client welfare. Quotes Principle VIII and Opinions 8.12 and 10.015. Cites Principles I and II and Opinions 10.01 and 10.015. Scott, *Doctors as Advocates, Lawyers as Healers, 29 Hamline J. Pub. L. Pol'y, 331, 340-41, 347, 371 (2008).*

Journal 2007 Addresses physician liability for an extramarital affair with a patient's spouse. Concludes that such an affair should be regarded as a breach of a fiduciary duty. Quotes Preamble, Principles I, II, and VIII, and Opinions 8.145, 9.04, 9.123, and 10.015. Demaine, *"Playing Doctor" With the Patient's Spouse: Alternative Conceptions of Health Professional Liability, 14 Va. J. Soc. Pol'y & L. 308, 325, 330-31, 331-32 (2007).*

Journal 2007 Argues that issuance of apologies from physicians who commit medical errors will diminish the number of malpractice suits brought. Concludes that patients desire apologies in the case of medical errors and are less likely to sue when they are given. Cites Principles I, II, III, and IV and Opinion 8.12. Tabler, *Should Physicians Apologize for Medical Errors? 19 Health Lawyer 23, 25 (Jan. 2007).*

Journal 2007 Discusses military policies on the ethical treatment of enemy combatants. Concludes that military medical personnel should adhere to the ethical standards of their profession at all times. References Principle II. Xenakis, *How Should We Respond? Seton Hall University School of Law Guantanamo Teach-In, 37 Seton Hall L. Rev. 703, 709 (2007).*

Journal 2006 Evaluates the constitutionality of federal faith-based initiative programs. Concludes that such programs violate the First Amendment under the combined Lemon and Zelman test. Cites Principles II and VIII. Boden, *Compassion Inaction: Why President Bush's Faith-Based Initiatives Violate the Establishment Clause, 29 Seattle U. L. Rev. 991, 1023 (2006).*

Journal 2006 Explores conscience clause legislation relating to the dispensing of oral contraceptives. Concludes that such legislation must balance the interests of the patient and the health care provider. Cites Principles I, II, III, IV, V, VI, VII, VIII, and IX. Collins, *Conscience Clauses and Oral Contraceptives: Conscientious Objection or Calculated Obstruction? 15 Ann. Health L. 37, 54 (2006).*

Journal 2006 Examines physician criminal activity and subsequent disciplinary actions by state licensing boards. Concludes that licensing boards should impose greater penalties on physicians convicted of crimes. Quotes Principles II and III. Jung, Lurie, & Wolfe, *U.S. Physicians Disciplined for Criminal Activity, 16 Health Matrix 335, 335 (2006).*

Journal 2006 Reviews Supreme Court decisions on protection of a public employee's freedom of speech. Concludes that the law should provide constitutional protection when an employee's speech is critical of his or her public employer. Quotes Principle II. Note, *Leading Cases–Public Employee Speech, 120 Harv. L. Rev. 125, 282 (2006).*

Journal 2005 Argues that disciplining physicians who give questionable expert testimony in medical malpractice cases may reduce insurance premiums for physicians. Concludes that state regulation of medical expert testimony is vital to tort liability reform. Cites Principle II. Gomez, *Silencing the Hired Guns: Ensuring Honesty in Medical Expert Testimony Through State Legislation, 26 J. Legal Med. 385, 399 (2005).*

Journal 2005 Examines issues surrounding tort reform proposals. Concludes that more can be done to correct the current tort system before moving toward a "one size fits all" approach. Quotes Principles I, II, III, IV, V, VI, VII, VIII, and IX. Messerly & Warwick, *Nowhere to Turn: A Glance at the Facts Behind the Supposed Need for Tort "Reform," 28 Hamline L. Rev. 489, 506 (2005).*

Journal 2003 Considers conflicts of interest and potential liability that a team physician faces when treating an injured athlete. Concludes that an athlete's health should be the team physician's primary concern in making treatment decisions. References Principles I and II. Landis, *The Team Physician: An Analysis of the Causes of Action, Conflicts, Defenses and Improvements, 1 DePaul J. Sports L. & Contemp. Probs. 139, 144 (2003).*

Journal 2003 Examines social norms, using public choice theory, to determine how certain groups in society use these norms to benefit their members. Concludes that the benefits provided by social norms may dissipate depending on various considerations. Quotes Principles II and VIII. Miller, *Norms and Interests, 32 Hofstra L. Rev. 637, 650, 670 (2003).*

Journal 2003 Considers the legal, medical, and ethical issues of physician-patient confidentiality in disclosure of paternity. Concludes that a balancing test should be applied to making determinations regarding disclosure of paternity. Quotes Principles I, IV, and V and Opinions 1.02, 5.055, and 10.01. Cites Principle II and Opinion 5.05. Richards & Wolf, *Medical Confidentiality and Disclosure of Paternity, 48 S. D. L. Rev. 409, 411, 412, 413 (2003).*

Journal 2003 Uses public policy arguments to support a preponderance standard for medical license revocations in situations involving false testimony by a medical expert witness. Concludes that medical licensing boards can more effectively protect the public by using a preponderance standard. Quotes Principles II, III, and IV and Opinions 1.02 and 9.07. Widmer, *South Dakota Should Follow Public Policy and Switch to the Preponderance Standard for Medical License Revocation After In Re the Medical License of Dr. Reuben Setliff, M.D., 48 S. D. L. Rev. 388, 396-97, 402 (2003).*

Journal 2002 Discusses therapeutic jurisprudence and the importance of trust in the structure of health care law. Concludes that understanding trust provides tools to formulate responses to new ethical, legal, and policy challenges. Quotes Principle Ch. I, Art. I, Sec. 4 (1847) [now Principle II and Opinion 8.12]. Hall, *Law, Medicine, and Trust, 55 Stan. L. Rev. 463, 471 (2002).*

Journal 2002 Analyzes the expanded use of the Civil False Claims Act in prosecuting health care fraud. Concludes that, in enforcing the law, government must balance its promises to beneficiaries, health care providers, and the public.

Quotes Principles I, II, and IV. Krause, *"Promises to Keep": Health Care Providers and the Civil False Claims Act,* 23 Cardozo L. Rev. 1363, 1365 (2002).

Journal 2002 Explores the development and current status of collective bargaining and unionization in the medical profession. Concludes that, because collective bargaining traditionally addresses conditions of employment, a focus on patient care will be difficult to ensure. References Principle II. Levy, *Collective Bargaining in the Elite Professions–Doctors' Application of the Labor Law Model to Negotiations With Health Plan Providers,* 13 U. Fla. J. L. & Pub. Pol'y 269, 277 (2002).

Journal 2002 Examines the origin and dynamics of the scope-of-practice laws governing health care providers. Concludes that the current system is not working and offers recommendations for change. Quotes Principles I and II. Safriet, *Closing the Gap Between Can and May in Health-Care Providers' Scopes of Practice: A Primer for Policymakers,* 19 Yale J. on Reg. 301, 311 (2002).

Journal 2002 Considers the case of *Ferguson v. City of Charleston.* Concludes that the Supreme Court's rationale in that case reflects insights from feminist legal theory. Quotes Opinion 10.01. Cites Principles II and IV. Taslitz, *A Feminist Fourth Amendment? Consent, Care, Privacy, and Social Meaning in Ferguson v. City of Charleston,* 9 Duke J. Gender L. & Pol'y 1, 18, 19 (2002).

Journal 2001 Discusses whether the medical profession needs a policy on honesty. Reviews ethical codes and concludes they fail to offer physicians meaningful guidance about what constitutes "the truth" and when and how to disclose it. Quotes Principle II and Opinions 8.12 and 10.01. DeVita, *Honestly, Do We Need a Policy on Truth?* 11 Kennedy Inst. Ethics J. 157, 158 (2001).

Journal 2001 Compares and contrasts certain ethical positions articulated by the legal and medical professions. Concludes that both professions generally agree on ethical principles, but sometimes differ in the manner of implementation. Quotes Principle II. Cites Opinion 5.02. Needell, *Legal Ethics in Medicine: Are Medical Ethics Different From Legal Ethics?* 14 St. Thomas L. Rev. 31, 35, 50 (2001).

Journal 2000 Considers whether government regulators should allow managed care organizations to cover the costs of alternative treatments. Concludes that legislation should be more attentive to its consumer protection role. Quotes Principle II. Boozang, *Is the Alternative Medicine? Managed Care Apparently Thinks So,* 32 Conn. L. Rev. 567, 606 (2000).

Journal 2000 Considers the rules governing expert testimony. Explores professional ethical standards affecting expert witnesses and concludes that codes of ethics have not succeeded in eliminating biased expert testimony. Recommends creation of an organization to assist courts in obtaining reliable expert witness testimony. Quotes Principle III and Opinion 6.01. Cites Principles I, II, and V

and Opinions 1.02 and 9.07. Murphy, *Expert Witnesses at Trial: Where Are the Ethics?* 14 Geo. J. Legal Ethics 217, 231-32 (2000).

Journal 2000 Discusses traditional medical ethics and the physician's duty to benefit patients. Concludes that in the 21st century, physicians will no longer be expected to determine on their own what will benefit their patients. Quotes Principle II and Opinion 8.08. Veatch, *Doctor Does Not Know Best: Why in the New Century Physicians Must Stop Trying to Benefit Patients,* 25 J. Med. & Phil. 701, 710, 711 (2000).

Journal 1999 Provides examples in which psychiatrists might use deception in their practice. Explains the motivations for such conduct and raises questions about possible blameworthiness for such conduct. Quotes Principles II and III. Haroun & Morris, *Weaving a Tangled Web: The Deceptions of Psychiatrists,* 10 J. Contemp. Leg. Issues 227, 235 (1999).

Journal 1999 Examines fraud and abuse throughout government health care programs, with emphasis on enforcement and available sanctions. Concludes that consideration of strategies for revising enforcement protocols is advisable. Quotes Principle II. Jost & Davies, *The Empire Strikes Back: A Critique of the Backlash Against Fraud and Abuse Enforcement,* 51 Ala. L. Rev. 239, 240 (1999).

Journal 1999 Describes historical and present views regarding medical diagnosis. Discusses pressures physicians face that may affect the diagnostic process. Suggests that legal institutions can reduce these pressures, which will enhance the physician-patient therapeutic relationship. Quotes Principle II and Opinion 9.07. Noah, *Pigeonholing Illness: Medical Diagnosis as a Legal Construct,* 50 Hastings L. J. 241, 301, 302 (1999).

Journal 1999 Analyzes the federal rules of evidence from a feminist perspective. Proposes a new "apology" evidence rule to serve as an exception to the general rule that statements by party opponents are admissible during trial. Suggests that physicians who commit medical errors may ease patients' anger by apologizing. The new evidence rule would permit physicians to be more forthcoming in this regard. Quotes Principles I and II. Orenstein, *Apology Excepted: Incorporating a Feminist Analysis Into Evidence Policy Where You Would Least Expect It,* 28 S.W. U. L. Rev. 221, 264 (1999).

Journal 1999 Evaluates changes in direct-to-consumer advertising of prescription pharmaceuticals. Discusses FDA regulation of this type of advertising. Recognizes the important role of the FDA in this context. Quotes Principles II and III. Terzian, *Direct-to-Consumer Prescription Drug Advertising,* 25 Am. J. Law & Med. 149, 165 (1999).

Journal 1998 Discusses gag provisions in physicians' contracts with managed care organizations. Examines effects of gag rules on physicians. Explores state legislation and proposed federal legislation pertaining to gag provisions. Cites

Principle II. Munoz, Nichols, Okata, Pitt, & Seager, *The Two Faces of Gag Provisions: Patients and Physicians in a Bind*, 17 Yale L. & Pol'y Rev. 249, 258 (1998).

Journal 1997 Reports on a study of physician attitudes regarding expert witnesses. Notes that a majority of physicians believe that medical expert testimony should be subject to peer review and, when appropriate, medical licensing board discipline. Quotes Principles II and VI and Opinion 9.07. Eitel, Hegeman, & Evans, *Medicine on Trial: Physicians' Attitudes About Expert Medical Witnesses, 18 J. Legal Med. 345, 355, 358 (1997).

Journal 1997 Discusses physician frustration with managed care plans caused by gag clauses and cost-containment mechanisms. Reviews the development of managed care organizations and federal attempts at limiting the use of gag clauses. Concludes that gag clauses are inherently flawed and compromise quality health care. Quotes Principles II and V, Fundamental Elements (1), and Opinion 8.13. Note, *Physicians, Bound and Gagged: Federal Attempts to Combat Managed Care's Use of Gag Clauses, 21 Seton Hall Legis. J. 567, 601-02 (1997).

Journal 1997 Discusses the need for balance between business ethics and medical ethics in the context of managed care. Explores two models for integrating ethics and managed care. Proposes the adoption of a collective responsibility model to improve quality of care. Quotes Principles I, II, III, IV, and V. Cites Preamble. References Opinion 8.13. Regan, *Regulating the Business of Medicine: Models for Integrating Ethics and Managed Care, 30 Colum. J. L. & Soc. Probs. 635, 651, 656, 657 (1997).

Journal 1996 Discusses the trend toward conserving resources expended on health care by withholding services absent a showing of necessity. Claims that the high standard of care physicians owe patients is jeopardized by medical treatment decisions based on coverage concerns. Concludes that the legal structure regarding health care plans should be changed. Quotes Preamble, Principles I, II, III, IV, V, VI, and VII, and Opinion 2.03. Hirshfeld & Thomason, *Medical Necessity Determinations: The Need for a New Legal Structure, 6 Health Matrix 3, 8-9 (1996).

Journal 1996 Considers the impact of gag clauses on the physician-patient relationship. Undertakes an extensive legal, ethical, and policy analysis. Concludes that gag clauses are violative of legal and ethical principles. Quotes Principles II, V, and VI and Fundamental Elements (1). Cites Preamble. Martin & Bjerknes, *The Legal and Ethical Implications of Gag Clauses in Physician Contracts, XXII Am. J. Law & Med. 433, 465-66 (1996).

Journal 1996 Examines the issue of attorney-client sexual relationships and the ethical problems inherent in such conduct. Recommends promulgation of a rule regulating such relationships. Quotes Principle II. Myers, Sonenshein, & Hofstein, *To Regulate or Not To Regulate Attorney-Client Sex? The Ethical Question in Pennsylvania, 69 Temp. L. Rev. 741, 780 (1996).

Journal 1996 Discusses the ethical implications of sexual misconduct in the medical field. Examines the current civil and criminal tools used to curb physician-patient misconduct. Notes the inadequacy of physician reporting. Proposes a statutory approach to discipline physicians who abuse their fiduciary duties. Quotes Principle II. References Opinion 8.14. Note, *Sexual Conduct Within the Physician-Patient Relationship: A Statutory Framework for Disciplining This Breach of Fiduciary Duty, 1 Widener L. Symp. J. 501, 507 (1996).

Journal 1994 Compares Texas law with Illinois law on the issue of ex parte communications between defense counsel and the patient/plaintiff's physician in civil litigation. Argues that preservation of the physician-patient relationship requires prohibition of such contact. Quotes Principles II and IV and Opinion 5.05. Comment, *From the Land of Lincoln a Healing Rule: Proposed Texas Rule of Civil Procedure Prohibiting Ex Parte Contact Between Defense Counsel and a Plaintiff's Treating Physician, 25 Tex. Tech L. Rev. 1081, 1081, 1082 (1994).

Journal 1994 Reviews the evolution of the physician-patient relationship, with attention to patient autonomy. Examines the changing health care delivery environment. Quotes Preamble, Principles I, II, III, IV, V, and VI, Fundamental Elements (1) and (2), and Opinions 1.02 and 8.07 (1981) [now Opinion 8.08]. Cites Opinion 1.01. Szczygiel, *Beyond Informed Consent, 21 Ohio N. U. L. Rev. 171, 217, 218, 220, 225, 226, 256 (1994).

Journal 1993 Discusses physicians' duty to disclose to patients medical treatment alternatives that are not readily available. Proposes that based on the historical development and legal requirements of the informed consent doctrine, physicians should be required to inform patients of non–readily available alternatives or face liability for breach of such obligation. Quotes Principles I, II, III, IV, and V and Opinion 8.08. Note, *Informed Choice: Physicians' Duty to Disclose Nonreadily Available Alternatives, 43 Case W. Res. L. Rev. 491, 491, 498-99, 508, 509 (1993).

Journal 1993 Discusses the problems physicians may encounter by exposing an errant colleague, such as harm to the reporting physician's reputation and the fear of litigation. States that problems involving physician competency and unethical behavior should be investigated, and that physicians should take personal responsibility for reporting problems they observe. References Principle II and Opinions 8.14 and 9.031. Morreim, *Am I My Brother's Warden? Responding to the Unethical or Incompetent Colleague, 23 Hastings Center Rep. 19, 23 (May/June 1993).

Journal 1993 Explores problems associated with parental requests to withhold diagnoses from children. Discusses the physician's conflict between a duty to respect parents' wishes and a duty to tell children the truth. Quotes Principle II. Sigman, Kraut, & La Puma, *Disclosure of a Diagnosis to Children and Adolescents When Parents Object, 147 Am. J. Diseases Children 764, 766 (1993).

Journal 1991 Examines the issues surrounding judicial use of professional ethics codes in private litigation. Concludes that judges should more extensively use professional ethics codes to define public policy, standards of care, and legal causes of action. Quotes Principle II and Opinion 2.19. Note, *Professional Ethics Codes in Court: Redefining the Social Contract Between the Public and the Professions, 25 Georgia L. Rev. 1327, 1335, 1351 (1991).*

Journal 1990 Examines the extent to which forensic psychiatrists are consulted in medical malpractice cases. Considers the appropriate standard of care, particularly for psychiatric malpractice cases, and the problems associated with its determination. References Principles II and IV. Modlin, *Forensic Psychiatry and Malpractice, 18 Bull. Am. Acad. Psychiatry Law 153, 161 (1990).*

Journal 1990 Discusses the moral dilemma in deciding whether to withdraw artificial nutrition and hydration from a patient and the appropriate role of the judiciary. Concludes that judicial decisions do not represent the moral viewpoint of society and that moral pronouncements should not be made in the courtroom. Quotes Preamble, Principles I, II, III, IV, V, VI, and VII, and Opinion 2.20. Peccarelli, *A Moral Dilemma: The Role of Judicial Intervention in Withholding or Withdrawing Nutrition and Hydration, 23 John Marshall L. Rev. 537, 539, 540, 541 (1990).*

Journal 1989 Discusses the history of the physician-patient privilege up through changes implemented under the Ohio Tort Reform Act of 1987. Aspects of the physician-patient privilege that are most significantly affected by this Tort Reform Act are highlighted, with recommendations for further refinement of the privilege in Ohio. Quotes Principles II and IV and Opinion 5.05. Note, *The Ohio Physician-Patient Privilege: Modified, Revised, and Defined, 49 Ohio St. L. J. 1147, 1167 (1989).*

Journal 1985 Initially describes how existing doctrines protect the value of autonomy in the context of the physician-patient relationship, then examines various problems in the current protective scheme. Concludes by recommending the creation of an independent articulable protected interest in patient autonomy. Quotes Principles II and IV. Cites Opinions 4.04 (1984) [now Opinions 8.03 and 8.032] and 6.03 (1984) [now Opinion 6.02]. Shultz, *From Informed Consent to Patient Choice: A New Protected Interest, 95 Yale L. J. 219, 275 (1985).*

Principle III

Ariz. 1965 Physician appealed denial of medical license which was based on alleged violations of local medical society rules and Principles 3, 5, and 10 (1957) [now Principles III and VII and Opinions 3.01, 8.11, and 9.06]. Alleged violations included treating a patient without first obtaining a prior treating physician's permission, inadequate patient care, performing operations without hospital privileges, and signing the medical record of a deceased patient who had been treated by interns. The court held that the evidence failed to show any clear violation of the Principles and that a local medical society had no right to prescribe a code of ethics for state licensing purposes. *Arizona State Bd. of Medical Examiners v. Clark, 97 Ariz. 205, 398 P.2d 908, 914-15, 915 n.3.*

Ky. App. 1978 Plaintiff-physician attempted to enjoin defendant medical society from expelling him for actions contrary to a variety of Principles, the most relevant to his alleged unethical behavior being Principle 4 (1957) [now Principles II and III]. After reviewing the procedures followed by the medical society in considering the evidence pertaining to the charges, the court affirmed judgment dismissing the action, concluding that plaintiff was not deprived of due process. *Kirk v. Jefferson County Medical Soc'y, 577 S.W.2d 419, 421.*

Ohio 1980 A physician, charged with violating the state medical licensing statute by distributing controlled substances without a proper license and writing prescriptions for narcotics in the name of one person when they were intended for another, challenged the state medical board's decision to suspend his license and place him on two years' probation. Under the statute, a physician could be disciplined for various activities including violation of any provision of a code of ethics of a national professional organization such as the AMA. The board found in part that the physician's actions violated Principles 4 and 7 (1957) [now Principles II and III and Opinions 8.06 and 9.04]. The trial court reversed, holding that the board had insufficient evidence for its decision, and the court of appeals affirmed. On appeal, the Supreme Court held that expert testimony was not required at a hearing before a medical licensing board because they were experts and could determine for themselves whether the Principles had been violated. *Arlen v. State, 61 Ohio St. 2d 168, 399 N.E.2d 1251, 1252, 1253-54.*

Journal 2011 Proposes fundamental reforms to the medical liability system based on the development of clinical practice guidelines by private, for-profit firms that in turn would bear the liability cost for providers who buy or license, and then follow the firm's prescribed guidelines. Quotes Principle III. Avraham, *Private Regulation, 34 Harv. J. L. & Pub. Pol'y 543, 614-15 (2011).*

Journal 2011 Reviews the use and current regulation of medical marijuana to alleviate pain in terminally ill patients. Focusing on patient autonomy, concludes that patients should have access to medical marijuana in controlled doses under controlled conditions. Quotes Principle III and Opinions 10.01, 10.015, and 10.02. References Principle VIII. Pfeifer, *Smoking Gun: The Moral and Legal Struggle for Medical Marijuana, 27 Touro L. Rev. 339, 340-41, 345-346 (2011).*

Journal 2010 Analyzes factors contributing to the emergence of medical repatriation and evaluates whether this practice comports with current legal and ethical standards. Proposes changes to federal regulations that govern hospitals and clarifications to medical ethical standards. Quotes the Preamble and Principles I, II, III, IV, V, VI, VII, VIII, and IX. Zoellner, *Medical Repatriation: Examining the Legal and Ethical Implications of an Emerging Practice*, 32 Wash. U. J. L. & Pol'y 515, 530-532 (2010).

Journal 2009 Discusses the interaction between statutes and case law governing the medical field and the core principles of medical professionalism. Concludes the legal framework of medical professionalism does not encompass all the elements required of a medical professional. Quotes Principles II, III, IV, V, VI, VII, and VIII. Fichter, *The Law of Doctoring: A Study of the Codification of Medical Professionalism*, 19 Health Matrix 317, 338, 339, 340, 343, 351 (2009).

Journal 2009 Discusses tobacco use in psychiatric institutions and its impact on the health and behavior of patients. Concludes legislative action should be taken to remove tobacco from psychiatric institutions to provide patients with the health and safety benefits of smoke-free facilities. Quotes Principles I and III. Hackett, *Smoke-Free State Psychiatric Facility Grounds: Is Legislation Necessary and Appropriate to Remove Tobacco From These Treatment Settings?* 53 N. Y. L. Sch. L. Rev. 99, 122-23 (2009).

Journal 2009 Explores the jurisprudential foundation of the fiduciary duty physicians owe their patients and discusses the failure of physicians to disclose to patients errors and other emergent medical risks. Concludes law should recognize the physician's duty to disclose such risks by enforcing a cause of action for breach of that duty. Quotes Principles III and VIII and Opinions 8.12, 10.015, and 10.02. References Opinion 8.12. Hafemeister, *Lean on Me: A Physician's Fiduciary Duty to Disclose an Emergent Medical Risk to the Patient*, 86 Wash. U. L. Rev. 1167, 1172-1173, 1178, 1182, 1185, 1188, 1209 (2009).

Journal 2008 Examines the development of bioethics and environmental ethics, as well as laws promoting the role of bioethicists in decision making. Concludes environmental ethicists must convince legislatures of the role of environmental ethics in order to have a greater impact on decision making. Quotes Principles I, II, III, IV, V, VI, VII, VIII, and IX. Robertson, *Seeking a Seat at the Table: Has Law Left Environmental Ethics Behind as It Embraces Bioethics?* 32 Wm. & Mary Envtl. L. & Pol'y Rev. 273, 307 (2008).

Journal 2007 Argues that issuance of apologies from physicians who commit medical errors will diminish the number of malpractice suits brought. Concludes that patients desire apologies in the case of medical errors and are less likely to sue when they are given. Cites Principles I, II, III, and IV and Opinion 8.12. Tabler, *Should Physicians Apologize for Medical Errors?* 19 Health Lawyer 23, 25 (Jan. 2007).

Journal 2007 Examines relative vs absolute rights to confidentiality for military detainees considering the utilitarian need to protect the public at large. Concludes that evolving standards may favor individual rights to confidentiality, even from a utilitarian perspective. Quotes Opinions 1.02 and 5.05. References Principle III. Wynia, *Breaching Confidentiality to Protect the Public: Evolving Standards of Medical Confidentiality for Military Detainees*, 7 Am. J. Bioethics 1, 2 (Aug. 2007).

Journal 2006 Explores conscience clause legislation relating to the dispensing of oral contraceptives. Concludes that such legislation must balance the interests of the patient and the health care provider. Cites Principles I, II, III, IV, V, VI, VII, VIII, and IX. Collins, *Conscience Clauses and Oral Contraceptives: Conscientious Objection or Calculated Obstruction?* 15 Ann. Health L. 37, 54 (2006).

Journal 2006 Discusses mentally incompetent inmates and capital punishment. Proposes that, to be permissible, involuntary medication of death-row inmates must represent the best medically appropriate treatment. Quotes Principles I, III, and VIII and Opinion 2.06. Gabos, *The Perils of Singleton v. Norris: Ethics and Beyond*, 32 Am. J. L. & Med. 117, 118, 125-26, 127 (2006).

Journal 2006 Examines physician criminal activity and subsequent disciplinary actions by state licensing boards. Concludes that licensing boards should impose greater penalties on physicians convicted of crimes. Quotes Principles II and III. Jung, Lurie, & Wolfe, *U.S. Physicians Disciplined for Criminal Activity*, 16 Health Matrix 335, 335 (2006).

Journal 2006 Examines a mental health professional's competing duties of confidentiality and reporting a patient's threats of violence. Suggests new legislation should clarify duty to report a threat. Quotes Preamble and Principles III, IV, and VIII. Cites Opinion 5.05. Mossman, *Critique of Pure Risk Assessment or, Kant Meets Tarasoff*, 75 U. Cin. L. Rev. 523, 579 (2006).

Journal 2005 Examines issues surrounding tort reform proposals. Concludes that more can be done to correct the current tort system before moving toward a "one size fits all" approach. Quotes Principles I, II, III, IV, V, VI, VII, VIII, and IX. Messerly & Warwick, *Nowhere to Turn: A Glance at the Facts Behind the Supposed Need for Tort "Reform,"* 28 Hamline L. Rev. 489, 506 (2005).

Journal 2005 Argues that medicating a criminal defendant to restore competency is ethical, even in capital cases. Concludes that principles justifying administration of punishment in the legal system give rise to an ethical imperative for physicians to provide competence-restoring medical therapy. Quotes Principle III and Opinion 2.06. Mossman, *Is Prosecution "Medically Appropriate?"* 31 New Eng. J. on Crim. & Civ. Confinement 15, 53-54, 59 (2005).

Journal 2003 Uses public policy arguments to support a preponderance standard for medical license revocations in situations involving false testimony by a medical expert witness. Concludes that medical licensing boards can more effectively protect the public by using a preponderance standard. Quotes Principles II, III, and IV and Opinions 1.02 and 9.07. Widmer, *South Dakota Should Follow Public Policy and Switch to the Preponderance Standard for Medical License Revocation After In Re the Medical License of Dr. Reuben Setliff, M.D.*, 48 S. D. L. Rev. 388, 396-97, 402 (2003).

Journal 2002 Explores the implications of withholding medical treatment when abortion results in a live birth. Concludes that, in these situations, abortive parents and physicians should not solely decide the child's best interest. Quotes Preamble, Principles I and III, and Opinions 2.035, 2.20, and 2.215. Casagrande, *Children Not Meant to Be: Protecting the Interests of the Child When Abortion Results in Live Birth*, 6 Quinnipiac Health L. J. 19, 44, 45, 47-48 (2002).

Journal 2002 Advocates in favor of disclosure of information regarding a physician's clinical experience when obtaining informed consent. Concludes that the physician's experience is material and patients who inquire should be given this information. Quotes Principle Ch. I, Art. I, Sec. 4 (1847) [now Principle II and Opinion 8.12]. Iheukwumere, *Doctor, Are You Experienced? The Relevance of Disclosure of Physician Experience to a Valid Informed Consent*, 18 J. Contemp. Health L. & Pol'y 373, 376-77 (2002).

Journal 2002 Considers the dilemma of informed consent in the context of prescribing psychotropic medication to patients with mental illness and mental retardation. Recognizes the need for substituted decision-making in certain situations. Concludes that legislation would help address this issue. Quotes Preamble, Principles I, III, IV, VIII, and IX, and Opinion 8.08. O'Sullivan & Borcherding, *Informed Consent for Medication in Persons With Mental Retardation and Mental Illness*, 12 Health Matrix 63, 75, 86, 87, 88 (2002).

Journal 2001 Considers whether it is ethical for physicians to prescribe, and pharmacists to dispense, syringes for use by injection drug users. Concludes that ethical considerations suggest such actions are permissible but not obligatory. Quotes Principle III and Opinion 1.02. References Opinion 5.05. Lazzarini, *An Analysis of Ethical Issues in Prescribing and Dispensing Syringes to Injection Drug Users*, 11 Health Matrix 85, 107, 119 (2001).

Journal 2000 Considers the rules governing expert testimony. Explores professional ethical standards affecting expert witnesses and concludes that codes of ethics have not succeeded in eliminating biased expert testimony. Recommends creation of an organization to assist courts in obtaining reliable expert witness testimony. Quotes Principle III and Opinion 6.01. Cites Principles I, II, and V and Opinions 1.02 and 9.07. Murphy, *Expert Witnesses at Trial: Where Are the Ethics?* 14 Geo. J. Legal Ethics 217, 231-32 (2000).

Journal 1999 States that current First Amendment opinions do not give clear guidelines on professional speech. Describes the US Supreme Court's approach to commercial speech. Examines Supreme Court opinions and points out similarities between the Court's stance on commercial and professional speech. Cites Principle III. Halberstam, *Commercial Speech, Professional Speech, and the Constitutional Status of Social Institutions*, 147 U. Pa. L. Rev. 771, 857 (1999).

Journal 1999 Provides examples in which psychiatrists might use deception in their practice. Explains the motivations for such conduct and raises questions about possible blameworthiness for such conduct. Quotes Principles II and III. Haroun & Morris, *Weaving a Tangled Web: The Deceptions of Psychiatrists*, 10 J. Contemp. Leg. Issues 227, 235 (1999).

Journal 1999 Evaluates changes in direct-to-consumer advertising of prescription pharmaceuticals. Discusses Food and Drug Administration (FDA) regulation of this type of advertising. Recognizes the important role of the FDA in this context. Quotes Principles II and III. Terzian, *Direct-to-Consumer Prescription Drug Advertising*, 25 Am. J. Law & Med. 149, 165 (1999).

Journal 1998 Examines the US Supreme Court's decision in *Zinermon v. Burch* in relation to other Supreme Court decisions regarding the role of the courts in mental health treatment determinations. Argues that the government must strike a balance between the duty to care for the mentally ill and the duty to respect individual liberty. Provides approaches legislatures could adopt regarding mental health issues. References Principles I and III. Nidich, *Zinermon v. Burch and Voluntary Admissions to Public Hospitals: A Common Sense Proposal for Compromise*, 25 N. Ky. L. Rev. 699, 710 (1998).

Journal 1997 Discusses the practice of physician deselection by managed care organizations. Suggests that deselection harms the physician-patient relationship and creates a conflict of interest. Argues that solutions to deselection should consider effects on the patient rather than on the physician. Quotes Principle III. Cites Principle I and Opinions 8.05 and 8.13. Liner, *Physician Deselection: The Dynamics of a New Threat to the Physician-Patient Relationship*, 23 Am. J. Law & Med. 511, 513, 527 (1997).

Journal 1997 Discusses the need for balance between business ethics and medical ethics in the context of managed care. Explores two models for integrating ethics and managed care. Proposes the adoption of a collective responsibility model to improve quality of care. Quotes Principles I, II, III, IV, and V. Cites Preamble. References Opinion 8.13. Regan, *Regulating the Business of Medicine: Models for Integrating Ethics and Managed Care*, 30 Colum. J. L. & Soc. Probs. 635, 651, 656, 657 (1997).

Journal 1996 Discusses the trend toward conserving resources expended on health care by withholding services absent a showing of necessity. Claims that the high standard of care physicians owe patients is jeopardized by medical treatment decisions based on coverage concerns. Concludes that the legal structure regarding health care plans should be changed. Quotes Preamble, Principles I, II, III, IV, V, VI, and VII, and Opinion 2.03. Hirshfeld & Thomason, *Medical Necessity Determinations: The Need for a New Legal Structure, 6 Health Matrix 3, 8-9 (1996).*

Journal 1995 Offers relevant historical perspectives and provides comprehensive ethical and legal discussion of physician-assisted suicide and euthanasia. Highlights important legislative developments, including the Oregon Death with Dignity Act, and analyzes significant judicial opinions. Quotes Principles III, IV, and VI and Opinions 2.21 and 9.12. Cites Opinions 2.20 and 8.11. Stone & Winslade, *Physician-Assisted Suicide and Euthanasia in the United States: Legal and Ethical Observations, 16 J. Legal Med. 481, 483, 490, 497, 498, 499 (1995).*

Journal 1994 Explores the ethical issues involved in a multidisciplinary team working with children in legal proceedings. Focuses on the relationships between professionals and the conflicts that arise regarding disclosure of confidential information and forced disclosure of nonprivileged information. Quotes Principles III and IV, Fundamental Elements (4), and Opinions 1.02 (1992) and 5.07 (1992) [now Opinion 5.05]. Cites Opinion 2.02. Glynn, *Multidisciplinary Representation of Children: Conflicts Over Disclosures of Client Communications, 27 J. Marshall L. Rev. 617, 625, 626, 630-32, 637, 639, 643 (1994).*

Journal 1994 Argues that physician aid-in-dying should be protected by the US Constitution and that patients should have a federal cause of action to challenge prohibitive state statutes. Considers how such a cause of action might affect public policy. Quotes Principles I and III. References Opinion 2.06. Note, *Toward a More Perfect Union: A Federal Cause of Action for Physician Aid-In-Dying, 27 U. Mich. J. L. Ref. 521, 538 (1994).*

Journal 1994 Reviews the evolution of the physician-patient relationship, with attention to patient autonomy. Examines the changing health care delivery environment. Quotes Preamble, Principles I, II, III, IV, V, and VI, Fundamental Elements (1) and (2), and Opinions 1.02 and 8.07 (1981) [now Opinion 8.08]. Cites Opinion 1.01. Szczygiel, *Beyond Informed Consent, 21 Ohio N. U. L. Rev. 171, 217, 218, 220, 225, 226, 256 (1994).*

Journal 1993 Discusses physicians' duty to disclose to patients medical treatment alternatives that are not readily available. Proposes that based on the historical development and legal requirements of the informed consent doctrine, physicians should be required to inform patients of non–readily available alternatives or face liability for breach of such obligation. Quotes Principles I, II, III, IV, and V and Opinion 8.08. Note, *Informed Choice: Physicians' Duty to Disclose Nonreadily Available Alternatives, 43 Case W. Res. L. Rev. 491, 491, 498-99, 508, 509 (1993).*

Journal 1991 Examines the wisdom and likely results of medicalizing psychoactive drugs of abuse. Concludes that although many physicians would consider prescribing psychoactive drugs of abuse for drug abusers in order to end dependence, few would be willing to prescribe such drugs for recreational purposes. Quotes Principle III. Levine, *Medicalization of Psychoactive Substance Use and the Doctor-Patient Relationship, 69 Milbank Quarterly 623, 624 (1991).*

Journal 1990 Discusses the moral dilemma in deciding whether to withdraw artificial nutrition and hydration from a patient and the appropriate role of the judiciary. Concludes that judicial decisions do not represent the moral viewpoint of society and that moral pronouncements should not be made in the courtroom. Quotes Preamble, Principles I, II, III, IV, V, VI, and VII, and Opinion 2.20. Peccarelli, *A Moral Dilemma: The Role of Judicial Intervention in Withholding or Withdrawing Nutrition and Hydration, 23 John Marshall L. Rev. 537, 539, 540, 541 (1990).*

Principle IV

10th Cir. 2001 Plaintiffs, former employees of a public medical center, brought suit against medical director under 42 USC § 1983, based upon medical director's racially and sexually harassing actions and statements. The district court awarded compensatory and punitive damages against the medical director. Affirming the award of damages, the court quoted Principles I and IV and concluded that the medical director's behavior impacted not only plaintiffs, but the overall public health. *Nieto v. Kapoor, 268 F.3d 1208, 1223 n. 12.*

D. Kan. 1991 With apparent reliance on Principle IV and Opinion 5.05, plaintiff claimed that other than in discovery or judicial proceedings, the physician-patient privilege is absolute and precludes ex parte communications with

defense counsel. While recognizing the confidential nature of the physician-patient relationship, the court held that the ethical standards promulgated by the AMA are not binding law and that, where a litigant-patient has placed his or her medical status in issue, the physician is released from the constraints imposed by the physician-patient relationship for the purposes of the litigation. *Bryant v. Hilst, 136 F.R.D. 487, 490.*

E.D. La. 2005 Plaintiff filed a motion to modify the district court's order requiring five days' notice to opposing counsel before interviewing plaintiff's prescribing physician. The court quoted Opinion 5.05 and cited Principle IV when discussing the physician-patient relationship and the physician's duty to protect confidences revealed by a patient. The court granted the plaintiff's motion and modified the order to ensure that defendants were faced with the same restrictions as the plaintiff and that plaintiff could conduct ex parte interviews with physicians not named as defendants. *In re Vioxx Products Liability Litigation, 230 F.R.D. 473, 476 n. 17.*

N.D. Ohio 1965 Plaintiff-patient alleged that the defendant–malpractice insurer induced physician to reveal confidential information about plaintiff on pretext that plaintiff filed a malpractice suit. In denying defendant's motion for reconsideration of the court's earlier opinion, the court confirmed its holding that actions of a third party inducing a physician to divulge confidential information may result in liability to the patient. In so holding, the court quoted (with incorrect citation to Ch. II, Sec.1) Principles Ch. I, Sec. 2 (1912) [now Principle IV and Opinion 5.08], to emphasize the medical profession's established views regarding confidentiality. *Hammonds v. Aetna Casualty & Sur. Co., 243 F. Supp. 793, 803.*

M.D. Pa. 1987 Plaintiff in a medical malpractice action sought to preclude his treating physicians from serving as defendant's expert witnesses at trial. The court held that defense counsel's failure to provide prior notice of ex parte communication with plaintiff's treating physicians barred their use as defense experts. Referring to *Petrillo v. Syntex Laboratories, Inc.,* 148 Ill. App. 3d 581, 499 N.E.2d 952 (1986), the court noted that the court there favorably cited Principle IV and Opinions 5.05, 5.06, and 5.07 (1984) in support of a public policy protecting confidentiality between physician and patient and against ex parte discussion. *Manion v. N.P.W. Medical Ctr. of N.E. Pa., Inc., 676 F.Supp. 585, 591.*

Ala. 1973 Physician revealed patient information to the patient's employer, contrary to instructions of patient. Patient sued for breach of fiduciary duty. Citing Principle 9 (1957) [now Principle IV and Opinion 5.05], as well as cases from other states, the court held that even in the absence of a testimonial privilege statute, as a matter of public policy, a physician has a fiduciary duty not to make extrajudicial disclosures of patient information acquired in the course of treatment unless the public interest or the private interest of the patient demands otherwise. In holding that the physician had breached his contract with patient, the court found the Principles together with state licensing requirements sufficient to establish the public policy of confidentiality. *Horne v. Patton, 291 Ala. 701, 287 So. 2d 824, 829, 832.*

Alaska 1977 Physician–school board member failed to fully comply with state's conflict of interest law by refusing to reveal the names of patients from whom he had received over $100 in income. The physician claimed a legal privilege or ethical duty not to disclose the information under Principle 9 (1957) [now Principle IV and Opinion 5.05] and, alternatively, that the conflict of interest law unconstitutionally invaded a patient's right to privacy. The court held that disclosure was not barred by a legal privilege or ethical mandate, but that the conflict of interest law unconstitutionally

invaded patient privacy due to the absence of protective regulations. In ruling on the ethical duty issue, the court noted that under Alaska law, a physician's license may be revoked for violating the Principles. However, the court found this licensing provision irrelevant to the privileged relationship exception in the conflict of interest law. The court found that otherwise the privilege exception in the statute could be changed by the AMA, a private organization, simply by amending the Principles. *Falcon v. Alaska Pub. Offices Comm'n, 570 P.2d 469, 474 n.13.*

Ariz. App. 1992 Employer argued that workers' compensation statute abrogated the physician-patient privilege statute, permitting ex parte communications with employee's treating physician. Recognizing that a physician is ethically bound to protect the confidentiality of privileged information pursuant to Principle IV, yet lacks the legal training to distinguish between privileged and unprivileged information, the court held that a claimant has the right to insist that his attorney be present when his employer interviews the employee's physician. *Salt River Project v. Industrial Comm'n, 1992 Ariz. App. LEXIS 323, 129 Ariz. Adv. Rep. 39.*

Ariz. App. 1989 In a medical malpractice action, defense counsel interviewed several of plaintiff's treating physicians ex parte and notified plaintiff of this in preparation for a medical liability review panel hearing. Plaintiff moved to bar all testimony by those physicians and to disqualify defense counsel from representing defendants. The appellate court noted a physician's obligation of confidentiality pursuant to Principle IV and Opinion 5.05 and held that defense counsel in a medical malpractice action may not engage in nonconsensual ex parte communications with plaintiff's treating physicians. *Duquette v. Superior Court, 161 Ariz. 269, 778 P.2d 634, 641.*

Cal. 1976 Parents sued psychotherapists to recover for murder of daughter by psychiatric patient, alleging that failure to warn victim of patient's violent threat was a proximate cause of her death. In considering whether such a revelation would have been a violation of professional ethics, the Court noted that Principle 9 (1957) [now Principle IV and Opinion 5.05] recognized that the confidential nature of a physician-patient communication must yield when disclosure is necessary to protect an individual or community as a whole. The court concluded that, in the circumstances of this case, disclosure would not have violated medical ethics and held that psychotherapists are under a duty to warn when they determine or should determine that a patient poses a serious danger of violence to someone else. *Tarasoff v. Regents of Univ. of Cal., 17 Cal.3d 425, 551 P.2d 334, 347, 131 Cal. Rptr. 14, 27.*

Cal. 1970 Psychiatrist-witness in civil assault case applied for writ of habeas corpus after being held in contempt of court for refusing to produce patient's psychiatric records. Patient, plaintiff in the assault action, neither expressly claimed nor waived the statutory psychotherapist-patient privilege. The court held that the litigant-patient exception to the statutory psychotherapist-patient privilege does not unconstitutionally infringe rights of privacy of either psychotherapists or their patients. The court noted that in such a context a psychiatrist does not violate Principle 9 (1957) [now Principle IV and Opinion 5.05] since the Principle allows for legally compelled disclosure. *In re Lifschutz, 2 Cal. 3d 415, 467 P.2d 557, 565-66 n.9, 85 Cal. Rptr. 829, 837-38 n.9.*

Cal. App. 1982 Defendant was convicted of lewd act with a child and child molestation or annoyance, after licensed clinical psychologist reported defendant's admission of sexual conduct to authorities. The court held that the psychologist's testimony was properly admitted since a statute requiring the reporting of actual or suspected child abuse expressly made the psychotherapist-patient privilege inapplicable. The court quoted Principle 9 (1957) [now Principle IV and Opinions 2.02 and 5.05] in concluding the disclosure was not a breach of professional ethics. *People v. Stritzinger, 137 Cal. App. 3d 126, 186 Cal. Rptr. 750, 752 rev'd, 34 Cal.3d 505, 668 P.2d 738, 194 Cal. Rptr. 431 (1983).*

Colo. 1989 Spouse of police officer killed by released psychiatric patient sued state mental hospital and psychiatrist for negligence. Patient had blamed police for his misfortunes during repeated involuntary commitments for paranoid schizophrenia, and psychiatrist knew that patient would have access to a gun after release. The court held that a psychiatrist owed a duty of care in determining whether patient had propensity for violence and posed unreasonable risk of serious bodily harm to others. In so holding, the court cited Principle 9 (1957) [now Principle IV and Opinion 5.05], in support of the view that there are situations in which the need to protect an individual or the community from the threat of harm from a patient may outweigh the strong policy in favor of nondisclosure of patient confidences. *Perreira v. State, 768 P.2d 1198, 1210 n.7.*

Del. Super. 1993 Plaintiff-patient brought action for invasion of privacy, breach of confidentiality, and breach of implied contract against defendants, a physician and nurse. Plaintiff alleged that defendant-nurse, without plaintiff's consent, informed plaintiff's mother and grandmother that she was pregnant. Plaintiff also alleged that defendant-physician was liable for the nurse's conduct based on respondeat superior. The defendants questioned whether plaintiff had stated a cause of action and, if so, whether the cause should be treated as a medical malpractice action. Quoting Principle IV and noting that the legislature and the courts had recognized the duty of confidentiality, the court held that plaintiff had a cause of action for breach of confidentiality. *Martin v. Baehler, 1993 WL 258843, 3.*

D.C. App. 2005 Appellant widow filed suit against appellee hospital for negligence in relation to her husband's suicide after his release from hospital. The district court granted appellee's motion for summary judgment, finding that patient suicide occurring six hours after release was not foreseeable. The appellate court affirmed. In the dissenting opinion, Principle IV is quoted to support the position

that the hospital, although the information was confidential, should have told appellant of her husband's suicidal tendencies because of the risk he posed to himself. *Garby v. George Washington University Hosp., 886 A.2d 510, 526.*

D.C. App. 1985 Patient sued plastic surgeon for breach of confidential physician-patient relationship following surgeon's use of before and after photographs of her plastic surgery in a department store presentation. In considering whether such a breach was an actionable tort, the court made reference to an earlier case quoting Principles Ch. II, Sec. 2 (1947) [erroneously cited in the earlier case as Ch. II, Sec. 1 (1943)] [now Principle IV and Opinion 5.05] as evidence of the strong public policy which exists in favor of maintaining a patient's confidences. *Vassiliades v. Garfinckel's, Brooks Bros., 492 A.2d 580, 590, 591.*

Fla. App. 1995 The court considered the issue of the effect of § 455.241(2) of the Florida Statutes on right of defense in a medical malpractice action to engage in ex parte communications with plaintiff's nonparty treating physician. The court held that a 1988 amendment to § 455.241(2) negated the applicability of the statute to medical malpractice cases. The dissent, citing *Petrillo v. Syntex Laboratories, Inc.,* 148 Ill. App. 3d 581, 499 N.E.2d 952 (1986), quoted Principles II and IV and Opinions 5.05, 5.06, and 5.08 as strong public policy support for its position that ex parte communications should be barred altogether. *Castillo-Plaza v. Green, 655 So. 2d 197, 206 n.4.*

Ill. 1997 Trial court held various statutory sections, including those permitting unlimited disclosure of a patient's medical records, unconstitutional. On appeal, state Supreme Court affirmed. Regarding provisions mandating consent to the disclosure of medical records, the court noted, with reference to Principle IV and Opinion 5.05, the crucial importance of confidentiality in the physician-patient relationship. *Best v. Taylor Machine Works, 179 Ill. 2d 367, 689 N.E. 2d 1057, 1099.*

Ill. 1997 Plaintiffs brought action for medical malpractice and loss of consortium against physicians. Defendants sought the release of medical information according to a statute providing for unlimited access to a plaintiff's medical records. The trial court found this provision unconstitutional as a violation of separation of powers and of patients' privacy rights. On appeal, the court agreed that the statute violated separation of powers. Further, with apparent reference to Principle IV, the court noted the ethical duty of physicians to maintain patient confidentiality. The court, in turn, held that the statute violated the right to privacy, as patients hold confidentiality of personal medical information to be an integral part of privacy interests. *Kunkel v. Walton, 179 Ill. 2d 519, 689 N.E. 2d 1047, 1055.*

Ill. App. 1987 In appeal of malpractice action, an issue was whether expert testimony of plaintiff's treating physician, based upon discussions with the defense counsel without patient's consent, was admissible. The court held that ex parte communications between a plaintiff's treating physician and legal adversary violated public policy. In determining the existence of such a policy favoring the sanctity of the doctor-patient relationship, the court noted *Petrillo v. Syntex Laboratories Inc.,* 148 Ill. App. 3d 581, 499 N.E.2d 952 (1st Dist. 1986) and its reference to the Principles and Opinions, namely Principle IV and Opinion 5.05 (1984), which establish an ethical obligation to keep physician-patient communications confidential, generally requiring a patient's consent before information is released. *Yates v. El-Deiry,* 160 Ill. App. 3d 198, 513 N.E.2d 519, 522.

Ill. App. 1986 Defense attorney in product liability suit was held in contempt of court for conducting ex parte discussions with plaintiff-patient's treating physician without patient's consent and contrary to authorized methods of discovery. The court held that the strong public policy favoring physician-patient confidentiality articulated in Principles II and IV and Opinions 5.05, 5.06, 5.07, and 5.08 (1984) justified a rule against such ex parte discussions. Further, the court held that the public has the right to rely on physicians to faithfully execute their ethical obligations. *Petrillo v. Syntex Laboratories, Inc.,* 148 Ill. App. 3d 581, 499 N.E.2d 952, 957, 958, 959 cert. denied, 483 US 1007 (1987).

Ill. App. 1979 Patient filed suit against physician for breach of contract and breach of confidential relationship after physician's employee disclosed patient's name to police. Patient alleged that implied contract arose out of a statutory physician-patient privilege, and provisions of the Code of Medical Ethics, with apparent reference to Principle 9 (1957) [now Principle IV and Opinion 5.05]. The court held that disclosure of patient's name alone by a physician or the physician's agents is insufficient to state a cause of action in contract and does not violate the physician-patient privilege. *Geisberger v. Willuhn,* 72 Ill. App. 3d 435, 390 N.E.2d 945, 946, 948.

Ind. App. 1996 A patient filed suit against a mental health counseling center for disclosing to a third party death threats made by the patient during therapy. The patient claimed this was a breach of the standard of care owed to her. The trial court found that the counseling center was not statutorily prohibited from disclosing death threats the patient made. On appeal, the court affirmed the decision. It noted, with apparent reference to Principle IV and Opinion 5.05, that physicians may disclose confidential information to ensure the safety of the public or of individuals. In clarifying its holding, the court observed that while free and frank communication should be promoted to aid proper diagnosis and treatment, public policy supports disclosure of confidential information when appropriate. *Rocca v. Southern Hills Counseling Center, Inc.,* 671 N.E. 2d 913, 916.

Me. 1999 Physician appealed decision of the Board of Licensure in Medicine imposing a civil penalty for his failure to release medical records to patient's physicians. Physician argued that the Board did not specify the ethical standards that his conduct violated. The court vacated the Board's decision on the grounds that the physician was denied the opportunity to refute evidence of a violation of professional standards or to develop a defense predicated on those standards. The Board, in defense of its decision, presented Opinions 7.01 and 7.02 to the court. The court, in vacating the decision, pointed out that the hearing record did not demonstrate which Opinions the Board applied. Furthermore, the court, quoting Principle IV, stated that the physician had a responsibility to protect the patient's medical records. *Balian v. Board of Licensure in Medicine,* 722 A.2d 364, 368.

Md. App. 2007 In an espionage case, a psychiatrist was engaged to evaluate defendant's competency. Defendant disclosed confidential information which the psychiatrist later disclosed to defendant's wife and the media. Defendant and his wife filed a complaint for breach of confidentiality with the State Board of Physicians, which revoked the psychiatrist's medical license. On appeal, the psychiatrist denied any unprofessional conduct. The court, quoting Principle IV, found the psychiatrist's behavior was unethical and unprofessional. With apparent reference to Opinion 5.05, the psychiatrist argued there was an exception to the duty of confidentiality when disclosure would protect the "community interest." The court found no such "community interest" exception. *Salerian v. Maryland State Board of Physicians,* 176 Md. App. 231, 932 A.2d 1225, 1235-36, 1241-42.

Md. Att'y Gen. 1989 Except as required by statute, physicians are not legally obligated to report that an adult has been sexually assaulted. Quoting Principle IV regarding the safeguarding of patient confidences within the constraints of the law, the opinion concludes that a physician must consider the confidential nature of the physician-patient relationship when deciding whether to report that a patient has been sexually assaulted. *Maryland Att'y Gen. Op. No. 89-022.*

Md. Att'y Gen. 1986 State attorney general opined that statute authorized physicians to report to the Motor Vehicle Administration patients with certain disorders that would impair their ability to drive. The opinion cites Principle IV in support of the conclusion that, where required by law, a physician's disclosure of patient information is proper. *Maryland Att'y Gen. Op. No. 86-030 71 Op. Att'y. Gen. 407, 410.*

Md. Att'y Gen. 1977 Opinion addresses the obligation of a psychiatrist to report child abuse information obtained from a parent-patient. Referring to state statutes and to Principle 9 (1957) [now Principle IV and Opinions 2.02 and 5.05], the opinion concludes that the question of whether to disclose suspected child abuse is a matter left to the individual psychiatrist's professional and moral judgment. *Maryland Att'y. Gen. Opinion, 62 Op. Att'y Gen. 157, 160.*

Mass. 1989 Physician appealed after being disciplined for discussing anticipated deposition testimony with malpractice defendant's attorney one day prior to scheduled deposition. The court, referring to Principle IV, noted that the AMA's ethical standards did not specifically address situation presented. After weighing the fact that physician had specifically asked attorney whether discussion was appropriate, the court held that the physician's behavior did not constitute gross misconduct and thus he could not be disciplined under licensing statute. *Hellman v. Board of Registration in Medicine, 404 Mass. 800, 537 N.E.2d 150, 153 n.4.*

Mass. 1984 Employee sued employer for libel and invasion of privacy following disclosure of medical facts about employee to other employees. In part, claim involved disclosure of opinion about employee's mental state to his supervisor by physician retained by employer. Citing Principle 9 (1957) [now Principle IV and Opinions 5.05 and 5.09], the court held that a physician retained by an employer may disclose to the employer information concerning an employee if receipt of the information is reasonably necessary to serve a substantial and valid business interest of the employer. *Bratt v. Intn'l Business Mach. Corp., 392 Mass. 508, 467 N.E.2d 126, 137 n.23.*

Minn. 1976 Plaintiff-patient in malpractice action appealed trial court's order to provide authorization for private, informal interview between defense counsel and patient's treating physician. In holding that formal pretrial discovery provided the exclusive procedure by which defendant could obtain medical testimony, the court noted, without deciding the issue, that a physician who discloses confidential patient information in a private interview may be subject to tort liability for breach of patient's right to privacy or professional discipline for unprofessional conduct, citing Principle 9 (1957) [now Principle IV and Opinion 5.05]. *Wenninger v. Muesing, 240 N.W.2d 333, 337 n.3.*

Mo. 1998 Defendant convicted of first-degree murder claimed that a physician's testimony at trial violated Principle IV and the statutory physician-patient privilege because the physician contacted the press, provided interviews about his examination of defendant, and testified for the prosecution to rebut defendant's posttraumatic stress disorder defense. The court stated that the defendent waived any privilege and that it was not its place to enforce professional ethical standards. *State v. Johnson, 968 S.W.2d 123, 131.*

Mo. 1993 Patient sued physicians alleging a breach of fiduciary duty of confidentiality for participating in an unauthorized ex parte discussion with defendant's attorney. While recognizing this duty, the court held that, where the plaintiff's medical condition is in issue, this constitutes a waiver of both the testimonial privilege and the physician's fiduciary duty insofar as the information is related to the medical issues. Quoting Opinion 5.05 and citing Principle IV, the court stated that courts may apply ethical principles to frame the specific limits of the legal duty of confidentiality. *Brandt v. Medical Defense Assoc., 856 S.W.2d 667, 671 n.1.*

Mo. 1989 In a personal injury suit, plaintiff challenged trial court's authority to compel plaintiff to authorize ex parte meetings between defendant insurance company and plaintiff's treating physician. Applying a balancing test between preserving the physician-patient confidential and fiduciary

relationship, the physician-patient testimonal privilege, and the quest for truth in civil litigation, the court held that such information could be obtained through the methods of formal discovery. The court quoted Principle IV and Opinion 5.05 (1984) as statements of the policy underlying medical confidentiality and a basis for a patient's affirmative right to rely on the confidential nature of disclosures to a treating physician. *State ex. rel. Woytus v. Ryan, 776 S.W.2d 389, 392-93.*

Mo. App. 1985 In a prohibition proceeding arising from a medical malpractice action, defense attorneys sought order compelling plaintiff to authorize a private interview between defense attorneys and physician who treated plaintiff for injuries allegedly caused by defendant-physician. The appellate court, after discussing Principle IV and Opinion 5.05 (1984), held that the defense attorneys had the right to seek an ex parte interview with the treating physician, subject to the willingness of the physician to grant the interview. Furthermore, the court noted that Opinion 5.05 prevents a physician from revealing a patient's confidences only where there is a lack of consent from the patient and found that consent did exist here in the form of a medical authorization executed by plaintiff during pendency of the malpractice action. *State ex rel. Stufflebam v. Appelquist, 694 S.W.2d 882, 886, 888 n.7, overruled by State ex. rel. Woytus v. Ryan, 776 S.W.2d 389 (Mo. 1989).*

N.J. 1985 Plaintiff provided authorization for release of decedent's medical records from former treating physicians but refused to consent to depositions or interviews between defense counsel and physicians. The court noted physicians' ethical duty to avoid unauthorized disclosure, as stated in Principle 9 (1957) [now Principle IV and Opinion 5.05], but recognized that a patient's right to confidentiality was not absolute. After balancing the competing interests involved, the court held that defense counsel had a right to seek ex parte interviews of decedent's other treating physicians regarding litigation matters, provided procedural safeguards were met including clear statements that participation in such an interview is voluntary on the part of a physician. *Stempler v. Speidell, 100 N.J. 368, 495 A.2d 857, 860, cert. denied, 483 US 1007 (1987).*

N.J. 1979 In wrongful death action against a psychiatrist whose patient murdered plaintiff's decedent, the court concluded, in accord with Principle 9 (1957) [now Principle IV], that a psychiatrist may owe a duty to warn potential victims of possible danger from psychiatrist's patient despite the general emphasis on confidentiality. The court also noted the Preamble and Principles 1 and 3 (1957) [now revised Preamble, Principle I, and Opinion 5.05] in discussing the psychiatrist-patient relationship. *McIntosh v. Milano, 168 N.J. Super. 466, 403 A.2d 500, 510, 512-13.*

N.J. 1962 Parents sued pediatrician for unauthorized disclosure to life insurer of deceased infant's congenital heart defect. The court quoted Principle 9 (1957) [now Principle IV and Opinion 5.05] as an articulation of a physician's legal duty to his or her patient subject to exceptions of compelling social or patient interests. The court held that the parents had lost their limited right to nondisclosure by filing an insurance claim. *Hague v. Williams*, 37 N.J. 328, 181 A.2d 345, 347.

N.J. Super. 2002 Patient brought suit against physician for releasing her medical records to opposing counsel in a divorce action without her authorization or consent. The lower court dismissed the complaint for failure to state a claim and ruled the records were discoverable. The New Jersey Superior Court reversed, holding that the patient had a cause of action against both the physician and opposing counsel. Quotes Principle IV. *Crescenzo v. Crane*, 350 N.J. Super. 531, 796 A.2d 283, 290.

N.J. Super. 1991 Physician's estate sued hospital alleging that it violated state law against discrimination by restricting the physician's surgery privileges and requiring him to inform patients of his HIV-infected status before performing invasive procedures. The defendant hospital was also alleged to have breached its duty to maintain confidentiality of his seropositive diagnosis. The court held that the hospital had not discriminated against the physician since the hospital had relied on ethical and professional standards, including a report of the Council on Ethical and Judicial Affairs of the AMA dealing with the issue of AIDS [now Opinions 9.13 and 9.131]. However, the hospital was held to have breached its fiduciary duty to maintain the confidentiality of the physician's medical records. Referring to *McIntosh v. Milano*, 168 N.J. Super. 466, 403 A.2d 500 (1979), which had quoted AMA Principles of Medical Ethics sec. 9 (1957) [now Principle IV and Opinion 5.05] in applying the "duty to warn" exception, the court noted that the disclosure in this case went far beyond the medical personnel directly involved in the treatment of the physician and those patients entitled to informed consent. *Estate of Behringer v. Medical Ctr.*, 249 N.J. Super. 597, 614, 633, 592 A.2d 1251, 1259, 1268.

N.J. Super. 1988 Several portions of state department of corrections regulations concerning exceptions to privileged communications between psychologist and inmates were invalidated by appellate court because they permitted disclosure of confidences that did not present clear and imminent danger to the inmate or others, or failed to identify any intended victim. Court made general reference (with erroneous quotation) to Principle 9 (1957) [now Principle IV and Opinion 5.05]. *In re Rules Adoption*, 224 N.J. Super. 252, 540 A.2d 212, 215.

N.J. Super. 1987 Defendant in a personal injury suit sought to offer testimony from plaintiff's treating physician regarding plaintiff's prognosis. The court denied plaintiff's motion to exclude that evidence, despite the ethical obligation of physicians to uphold patients' communications as confidential under Principle 9 (1957) [now Principle IV and Opinion 5.05]. The court's decision was based on New Jersey case law permitting disclosure of a patient's medical condition to someone having a legitimate interest where the physical condition of the patient is made an element of a claim. *Kurdek*

v. West Orange Bd. of Educ., 222 N.J. Super. 218, 536 A.2d 332, 335.

N.J. Super. 1967 In a suit for separate maintenance, communications between plaintiff-wife and her psychiatrist were not protected from disclosure during depositions, despite Principle 9 (1957) [now Principle IV and Opinion 5.05], which prohibited physicians from disclosing patient confidences except where necessary to protect the welfare of the individual or of the community. The court concluded that the patient had only a limited right of nondisclosure, subject to exceptions created by supervening interest of society, and that the institution of litigation by the patient constituted a vitiation of that right. *Ritt v. Ritt*, 98 N.J. Super. 590, 238 A.2d 196, 199 rev'd, 52 N.J. 177, 244 A.2d 497 (1968).

N.Y. Sup. 2000 Physician brought wrongful discharge claim against corporate employer. The physician alleged she was discharged because she refused to reveal confidential medical information regarding employees. With apparent reference to Principle IV and Opinions 5.05 and 5.09, the affidavit filed by the physician claimed she had an ethical and legal duty to protect patient confidentiality. The court found termination of an employee at will based upon such grounds is sufficient to state a cause of action for breach of contract. The court ruled that obligations of good faith and fair dealing may be implied in a contract for the employment of a physician and that no physician should be placed in the position of choosing between retaining employment and violating ethical standards. *Horn v. New York Times*, 186 Misc. 2d 469, 719 N.Y.S. 2d 471, 474.

N.Y. Sup. 1977 Plaintiff, a psychiatric patient, sued her psychiatrist and the psychiatrist's spouse for violating several state statutes and her privacy rights by publishing a book about the intimate details of plaintiff's psychotherapy. The court found for plaintiff, basing its decision in part upon Principle 9 (1957) [now Principle IV and Opinion 5.05], which requires a physician to uphold the confidences of a patient. *Doe v. Roe*, 93 Misc. 2d 201, 400 N.Y.S.2d 668, 674.

N.Y. Surr. 1977 In a discovery proceeding, respondent-psychiatrist, who had treated some patients of deceased psychiatrist subsequent to his death, allegedly misappropriated decedent's patient records. Estate petitioned court for return of records and damages for injury to value of decedent's practice. Respondent sought dismissal of claim, arguing that estate could not sell patient records. The court rejected respondent's request. In so ruling, the court noted that under Principle 9 (1957) [now Principle IV and Opinion 5.05] prohibiting physicians from revealing patient confidences, various guidelines had been issued regarding sale of a medical practice [now Opinion 7.04]. Whether respondent's actions had interfered with the estate's efforts to dispose of decedent's practice in keeping with these guidelines presented the court with factual issues for later resolution. *Estate of Finkle*, 90 Misc. 2d 550, 395 N.Y.S.2d 343, 346.

N.C. 1990 Plaintiff in a malpractice case was granted an order prohibiting ex parte conferences between defendant's attorney and nonparty treating physicians. The court noted that both the Principles of Medical Ethics and Current Opinions affirm the physician's duty to protect patient confidentiality, in apparent reference to Principle IV and Opinion 5.05. In consideration of (1) the patient's right to privacy, (2) physician-patient confidentiality, (3) the adequacy of formal discovery procedures, and (4) the dilemma in which nonparty treating physicians are placed by ex parte conferences, the court held that an attorney may not interview a patient's nonparty treating physicians privately without express authorization. *Crist v. Moffatt, 326 N.C. 326, 333, 389 S.E.2d 41, 46.*

Ohio 2009 Physician appealed from a judgment affirming an order of the state medical board that permanently revoked appellant's certificate to practice medicine. The board found that appellant's sexual contact with patients violated Ohio statutes governing physician conduct and the AMA's Code of Medical Ethics, citing Principles I, II, IV, and VIII. The Court of Appeals held that Ohio state law allows the board to revoke a physician's certificate if it finds that the person violated any provision of the AMA's Code of Medical Ethics. *D'Souza v. State Med. Bd. of Ohio, 2009 WL 5108774, 6.*

Ohio 1999 Patients brought a class action suit against hospital on grounds that the hospital disclosed patients' confidential medical information to the hospital's law firm, in order to determine whether the patients were eligible for government benefits to pay for unpaid hospital bills. The trial court granted defendants' motion for summary judgment. On appeal, the court held that a physician or a hospital can be held liable for unauthorized out-of-court disclosure of patients' confidential information. In addition, the court found that an independent tort exists for unauthorized, unprivileged disclosure of patients' private medical information to a third party. The court cited Principle 9 (1957) [now Principle IV and Opinion 5.05], noting that courts have looked to such sources in providing a cause of action for breach of patient confidentiality. *Biddle v. Warren General Hospital, 86 Ohio St. 3d 395, 715 N.E.2d 518, 523.*

Ohio 1997 Estates of victims who were killed by their mentally ill son brought suit against son's psychotherapist for failing to disclose potential for violence. Son had been institutionalized and treated for schizophrenia. After release, he continued to take medication and see a psychotherapist. Despite parents' objections and attempts to have him involuntarily recommitted, psychotherapist reduced his medication and continued to recommend outpatient treatment. The court held that the psychotherapist had a duty to exercise reasonable care to control the son so as to prevent him from causing harm to his family. The court expressed concern for safeguarding the confidentiality of psychotherapeutic communications but noted that Principle 9 (1957) [now Principle IV and Opinion 5.05] has long allowed breaches of confidence when it becomes necessary to protect

the welfare of the individual or the community. *Estates of Morgan v. Fairfield Family Counseling Center, 77 Ohio St. 3d 284, 303, 673 N.E.2d 1311, 1326.*

Ohio 1991 State medical board revoked license of physician who had consensual sexual relations with his patient. The court upheld the board's ruling that this violated Principles I, II, and IV. Dissenting judge, citing AMA Council on Ethical and Judicial Affairs, Sexual Misconduct in the Practice of Medicine, 266 *JAMA* 2741 [now Opinion 8.14], argued that until 1991, the AMA did not clearly deem sexual contact with a patient unethical. *Pons v. Ohio State Medical Bd., 66 Ohio St. 3d 619, 623, 625, 614 N.E.2d 748, 752, 753.*

Ohio 1988 Administrator sued psychiatrist for wrongful death after recently discharged patient killed her infant daughter. In determining whether a professional judgment rule should be adopted in the malpractice standard of care where the prediction of violent behavior is involved, the court referred favorably to Principle 9 (1957) [now Principle IV and Opinion 5.05], which allows breaches of patient confidences when necessary to protect potential victims. *Littleton v. Good Samaritan Hosp., 39 Ohio St. 3d 86, 529 N.E.2d 449, 459 n.19.*

Ohio App. 2005 The Ohio State Medical Board permanently revoked the license of the appellant, a psychiatrist, for having inappropriate physical and sexual contact with a female patient. The trial court affirmed the board's ruling, and the appellant appealed. The board claimed that the appellant's relationship with his patient violated the AMA's Code of Medical Ethics, citing Principles I, II, and IV. The appellate court affirmed, stating that permanent revocation of the appellant's license was not excessive and was not a violation of due process as the board may revoke the appellant's license if treatment did not meet minimal standards of care and violated any provision of the AMA's Code of Medical Ethics. *Schechter v. Ohio State Med. Bd., 2005 WL 1869733, 9.*

Ohio App. 1999 Physician appealed trial court's affirmation of state medical board's decision to suspend his medical license because the physician engaged in sexual relationships with mothers of his pediatric patients. On appeal, the physician claimed that he was denied due process because physicians were not adequately notified that having sexual relations with parents of pediatric patients was unethical. The physician also claimed that the board had not presented adequate evidence that AMA's Code of Medical Ethics Principles I and IV extend to the parents of pediatric patients. The court quoted Principles I and IV, and stated that medical experts who testified were of the opinion that having sexual relationships with parents of pediatric patients constituted ethical violations. *Gladieux v. Ohio State Medical Board, 1999 WL 770959, *2, *4.*

Okla. 1988 In response to a police request, physician reported patient treated for a penile bite. Patient sued physician for negligence after information furnished by physician led to patient's arrest and conviction for rape. Patient alleged a tortious breach of the physician-patient confidential relationship, breach of contract, violation of licensing statute, and breach of Principle 9 (1957) [now Principle IV and Opinion 5.05]. The court reasoned that the benefit of the divulgence inured to the public at large and thus fell within the public policy exception to the testimonial privilege, created no liability in tort or contract, and was not a breach of medical ethics under the licensing statute or the Principles. *Bryson v. Tillinghast, 749 P.2d 110, 113, 114.*

Pa. 1973 Plaintiff in personal injury suit resulting from auto accident claimed that trial court should have allowed showing on cross-examination that defendant's expert medical witness, who had treated plaintiff, violated Principle 9 (1957) [now Principle IV and Opinion 5.05] by ex parte communications with defense counsel, in order to impeach his medical testimony. The court held that any connection between an alleged breach of medical ethics and the credibility of a physician on the witness stand was tenuous. Therefore, the trial court's decision barring further inquiry in this regard was proper. *Downey v. Weston, 451 Pa. 259, 301 A.2d 635, 638.*

Pa. Super. 1988 Plaintiff-patient sued her physician for breach of confidentiality when physician conferred with defense counsel in plaintiff's malpractice suit against the hospital (physician's employer). In its majority opinion, the court cited Principle IV, commenting that it gave very little guidance to physicians but nonetheless was not violated by the physician. The court also noted Opinion 5.07 (1986), finding that the plaintiff's suit minimized her expectations of confidentiality. The dissent, however, interpreted these same provisions, along with Opinion 5.05 (1986), as protecting plaintiff's expectations of confidentiality. *Moses v. McWilliams, 379 Pa. Super. 150, 549 A.2d 950, 956, 962 (dissent), appeal denied, 521 Pa. 630, 558 A.2d 532 (1989).*

S.C. 2003 Worker's Compensation Commission ordered injured employee's attorney to stop obstructing ex parte contacts between rehabilitative nurse hired by employer and treating physicians regarding employee's medical condition. The South Carolina Supreme Court reversed and held that the Worker's Compensation Act did not authorize such ex parte communication. Quotes Principle IV. *Brown v. Bi-Lo, Inc, 354 S.C. 436, 581 S.E.2d 836, 840, n. 5.*

S.C. App. 1997 Patient sued physician for breaching duty of confidentiality after physician divulged patient's emotional health status in a letter which was introduced during patient's divorce proceeding. The trial court dismissed the action for failure to state a cause of action, finding state law did not support a duty of confidentiality. The appeals court reversed. In part, it found a basis for such an action in medical and ethical principles, with apparent reference to Principle IV. Absent a compelling public interest in disclosure, confidences must be preserved. The court remanded to consider whether the disclosure was essential to the best interests of the patient or others. *McCormick v. England, 328 S.C. 627, 494 S.E. 2d 431, 435.*

Tenn. App. 1994 Plaintiff sought damages for wrongful death from defendant-surgeon. Defendant requested that the court require plaintiff to sign a form authorizing release of medical records and information to defense counsel. Trial court denied defendant's motion, noting, with apparent reference to Principle IV and Opinion 5.05, that confidential relationship exists between physician and patient. Appellate court affirmed although it did not reach the ethical issue of the propriety of disclosures by a physician. *Wright v. Wasudev, 1994 Tenn. App. LEXIS 657.*

Utah Att'y Gen. 1978 A physician who, acting in good faith, discloses confidential information to proper authorities concerning a patient's unfitness to drive is not liable for doing so. Reference is made to Principle 9 (1957) [now Principle IV and Opinion 5.05] to support propriety of such disclosure where the public interest is involved. *Utah Att'y Gen. Op. No. 77-294.*

Wash. 1988 Personal representative brought wrongful death action against decedent's physicians. At issue was whether defense counsel in a personal injury action may communicate ex parte with plaintiff's treating physician where plaintiff has waived the physician-patient relationship. In holding that defense counsel may not engage in ex parte communication, and is limited to formal discovery methods, the court cited Principle IV and Opinion 5.05 (1986) with approval, reasoning that the mere threat of disclosure of private conversations between a physician and defense counsel would chill the physician-patient relationship and hinder further treatment. *Loudon v. Mhyre, 110 Wash. 2d 675, 756 P.2d 138, 141, 141 n.3.*

Wash. App. 2000 Patient sued a physician under medical malpractice statute, seeking damages for emotional distress resulting from the physician's disclosure of confidential information to the patient's ex-husband. Trial court granted the defendant's motion for summary judgment. On appeal, the court held that a tort action did exist under the statute for damages resulting from the unauthorized disclosure of confidential information related to health care obtained within the physician-patient relationship. The court quoted Principle IV, stating that the accepted standard of care includes a duty to maintain confidentiality with respect to patient information. *Berger v. Sonneland, 101 Wash. App. 141, 1 P.3d 1187, 1192.*

W. Va. 1993 Plaintiff, in a malpractice action, sought a writ of prohibition to prevent the enforcement of a trial court order allowing ex parte interviews. The court, in granting the writ, held that any benefit from ex parte interviews that occurs is minimal compared to the danger that they will undermine the confidential nature of the physician-patient relationship. Quoting Principles of Medical Ethics Ch. II, sec. 1 (1943) [now Principle IV and Opinion 5.05], the court noted that the medical profession is well aware of the importance of patient confidentiality. *State ex. rel. Kitzmiller v. Henning, 437 S.E.2d 452, 454.*

W. Va. 1988 Patient-wife sued psychiatrist who disclosed subpoenaed confidential information to her husband's attorney in divorce proceedings. The court held that a tort action lies when confidential communications regarding mental health patients are released, except under limited circumstances such as a binding court order. The court, however, declined to recognize an enforceable contractual right to confidentiality, although it noted that some states have recognized such a right based upon Principle IV. *Allen v. Smith, 368 S.E.2d 924, 928.*

Wis. 1995 In medical malpractice suit, the court held that (1) subject to restrictions, defense counsel may engage in ex parte communications with plaintiff's treating physician if the communications do not involve disclosure of confidential information; (2) outside a judicial proceeding, defendant-physician may communicate ex parte with plaintiff's treating physician subject to a physician's duty of confidentiality; and (3) if defense counsel elicits confidential information from a treating physician during ex parte communications, the appropriate sanction is within the discretion of the court. The court expressly overruled *State ex rel. Klieger v. Alby,* 125 Wis. 2d 468, 373 N.W.2d 57 (Ct. App. 1985) and the cases applying it. The majority and concurring opinions referred to Principle IV and Opinion 5.05. *Steinberg v. Jensen, 194 Wis. 2d 440, 534 N.W.2d 361, 370, 377.*

Wis. App. 1994 In medical malpractice suit, defense counsel engaged in ex parte communications with plaintiff's consulting physicians. Plaintiff amended her complaint seeking punitive damages for breach of confidentiality. The court concluded that the rule of *State ex rel. Klieger v. Alby,* 125 Wis. 2d 468, 373 N.W.2d 57 (Ct. App. 1985), which prohibits ex parte communications that have the potential to breach physician-patient confidentiality, was violated and sanctions were required. The court referred to *Petrillo v. Syntax Labs., Inc., 148 Ill. App. 3d 581, 499 N.E.2d 952 (1986)* and its use of Principle IV and Opinion 5.05. *Steinberg v. Jensen, 186 Wis. 2d 237, 519 N.W.2d 753, 761 n.9, rev'd, 194 Wis. 2d 440, 534 N.W.2d 361 (1995).*

Wis. Att'y Gen. 1987 Physicians may report cases of suspected child abuse or neglect when a patient discloses that he or she has abused a child in some manner. Where report is made in good faith, physicians are immune from any civil or criminal liability. Passing reference is made to Principle 9 (1957) [now Principle IV and Opinions 2.02 and 5.05] in support of this position. *Wisconsin Att'y Gen. Op. 10-87 (Mar. 16, 1987) (LEXIS, States library, Wis. file).*

Journal 2010 Examines published resources within the medical and legal fields that focus on confidentiality and evaluates those resources to determine if they help clarify confidentiality issues. Further, discusses differences between these professions that may be hindrances when serving the same patient or client. Concludes that, while both professions guard against disclosure of patient/client communications, they also allow for disclosure in certain instances such as imminent death, harm, or injury.

References Principle IV and cites Opinions 2.02, 2.23, 2.24, and 5.05. Johns, *Multidisciplinary Practice and Ethics Part II—Lawyers, Doctors, and Confidentiality, 6 NAELA J. 55, 57-65, 68 (2010).*

Journal 2010 Discusses the effects of using deidentified health information on privacy and considers the dangers of nonconsensual use of health information. Concludes deidentification of health information is a necessary though insufficient protection of privacy, and further research and regulations should be developed to demonstrate respect for individuals without unduly burdening research. Quotes Principle IV and Opinions 5.05 and 7.025. Rothstein, *Is Deidentification Sufficient to Protect Health Privacy in Research? 10 Am. J. Bioethics 3, 5 (Sept. 2010).*

Journal 2010 Analyzes factors contributing to the emergence of medical repatriation and evaluates whether this practice comports with current legal and ethical standards. Proposes changes to federal regulations that govern hospitals and clarifications to medical ethical standards. Quotes the Preamble and Principles I, II, III, IV, V, VI, VII, VIII, and IX. Zoellner, *Medical Repatriation: Examining the Legal and Ethical Implications of an Emerging Practice, 32 Wash. U. J. L. & Pol'y 515, 530-532 (2010).*

Journal 2009 Explores the history of the debate over when lawyers may or must disclose client confidences. Concludes a lawyer's duty to keep client confidences involves a philosophical question of the lawyer's role in society. Quotes Principle 9 (1957) [now Principle IV]. Ariens, *"Playing Chicken": An Instant History of the Battle Over Exceptions to Client Confidences, 33 J. Legal Prof. 239, 255 (2009).*

Journal 2009 Discusses the interaction between statutes and case law governing the medical field and the core principles of medical professionalism. Concludes the legal framework of medical professionalism does not encompass all the elements required of a medical professional. Quotes Principles II, III, IV, V, VI, VII, and VIII. Fichter, *The Law of Doctoring: A Study of the Codification of Medical Professionalism, 19 Health Matrix 317, 338, 339, 340, 343, 351 (2009).*

Journal 2009 Discusses whether patients have a right to pain management. Concludes that no physician duty is established by law or ethics to provide pain management outside the traditional physician-patient relationship. Cites Principles I, II, IV, and VIII. Hall & Boswell, *Ethics, Law, and Pain Management as a Patient Right, 12 Pain Physician 499, 500 (2009).*

Journal 2009 Discusses the judicial standard for reviewing physician noncompete covenants. Concludes courts should apply a strict standard to such covenants, rather than declare the covenants per se invalid. Quotes Principles IV and VII, Principles of Medical Ethics §5 (1957) [now Principle VI], Code of Medical Ethics Ch. II, Art. I §3 (1847) [now Opinion 5.02], Opinion 9.02, and Code of Medical Ethics Ch. II, Art. I §4 (1847) [now Opinion 9.09]. Cites Opinions 8.041, 8.115, 9.02, 9.06, 9.065, 9.067, 10.01, and 10.015.

Koons, *Physician Employee Non-Compete Agreements on the Examining Table: The Need to Better Protect Patients' and the Public's Interests in Indiana,* 6 Ind. Health L. Rev. 253, 272-77, 280-81 (2009).

Journal 2009 Examines genetic discrimination, the Genetic Information Nondiscrimination Act, and the social fairness ideas behind its categorical protections for genetic information. Concludes genetic antidiscrimination acts based on broad categorical protections may be misguided. Cites Code of Ethics of the AMA § 8 (1848) [now Principle IV]. Morrow, *Insuring Fairness: The Popular Creation of Genetic Antidiscrimination,* 98 Geo. L. J. 215, 237 (2009).

Journal 2009 Examines a new Internal Revenue Service program for "whistleblower awards" given to informants who identify noncompliant taxpayers. Concludes that while whistleblowers may be useful for discovering noncompliance, Congress should prohibit awards given to those who breach confidential relationships. Quotes Principle IV. Morse, *Whistleblowers and Tax Enforcement: Using Inside Information to Close the "Tax Gap,"* 24 Akron Tax J. 1, 33 (2009).

Journal 2009 Examines Health Information Portability and Accountability Act (HIPAA) and the common law doctrine of informed consent with respect to electronic health record programs and the duty to obtain informed consent before allowing use of electronic health record services. Concludes that in order to protect individual privacy, electronic health record service providers should obtain informed consent before allowing their users to post their medical histories. Cites Principle IV. Prasse, *Hippocrates Would Roll Over in His Grave: An Examination of Why Internet Health Care Programs Should Obtain Informed Consent From Their Users,* 42 Creighton L. Rev. 733, 746 (2009).

Journal 2009 Explores the process of an attorney advising a client to seek mental health treatment and how that recommendation impacts the attorney-client relationship. Concludes attorneys must be willing to advise clients to seek treatment if appropriate. Quotes Principle IV. Suzuki, *When Something Is Not Quite Right: Considerations for Advising a Client to Seek Mental Health Treatment,* 6 Hastings Race & Poverty L. J. 209, 250 (2009).

Journal 2008 Discusses ex parte interviews with a treating physician in discovery before and after the HIPAA Privacy Rule and the issues facing physicians contacted for such interviews. Concludes courts and attorneys should work together to allow for efficient discovery while protecting physicians. Quotes Principles IV and VIII and Opinions 5.05 and 10.01. Burnette & Morning, *HIPAA and Ex Parte Interviews—the Beginning of the End?* 1 J. Health & Life Sci. L. 73, 100-01 (2008).

Journal 2008 Argues a general physician-patient privilege is needed in West Virginia and outlines the manner in which the privilege could be adopted. Concludes that the privilege will allow physicians to maintain their fiduciary role, foster open communication between patient and physician,

and encourage patients to freely seek medical treatment. Quotes Principle IV and Opinion 5.05. Johnson, *"I Will Not Divulge": How to Resolve the "Mass of Legal Confusion" Surrounding the Physician-Patient Relationship in West Virginia,* 110 W. Va. L. Rev. 1231, 1247 (2008).

Journal 2008 Examines the pattern of school shootings perpetuated by mentally unstable individuals, focusing on the shooter at Virginia Tech and the failings of the mental health system in that situation. Concludes schools and universities should implement new policies to protect the privacy of mental health records while ensuring a safe learning environment for all students. Quotes Principle IV. Muñoz, *Privacy at the Cost of Public Safety: Reevaluating Mental Health Laws in the Wake of the Virginia Tech Shootings,* 18 S. Cal. Interdisc. L. J. 161, 172 (2008).

Journal 2008 Examines the development of bioethics and environmental ethics, as well as laws promoting the role of bioethicists in decision making. Concludes environmental ethicists must convince legislatures of the role of environmental ethics in order to have a greater impact on decision making. Quotes Principles I, II, III, IV, V, VI, VII, VIII, and IX. Robertson, *Seeking a Seat at the Table: Has Law Left Environmental Ethics Behind as it Embraces Bioethics?* 32 Wm. & Mary Envtl. L. & Pol'y Rev. 273, 307 (2008).

Journal 2007 Reviews American Bar Association (ABA) Model Rule of Professional Conduct 3.6, governing the speech of attorneys while involved in trials, and analyzes how it applies distinctly to speech directed at judges, prosecutors, and the court system. Concludes that Rule 3.6 affords more protection to judges than to prosecutors or the court system. Quotes Principle IV. Hinkie, *Free Speech and Rule 3.6: How the Object of Attorney Speech Affects the Right to Make Public Criticism,* 20 Geo. J. Legal Ethics 695, 695 (2007).

Journal 2007 Discusses confidentiality privileges under the law. Concludes that the short story "Mr. Prinzo's Breakthrough" is a valuable tool for teaching students about exceptions to confidentiality privileges. Quotes Principle IV. Moore, *Mr. Prinzo's Breakthrough and the Limits of Confidentiality,* 51 St. Louis L. J. 1059, 1064 (2007).

Journal 2007 Argues that issuance of apologies from physicians who commit medical errors will diminish the number of malpractice suits brought. Concludes that patients desire apologies in the case of medical errors and are less likely to sue when they are given. Cites Principles I, II, III, and IV and Opinion 8.12. Tabler, *Should Physicians Apologize for Medical Errors?* 19 Health Lawyer 23, 25 (Jan. 2007).

Journal 2006 Analyzes cases where a patient's right to refuse care conflicts with the physician's obligation to protect that patient's well-being. Concludes health care providers should seek a compromise that best promotes both patient autonomy and well-being. Quotes Principle IV and Ch. I, Art. II, Sec. 6 (May 1847) [now Opinion 10.01]. Carrese, *Refusal of Care: Patients' Well-being and*

Physicians' Ethical Obligations, 296 JAMA 691, 692, 693 (2006).

Journal 2006 Explores conscience clause legislation relating to the dispensing of oral contraceptives. Concludes that such legislation must balance the interests of the patient and the health care provider. Cites Principles I, II, III, IV, V, VI, VII, VIII, and IX. Collins, *Conscience Clauses and Oral Contraceptives: Conscientious Objection or Calculated Obstruction? 15 Ann. Health L. 37, 54 (2006).*

Journal 2006 Analyzes the ethical and legal problems of confidentiality which arise in the context of genetic testing. Concludes that the disclosure of a patient's genetic disease to others is only allowable when the patient is a minor and the family has a right to know. Quotes Principle IV and references Principle 9 (1957) [now Principle IV and Opinion 5.05]. Denbo, *What Your Genes Know Affects Them: Should Patient Confidentiality Prevent Disclosure of Genetic Test Results to a Patient's Biological Relatives? 43 Am. Bus. L. J. 561, 572, 577 (2006).*

Journal 2006 Evaluates the influence that Justice Blackmun's experience at the Mayo Clinic had on his opinions related to medicine. Concludes that Blackmun's experience had less of an impact on his opinions than is traditionally assumed. Quotes Principle 9 (1957) [now Principle IV and Opinion 5.05]. Hunter, *Justice Blackmun, Abortion, and the Myth of Medical Independence, 72 Brooklyn L. Rev. 147, 190-91 (2006).*

Journal 2006 Examines a mental health professional's competing duties of confidentiality and reporting a patient's threats of violence. Suggests new legislation should clarify duty to report a threat. Quotes Preamble and Principles III, IV, and VIII. Cites Opinion 5.05. Mossman, *Critique of Pure Risk Assessment or, Kant Meets Tarasoff, 75 U. Cin. L. Rev. 523, 579 (2006).*

Journal 2006 Analyzes the privacy risks associated with introducing a system of electronic medical records. Concludes that cost and confidentiality concerns mandate that security must be built into the initial system. Cites Ch. I, Art. I, Sec. 2 (May 1847) [now Principle IV and Opinion 5.05]. Rothstein & Talbott, *Compelled Disclosure of Health Information: Protecting Against the Greatest Potential Threat to Privacy, 295 JAMA 2882, 2883 (2006).*

Journal 2006 Examines situations where physician-patient confidentiality may be breached to prevent violations of human rights. Suggests that new laws should be enacted to specify when a physician may testify about a violation of human rights. Quotes Principle IV and Opinion 5.05. Weissbrodt & Wilson, *Piercing the Confidentiality Veil: Physician Testimony in International Criminal Trials Against Perpetrators of Torture, 15 Minn. J. Int'l L. 43, 68, 68-69 (2006).*

Journal 2005 Discusses the current "market approach" regarding who controls personal genetic information. Concludes that, consistent with principles of individualism,

American citizens should have the right to their own genetic information. Quotes Principle IV. Cole, *Authentic Democracy: Endowing Citizens With a Human Right in Their Genetic Information, 33 Hofstra L. Rev. 1241, 1251 (2005).*

Journal 2005 Examines issues surrounding tort reform proposals. Concludes that more can be done to correct the current tort system before moving toward a "one size fits all" approach. Quotes Principles I, II, III, IV, V, VI, VII, VIII, and IX. Messerly & Warwick, *Nowhere to Turn: A Glance at the Facts Behind the Supposed Need for Tort "Reform," 28 Hamline L. Rev. 489, 506 (2005).*

Journal 2004 Argues that courts should put safeguards in place to protect the confidential relationship between at-risk children and health care professionals. Concludes that such protection may limit disclosure of private information in court proceedings, enhance the dignity of minors, and facilitate their well-being. Quotes Principle IV. Katner, *Confidentiality and Juvenile Mental Health Records in Dependency Proceedings, 12 Wm. & Mary Bill of Rts. J. 511, 529 (2004).*

Journal 2004 Argues that the privacy model rather than the property model is the most appropriate way to protect an individual's interest in genetic information. Concludes that privacy interests must nevertheless be balanced against other societal factors. References Principle IV and Opinion 5.05. Suter, *Disentangling Privacy From Property: Toward a Deeper Understanding of Genetic Privacy, 72 Geo. Wash. L. Rev. 737, 787 (2004).*

Journal 2003 Considers the legal, medical, and ethical issues of physician-patient confidentiality in disclosure of paternity. Concludes that a balancing test should be applied to making determinations regarding disclosure of paternity. Quotes Principles I, IV, and V and Opinions 1.02, 5.055, and 10.01. Cites Principle II and Opinion 5.05. Richards & Wolf, *Medical Confidentiality and Disclosure of Paternity, 48 S. D. L. Rev. 409, 411, 412, 413 (2003).*

Journal 2003 Uses public policy arguments to support a preponderance standard for medical license revocations in situations involving false testimony by a medical expert witness. Concludes that medical licensing boards can more effectively protect the public by using a preponderance standard. Quotes Principles II, III, and IV and Opinions 1.02 and 9.07. Widmer, *South Dakota Should Follow Public Policy and Switch to the Preponderance Standard for Medical License Revocation After In Re the Medical License of Dr. Reuben Setliff, M.D., 48 S. D. L. Rev. 388, 396-97, 402 (2003).*

Journal 2002 Analyzes the expanded use of the Civil False Claims Act in prosecuting health care fraud. Concludes that, in enforcing the law, government must balance its promises to beneficiaries, health care providers, and the public. Quotes Principles I, II, and IV. Krause, *"Promises to Keep": Health Care Providers and the Civil False Claims Act, 23 Cardozo L. Rev. 1363, 1365 (2002).*

Journal 2002 Considers the dilemma of informed consent in the context of prescribing psychotropic medication to patients with mental illness and mental retardation. Recognizes the need for substituted decision-making in certain situations. Concludes that legislation would help address this issue. Quotes Preamble, Principles I, III, IV, VIII, and IX, and Opinion 8.08. O'Sullivan & Borcherding, *Informed Consent for Medication in Persons With Mental Retardation and Mental Illness,* 12 Health Matrix 63, 75, 86, 87, 88 (2002).

Journal 2002 Considers the ethical and legal issues regarding breach of confidentiality in situations where a patient is pregnant and uses teratogenic substances. Concludes that a breach of confidentiality causes damage to the physician-patient relationship. Quotes Principle IV and Opinion 10.01. Plambeck, *Divided Loyalties: Legal and Bioethical Considerations of Physician–Pregnant Patient Confidentiality and Prenatal Drug Abuse,* 23 J. Legal Med. 1, 8, 25 (2002).

Journal 2002 Analyzes the role of prognostication in physician-patient communication. Concludes that the patient-physician model of shared decision-making offers the best hope for reestablishing prognostication. Quotes Principles Ch. I, Art. I, Sec. 2 and 4 (1846) [now Principle IV and Opinions 8.12 and 10.01]. Cites Opinion 8.08. Rich, *Prognostication in Clinical Medicine: Prophecy or Professional Responsibility?* 23 J. Legal Med. 297, 299, 318, 327 (2002).

Journal 2002 Considers the case of *Ferguson v. City of Charleston.* Concludes that the Supreme Court's rationale in that case reflects insights from feminist legal theory. Quotes Opinion 10.01. Cites Principles II and IV. Taslitz, *A Feminist Fourth Amendment? Consent, Care, Privacy, and Social Meaning in Ferguson v. City of Charleston,* 9 Duke J. Gender L. & Pol'y 1, 18, 19 (2002).

Journal 2001 Discusses issues surrounding the privacy of genetic information. Considers the social, ethical, and legal responses to problems that arise in this context. Concludes with a unique view of privacy that would protect the right of individuals not to know genetic information about themselves. Quotes Principle IV and Opinion 10.01. Laurie, *Challenging Medical-Legal Norms: The Role of Autonomy, Confidentiality, and Privacy in Protecting Individual and Familial Group Rights in Genetic Information,* 22 J. Legal Med. 1, 24 (2001).

Journal 2001 Considers ethical aspects of physician conflicts of interest in the context of human subjects research. Focuses on conflicts that are associated with clinical trials of new drugs and devices. Concludes by discussing the impact of these conflicts of interest on trust in the physician-patient relationship. References Principle IV and Opinion 8.032. Miller, *Trusting Doctors: Tricky Business When It Comes to Clinical Research,* 81 B. U. L. Rev. 423, 427-28 (2001).

Journal 2001 Considers conflicts of interest in clinical research and other types of medical practice. Compares the way in which physicians and lawyers address conflicts of interest in professional practice. Concludes that physicians are unaware of the need to create a meaningful conflict-of-interest doctrine for medical practice. Quotes Preamble, Principle IV, and Opinions 2.07, 8.03, 8.031, and 10.01. Moore, *What Doctors Can Learn From Lawyers About Conflicts of Interest,* 81 B. U. L. Rev. 445, 447, 449-50 (2001).

Journal 2001 Discusses linkages between governmental regulation of medical privacy and reduced medical error. Concludes that protection of patient privacy and the reduction of medical error will be important aspects of health care reform and will spur structural changes in health care delivery that will positively affect evolution of medical malpractice law. Quotes Principle IV. Terry, *An eHealth Diptych: The Impact of Privacy Regulation on Medical Error and Malpractice Litigation,* 27 Am. J. L. & Med. 361, 402 (2001).

Journal 2000 Discusses the development and history of the ethical doctrine of informed consent. Examines the current state of the law in Pennsylvania and concludes it does not adequately fulfill the goals of ethical and legal doctrines. Quotes Principle IV and Opinion 10.01. References Opinion 8.08. Warren, *Pennsylvania Medical Informed Consent Law: A Call to Protect Patient Autonomy Rights by Abandoning the Battery Approach,* 38 Duq. L. Rev. 917, 925 (2000).

Journal 1999 Examines reporting of AIDS and HIV under Texas law. Discusses limitations on a physician's ability to warn potentially at-risk third parties. Concludes that Texas law should be changed to place a duty upon physicians to notify at-risk third parties of a patient's HIV-positive status. Quotes Principle IV and Opinion 10.01. Acosta, *The Texas Communicable Disease Prevention and Control Act: Are We Offering Enough Protection to Those Who Need It Most?* 36 Hous. L. Rev. 1819, 1822, 1830, 1831 (1999).

Journal 1999 Discusses whether a physician has the duty to disclose cancer-related gene mutations to a patient's children. Reviews current legislation regarding disclosure of genetic information. Argues that the potential for harm outweighs imposition of a duty to disclose. Quotes Principle IV. Brownrigg, *Mother Still Knows Best: Cancer-Related Gene Mutations, Familial Privacy, and a Physician's Duty to Warn,* 26 Fordham Urb. L. J. 247 (1999).

Journal 1999 Discusses the use of expert witnesses. Points out that, although some professions have a code of ethics, there is not a single source that defines professional ethics for expert witnesses. Argues that ethical and professional standards for expert witnesses must be defined. Cites Principle IV. Lubet, *Expert Witnesses: Ethics and Professionalism,* 12 Geo. J. Legal Ethics 465, 466 (1999).

Journal 1999 Discusses the practice of male circumcision in the US. Examines situations where the state may intervene in parental decision-making affecting minor children. Argues that males should be afforded the same protection as females in statutes prohibiting the mutilation of genital organs. Quotes Principle IV. Povenmire, *Do Parents Have the Legal Authority to Consent to the Surgical Amputation of Normal, Healthy Tissue From Their Infant Children? The Practice of Circumcision in the United States, 7 Am. U. J. Gender Soc. Pol. & L. 87, 96 (1999).*

Journal 1999 Discusses the need for physicians to advocate on behalf of patients' rights in the context of health care delivery. Evaluates the nature and scope of the physician's role as advocate, noting that physicians cannot be expected to engage in attorney-like advocacy. Quotes Principles IV and VI, Fundamental Elements (2), (4), and (6) [now Opinion 10.01], Patient Responsibilities 5 [now Opinion 10.02], and Opinions 2.03, 2.07, 2.09, 2.16, 2.19, 3.06, 4.01, 4.04, 6.01, 7.02, 8.02, 8.03, 8.13, 8.132, 9.06, 9.07, and 9.131. Cites Opinions 5.05, 5.09, 7.01, 8.135, and 9.02. Sage, *Physicians as Advocates, 35 Hous. L. Rev. 1529, 1537, 1541, 1542, 1552-53, 1554, 1556, 1557, 1559, 1561-62, 1564, 1571, 1574, 1576, 1580 (1999).*

Journal 1999 Discusses the Department of Health and Human Services recommendations for federal legislation regarding confidentiality of health information. Points out that the recommendations include an exception for law enforcement access to medical records. Argues that such an exception must be narrow and clearly defined. Quotes Principle IV. Van Der Goes, *Opportunity Lost: Why and How to Improve the HHS-Proposed Legislation Governing Law Enforcement Access to Medical Records, 147 U. Pa. L. Rev. 1009, 1063 (1999).*

Journal 1999 Explores Model Rules of Professional Conduct focusing on the attorney-client relationship. Compares confidentiality provisions in the Model Rules with the rules of confidentiality governing the medical profession. Observes that existing confidentiality rules are incomplete and ambiguous. Concludes that one remedy is to embrace a discretionary confidentiality rule. Quotes Opinion 5.05. Cites Principle IV and Opinion 5.07. Zer-Gutman, *Revising the Ethical Rules of Attorney-Client Confidentiality: Towards a New Discretionary Rule, 45 Loy. L. Rev. 669, 683-84, 699, 709, 718 (1999).*

Journal 1998 Discusses issues of privacy arising out of collection and dissemination of genetic information about specific individuals. Emphasizes the need for privacy and confidentiality in this context. Suggests that future public policy should accommodate this need. Quotes Principle IV. Balint, *Issues of Privacy and Confidentiality in the New Genetics, 9 Alb. L. J. Sci. & Tech. 27, 32 (1998).*

Journal 1998 Recommends the passage of Ohio's proposed bill that would recognize an accountant-client privilege. Describes current recognized privileges, including the physician-patient privilege. Quotes Principle IV. Canning, *Privileged Communications in Ohio and What's New on the Horizon: Ohio House Bill 52 Accountant-Client Privilege, 31 Akron L. Rev. 505, 550 (1998).*

Journal 1998 Suggests that professional ethics correspond well to many governmental areas. Argues that the professional rules are more difficult for politically appointed attorneys. Indicates that ethical questions for government-appointed attorneys are often resolved through personal ethics rather than professional codes. Cites Principle IV. Lund, *The President as Client and the Ethics of the President's Lawyers, 61 L. & Contemp. Probs. 65, 68 (1998).*

Journal 1998 Discusses issues of patient consent regarding disclosure of medical information. Points out that recent changes in the health care system have presented medical record privacy concerns. Discloses findings of a study regarding hospital consent forms and calls for more research to be conducted. Cites Principle IV and Opinion 5.05. Merz, Sankar, & Yoo, *Hospital Consent for Disclosure of Medical Records, 26 J. Law Med. & Ethics 241, 248 (1998).*

Journal 1998 Examines the transition from paper medical records to electronic medical records. Identifies issues of confidentiality and privacy that arise as a result of the move to electronic medical records. Concludes that federal protection is needed to safeguard personal medical information. Quotes Principle IV and Opinions 5.07 and 5.075. Cites Opinion 8.061. Tsai, *Cheaper and Better: The Congressional Administrative Simplification Mandate Facilitates the Transition to Electronic Medical Records, 19 J. Legal Med. 549, 570, 581 (1998).*

Journal 1998 Explores the increased use and benefits of telemedicine. Points out that there is inadequate protection of privacy rights regarding electronic medical information. Concludes that federal law does not uniformly address medical record privacy and that Missouri law lacks adequate specificity. Quotes Principle IV. References Opinion 5.05. Young, *Telemedicine: Patient Privacy Rights of Electronic Medical Records, 66 UMKC L. Rev. 921, 926 (1998).*

Journal 1997 Discusses the Massachusetts statute that prohibits disclosure of a person's HIV status without obtaining informed consent. Suggests that legislation should be enacted mandating reporting of HIV to the department of public health. Quotes Principle IV. Agnello, *Advocating for a Change in the Massachusetts HIV Statute: Putting an End to Physician Uncertainty, 2 J. Trial App. Advoc. 105, 107 (1997).*

Journal 1997 Discusses the need for health care providers to have accurate medical information to treat patients effectively. Explains the benefits of computerized patient medical records and the privacy and confidentiality concerns raised. Concludes that patient privacy needs to be assured to improve service. Quotes Principle IV. Cuzmanes & Orlando, *Automation of Medical Records: The Electronic Superhighway and Its Ramifications for Health Care Providers, 6 J. Pharmacy & L. 19, 27 (1997).*

Journal 1997 Discusses principles of autonomy in the physician-patient relationship. Notes that rights to privacy and confidentiality are grounded in patient autonomy. Concludes that patients may be harmed when privacy rights are breached. Quotes Principle IV. Doyal, *Human Need and the Right of Patients to Privacy, 14 J. Contemp. Health L. & Pol'y 1, 3 (1997).*

Journal 1997 Considers principles of confidentiality in the physician-patient relationship. Notes the current trend emphasizing public reporting obligations of physicians to protect members of society. Emphasizes need for balance between patient rights and societal interests. Quotes Principle IV and Opinion 5.05. References Preamble. Jozefowicz, *The Case Against Having Professional Privilege in the Physician-Patient Relationship, 16 Med. & L. 385, 386-87, 391 (1997).*

Journal 1997 Suggests that ex parte conferences between treating physicians and opposing counsel undermine the physician-patient relationship. Notes that there are no significant benefits within the fact-finding process that justify the conflicts of interest created. Concludes that ex parte conferences are unnecessary. Quotes Principle IV and Opinion 5.05. Kassel, *Counterpoint . . . Defense Counsel's Ex Parte Communication with Plaintiff's Doctors: A Bad One-Sided Deal, 9 S. C. Law. 42, 43 (Sept./Oct. 1997).*

Journal 1997 Discusses the need for balance between business ethics and medical ethics in the context of managed care. Explores two models for integrating ethics and managed care. Proposes the adoption of a collective responsibility model to improve quality of care. Quotes Principles I, II, III, IV, and V. Cites Preamble. References Opinion 8.13. Regan, *Regulating the Business of Medicine: Models for Integrating Ethics and Managed Care, 30 Colum. J. L. & Soc. Probs. 635, 651, 656, 657 (1997).*

Journal 1997 Explores confidentiality problems that arise as a result of new health information systems. Examines legal aspects of medical records confidentiality. Advocates legislation at the national level to protect privacy of personal health information. Cites Principles of Medical Ethics § 9 (1957) [now Principle IV]. Turkington, *Medical Record Confidentiality Law, Scientific Research, and Data Collection in the Information Age, 25 J. Law Med. & Ethics 113, 126 (1997).*

Journal 1996 Explores whether patients have a duty to disclose their HIV status to treating physicians. Suggests that recognizing such a duty may subject patients to a lower standard of care and provide a disincentive to be tested. Concludes that courts should not impose a duty to disclose on patients. Quotes Principle 9 (1957) [now Principle IV] and Opinion 9.131. DeNatale & Parrish, *Health Care Workers' Ability to Recover in Tort for Transmission or Fear of Transmission of HIV From a Patient, 36 Santa Clara L. Rev. 751, 782-83, 787 (1996).*

Journal 1996 Discusses the trend toward conserving resources expended on health care by withholding services absent a showing of necessity. Claims that the high standard of care physicians owe patients is jeopardized by medical treatment decisions based on coverage concerns. Concludes that the legal structure regarding health care plans should

be changed. Quotes Preamble, Principles I, II, III, IV, V, VI, and VII, and Opinion 2.03. Hirshfeld & Thomason, *Medical Necessity Determinations: The Need for a New Legal Structure, 6 Health Matrix 3, 8-9 (1996).*

Journal 1996 Discusses sexual abuse litigation in which accusers have recovered memories of molestation in psychotherapy sessions. Observes that to successfully defend against such claims, it is necessary for the accused to have access to the clinical record. Posits that confidentiality problems can be eliminated with in camera record inspections. References Principle IV and Opinion 5.05. Loftus, Paddock, & Guernsey, *Patient-Psychotherapist Privilege: Access to Clinical Records in the Tangled Web of Repressed Memory Litigation, 30 U. Rich L. Rev. 109, 127 (1996).*

Journal 1996 Reviews two Washington State Supreme Court decisions in which subsequent treating physicians testified against their patients and on behalf of defendant physicians in malpractice litigation. Observes that these decisions erode the physician-patient privilege. Posits that the decisions are inconsistent with current medical ethics and proposes a statutory enactment as a solution. Quotes Opinion 5.05. Cites Principle 9 (1957) [now Principle IV]. Oppenheim, *Physicians as Experts Against Their Own Patients? What Happened to the Privilege? 63 Def. Couns. J. 254, 257, 261 (1996).*

Journal 1996 Considers prearraignment forensic evaluations. Notes the prohibition against use of such evaluations. Examines underlying ethical precepts. Observes that principles of beneficence are misapplied to forensic psychiatry in this context. Advocates a new ethical framework. Quotes Preamble. References Principle IV and Opinion 5.05. Ornish, Mills, & Ornish, *Prearraignment Forensic Evaluations: Toward a New Policy, 24 Bull. Am. Acad. Psychiatry Law 453, 454, 469 (1996).*

Journal 1996 Examines the psychiatrist-patient duty of confidentiality. Notes that Principles of Medical Ethics prohibit the disclosure of patient confidences and medical records. Observes that exceptions to this prohibition exist when required by law or to protect the community. Quotes Principle 9 (1957) [now Principle IV and Opinion 5.05]. Sadoff, *Ethical Obligations for the Psychiatrist: Confidentiality, Privilege, and Privacy in Psychiatric Treatment, 29 Loy. L.A. L. Rev. 1709, 1710, 1711 (1996).*

Journal 1996 Examines the theories courts have used when evaluating claims for emotional distress damages arising from HIV misdiagnosis. Observes that the physical injury requirement is outdated but notes that alternatives may give rise to potentially unlimited liability. Concludes that physicians should be afforded good faith immunity from suits. Quotes Principle 9 (1957) [now Principle IV]. Schmid, *Protecting the Physician in HIV Misdiagnosis Cases, 46 Duke L. J. 431, 458 (1996).*

Journal 1995 Discusses the belief of health care providers that they have an ethical obligation to warn the partners of HIV-positive patients. Examines both the scope of a

Massachusetts statute that prevents providers from releasing HIV test results of patients and possible defenses that providers may assert. Quotes Principle IV and Opinion 5.05. Friedland, *HIV Confidentiality and the Right to Warn—The Health Care Provider's Dilemma*, 80 Mass. L. Rev. 3, 4 (March 1995).

Journal 1995 Examines federal legislative proposals intended to protect confidentiality of computerized medical records. Concludes that proposed legislation will significantly undermine confidentiality. Cites Opinion 5.07. References Principle IV. Hoge, *Proposed Federal Legislation Jeopardizes Patient Privacy*, 23 Bull. Am. Acad. Psychiatry Law 495, 498, 500 (1995).

Journal 1995 Offers relevant historical perspectives and provides comprehensive ethical and legal discussion of physician-assisted suicide and euthanasia. Highlights important legislative developments, including the Oregon Death with Dignity Act, and analyzes significant judicial opinions. Quotes Principles III, IV, and VI and Opinions 2.21 and 9.12. Cites Opinions 2.20 and 8.11. Stone & Winslade, *Physician-Assisted Suicide and Euthanasia in the United States: Legal and Ethical Observations*, 16 J. Legal Med. 481, 483, 490, 497, 498, 499 (1995).

Journal 1994 Compares Texas law with Illinois law on the issue of ex parte communications between defense counsel and the patient/plaintiff's physician in civil litigation. Argues that preservation of the physician-patient relationship requires prohibition of such contact. Quotes Principles II and IV and Opinion 5.05. Comment, *From the Land of Lincoln a Healing Rule: Proposed Texas Rule of Civil Procedure Prohibiting Ex Parte Contact Between Defense Counsel and a Plaintiff's Treating Physician*, 25 Tex. Tech L. Rev. 1081, 1081, 1082 (1994).

Journal 1994 Considers whether an exception should be made to physician-patient confidentiality that would allow a physician to reveal parental medical history to a child. Concludes that such an exception would not completely erode physician-patient confidentiality. Quotes Principle IV, Fundamental Elements (4), and Opinion 5.05. Cites Principle I and Fundamental Elements (1). Friedland, *Physician-Patient Confidentiality: Time to Re-examine a Venerable Concept in Light of Contemporary Society and Advances in Medicine*, 15 J. Legal Med. 249, 257, 264, 276 (1994).

Journal 1994 Explores the ethical issues involved in a multidisciplinary team working with children in legal proceedings. Focuses on the relationships between professionals and the conflicts that arise regarding disclosure of confidential information and forced disclosure of nonprivileged information. Quotes Principles III and IV, Fundamental Elements (4), and Opinions 1.02 (1992) and 5.07 (1992) [now Opinion 5.05]. Cites Opinion 2.02. Glynn, *Multidisciplinary Representation of Children: Conflicts Over Disclosures of Client Communications*, 27 J. Marshall L. Rev. 617, 625, 626, 630-32, 637, 639, 643 (1994).

Journal 1994 Discusses physician-patient confidentiality and the exception that permits breach of a patient's confidence if required by law. Argues that this is always a legitimate exception to the confidentiality rule. Quotes Principle IV and Fundamental Elements (4). McConnell, *Confidentiality and the Law*, 20 J. Med. Ethics 47, 47 (1994).

Journal 1994 Reviews the evolution of the physician-patient relationship, with attention to patient autonomy. Examines the changing health care delivery environment. Quotes Preamble, Principles I, II, III, IV, V, and VI, Fundamental Elements (1) and (2), and Opinions 1.02 and 8.07 (1981) [now Opinion 8.08]. Cites Opinion 1.01. Szczygiel, *Beyond Informed Consent*, 21 Ohio N. U. L. Rev. 171, 217, 218, 220, 225, 226, 256 (1994).

Journal 1994 Discusses the importance of confidentiality in the physician-patient relationship and under what circumstances patient information may be released. Examines unique considerations that apply when a physician provides medical care to a minor or an HIV-infected individual. Quotes Principle IV and Fundamental Elements (4). Weiner & Wettstein, *Confidentiality of Patient-Related Information*, 112 Arch. Ophthalmology 1032, 1033 (1994).

Journal 1993 Discusses family privacy rights and considers the meaning of justice, self-respect, and the fundamental principles of physician ethics. Concludes that physicians have an ethical duty to intervene in domestic violence so long as such intervention does not breach confidentiality or violate patient autonomy. Quotes Principle IV and Opinion 5.05. References Opinions 8.14 and 9.131. Jecker, *Privacy Beliefs and the Violent Family: Extending the Ethical Argument for Physician Intervention*, 269 JAMA 776, 778, 779 (1993).

Journal 1993 Discusses physicians' duty to disclose to patients medical treatment alternatives that are not readily available. Proposes that based on the historical development and legal requirements of the informed consent doctrine, physicians should be required to inform patients of non–readily available alternatives or face liability for breach of such obligation. Quotes Principles I, II, III, IV, and V and Opinion 8.08. Note, *Informed Choice: Physicians' Duty to Disclose Nonreadily Available Alternatives*, 43 Case W. Res. L. Rev. 491, 491, 498-99, 508, 509 (1993).

Journal 1993 Explores the idea of reverse informed consent, which would impose a duty on patients to inform health care professionals of their infectious status. Concludes that such a duty is justified. Quotes Principles IV and VI and Opinions 8.11 and 9.131. Oddi, *Reverse Informed Consent: The Unreasonably Dangerous Patient*, 46 Vand. L. Rev. 1417, 1449, 1463, 1465, 1479 (1993).

Journal 1993 Discusses the issues surrounding the confidentiality of electronic and computerized medical records. Concludes that any legal standard addressing this problem should balance the need to protect patient confidentiality with the practical constraints, such as cost and accessibility limiting ideal security. References Principle IV and Opinion 5.07. Waller & Fulton, *The Electronic Chart: Keeping It Confidential and Secure, 26 J. Health & Hosp. L. 104, 105 (April 1993).*

Journal 1992 Discusses legal issues in the context of disclosing health information in adoptions. Presents the arguments for and against disclosure, including the traditional view favoring nondisclosure. References Principle IV. Blair, *Lifting the Genealogical Veil: The Blueprint for Legislative Reform of the Disclosure of Health-Related Information in Adoption, 70 No. Carolina L. Rev. 681, 692 (1992).*

Journal 1991 Discusses the case of *Crist v. Moffat,* which prohibits ex parte communications with a plaintiff's treating physician in North Carolina. Examines the physician-patient privilege and looks at various jurisdictions that permit and forbid ex parte communications. Quotes Principle IV and Opinion 5.06. Comment, *Shielding the Plaintiff and Physician: The Prohibition of Ex Parte Contacts With a Plaintiff's Treating Physician, 13 Campbell L. Rev. 233, 243, 248 (1991).*

Journal 1990 Examines the relationship between professional ethics and professional autonomy, perceived problems of health care rationing under a prospective payment vs a fee-for-service system, and the relationship between professional ethics and the problem of rationing. Concludes that rationing is inevitable, forcing important ethical questions to be addressed. Quotes Principles IV and VI. Agich, *Rationing and Professional Autonomy, 18 Law Med. & Health Care 77, 79, 82 (1990).*

Journal 1990 Examines the extent to which forensic psychiatrists are consulted in medical malpractice cases. Considers the appropriate standard of care, particularly for psychiatric malpractice cases, and the problems associated with its determination. References Principles II and IV. Modlin, *Forensic Psychiatry and Malpractice, 18 Bull. Am. Acad. Psychiatry Law 153, 161 (1990).*

Journal 1990 Discusses the moral dilemma in deciding whether to withdraw artificial nutrition and hydration from a patient and the appropriate role of the judiciary. Concludes that judicial decisions do not represent the moral viewpoint of society and that moral pronouncements should not be made in the courtroom. Quotes Preamble, Principles I, II, III, IV, V, VI, and VII, and Opinion 2.20. Peccarelli, *A Moral Dilemma: The Role of Judicial Intervention in Withholding or Withdrawing Nutrition and Hydration, 23 John Marshall L. Rev. 537, 539, 540, 541 (1990).*

Journal 1990 Presents current issues, policies, legislation, and judicial decisions regarding impaired physicians. Concludes by proposing enhanced confidentiality requirements in disciplinary proceedings and nationwide adoption of a uniform law in this area. Quotes Opinion 4.07. References Principle IV. Walzer, *Impaired Physicians: An Overview and Update of the Legal Issues, 11 J. Legal Med. 131, 174, 192 (1990).*

Journal 1989 Discusses the history of the physician-patient privilege up through changes implemented under the Ohio Tort Reform Act of 1987. Aspects of the physician-patient privilege that are most significantly affected by this Tort Reform Act are highlighted, with recommendations for further refinement of the privilege in Ohio. Quotes Principles II and IV and Opinion 5.05. Note, *The Ohio Physician-Patient Privilege: Modified, Revised, and Defined, 49 Ohio St. L. J. 1147, 1167 (1989).*

Journal 1985 Initially describes how existing doctrines protect the value of autonomy in the context of the physician-patient relationship, then examines various problems in the current protective scheme. Concludes by recommending the creation of an independent articulable protected interest in patient autonomy. Quotes Principles II and IV. Cites Opinions 4.04 (1984) [now Opinions 8.03 and 8.032] and 6.03 (1984) [now Opinion 6.02]. Shultz, *From Informed Consent to Patient Choice: A New Protected Interest, 95 Yale L. J. 219, 275 (1985).*

Journal 1983 Examines the evolution and impact of decisions in *Tarasoff v. Regents of the University of California,* 131 Cal. Rptr. 14 (Cal. 1976), and *McIntosh v. Milano,* 403 A.2d 500 (N.J. Super. 1979), which established a duty on the part of a physician or psychotherapist to warn third parties foreseeably endangered by a patient. In establishing such a duty, the courts endeavored to balance the physician's duty to warn endangered third parties with the duty to maintain confidentiality within the physician-patient relationship. Quotes Principle IV. Roth & Levin, *Dilemma of Tarasoff: Must Physicians Protect the Public or Their Patients? 11 Law Med. & Health Care 104, 106 (1983).*

Journal 1981 Observes that a reevaluation of medicine and the medical profession is occurring on at least three levels: theoretical, educational, and professional. Notes that physicians are facing various challenges to the exercise of many of their societal functions and emphasizes that physicians view law and the medical profession as the source most responsible for these challenges. Quotes Principle IV. Schwartz & Gibson, *Defining the Role of the Physician: Medical Education, Tradition, and the Legal Process, 18 Houston L. Rev. 779, 791 (1981).*

Principle V

S.D. Ind. 1992 Drug manufacturer sought protective order to prevent disclosure of patients' and physicians' names from adverse drug reaction reports. Plaintiff, quoting Principle V, which requires that physicians "make relevant information available to . . . the public," argued that requiring the disclosure of physicians' names would not deter physicians from reporting adverse drug reactions. The court held that the Principle notwithstanding, disclosure of physicians' names would seriously undermine the FDA's voluntary reporting system. *In re Eli Lilly & Co., 142 F.R.D. 454, 458.*

D.S.C. 1968 Military dependent sued government physicians under Federal Tort Claims Act where child with acute abdominal pain was twice referred to naval hospital with diagnosis of possible appendicitis and twice sent home without treatment, eventually suffering ruptured appendix and serious complications. In finding for the plaintiff, the court quoted Principle 8 (1957) [now Principle V and Opinion 8.04] in considering whether the physicians had a duty to seek consultation in such a situation. *Steeves v. United States, 294 F. Supp. 446, 454.*

Cal. App. 2004 Trial court sustained a demur to the appellants' first amended complaint. The appellate court quoted Principles II and V in concluding the coroner's practice of hiring a pathologist who had a close working relationship with a company which treats individuals whose death the pathologist may be required to investigate was a questionable policy due to the pathologist's wide discretion. The appellate court, however, affirmed the trial court's decision that appellants had not stated any viable claims. *Miller v. Rupf, 2004 WL 2092015, 11 n. 9.*

Minn. 1999 Plaintiffs sought declaratory relief against hospital for its refusal to grant plaintiffs access to peer review materials. The trial court granted the defendant's motion for summary judgment. On appeal the Minnesota Supreme Court held that physicians' private right to access a hospital's peer review materials did not outweigh public interest in quality health care. The court stated that quality care could be jeopardized if physicians had access to peer review material. The court also cited Principle V, stating that physicians have an ethical duty to participate in the peer review process. *Amaral v. Saint Cloud Hospital, 598 N.W.2d 379, 388.*

Tex. 1993 Estate of man who committed suicide after taking drug filed suit against manufacturer and sought adverse reaction or drug experience reports submitted to the FDA. These reports are voluntarily submitted by physicians and other health care providers and, according to 21 CFR § 314.430(e)(4)(ii), the FDA must keep the identity of the reporters and the patients confidential. Noting the public interest in the voluntary reporting system and that the trial court had ordered disclosure of confidential information without applying the standard of relevance and need, the court denied disclosure of the reporters' identities. Quoting Principle V, the dissent declared that the decision adversely affected public health and safety by leaving drug manufacturers free to conceal important information. *Eli Lilly & Co. v. Marshall, 850 S.W.2d 155, 163.*

Journal 2011 Examines ethical reasons for excluding medical methods from patent protection and discusses whether they are appropriate. Compares the treatment of medical methods under the Japanese patent system with laws in Europe and the US. Concludes the ethical issues surrounding Japan's patent system should be viewed from the standpoint of whether the patent system can be socially justified and would lead to industrial development. Quotes Principle 2 (1957) [now Principle V]. Liu & Sato, *Patent Protection of Medical Methods—Focusing on Ethical Issues, 20 Pac. Rim. L. & Pol'y J. 125, 135 (2011).*

Journal 2011 Argues that regulation of physicians' off-label use of prescription medications is necessary to prevent harm to both the patient and to society via unnecessary increases in health care spending. Concludes the state should intervene in the physician-patient relationship when physicians prescribe medicine off-label that is not justified by high-quality evidence of safety and efficacy. Quotes Principles I and V. Rosoff & Coleman, *The Case for Legal Regulation of Physicians' Off-Label Prescribing, 86 Notre Dame L. Rev. 649, 675 (2011).*

Journal 2010 Analyzes factors contributing to the emergence of medical repatriation and evaluates whether this practice comports with current legal and ethical standards. Proposes changes to federal regulations that govern hospitals and clarifications to medical ethical standards. Quotes the Preamble and Principles I, II, III, IV, V, VI, VII, VIII, and IX. Zoellner, *Medical Repatriation: Examining the Legal and Ethical Implications of an Emerging Practice, 32 Wash. U. J. L. & Pol'y 515, 530-532 (2010).*

Journal 2009 Explores emerging issues in conflict management systems design (CMSD). Concludes as the practice of CMSD in the organizational context continues to expand, practitioners should openly discuss the emerging issues of the field. References Principles I, II, V, and VIII. Costantino, *Second Generation Organizational Conflict Management Systems Design: A Practitioner's Perspective on Emerging Issues, 14 Harv. Negot. L. Rev. 81, 95 (2009).*

Journal 2009 Discusses the interaction between statutes and case law governing the medical field and the core principles of medical professionalism. Concludes the legal framework of medical professionalism does not encompass all the elements required of a medical professional. Quotes Principles II, III, IV, V, VI, VII, and VIII. Fichter, *The Law of Doctoring: A Study of the Codification of Medical Professionalism, 19 Health Matrix 317, 338, 339, 340, 343, 351 (2009).*

Journal 2008 Considers whether certain medical and surgical procedures should be removed from the scope of patentability. Concludes "pure" medical and surgical techniques should not be patentable while granting medical process patents for other procedures. Quotes Principle V and Opinion 9.08. Peschel, *Revisiting the Compromise of 35 USC § 287(c), 16 Tex. Intell. Prop. L. J. 299, 315 (2008).*

Journal 2008 Examines the development of bioethics and environmental ethics, as well as laws promoting the role of bioethicists in decision making. Concludes environmental ethicists must convince legislatures of the role of environmental ethics in order to have a greater impact on decision making. Quotes Principles I, II, III, IV, V, VI, VII, VIII, and IX. Robertson, *Seeking a Seat at the Table: Has Law Left Environmental Ethics Behind as It Embraces Bioethics? 32 Wm. & Mary Envtl. L. & Pol'y Rev. 273, 307 (2008).*

Journal 2007 Compares the role of conscience clauses in various professions. Concludes that conscience clauses in the area of health care must not impede access to care. Quotes Preamble and Principles V, VI, and VIII. Chudoba, *Conscience in America: The Slippery Slope of Mixing Morality With Medicine, 36 Sw. U. L. Rev. 85, 86, 103, 104, 105 (2007).*

Journal 2007 Examines ethical issues raised by advances in computed tomography (CT) imaging technology. Concludes that widespread cooperation and patient advocacy are needed to ensure ethical use of CT. Quotes Principle V. Wann, Nassef, Jeffrey, Messer, Wilke, Duerinckx, Blankenship, Rosenberg, & Dembo, *Ethical Considerations in CT Angiography, 23 Int. J. Cardiovasc. Imaging 379, 384 (2007).*

Journal 2006 Examines ethical dilemmas physicians may face as providers of pay-for-performance medical care. Concludes that this strategy offers a benefit to patients as long as physicians uphold stringent ethical standards and work together to ensure optimum patient care. Cites Principles I, V, VIII, and IX and Opinions 2.035, 2.095, 6.01, 8.021, 8.03, 8.0501, 8.053, 8.054, and 8.121. Bostick, Sade, & McMahon, *Report of the Council on Ethical and Judicial Affairs: Physician Pay-for-Performance Programs, 3 Ind. Health L. Rev. 429, 430, 431, 432-33, 434, 435, 436 (2006).*

Journal 2006 Explores conscience clause legislation relating to the dispensing of oral contraceptives. Concludes that such legislation must balance the interests of the patient and the health care provider. Cites Principles I, II, III, IV, V, VI, VII, VIII, and IX. Collins, *Conscience Clauses and Oral Contraceptives: Conscientious Objection or Calculated Obstruction? 15 Ann. Health L. 37, 54 (2006).*

Journal 2005 Examines issues surrounding tort reform proposals. Concludes that more can be done to correct the current tort system before moving toward a "one size fits all" approach. Quotes Principles I, II, III, IV, V, VI, VII, VIII, and IX. Messerly & Warwick, *Nowhere to Turn: A Glance at the Facts Behind the Supposed Need for Tort "Reform," 28 Hamline L. Rev. 489, 506 (2005).*

Journal 2004 Discusses the need for a greater understanding of and openness to religious values by the professions.

Concludes that, although such openness is important, problems may arise when professional values and religious values clash. Quotes Opinion 5.05. References Principle V. Sullivan, *Naked Fitzies and Iron Cages: Individual Values, Professional Virtues, and the Struggle for Public Space, 78 Tul. L. Rev. 1687, 1702, 1703 (2004).*

Journal 2003 Examines policy options for integration of traditional and modern medicine. Concludes that solid cross-sectoral linkages between different traditions can stabilize an integrated health care system. Quotes Preamble and Principle V. Holliday, *Traditional Medicines in Modern Societies: An Exploration of Integrationist Options Through East Asian Experience, 28 J. Med. & Phil. 373, 387 (2003).*

Journal 2003 Considers the legal, medical, and ethical issues of physician-patient confidentiality in disclosure of paternity. Concludes that a balancing test should be applied to making determinations regarding disclosure of paternity. Quotes Principles I, IV, and V and Opinions 1.02, 5.055, and 10.01. Cites Principle II and Opinion 5.05. Richards & Wolf, *Medical Confidentiality and Disclosure of Paternity, 48 S. D. L. Rev. 409, 411, 412, 413 (2003).*

Journal 2002 Reviews how changes in the health care delivery system underscore the importance of information in patient empowerment. Concludes that patients should use information to take charge of their health care. Quotes Principle V and Opinion 10.02. Cites Opinion 10.01. Kane, *Information Is the Key to Patient Empowerment, 11 Annals Health L. 25, 29-30, 44 (2002).*

Journal 2002 Evaluates pain management treatment for prisoners. Concludes that withholding treatment for, or failing to adequately treat, pain violates the Eighth Amendment. Quotes Principle V and Opinion 2.20. McGrath, *Raising the "Civilized Minimum" of Pain Amelioration for Prisoners to Avoid Cruel and Unusual Punishment, 54 Rutgers L. Rev. 649, 657, 660 (2002).*

Journal 2002 Evaluates the application of biomedical knowledge in clinical practice. Concludes that serious inadequacies exist in the current practice of evidence-based medicine. Quotes Principle V and Opinion 9.08. References Opinion 9.095. Noah, *Medicine's Epistemology: Mapping the Haphazard Diffusion of Knowledge in the Biomedical Community, 44 Ariz. L. Rev. 373, 404, 447, 448 (2002).*

Journal 2000 Discusses patent law and policy. Examines whether those who practice medicine should be excused from patent laws because of the conflict that medical procedure patents create with respect to the practice of medicine. Concludes that Congress should repeal section 287(c) of the Patent Act. Quotes Principle V and Opinions 9.08 and 9.09. Cites Opinion 8.03. References Opinion 10.01. Ho, *Patents, Patients, and Public Policy: An Incomplete Intersection at 35 USC § 287(c), 33 U.C. Davis L. Rev. 601, 603, 623, 624, 625, 631 (2000).*

Journal 2000 Considers the rules governing expert testimony. Explores professional ethical standards affecting expert witnesses and concludes that codes of ethics have not succeeded in eliminating biased expert testimony. Recommends creation of an organization to assist courts in obtaining reliable expert witness testimony. Quotes Principle III and Opinion 6.01. Cites Principles I, II, and V and Opinions 1.02 and 9.07. Murphy, *Expert Witnesses at Trial: Where Are the Ethics? 14 Geo. J. Legal Ethics 217, 231-32 (2000).*

Journal 2000 Describes possible solutions designed to improve postapproval regulation of prescription drugs so that fewer patients will suffer from adverse drug reactions. Concludes that the FDA along with physicians and clinical researchers should rethink the existing approach to monitoring of unexpected side effects. Quotes Principle V and Opinion 9.032. Cites Opinion 5.05. Noah, *Adverse Drug Reactions: Harnessing Experimental Data to Promote Patient Welfare, 49 Cath. U. L. Rev. 449, 477, 497-98 (2000).*

Journal 2000 Evaluates the regulatory framework governing prescription drugs. Considers problems faced by elderly patients when taking FDA-approved medications. Concludes that in order to optimize patient safety, the existing regulatory system must undergo important structural changes. Quotes Principle V and Opinion 9.032. Noah & Brushwood, *Adverse Drug Reactions in Elderly Patients: Alternative Approaches to Postmarket Surveillance, 33 J. Health L. 383, 400, 445 (2000).*

Journal 1997 Discusses physician frustration with managed care plans caused by gag clauses and cost-containment mechanisms. Reviews the development of managed care organizations and federal attempts at limiting the use of gag clauses. Concludes that gag clauses are inherently flawed and compromise quality health care. Quotes Principles II and V, Fundamental Elements (1), and Opinion 8.13. Note, *Physicians, Bound and Gagged: Federal Attempts to Combat Managed Care's Use of Gag Clauses, 21 Seton Hall Legis. J. 567, 601-02 (1997).*

Journal 1997 Discusses the need for balance between business ethics and medical ethics in the context of managed care. Explores two models for integrating ethics and managed care. Proposes the adoption of a collective responsibility model to improve quality of care. Quotes Principles I, II, III, IV, and V. Cites Preamble. References Opinion 8.13. Regan, *Regulating the Business of Medicine: Models for Integrating Ethics and Managed Care, 30 Colum. J. L. & Soc. Probs. 635, 651, 656, 657 (1997).*

Journal 1996 Discusses the trend toward conserving resources expended on health care by withholding services absent a showing of necessity. Claims that the high standard of care physicians owe patients is jeopardized by medical treatment decisions based on coverage concerns. Concludes that the legal structure regarding health care plans should be changed. Quotes Preamble, Principles I, II, III, IV, V, VI, and VII, and Opinion 2.03. Hirshfeld & Thomason, *Medical Necessity Determinations: The Need for a New Legal Structure, 6 Health Matrix 3, 8-9 (1996).*

Journal 1996 Considers the impact of gag clauses on the physician-patient relationship. Undertakes an extensive legal, ethical, and policy analysis. Concludes that gag clauses are violative of legal and ethical principles. Quotes Principles II, V, and VI and Fundamental Elements (1). Cites Preamble. Martin & Bjerknes, *The Legal and Ethical Implications of Gag Clauses in Physician Contracts, XXII Am. J. Law & Med. 433, 465-66 (1996).*

Journal 1994 Reviews the evolution of the physician-patient relationship, with attention to patient autonomy. Examines the changing health care delivery environment. Quotes Preamble, Principles I, II, III, IV, V, and VI, Fundamental Elements (1) and (2), and Opinions 1.02 and 8.07 (1981) [now Opinion 8.08]. Cites Opinion 1.01. Szczygiel, *Beyond Informed Consent, 21 Ohio N. U. L. Rev. 171, 217, 218, 220, 225, 226, 256 (1994).*

Journal 1993 Discusses physicians' duty to disclose to patients medical treatment alternatives that are not readily available. Proposes that based on the historical development and legal requirements of the informed consent doctrine, physicians should be required to inform patients of non–readily available alternatives or face liability for breach of such obligation. Quotes Principles I, II, III, IV, and V and Opinion 8.08. Note, *Informed Choice: Physicians' Duty to Disclose Nonreadily Available Alternatives, 43 Case W. Res. L. Rev. 491, 491, 498-99, 508, 509 (1993).*

Journal 1990 Discusses the moral dilemma in deciding whether to withdraw artificial nutrition and hydration from a patient and the appropriate role of the judiciary. Concludes that judicial decisions do not represent the moral viewpoint of society and that moral pronouncements should not be made in the courtroom. Quotes Preamble, Principles I, II, III, IV, V, VI, and VII, and Opinion 2.20. Peccarelli, *A Moral Dilemma: The Role of Judicial Intervention in Withholding or Withdrawing Nutrition and Hydration, 23 John Marshall L. Rev. 537, 539, 540, 541 (1990).*

Principle VI

2d Cir. 1980 Appeal by hospital of National Labor Relations Board order to employ two part-time staff physicians on a full-time basis and to consider their applications for permanent admitting privileges. Physicians had joined picket line in sympathy with striking union employees without giving advance notice and were allegedly denied full-time positions in retaliation. The court held that support of the strike was activity protected by the National Labor Relations Act but that the physicians lost protection when they told patients the facility was unable to provide adequate care, in careless disregard of the truth. Further, the court noted that the failure to give notice before striking raised ethical questions under Principle 5 (1957) [now Principle VI]. *Montefiore Hosp. & Medical Ctr. v. NLRB, 621 F.2d 510, 516.*

4th Cir. 1984 Prisoner sued private physician under 42 USC § 1983 for failure to provide medical treatment in violation of his Eighth Amendment rights. The court held that the exercise of the physician's medical judgment did not constitute action under color of state law. While not specifically referring to Principle VI (1980), the court cited the Principles for the general proposition that the physician-patient relationship is independent of state administrative supervision. This concept is apparently embodied in Principle VI. *Calvert v. Sharp, 748 F.2d 861, 863, cert. denied, 471 US 1132 (1975).*

6th Cir. 1989 Plaintiff, a chiropractic association, alleged that the AMA and several other professional associations violated antitrust law by conspiring to contain and ultimately eliminate the practice of chiropractic. The court provided a historical overview of the AMA's gradual, but incomplete, recognition of chiropractors and limited licensed practitioners, referring specifically to Principle 3 (1957) as well as to the Opinions and Reports of the Judicial Council Sec. 3, Para. 8 (1969), and to the Opinions and Reports 3.60 and 3.70 (1977) [now Principle VI and Opinions 3.01 and 3.04]. Based on its reading of these Principles and Opinions, the court reversed the trial court's grant of summary judgment to the AMA because there remained a material issue of fact of whether it had continued to illegally boycott chiropractic. *Chiropractic Coop. Ass'n v. AMA, 867 F.2d 270, 272-75.*

W.D. Ark. 1989 Physician sued hospital alleging that it had acted in bad faith when it terminated his employment for failure to accept responsibility for "medical" as opposed to "surgical" patients. Plaintiff argued that the incorporation of the AMA's Principles of Medical Ethics into the hospital's bylaws gave him the right to choose which patients to serve, in apparent reference to Principle VI. While recognizing this right, the court held that the hospital had a corresponding right to consider such a refusal in its employment decisions. *Maxey v. United States, 1989 US Dist. LEXIS 5827.*

N.D. Ga. 1981 Decedent's widow brought wrongful death action against hospital, treating physician, and physician supervising a group of emergency room physicians who had independent contracts with the hospital. Plaintiff claimed the supervising physician was vicariously liable in damages to her under the doctrine of respondeat superior. The court noted that the traditional control test used to identify agency relationships is ineffective in the context of physician-hospital relationships because physicians are bound by Principle 6 (1957) [now most closely embodied by the independent judgment aspects of Principle VI], which requires physicians to practice medicine according to their independent professional judgment. *Stewart v. Midani, 525 F. Supp. 843, 848-49.*

E.D. Mich. 1986 Plaintiff-chiropractors claimed violation of the Sherman Antitrust Act, alleging that the AMA conspired with others to injure them professionally and financially. In support of their claim, plaintiffs cited Principle 3 (1957) and the Opinions and Reports of the Judicial Council Sec. 3, Para. 8 (1969) [now Principle VI and Opinions 3.01 and 3.04]. The court, noting the 1977 change in the AMA's position regarding chiropractic reflected in the Opinions and Reports of the Judicial Council 3.60 and 3.70 (1977) [now Opinion 3.04], held that plaintiffs failed to demonstrate evidence of an overt act by the AMA within the statutory limitations period. Summary judgment entered for AMA. *Chiropractic Coop. Ass'n v. AMA, 1986-2 Trade Cas. (CCH) & 67,294, aff'd in part and rev'd in part, 867 F.2d 270 (6th Cir. 1989).*

E.D. Mich. 1985 In an antitrust case brought by plaintiff-chiropractic association against the AMA, plaintiffs presented the court with a motion in limine asking that the court strike defendant's affirmative defense of a good faith concern with public health and patient care. Plaintiffs argued that the defense was unprecedented, in conflict with existing law, and dramatically wrong. Plaintiffs referred to Principle 3 (1957) [now Principle VI and Opinions 3.01 and 3.04] as the source of the AMA's antitrust violations. The court denied plaintiffs' motion to strike, stating that under the rule of reason test, the AMA had the right to present evidence that its actions furthered the public interest and patient care. *Chiropractic Coop. Ass'n v. AMA, 617 F. Supp. 264, 266, aff'd in part and rev'd in part, 867 F.2d 270 (6th Cir. 1989).*

D.N.M. 1987 In an antitrust action against major health insurance provider and state medical society, group of chiropractors alleged that a conspiracy existed in which the insurer refused to provide health cost reimbursement coverage for chiropractic services. Plaintiffs urged court to apply a per se analysis, rather than the rule of reason analysis, to determine the legality of defendants' restrictive practices. The court declined to apply the per se test. In part, court's conclusion was based on view that concerns of defendant-physicians about relationship with chiropractors because of ethical restrictions imposed by Principle 3 (1957) [now Principle VI and Opinions 3.01 and 3.04] deserved more consideration than the per se test would afford. *Johnson v. Blue Cross/Blue Shield, 677 F. Supp. 1112, 1118.*

D. Vt. 1986 Prisoner sued prison officials and private physician under section 42 USC § 1983, claiming cruel and unusual punishment in violation of his constitutional rights after physician allegedly frightened the prisoner while he was physically restrained, performed a colonoscopy with the examining room door open to a main hallway, and allowed guards to participate in the exam. The court held that although state law required the provision of medical care to inmates, the ethical canons upon which the physician-patient relationship was based were not derived from state law and the physician's actions did not constitute state action. In so holding, the court relied on *Calvert v. Sharpe, 748 F.2d 861 (4th cir. 1984),* which generally cites the Principles for the proposition that the physician-patient relationship is independent of state supervision. Principle VI reflects this concept. *Nash v. Wennar, 645 F.Supp. 238, 242.*

Ariz. 1984 Mother sued hospital and physicians after minor son was transferred to another facility for solely financial reasons although emergency surgical care was medically indicated. In holding that the hospital's transfer policy pre-empted further care by the physicians and that the record revealed no physician negligence, the court stated that generally the standard of care for physicians is determined by what is usually done by members of the profession. The court then cited Principle VI, apparently for the proposition that in emergency situations there may be an ethical, rather than legal, obligation to provide care. *Thompson v. Sun City Community Hosp., Inc., 141 Ariz. 597, 688 P.2d 605, 612 n.7.*

Ariz. App. 2009 Outpatient treatment center, which was not owned by a licensed physician or other licensed medical professional, sued automobile insurer for refusal to reimburse injured persons treated by the center. The court quoted Principle VI and discussed the changes made to the Principle to comply with federal antitrust law. The court explained that Principle VI permits physicians to practice in a variety of business structures consistent with the lack of any restriction as to corporate ownership of an outpatient treatment center. The appeals court held that the center was legally licensed. *Midtown Medical Group, Inc. v. State Farm Mutual Automobile Insurance Co., 220 Ariz. 341, 206 P.3d 790, 797-98.*

Ariz. App. 1980 Malpractice suit against a paid on-call physician for refusal to treat decedent resulting in delay in treatment. The court quoted Principle 5 (1957) [now Principle VI and Opinion 8.11] as establishing an ethical duty to provide emergency care. However, court distinguished any such ethical obligation from its holding that physician had a contractual duty to treat emergency patients to the best of his ability. *Hiser v. Randolph, 126 Ariz. 608, 617 P.2d 774, 776 n.1, 777, 778.*

Cal. App. 2003 Patient and her husband sued medical clinic for terminating care after the patient filed malpractice claims against two clinic physicians. Clinic's policy required termination of all medical care for patients and their families in such a situation. Appeals court upheld summary judgment for the clinic on several claims, but denied summary judgment on claims for interference with contractual relations, negligent infliction of emotional distress, and breach of fiduciary duty. Quotes Principles VI and VIII. *Scripps Clinic v. Superior Court, 108 Cal. App.4th 917, 134 Cal. Rptr. 2d 101, 117.*

Cal. App. 1978 Surviving spouse sued physicians who were on emergency surgical call panel for malpractice where patient died during surgery. Although defendants claimed immunity under state Good Samaritan statute, the court held the statute inapplicable since the legislative purpose was to encourage physicians to render care on an irregular basis

to unattended persons discovered by chance at the scene of an emergency. In so holding, the court noted that Principle 5 (1957) [now Principle VI and Opinions 8.11 and 9.06] imposed an ethical duty to render emergency medical care. *Colby v. Schwartz, 78 Cal. App. 3d 885, 144 Cal. Rptr. 624, 627 n.2.*

Ky. App. 1989 Malpractice suit was initiated against physician for failure to treat plaintiff's brother where defendant had repeatedly rebuffed plaintiff's request for emergency assistance and told him to get in line or sign in. Plaintiff removed his brother to another hospital where he subsequently died of heart attack. Plaintiff argued that defendant was under a duty to treat based upon, inter alia, the AMA Code of Ethics [apparently Principle VI and Opinion 8.11]. The court rejected the argument, finding that a breach of ethical standards may establish grounds for professional discipline, but not a civil cause of action, and held that defendant was under no legal duty to treat. *Noble v. Sartori, 1989 Ky. App. LEXIS 67.*

Minn. 2005 Respondents, providers of massage services, physical therapy, and chiropractic care, attempted to recover benefits from automobile insurers. The trial court dismissed respondents' complaint because it found they violated the corporate practice of medicine doctrine. The appellate court later reversed. The Minnesota Supreme Court affirmed in part and reversed in part. In a separate opinion, concurring in part and dissenting in part, three justices quoting Principle VI would have overruled *Granger v. Adson*, 190 Minn. 23, 250 N.W. 722 (1933), to the extent that it made the corporate practice of medicine doctrine part of Minnesota common law, and found that a ban on the corporate practice of medicine is no longer sound public policy. *Isles Wellness, Inc. v. Progressive N. Ins. Co., 703 N.W.2d 513, 528.*

N.J. Super. 1994 Plaintiff-physician alleged that nursing home violated public policy when it terminated his at-will employment in retaliation for his refusal to see and treat patients in excess of his original workload. With apparent reference to Principle VI, physician argued that caring for excessive numbers of patients violated his ethical responsibilities and public policy. The court held that even though physician's objections to nursing home's practices may have supported a reasonable belief that public policy was violated, there was insufficient evidence that objections contributed to termination. *Fineman v. New Jersey Dept. of Human Servs., 272 N.J. Super. 606, 640 A.2d 1161, 1163, 1166, 1169-70, cert. denied, 138 N.J. 267, 649 A.2d 1287 (1994).*

N.J. Super. 1960 Plaintiff, a graduate of a school of osteopathy and licensed to practice medicine and surgery in New Jersey, sought to compel the defendant medical society to admit him to full membership. Defendant claimed as an affirmative defense that to admit plaintiff would violate Principle 3 (1957) [now Principle VI and Opinion 3.01] because plaintiff possessed a degree in osteopathy rather than an M.D. The court noted that the defendant society had virtually monopolistic control of medical practice in the state and that exclusion from membership caused substantial injury. In view of this, the court ordered the defendant society to admit plaintiff to its membership. To bar membership of a licensed graduate of an approved school of osteopathy would, the court held, violate public policy. *Falcone v. Middlesex County Medical Soc'y, 62 N.J. Super. 184, 162 A.2d 324, 328-29, aff'd, 34 N.J. 582, 170 A.2d 791 (1961).*

N.Y. Sup. 1993 Defendant was charged with violating state statute imposing criminal sanction on a physician who refuses to treat a person seeking emergency medical care. Defendant sought dismissal of the charge, challenging the constitutionality of the statute and arguing that it requires mens rea. The court denied defendant's motion for dismissal, concluding that the statute was constitutional and that the legislature clearly imposed strict liability. The court quoted Principle VI in support of its strict liability conclusion. *People v. Anyakora, 162 Misc. 2d 47, 616 N.Y.S.2d 149, 155.*

Ohio App. 1991 Medical corporation sought an injunction to enforce a covenant not to compete against defendant-physician. The lower court granted summary judgment based on a referee's report which concluded that under Principle VI and Opinions 6.11, 9.02, and 9.06 (1989), restrictive covenants were per se unenforceable as a matter of public policy. While recognizing a strong public interest in allowing open access to health care, the appellate court in reversing held that Opinion 9.02, which applied specifically to restrictive covenants, only "discouraged" such covenants. *Ohio Urology, Inc. v. Poll, 72 Ohio. App. 446, 450, 451, 594 N.E.2d 1027, 1030, 1031.*

Wash. 1951 Plaintiff, a charitable, not-for-profit medical corporation, offered prepaid health care services to members and their families. Suit was filed against county medical society and others for damages and injunction for defendants' alleged efforts to monopolize prepaid medical care in area and unlawfully restrain competition by plaintiff and its physicians. Defendants alleged as affirmative defense that their efforts were designed to curb unethical prepaid contract practice by plaintiff. Court examined at length AMA's position regarding contract practice including Principles Ch. III, Art. VI, Secs. 3 and 4 (1947) [now Principle VI and Opinions 8.05 and 9.06], concluding nothing in plaintiff's practice violated the AMA's ethical guidelines. Further, quoting Principles Ch. III, Art. III, Sec.1 (1947) [now Opinion 8.04] dealing with consultations, court noted that defendants' efforts impeded plaintiff's physicians from obtaining consultations. Court concluded that defendants' actions constituted unlawful, monopolistic behavior and issued an injunction, although it declined to award damages. *Group Health Coop. v. King County Medical Soc'y, 39 Wash. 2d 586, 237 P.2d 737, 744, 750-51, 759-60.*

Wash. App. 1984 Plaintiff-pathologist sued his corporate employer and one of its subsidiaries for breach of his employment contract; defendants counterclaimed, alleging that plaintiff had tortiously interfered with defendants' business relationships. Plaintiff had discouraged the transfer of laboratory specimens for analysis at a distant lab because he allegedly believed that to do so would be a violation of

medical ethics, particularly Principle 6 (1957) [now Principle VI]. In finding for plaintiff, the court acknowledged that a physician was bound to uphold duly prescribed medical ethical principles despite his employment status, especially where such a principle coincided with a public policy favoring acts that tend to prevent a deterioration of the quality of medical care. *Wood v. Upjohn Co., No. 6093-1-II (Sept. 4, 1984) (LEXIS, States library, Wash. file).*

Journal 2011 Discusses the development of lethal autonomous robots, as well as issues raised by this new military technology. Concludes discussion on the advancement and acceptance of lethal autonomous robots is needed on the national and international levels in order to successfully manage advancements in robotic technology. Cites Preamble and Principles I and VI. Allenby, Arkin, Barrett, Borenstein, Gaudet, Kittrie, Lin, Lucas, Marchant, O'Meara, & Silberman, *International Governance of Autonomous Military Robots, 12 Colum. Sci. & Tech. L. Rev. 272, 291 (2011).*

Journal 2011 Examines barriers to seeking services for communication impairments perceived by lesbian, gay, bisexual, and transgender (LGBT) people. Concludes assumptions of heterosexuality are perceived as prejudices by LGBT patients and impair the delivery of speech pathologist or audiologist services. References Principle VI. Kelly & Robinson, *Disclosure of Membership in the Lesbian, Gay, Bisexual, and Transgender Community by Individuals With Communication Impairments: A Preliminary Web-Based Survey, 20 Am. J. Speech-Language Pathology 86, 90 (2011).*

Journal 2010 Discusses the inadequacy of sexual minority health care education in medical school curricula and the disparities that exist in medical access for sexual minorities. Concludes medical schools should reevaluate their curricula to improve student understanding of sexual minority health care. Quotes Principle VI. Kolder & Julian, *Teaching About Sexual Minorities: An Iowa Experience, 1 Proc. Obstetrics Gynecology 1, 1 (April 2010, Article 10).*

Journal 2010 Analyzes factors contributing to the emergence of medical repatriation and evaluates whether this practice comports with current legal and ethical standards. Proposes changes to federal regulations that govern hospitals and clarifications to medical ethical standards. Quotes the Preamble and Principles I, II, III, IV, V, VI, VII, VIII, and IX. Zoellner, *Medical Repatriation: Examining the Legal and Ethical Implications of an Emerging Practice, 32 Wash. U. J. L. & Pol'y 515, 530-532 (2010).*

Journal 2009 Examines the role of physicians during natural and man-made disasters. Concludes hospitals must make plans to define disaster response procedures that shift responsibility for survival from the physician to the community. Quotes Code of Ethics, Ch. III, Art. I §1 (1847) [now Opinion 9.067], Principle 5 (1957) [now Principle VI], Principle VI, and Opinions 2.23, 9.067, and 9.131. Cites Opinions 9.06, 9.067, and 9.12. Ahronheim, *Service by*

Health Care Providers in a Public Health Emergency: The Physician's Duty and the Law, 12 J. Health Care L. & Pol'y 195, 209-11, 215, 225 (2009).

Journal 2009 Discusses the interaction between statutes and case law governing the medical field and the core principles of medical professionalism. Concludes the legal framework of medical professionalism does not encompass all the elements required of a medical professional. Quotes Principles II, III, IV, V, VI, VII, and VIII. Fichter, *The Law of Doctoring: A Study of the Codification of Medical Professionalism, 19 Health Matrix 317, 338, 339, 340, 343, 351 (2009).*

Journal 2009 Discusses the judicial standard for reviewing physician noncompete covenants. Concludes courts should apply a strict standard to such covenants, rather than declare the covenants per se invalid. Quotes Principles IV and VII, Principles of Medical Ethics §5 (1957) [now Principle VI], Code of Medical Ethics Ch. II, Art. I §3 (1847) [now Opinion 5.02], Opinion 9.02, and Code of Medical Ethics Ch. II, Art. I §4 (1847) [now Opinion 9.09]. Cites Opinions 8.041, 8.115, 9.02, 9.06, 9.065, 9.067, 10.01, and 10.015. Koons, *Physician Employee Non-Compete Agreements on the Examining Table: The Need to Better Protect Patients' and the Public's Interests in Indiana, 6 Ind. Health L. Rev. 253, 272-77, 280-81 (2009).*

Journal 2008 Discusses the ethics of physicians offering diagnoses reached through observation of signs in a person who has not approached them for medical advice. Concludes that diagnosis of a nonpatient may be ethical based on considerations of relationship, urgency, risk of harm, and accuracy. Quotes Principle VI. Mitchell, *The Ethics of Passer-By Diagnosis, 371 Lancet 85, 87 (2008).*

Journal 2008 Explores the legal, ethical, and policy implications of concierge medicine. Argues physicians engaged in concierge care must strive to meet ethical and legal standards, and take care to communicate clearly with patients about services and fees. Quotes Opinion 8.055. Cites Principles II and VI and Opinion 8.055. Portman & Romanow, *Concierge Medicine: Legal Issues, Ethical Dilemmas, and Policy Challenges, 1 J. Health & Life Sci. L. 1, 4, 28-29 (2008).*

Journal 2008 Examines the development of bioethics and environmental ethics, as well as laws promoting the role of bioethicists in decision making. Concludes environmental ethicists must convince legislatures of the role of environmental ethics in order to have a greater impact on decision making. Quotes Principles I, II, III, IV, V, VI, VII, VIII, and IX. Robertson, *Seeking a Seat at the Table: Has Law Left Environmental Ethics Behind as It Embraces Bioethics? 32 Wm. & Mary Envtl. L. & Pol'y Rev. 273, 307 (2008).*

Journal 2008 Examines the benefits and costs of adopting a tort duty to affirmatively aid and the implications of a criminal law duty to aid. Concludes the absence in American tort and criminal law of an affirmative duty to aid is appropriate despite its contradiction of social and moral values. Quotes

Principle VI. Scordato, *Understanding the Absence of a Duty to Reasonably Rescue in American Tort Law, 82 Tul. L. Rev. 1447, 1486 (2008).*

Journal 2007 Compares the role of conscience clauses in various professions. Concludes that conscience clauses in the area of health care must not impede access to care. Quotes Preamble and Principles V, VI, and VIII. Chudoba, *Conscience in America: The Slippery Slope of Mixing Morality With Medicine, 36 Sw. U. L. Rev. 85, 86, 103, 104, 105 (2007).*

Journal 2007 Considers how a physician should treat a patient who has suffered a bad outcome from care provided via "medical tourism." Concludes that the ethical response is to provide care for the patient as for any other. Quotes Principle VI. Jones & McCullough, *What to Do When a Patient's International Medical Care Goes South, 46 J. of Vascular Surgery 1077, 1078 (2007).*

Journal 2007 Questions whether it is ethical for a physician to provide medical care to a family member. Concludes that providing such care becomes increasingly problematic as the likelihood of complications increases. Quotes Principle VI and Opinion 8.19. Oberheu, Jones, & Sade, *A Surgeon Operates on His Son: Wisdom or Hubris? 84 Ann. Thorac. Surg. 723, 725, 726 (2007).*

Journal 2006 Explores the legal and ethical issues surrounding concierge medicine. Concludes that concierge medicine is best restricted to a small class of wealthy individuals. Quotes Principle IX and Opinion 8.055. Cites Principle VI and Opinions 8.055, 8.11, 8.115, 9.065, and 10.05. Carnahan, *Law, Medicine, and Wealth: Does Concierge Medicine Promote Health Care Choice, or is it a Barrier to Access? 17 Stan. L. & Pol'y Rev. 121, 149-50, 151, 152, 153-54 (2006).*

Journal 2006 Explores conscience clause legislation relating to the dispensing of oral contraceptives. Concludes that such legislation must balance the interests of the patient and the health care provider. Cites Principles I, II, III, IV, V, VI, VII, VIII, and IX. Collins, *Conscience Clauses and Oral Contraceptives: Conscientious Objection or Calculated Obstruction? 15 Ann. Health L. 37, 54 (2006).*

Journal 2005 Examines issues surrounding tort reform proposals. Concludes that more can be done to correct the current tort system before moving toward a "one size fits all" approach. Quotes Principles I, II, III, IV, V, VI, VII, VIII, and IX. Messerly & Warwick, *Nowhere to Turn: A Glance at the Facts Behind the Supposed Need for Tort "Reform," 28 Hamline L. Rev. 489, 506 (2005).*

Journal 2003 Discusses whether compassion represents an adequate ethical response when an individual is suffering. Concludes that compassion may not have a proper role in social or legal decision-making because of its potential to ignore those who are in need. Quotes Principle VI. Shepherd, *Face to Face: A Call for Radical Responsibility in Place of Compassion, 77 St. John's L. Rev. 445, 472 (2003).*

Journal 2001 Discusses the prohibition on nonlawyer ownership of legal service providers. Considers how ethical rules and standards governing physicians have been directed toward preserving independent judgment. Concludes that ethical conflicts created by abandoning the prohibition on nonlawyer ownership of legal service providers may be managed by following the medical ethics model. Quotes Principle VI and Opinions 2.03, 2.09, 8.02, 8.021, 8.03, 8.05, 8.051, 8.054, 8.13, and 8.132. Harris & Foran, *The Ethics of Middle-Class Access to Legal Services and What We Can Learn From the Medical Profession's Shift to a Corporate Paradigm, 70 Fordham L. Rev. 775, 817, 821, 822, 823, 824 (2001).*

Journal 2000 Examines the ethical, social, and moral dilemmas faced by gays and lesbians who desire to have genetically related children. Discusses assisted reproductive technologies most commonly used by gays and lesbians. Explores the barriers associated with access to reproductive technologies by these individuals. Quotes Principle VI. DeLair, *Ethical, Moral, Economic and Legal Barriers to Assisted Reproductive Technologies Employed by Gay Men and Lesbian Women, 4 DePaul J. Health Care L. 147, 150 (2000).*

Journal 2000 Discusses and evaluates different systems for addressing consumer concerns about managed health care. Asserts that current legal systems for identifying and resolving consumer concerns are not understood by most consumers and are not accessible by many, especially the uninsured. Concludes that several immediate steps are realistic for moving toward reform. Cites Principle VI. References Opinions 8.13 and 9.065. Kinney, *Tapping and Resolving Consumer Concerns About Health Care, 26 Am. J. Law & Med. 335, 337, 375 (2000).*

Journal 2000 Discusses managed care in terms of problems, responses, and accomplishments. Demonstrates how a physician union's collective bargaining process can benefit patients and physicians in addressing problems with managed care. Concludes that barriers preventing such unions should be removed. Quotes Principles VI and VII and Opinion 10.01. Rugg, *An Old Solution to a New Problem: Physician Unions Take the Edge Off Managed Care, 34 Colum. J. L. & Soc. Probs. 1, 41 (2000).*

Journal 2000 Examines current laws prohibiting discrimination in the context of access to health care, placing emphasis on people with HIV/AIDS. Considers the implications of *Bragdon v. Abbott.* Concludes that everyone should be entitled to health care in the absence of an acceptable justification for its denial. Quotes Preamble, Principle VI, and Opinion 9.131. Shepherd, *HIV, the ADA, and the Duty to Treat, 37 Hous. L. Rev. 1055, 1061, 1083-84 (2000).*

Journal 1999 Discusses potential conflicts between a criminal defense attorney's religious beliefs and representation of the client. Explores theories that would allow an attorney to put religious beliefs over the client's interest. Offers analogies within the physician-patient relationship. Concludes that

a defense attorney is bound by duty and must set aside conflicting religious beliefs. Quotes Principle VI and Opinions 8.11, 9.06, and 9.12. Reza, *Religion and the Public Defender, 26 Fordham Urb. L. J. 1051, 1062, 1063 (1999).*

Journal 1999 Discusses the need for physicians to advocate on behalf of patients' rights in the context of health care delivery. Evaluates the nature and scope of the physician's role as advocate, noting that physicians cannot be expected to engage in attorney-like advocacy. Quotes Principles IV and VI, Fundamental Elements (2), (4), and (6) [now Opinion 10.01], Patient Responsibilities 5 [now Opinion 10.02], and Opinions 2.03, 2.07, 2.09, 2.16, 2.19, 3.06, 4.01, 4.04, 6.01, 7.02, 8.02, 8.03, 8.13, 8.132, 9.06, 9.07, and 9.131. Cites Opinions 5.05, 5.09, 7.01, 8.135, and 9.02. Sage, *Physicians as Advocates, 35 Hous. L. Rev. 1529, 1537, 1541, 1542, 1552-53, 1554, 1556, 1557, 1559, 1561-62, 1564, 1571, 1574, 1576, 1580 (1999).*

Journal 1999 Discusses whether health care professionals have the right to refuse to treat patients under common law and federal statutes and regulations. Explores the impact of the Americans with Disabilities Act and the US Supreme Court decision in *Bragdon v. Abbott* on the duties of health care professionals in the context of providing treatment to HIV-positive patients. Quotes Principle VI and Opinions 2.23 and 9.131. White, *Health Care Professionals and Treatment of HIV-Positive Patients, 20 J. Legal Med. 67, 86 (1999).*

Journal 1998 Discusses the development and existence of the corporate practice of medicine doctrine. Points out that the doctrine is inconsistent with recent changes in the health care system. Suggests that the ban on corporate practice should be eliminated. Cites Principle VI. Freiman, *The Abandonment of the Antiquated Corporate Practice of Medicine Doctrine: Injecting a Dose of Efficiency Into the Modern Health Care Environment, 47 Emory L. J. 697, 712 (1998).*

Journal 1998 Focuses on conflicts of interest and pressures physicians face when treating professional athletes. Discusses case law regarding team physician liability. Concludes that team physicians and their attorneys need to be aware of conflicts of interest that may arise from treatment of professional athletes. Quotes Principle VI (1957) [now most closely embodied by the independent judgment aspects of Principle VI]. Polsky, *Winning Medicine: Professional Sports Team Doctors' Conflicts of Interest, 14 J. Contemp. Health L. & Pol'y 503, 505 (1998).*

Journal 1997 Reports on a study of physician attitudes regarding expert witnesses. Notes that a majority of physicians believe that medical expert testimony should be subject to peer review and, when appropriate, medical licensing board discipline. Quotes Principles II and VI and Opinion 9.07. Eitel, Hegeman, & Evans, *Medicine on Trial: Physicians' Attitudes About Expert Medical Witnesses, 18 J. Legal Med. 345, 355, 358 (1997).*

Journal 1997 Analyzes the prohibition against employment agreements between corporations and licensed physicians. Discusses the origins and development of the corporate practice of medicine doctrine. Proposes that state legislatures should adopt doctrinal modifications to aid in the movement toward managed care. Quotes Principle VI. Mars, *The Corporate Practice of Medicine: A Call for Action*, 7 Health Matrix 241, 267 (1997).

Journal 1996 Discusses the trend toward conserving resources expended on health care by withholding services absent a showing of necessity. Claims that the high standard of care physicians owe patients is jeopardized by medical treatment decisions based on coverage concerns. Concludes that the legal structure regarding health care plans should be changed. Quotes Preamble, Principles I, II, III, IV, V, VI, and VII, and Opinion 2.03. Hirshfeld & Thomason, *Medical Necessity Determinations: The Need for a New Legal Structure*, 6 Health Matrix 3, 8-9 (1996).

Journal 1996 Considers the impact of gag clauses on the physician-patient relationship. Undertakes an extensive legal, ethical, and policy analysis. Concludes that gag clauses are violative of legal and ethical principles. Quotes Principles II, V, and VI and Fundamental Elements (1). Cites Preamble. Martin & Bjerknes, *The Legal and Ethical Implications of Gag Clauses in Physician Contracts*, XXII Am. J. Law & Med. 433, 465-66 (1996).

Journal 1996 Discusses commercialization of the medical industry. Addresses ethical and policy considerations that form the basis for the corporate practice of medicine doctrine. Observes that the doctrine is now outdated. Quotes Principle VI. Parker, *Corporate Practice of Medicine: Last Stand or Final Downfall?* 29 J. Health & Hosp. L. 160, 167, 173 (1996).

Journal 1996 Examines the recent trend in health care laws and ethics to focus on the alleviation of suffering. Expresses concern that such a focus may result in the valuation of one life over another. Emphasizes the need to evaluate multiple, diverse responses to suffering. Quotes Principle VI. References Opinion 2.162. Shepherd, *Sophie's Choices: Medical and Legal Responses to Suffering*, 72 Notre Dame L. Rev. 103, 106, 133 (1996).

Journal 1995 Examines the rights of health care professionals to refuse to participate in patient care on the basis of conscientious objection. Suggests steps that health care facilities may take when dealing with health care professionals who object to participating in patient care. Quotes Principles I and VI and Opinions 1.02, 2.035, and 9.055. Dellinger & Vickery, *When Staff Object to Participating in Care*, 28 J. Health & Hospital Law 269, 272, 276 (1995).

Journal 1995 Offers relevant historical perspectives and provides comprehensive ethical and legal discussion of physician-assisted suicide and euthanasia. Highlights important legislative developments, including the Oregon Death with Dignity Act, and analyzes significant judicial opinions. Quotes Principles III, IV, and VI and Opinions 2.21 and 9.12. Cites Opinions 2.20 and 8.11. Stone & Winslade, *Physician-Assisted Suicide and Euthanasia in the United States: Legal and Ethical Observations*, 16 J. Legal Med. 481, 483, 490, 497, 498, 499 (1995).

Journal 1995 Examines the history of Medicaid physician reimbursement and physician participation. Concludes that states should facilitate tie-ins among Medicaid patients and privately insured patients rather than raising physician fees. Cites Principle VI. Watson, *Medicaid Physician Participation: Patients, Poverty, and Physician Self-interest*, XXI Am. J. Law & Med. 191, 218 (1995).

Journal 1994 Analyzes the corporate practice of medicine doctrine. Asserts that viability of the doctrine is questionable in the modern health care industry. Quotes Principle VI. Dowell, *The Corporate Practice of Medicine Prohibition: A Dinosaur Awaiting Extinction*, 27 J. Health & Hospital Law 369, 370 (1994).

Journal 1994 Explores how the Americans with Disabilities Act has created, through federal civil rights mechanisms, a legal duty to treat HIV-infected patients. Discusses previous attempts to create a professional obligation to treat patients with AIDS. Quotes Principle VI and Opinion 9.131. Cites Opinion 9.12. Halevy & Brody, *Acquired Immunodeficiency Syndrome and the Americans with Disabilities Act: A Legal Duty to Treat*, 96 Am. J. Med. 282, 283, 284 (1994).

Journal 1994 Reviews the evolution of the physician-patient relationship, with attention to patient autonomy. Examines the changing health care delivery environment. Quotes Preamble, Principles I, II, III, IV, V, and VI, Fundamental Elements (1) and (2), and Opinions 1.02 and 8.07 (1981) [now Opinion 8.08]. Cites Opinion 1.01. Szczygiel, *Beyond Informed Consent*, 21 Ohio N. U. L. Rev. 171, 217, 218, 220, 225, 226, 256 (1994).

Journal 1993 Explores the traditional view that lawyers have unfettered discretion to select clients and New York's antidiscrimination disciplinary rule, statutes, and case law. Concludes that the legal profession should prohibit invidious or improper discrimination. Quotes Principle VI and Opinions 9.12 and 9.131. Begg, *Revoking the Lawyers' License to Discriminate in New York: The Demise of a Traditional Professional Prerogative*, 7 Geo. J. Legal Ethics 275, 298, 299 (1993).

Journal 1993 Addresses both patient rights under California consent and confidentiality laws relating to AIDS and prohibitions on unreasonable searches and seizures under the US Constitution. Concludes that any health care worker who can document an exposure to blood or body fluids should have the option of compelling a nonconsenting patient to be tested for HIV. Quotes Principle VI and Opinion 9.131. Comment, *Nonconsensual HIV Testing in the Health Care Setting: The Case for Extending the Occupational Protections of California Proposition 96 to Health Care Workers*, 26 Loy. L. A. L. Rev. 1251, 1269 (1993).

Journal 1993 Discusses physicians' duty to disclose to patients medical treatment alternatives that are not readily available. Proposes that based on the historical development and legal requirements of the informed consent doctrine, physicians should be required to inform patients of non–readily available alternatives or face liability for breach of such obligation. Quotes Principles I, II, III, IV, and V and Opinion 8.08. Note, *Informed Choice: Physicians' Duty to Disclose Nonreadily Available Alternatives, 43 Case W. Res. L. Rev. 491, 491, 498-99, 508, 509 (1993).*

Journal 1993 Explores the idea of reverse informed consent, which would impose a duty on patients to inform health care professionals of their infectious status. Concludes that such a duty is justified. Quotes Principles IV and VI and Opinions 8.11 and 9.131. Oddi, *Reverse Informed Consent: The Unreasonably Dangerous Patient, 46 Vand. L. Rev. 1417, 1449, 1463, 1465, 1479 (1993).*

Journal 1992 Discusses the plight of undocumented aliens and their need for access to medical care. Considers existing systems for providing such care, as well as barriers to the receipt of medical attention. Cites Principles VI and VII. Loue, *Access to Health Care and the Undocumented Alien, 13 J. Legal Med. 271, 291 (1992).*

Journal 1991 Considers whether physicians have an obligation to provide medical care to HIV-infected patients. Examines various sources for such a duty, including a moral obligation not to discriminate and a social responsibility to provide access to health care. Quotes Opinion 9.131. Cites Principle VI. Daniels, *Duty to Treat or Right to Refuse? 21 Hastings Center Rep. 36, 37, 42 (March/April 1991).*

Journal 1991 Discusses the problem of noncompliant patients and whether a physician may deny treatment to these individuals. Concludes that physicians are not relieved of their duty to treat noncompliant patients, especially because these patients may not be able to adequately control their behavior. Cites Principle VI and Opinion 9.12. Orentlicher, *Denying Treatment to the Noncompliant Patient, 265 JAMA 1579, 1581 (1991).*

Journal 1990 Examines the relationship between professional ethics and professional autonomy, perceived problems of health care rationing under a prospective payment vs a fee-for-service system, and the relationship between professional ethics and the problem of rationing. Concludes that rationing is inevitable, forcing important ethical questions to be addressed. Quotes Principles IV and VI. Agich, *Rationing and Professional Autonomy, 18 Law Med. & Health Care 77, 79, 82 (1990).*

Journal 1990 Considers the propriety of HIV testing for hospital patients prior to nonemergency surgery. Concludes that testing of patients should be permitted so long as it is not done with the intent, nor the effect, of discriminating against individual patients. Quotes Principle VI and Opinion 9.131. Naccasha, *The Permissibility of Routine AIDS Testing in the Health Care Context, 5 Notre Dame J. L. Ethics & Pub. Pol'y, 223, 241 (1990).*

Journal 1990 Discusses a physician's duty to treat AIDS patients. Concludes that there is a weak basis for imposing an ethical duty to treat, but suggests that a legal duty may be fashioned. Quotes Principle V (1980) [now Principle VI]. Note, *Ethics and AIDS: A Summary of the Law and a Critical Analysis of the Individual Physician's Ethical Duty to Treat, XVI Am. J. Law & Med. 249, 262 (1990).*

Journal 1990 Discusses the moral dilemma in deciding whether to withdraw artificial nutrition and hydration from a patient and the appropriate role of the judiciary. Concludes that judicial decisions do not represent the moral viewpoint of society and that moral pronouncements should not be made in the courtroom. Quotes Preamble, Principles I, II, III, IV, V, VI, and VII and Opinion 2.20. Peccarelli, *A Moral Dilemma: The Role of Judicial Intervention in Withholding or Withdrawing Nutrition and Hydration, 23 John Marshall L. Rev. 537, 539, 540, 541 (1990).*

Journal 1989 Discusses the legal and ethical challenges that AIDS poses for health care providers. Proposes that health care providers actively participate in preventing HIV infection, providing care for HIV-infected individuals, and fighting AIDS and its associated stigma. Quotes Principle VI and Opinion 9.131. Forrester, *AIDS: The Responsibility to Care, 34 Vill. L. Rev. 799, 811 (1989).*

Journal 1989 Discusses common law developments in the 1960s and 1970s that established a duty to provide emergency care and treatment. Observes that the common law met with only limited success in this regard and concludes that the Consolidated Omnibus Budget Reconciliation Act of 1985 offers the greatest likelihood for creating a nationally enforceable legal duty to provide emergency care. Quotes Principle VI. Rothenberg, *Who Cares? The Evolution of the Legal Duty to Provide Emergency Care, 26 Houston L. Rev. 21, 22 (1989).*

Journal 1988 Noting that safety precautions have been recommended by Centers for Disease Control and Prevention (CDC) and Occupational Safety and Health Administration (OSHA), observes that, despite these measures, if health care providers believe that a risk of contagion exists when caring for HIV-seropositive patients, they may take steps to limit exposure by reducing care. Against this background, it is suggested that policies be developed to help ensure that the threat of AIDS does not limit access to care for such patients. Quotes Principle 5 (1980) [sic] [now Principle VI]. Brennan, *Ensuring Adequate Health Care for the Sick: The Challenge of the Acquired Immunodeficiency Syndrome as an Occupational Disease, 1988 Duke L. J. 29, 47.*

Journal 1988 Discusses the question of whether health professionals are obligated to subject themselves to the risks that attend treating patients with communicable diseases, particularly AIDS. Examines the ethical pronouncements and codes of the nursing and medical professions in this respect, noting that the most recent statements of professional values imply the existence of an obligation to treat HIV-infectious patients. Quotes Opinion 8.10 (1986) [now

Opinion 8.11] and Principle VI. Cites Opinion 9.11 (1986) [now Opinion 9.12]. Freedman, *Health Professions, Codes, and the Right to Refuse to Treat HIV-Infectious Patients, 18 Hastings Center Rep. 20 (Supp.), 23, 24 (April/May 1988).*

Journal 1986 Examines common law and statutory law applicable to patient dumping, and emphasizes the anti-dumping provisions of Consolidated Omnibus Budget

Reconciliation Act (COBRA). Weaknesses in this federal legislative scheme are highlighted, and recommendations for strengthening the statute and maximizing access to emergency medical care are offered. Quotes Principle VI and Opinion 8.10 (1986) [now Opinion 8.11]. Note, *Preventing Patient Dumping: Sharpening the COBRA's Fangs, 61 N. Y. U. L. Rev. 1186, 1189-90 (1986).*

Principle VII

Ariz. 1965 Physician appealed denial of medical license which was based on alleged violations of local medical society rules and Principles 3, 5, and 10 (1957) [now Principles III and VII and Opinions 3.01, 8.11, and 9.06]. Alleged violations included treating a patient without first obtaining a prior treating physician's permission, inadequate patient care, performing operations without hospital privileges, and signing the medical record of a deceased patient who had been treated by interns. The court held that the evidence failed to show any clear violation of the Principles and that a local medical society had no right to prescribe a code of ethics for state licensing purposes. *Arizona State Bd. of Medical Examiners v. Clark, 97 Ariz. 205, 398 P.2d 908, 914-15, 915 n.3.*

Journal 2010 Examines the physicians' "Right of Conscience" (ROC) and professional integrity within the context of the patient-physician relationship. Discusses the evolution of the patient-physician relationship and the legal transition of empowering patient autonomy. Concludes physicians should be allowed limited ROC to prevent marginalization of physicians' morals and values while ultimately strengthening the patient-physician relationship. Quotes Principle VII. Gold, *Physicians' "Right of Conscience"—Beyond Politics, 38 J. L. Med & Ethics, 134, 138 (2010).*

Journal 2010 Analyzes factors contributing to the emergence of medical repatriation and evaluates whether this practice comports with current legal and ethical standards. Proposes changes to federal regulations that govern hospitals and clarifications to medical ethical standards. Quotes the Preamble and Principles I, II, III, IV, V, VI, VII, VIII, and IX. Zoellner, *Medical Repatriation: Examining the Legal and Ethical Implications of an Emerging Practice, 32 Wash. U. J. L. & Pol'y 515, 530-532 (2010).*

Journal 2009 Discusses the interaction between statutes and case law governing the medical field and the core principles of medical professionalism. Concludes the legal framework of medical professionalism does not encompass all the elements required of a medical professional. Quotes Principles II, III, IV, V, VI, VII, and VIII. Fichter, *The Law of Doctoring: A Study of the Codification of Medical Professionalism, 19 Health Matrix 317, 338, 339, 340, 343, 351 (2009).*

Journal 2009 Discusses the essential role of professionals in the community and the conflicting moral obligations facing professionals. Concludes the legal profession's insistence that priority be given exclusively to the client's interests prevents it from successfully addressing ethical problems. Cites Preamble and Principle VII. Greenstein, *Against Professionalism, 22 Geo. J. Legal Ethics 327, 349 (2009).*

Journal 2009 Discusses the judicial standard for reviewing physician noncompete covenants. Concludes courts should apply a strict standard to such covenants, rather than declare the covenants per se invalid. Quotes Principles IV and VII, Principles of Medical Ethics §5 (1957) [now Principle VI], Code of Medical Ethics Ch. II, Art. I §3 (1847) [now Opinion 5.02], Opinion 9.02, and Code of Medical Ethics Ch. II, Art. I §4 (1847) [now Opinion 9.09]. Cites Opinions 8.041, 8.115, 9.02, 9.06, 9.065, 9.067, 10.01, and 10.015. Koons, *Physician Employee Non-Compete Agreements on the Examining Table: The Need to Better Protect Patients' and the Public's Interests in Indiana, 6 Ind. Health L. Rev. 253, 272-77, 280-81 (2009).*

Journal 2008 Examines the development of bioethics and environmental ethics, as well as laws promoting the role of bioethicists in decision making. Concludes environmental ethicists must convince legislatures of the role of environmental ethics in order to have a greater impact on decision making. Quotes Principles I, II, III, IV, V, VI, VII, VIII, and IX. Robertson, *Seeking a Seat at the Table: Has Law Left Environmental Ethics Behind as it Embraces Bioethics? 32 Wm. & Mary Envtl. L. & Pol'y Rev. 273, 307 (2008).*

Journal 2008 Argues that as a matter of public health, physicians must control antibiotic administration to combat antibiotic resistance. Concludes that despite limited incentives for antibiotic conservation, physicians must acknowledge their important role in mitigating the public health threat of antibiotic resistance. Quotes Principles VII and VIII and Opinions 2.09 and 10.015. Cites Opinion 2.03. Saver, *In Tepid Defense of Population Health: Physicians and Antibiotic Resistance, 34 Am. J. L. & Med. 431, 457 (2008).*

Journal 2008 Questions why pediatricians are not more involved in community activities. Concludes that greater community involvement might boost morale in the profession. Quotes Principle VII. Wilson, *Dwindling Community*

Involvement: A Sign of Professional Failure to Thrive? 162 Arch. Pediatr. Adolesc. Med. 695, 695 (2008).

Journal 2007 Examines physicians' duty to treat victims of highly infectious diseases during an epidemic. Concludes that no clear duty exists, and that if physicians are compelled to provide care by law they must be afforded sufficient due process to protect their property interests in their medical licenses. Quotes Ch. III, Art. I, Sec. I (May 1847) [now Opinions 2.25 and 9.067], and Opinion 9.131. References Principle 10 (1957) [now Principle VII]. Schwartz, *Doubtful Duty: Physicians' Legal Obligation to Treat During an Epidemic, 60 Stan. L. Rev. 657, 662, 663 (2007).*

Journal 2006 Examines the legal and public health issues raised by increased rates of hepatitis C in prison populations. Concludes that reform is needed to provide adequate health care to prisoners and that courts have the power to require such care under the Eighth Amendment. Quotes Preamble, Principles VII, VIII, and IX, and Opinion 10.015. Brunsden, *Hepatitis C in Prisons: Evolving Toward Decency Through Adequate Medical Care and Public Health Reform, 54 UCLA L. Rev. 465, 500 (2006).*

Journal 2006 Explores conscience clause legislation relating to the dispensing of oral contraceptives. Concludes that such legislation must balance the interests of the patient and the health care provider. Cites Principles I, II, III, IV, V, VI, VII, VIII, and IX. Collins, *Conscience Clauses and Oral Contraceptives: Conscientious Objection or Calculated Obstruction? 15 Ann. Health L. 37, 54 (2006).*

Journal 2006 Considers the interaction of laws, rules, and guidelines in the area of health law. Suggests that the legislature should revise current laws to reflect local variability in practice. Quotes Preamble and Principles VII and IX. Heimer, *Responsibility in Health Care: Spanning the Boundary Between Law and Medicine, 41 Wake Forest L. Rev. 465, 498 (2006).*

Journal 2006 Examines methods of teaching law students about social justice. Concludes that a change in teaching methods would encourage students to place a higher value on furthering social justice. Quotes Principle VII. Rand, *An Interdisciplinary Search for Help Through Social Work's Empowerment Approach, 13 Clinical L. Rev. 459, 477 (2006).*

Journal 2005 Examines issues surrounding tort reform proposals. Concludes that more can be done to correct the current tort system before moving toward a "one size fits all" approach. Quotes Principles I, II, III, IV, V, VI, VII, VIII, and IX. Messerly & Warwick, *Nowhere to Turn: A Glance at the Facts Behind the Supposed Need for Tort "Reform," 28 Hamline L. Rev. 489, 506 (2005).*

Journal 2005 Examines the practice of "boutique medicine" and considers legal and ethical implications. Concludes that boutique medical services would be ethical only if physicians used retainer money from their boutique clients to augment health care costs of the poor. Quotes Principles VII

and IX and Opinion 8.055. Russano, *Is Boutique Medicine a New Threat to American Health Care or a Logical Way of Revitalizing the Doctor-Patient Relationship? 17 Wash. U. J. L. & Pol'y 313, 331, 332 (2005).*

Journal 2005 Discusses ethical, legal, and policy issues associated with treatment and research involving patients who are in a persistent vegetative or minimally conscious state. Concludes that patients in these states are at risk for therapeutic failures until physicians can more accurately determine which patients will benefit from treatment and accurately convey such information to families or surrogates. Quotes Principles VII and IX and Opinions 8.031, 8.0315, 9.065, 10.01, and 10.015. Tovino & Winslade, *A Primer on the Law and Ethics of Treatment, Research, and Public Policy in the Context of Severe Traumatic Brain Injury, 14 Ann. Health L. 1, 18, 38, 39, 40, 41 (2005).*

Journal 2004 Argues that the corporate practice of medicine doctrine is no longer practical in today's health care system. Concludes that federal legislation must be enacted to align the states on the issue and to ensure that physicians may practice in a way that benefits patients and the health care system. Quotes Principle VI. Huberfeld, *Be Not Afraid of Change: Time to Eliminate the Corporate Practice of Medicine Doctrine, 14 Health Matrix 243, 256 (2004).*

Journal 2003 Discusses conflicts of interest caused when managed care organizations provide financial incentives to physicians. Concludes that the focus of managed care is not well-suited for the doctor-patient relationship. Quotes Opinion 8.03. Cites Principle VII. References Opinion 8.051. Hall, *Bargaining With Hippocrates: Managed Care and the Doctor-Patient Relationship, 54 SC L. Rev. 689, 696, 735 (2003).*

Journal 2003 Considers a legislative plan allowing voluntary, consensual organ donation by condemned prisoners. Concludes that, in view of the current organ shortage, the benefits of such a plan outweigh the concerns. Quotes Principle VII and Opinion 2.06. Perales, *Rethinking the Prohibition of Death Row Prisoners as Organ Donors: A Possible Lifeline to Those on Organ Donor Waiting Lists, 34 St. Mary's L. J. 687, 721, 725 (2003).*

Journal 2001 Examines international ethical guidelines for psychiatrists. Observes that many psychiatrists are unaware of the relevant guidelines. Concludes that information about these guidelines should be more widely disseminated with a goal of increased compliance. Quotes Principle VII. Martens, *Necessity of Adapting Psychiatric Treatment to Relevant Ethical Guidelines, 20 Med. Law 393, 394 (2001).*

Journal 2000 Discusses managed care in terms of problems, responses, and accomplishments. Demonstrates how a physician union's collective bargaining process can benefit patients and physicians in addressing problems with managed care. Concludes that barriers preventing such unions should be removed. Quotes Principles VI and VII and Opinion 10.01. Rugg, *An Old Solution to a New Problem:*

Physician Unions Take the Edge Off Managed Care, 34 Colum. J. L. & Soc. Probs. 1, 41 (2000).

Journal 1996 Discusses the trend toward conserving resources expended on health care by withholding services absent a showing of necessity. Claims that the high standard of care physicians owe patients is jeopardized by medical treatment decisions based on coverage concerns. Concludes that the legal structure regarding health care plans should be changed. Quotes Preamble, Principles I, II, III, IV, V, VI, and VII, and Opinion 2.03. Hirshfeld & Thomason, *Medical Necessity Determinations: The Need for a New Legal Structure, 6 Health Matrix 3, 8-9 (1996).*

Journal 1996 Proposes an alternative method of capital punishment to allow for organ donation by executed prisoners. Provides justifications for this proposal. Concludes that physicians should be able to ethically participate in this process. Quotes Principle VII. Cites Opinion 2.06. References Opinion 2.162 (1994) [subsequently amended]. Patton, *A Call for Common Sense: Organ Donation and the Executed Prisoner, 3 Va. J. Soc. Pol'y & L. 387, 404, 405, 407-10 (1996).*

Journal 1995 Explores the debates and commentaries regarding patenting medical instruments and processes. Concludes that current patent law fails to address the ethical concerns of physicians and their patients. Quotes Principles of Medical Ethics §10 (1971) [now Principle VII] and Principle §2 (1971) [now Opinion 9.095] and Opinions 9.08

and 9.09. Reisman, *Physicians and Surgeons as Inventors: Reconciling Medical Process Patents and Medical Ethics, 10 High Tech. L. J. 355, 356, 368-70, 385 (1995).*

Journal 1992 Discusses the problem of discrimination based on HIV status, particularly among women and children. Examines medical and public health issues involving HIV. Cites Principle VII. References Opinion 9.131. Gittler & Rennart, *HIV Infection Among Women and Children and Antidiscrimination Laws: An Overview, 77 Iowa L. Rev. 1313, 1363 (1992).*

Journal 1992 Discusses the plight of undocumented aliens and their need for access to medical care. Considers existing systems for providing such care, as well as barriers to the receipt of medical attention. Cites Principles VI and VII. Loue, *Access to Health Care and the Undocumented Alien, 13 J. Legal Med. 271, 291 (1992).*

Journal 1990 Discusses the moral dilemma in deciding whether to withdraw artificial nutrition and hydration from a patient and the appropriate role of the judiciary. Concludes that judicial decisions do not represent the moral viewpoint of society and that moral pronouncements should not be made in the courtroom. Quotes Preamble, Principles I, II, III, IV, V, VI, and VII, and Opinion 2.20. Peccarelli, *A Moral Dilemma: The Role of Judicial Intervention in Withholding or Withdrawing Nutrition and Hydration, 23 John Marshall L. Rev. 537, 539, 540, 541 (1990).*

Principle VIII

Cal. App. 2003 Patient and her husband sued medical clinic for terminating care after the patient filed malpractice claims against two clinic physicians. Clinic's policy required termination of all medical care for patients and their families in such a situation. Appeals court upheld summary judgment for the clinic on several claims, but denied summary judgment on claims for interference with contractual relations, negligent infliction of emotional distress, and breach of fiduciary duty. Quotes Principles VI and VIII. *Scripps Clinic v. Superior Court, 108 Cal. App.4th 917, 134 Cal. Rptr. 2d 101, 117.*

Ohio 2009 Physician appealed from a judgment affirming an order of the state medical board that permanently revoked appellant's certificate to practice medicine. The board found that appellant's sexual contact with patients violated Ohio statutes governing physician conduct and the AMA's Code of Medical Ethics, citing Principles I, II, IV, and VIII. The Court of Appeals held that Ohio state law allows the board to revoke a physician's certificate if it finds that the person violated any provision of the Code of Ethics of the AMA. *D'Souza v. State Med. Bd. of Ohio, 2009 WL 5108774, 6.*

Journal 2011 Examines the way in which the actuary delivers services in the context of the pension funding crises that

exist in the United States. Concludes by offering proposals for self-regulatory mechanisms to address the practices within the profession that have been identified as factors that contributed to the crisis in pension funding. Cites Principle VIII. Gunz & Jennings, *A Proactive Proposal for Self-regulation of the Actuarial Profession: A Means of Avoiding the Audit Profession's Post-Enron Regulatory Fate, 48 Am. Bus. L.J. 641, 654 (2011).*

Journal 2011 Reviews the responsible conduct of research (RCR) domains of publication practices and authorship, conflicts of interest, and research misconduct. Concludes that because the accuracy, completeness, and value of the scientific record impact the health of society, scientists are obligated to use the highest possible standards of research conduct. Quotes Principle VIII and Opinion 8.031. Horner & Minifie, *Research Ethics III: Publication Practices and Authorship, Conflicts of Interest, and Research Misconduct, 54 J. Speech, Language, & Hearing Res. S346, S351, S352 (2011).*

Journal 2011 Reviews the use and current regulation of medical marijuana to alleviate pain in terminally ill patients. Focusing on patient autonomy, concludes that patients should have access to medical marijuana in controlled doses under controlled conditions. Quotes Principle III and Opinions 10.01, 10.015, and 10.02. References Principle VIII. Pfeifer, *Smoking Gun: The Moral and Legal Struggle for Medical Marijuana*, 27 Touro L. Rev. 339, 340-41, 345-346 (2011).

Journal 2010 Examines the growth and regulation of donor-assisted reproduction. Concludes reform is needed to permit children to access genetic and health information, with the goal of increasing the safety of donor-assisted reproduction while maintaining donor anonymity. Quotes Principle VIII. Luetkemeyer, *Who's Guarding the Henhouse and What Are They Doing With the Eggs (and Sperm)? A Call for Increased Regulation of Gamete Donation and Long-term Tracking of Donor Gametes*, 3 St. Louis U. J. Health L. & Pol'y 397, 414 (2010).

Journal 2010 Analyzes factors contributing to the emergence of medical repatriation and evaluates whether this practice comports with current legal and ethical standards. Proposes changes to federal regulations that govern hospitals and clarifications to medical ethical standards. Quotes the Preamble and Principles I, II, III, IV, V, VI, VII, VIII, and IX. Zoellner, *Medical Repatriation: Examining the Legal and Ethical Implications of an Emerging Practice*, 32 Wash. U. J. L. & Pol'y 515, 530-532 (2010).

Journal 2009 Explores emerging issues in conflict management systems design (CMSD). Concludes as the practice of CMSD in the organizational context continues to expand, practitioners should openly discuss the emerging issues of the field. References Principles I, II, V, and VIII. Costantino, *Second Generation Organizational Conflict Management Systems Design: A Practitioner's Perspective on Emerging Issues*, 14 Harv. Negot. L. Rev. 81, 95 (2009).

Journal 2009 Examines therapeutic uses of cannabis and the legal and social controversies surrounding its legalization. Concludes changes in the regulation of medical cannabis are necessary to better care for patients and better utilize resources that are currently directed toward the war on drugs. Quotes Principle VIII and Opinion 2.17. DiFonzo, *The End of the Red Queen's Race: Medical Marijuana in the New Century*, 27 Quinnipiac L. Rev. 673, 736, 737 (2009).

Journal 2009 Discusses the interaction between statutes and case law governing the medical field and the core principles of medical professionalism. Concludes the legal framework of medical professionalism does not encompass all the elements required of a medical professional. Quotes Principles II, III, IV, V, VI, VII, and VIII. Fichter, *The Law of Doctoring: A Study of the Codification of Medical Professionalism*, 19 Health Matrix 317, 338, 339, 340, 343, 351 (2009).

Journal 2009 Discusses the importance of trust in the physician-patient and in the attorney-client relationship. Notes the lack of an appropriate remedy for breaches of fiduciary duties. Concludes there should be a statutory remedy for breaches of trust in the professional relationship. Quotes Principle VIII. Forell & Sortun, *The Tort of Betrayal of Trust*, 42 U. Mich. J. L. Reform, 557, 603 (2009).

Journal 2009 Explores the jurisprudential foundation of the fiduciary duty physicians owe their patients and discusses the failure of physicians to disclose to patients errors and other emergent medical risks. Concludes law should recognize the physician's duty to disclose such risks by enforcing a cause of action for breach of that duty. Quotes Principles III and VIII and Opinions 8.12, 10.015, and 10.02. References Opinion 8.12. Hafemeister, *Lean on Me: A Physician's Fiduciary Duty to Disclose an Emergent Medical Risk to the Patient*, 86 Wash. U. L. Rev. 1167, 1172-1173, 1178, 1182, 1185, 1188, 1209 (2009).

Journal 2009 Explores the nature of the physician-patient relationship and the impact of increased availability of medical information on patient autonomy and physician responsibility to exercise independent judgment. Concludes physicians must treat patients in accordance with their fiduciary obligation to use their own judgment when confronted with a patient demanding unnecessary medical services. Quotes Preamble, Principles I and VIII, and Opinions 2.035, 8.03, and 10.015. Hafemeister, *The Fiduciary Obligation of Physicians to "Just Say No" if an "Informed" Patient Demands Services That Are Not Medically Indicated*, 39 Seton Hall L. Rev. 335, 372, 373, 374 (2009).

Journal 2009 Discusses whether patients have a right to pain management. Concludes that no physician duty is established by law or ethics to provide pain management outside the traditional physician-patient relationship. Cites Principles I, II, IV, and VIII. Hall & Boswell, *Ethics, Law, and Pain Management as a Patient Right*, 12 Pain Physician 499, 500 (2009).

Journal 2008 Discusses ex parte interviews with a treating physician in discovery before and after the HIPAA Privacy Rule and the issues facing physicians contacted for such interviews. Concludes courts and attorneys should work together to allow for efficient discovery while protecting physicians. Quotes Principles IV and VIII and Opinions 5.05 and 10.01. Burnette & Morning, *HIPAA and Ex Parte Interviews—The Beginning of the End?* 1 J. Health & Life Sci. L. 73, 100-01 (2008).

Journal 2008 Discusses legal and ethical considerations in making organ transplants available to qualified incarcerated individuals at public expense. Concludes legal and ethical norms suggest organ transplants should be made available to prisoners and new policies should be established to provide necessary transplant services. Apparent reference to Principle VIII. McKinney, Winslade, & Stone, *Offender Organ Transplants: Law, Ethics, Economics, and Health Policy*, 9 Hous. J. Health L. & Pol'y 39, 62 (2008).

Journal 2008 Discusses covenants not to compete and Kentucky cases dealing with physician noncompetition agreements. Concludes Kentucky should enact legislation permitting reasonable noncompetition agreements ancillary to sale of practice contracts to increase patient choice of physician. Quotes Principle VIII and Opinion 9.02. Naiser, *Physician Noncompetition Agreements in Kentucky:*

The Past Discounting of Public Interests and a Proposed Solution, 47 U. Louisville L. Rev. 195, 195, 200 (2008).

Journal 2008 Examines the development of bioethics and environmental ethics, as well as laws promoting the role of bioethicists in decision making. Concludes environmental ethicists must convince legislatures of the role of environmental ethics in order to have a greater impact on decision making. Quotes Principles I, II, III, IV, V, VI, VII, VIII, and IX. Robertson, *Seeking a Seat at the Table: Has Law Left Environmental Ethics Behind as It Embraces Bioethics? 32 Wm. & Mary Envtl. L. & Pol'y Rev. 273, 307 (2008).*

Journal 2008 Examines ethical issues related to broadcasting cardiothoracic surgeries for educational and media purposes. Concludes that seven ethical guidelines should be followed to ensure patient safety. Quotes Principle VIII and Opinion 8.121. Sade, *Broadcast of Surgical Procedures as a Teaching Instrument in Cardiothoracic Surgery, 86 Ann. Thorac. Surg. 357, 359 (2008).*

Journal 2008 Argues that as a matter of public health, physicians must control antibiotic administration to combat antibiotic resistance. Concludes that despite limited incentives for antibiotic conservation, physicians must acknowledge their important role in mitigating the public health threat of antibiotic resistance. Quotes Principles VII and VIII and Opinions 2.09 and 10.015. Cites Opinion 2.03. Saver, *In Tepid Defense of Population Health: Physicians and Antibiotic Resistance, 34 Am. J. L. & Med. 431, 457 (2008).*

Journal 2008 Explores the fiduciary relationship between physicians and patients, professional and ethical obligations of both physicians and lawyers, and the implications for conflict resolution in health care. Concludes physicians must put patient interests above their own and lawyers must work to discern clients' best interests and support client welfare. Quotes Principle VIII and Opinions 8.12 and 10.015. Cites Principles I and II and Opinions 10.01 and 10.015. Scott, *Doctors as Advocates, Lawyers as Healers, 29 Hamline J. Pub. L. Pol'y, 331, 340-41, 347, 371 (2008).*

Journal 2007 Compares the role of conscience clauses in various professions. Concludes that conscience clauses in the area of health care must not impede access to care. Quotes Preamble and Principles V, VI, and VIII. Chudoba, *Conscience in America: The Slippery Slope of Mixing Morality With Medicine, 36 Sw. U. L. Rev. 85, 86, 103, 104, 105 (2007).*

Journal 2007 Addresses physician liability for an extramarital affair with a patient's spouse. Concludes that such an affair should be regarded as a breach of a fiduciary duty. Quotes Preamble, Principles I, II, and VIII, and Opinions 8.145, 9.04, 9.123, and 10.015. Demaine, *"Playing Doctor" With the Patient's Spouse: Alternative Conceptions of Health Professional Liability, 14 Va. J. Soc. Pol'y & L. 308, 325, 330-31, 331-32 (2007).*

Journal 2007 Discusses the evolution of informed consent doctrine. Concludes that, in context of research, informed consent exceptions should be substantially narrowed. Quotes Ch. I, Art. I, Sec. 4 (May 1847) [now Opinion 8.082], and Ch. I, Art. I, Sec. 1 (May 1847) [now Principles I and VIII]. References Opinions 2.08 and 8.08. Grimm, *Informed Consent for All! No Exceptions, 37 N. M. L. Rev. 39, 39, 61 (2007).*

Journal 2007 Analyzes drafters' original intent for the Confrontation Clause as well as the contemporary interpretation under Crawford. Concludes that only statements taken by law enforcement agents should be considered testimonial in nature. Quotes Principle VIII. Harbinson, *Crawford v. Washington and Davis v. Washington's Originalism: Historical Arguments Showing Child Abuse Victims' Statements to Physicians Are Nontestimonial and Admissible as an Exception to the Confrontation Clause, 58 Mercer L. Rev. 569, 617 (2007).*

Journal 2007 Evaluates the added cost of extrarenal findings in CT imaging of kidney donors. Concludes that because incidental findings arise in 28% of cases, pertinent ethical issues should be considered. References Principle VIII. Maizlin, Barnard, Gourlayz, & Brown, *Economic and Ethical Impact of Extrarenal Findings on Potential Living Kidney Donor Assessment with Computed Tomography Angiography, 20 Transplant Int'l. 338, 341 (2007).*

Journal 2006 Evaluates the constitutionality of federal faith-based initiative programs. Concludes that such programs violate the First Amendment under the combined Lemon and Zelman test. Cites Principles II and VIII. Boden, *Compassion Inaction: Why President Bush's Faith-Based Initiatives Violate the Establishment Clause, 29 Seattle U. L. Rev. 991, 1023 (2006).*

Journal 2006 Examines ethical dilemmas physicians may face as providers of pay-for-performance medical care. Concludes that this strategy offers a benefit to patients as long as physicians uphold stringent ethical standards and work together to ensure optimum patient care. Cites Principles I, V, VIII, and IX and Opinions 2.035, 2.095, 6.01, 8.021, 8.03, 8.0501, 8.053, 8.054, and 8.121. Bostick, Sade, & McMahon, *Report of the Council on Ethical and Judicial Affairs: Physician Pay-for-Performance Programs, 3 Ind. Health L. Rev. 429, 430, 431, 432-33, 434, 435, 436 (2006).*

Journal 2006 Examines the legal and public health issues raised by increased rates of Hepatitis C in prison populations. Concludes that reform is needed to provide adequate health care to prisoners and that courts have the power to require such care under the Eighth Amendment. Quotes Preamble, Principles VII, VIII, and IX, and Opinion 10.015. Brunsden, *Hepatitis C in Prisons: Evolving Toward Decency Through Adequate Medical Care and Public Health Reform, 54 UCLA L. Rev. 465, 500 (2006).*

Journal 2006 Explores conscience clause legislation relating to the dispensing of oral contraceptives. Concludes that such legislation must balance the interests of the patient and the health care provider. Cites Principles I, II, III, IV, V, VI, VII, VIII, and IX. Collins, *Conscience Clauses and Oral Contraceptives: Conscientious Objection or Calculated Obstruction?* 15 Ann. Health L. 37, 54 (2006).

Journal 2006 Discusses mentally incompetent inmates and capital punishment. Proposes that, to be permissible, involuntary medication of death-row inmates must represent the best medically appropriate treatment. Quotes Principles I, III, and VIII and Opinion 2.06. Gabos, *The Perils of Singleton v. Norris: Ethics and Beyond,* 32 Am. J. L. & Med. 117, 118, 125-26, 127 (2006).

Journal 2006 Examines the practice of law firms employing their own in-house counsel. Concludes there will likely be an increase in firms that retain in-house counsel to represent them. Quotes Principle VIII. Gorman, *Empirical Studies of the Legal Profession: What Do We Know About Lawyers' Lives? Explaining the Spread of Law Firm In-House Counsel Positions: A Response to Professor Chambliss,* 84 N. C. L. Rev. 1577, 1585.

Journal 2006 Discusses the prevalence and cause of physicians' failure to provide proper care. Concludes that patients should be able to sue their physicians for breach of fiduciary duty. Quotes Principle VIII and Opinion 8.03. Mehlman, *Dishonest Medical Mistakes,* 59 Vand. L. Rev. 1137, 1144 (2006).

Journal 2006 Examines a mental health professional's competing duties of confidentiality and reporting a patient's threats of violence. Suggests new legislation should clarify duty to report a threat. Quotes Preamble and Principles III, IV, and VIII. Cites Opinion 5.05. Mossman, *Critique of Pure Risk Assessment or, Kant Meets Tarasoff,* 75 U. Cin. L. Rev. 523, 579 (2006).

Journal 2006 Examines the constitutionality of conscience clauses under the Fourteenth Amendment. Concludes that state involvement through the enactment of such clauses may violate the Fourteenth Amendment. Cites Principle VIII. Rozenek, *Whose Conscience Is It Anyway? The State's Role in Conscience Clause Creation and the Denial of Contraception,* 40 Suffolk U. L. Rev. 215, 220 (2006).

Journal 2006 Reviews conflicts which arise when a physician must choose between violating a law and adhering to an ethical principle. Concludes the physician must consider the needs of the patient and acknowledges that there are cases where violating a law may be justified. Quotes Principle VIII and Opinion 1.02. Schwartz, *The Ethical Health Lawyer: When Doing the Right Thing Means Breaking the Law: What Is the Role of the Health Lawyer?* 34 J. L. Med. & Ethics 624, 625, 626 (2006).

Journal 2005 Discusses physician responses to the medical malpractice liability crisis. Concludes that certain responses may violate ethical obligations that physicians owe to their patients and to society as a whole. Cites Opinions 9.025 and 10.015. References Principle VIII. Kachalia, Choudhry, & Studdert, *Physician Responses to the Malpractice Crisis:*

From Defense to Offense, 33 J. L. Med. & Ethics 416, 419, 421, 424 (2005).

Journal 2005 Argues that the Eighth Circuit's ruling in *Singleton v. Norris* failed to consider the ethical standards of the medical community. Concludes that, as a result, physicians may be placed in an untenable position regarding treatment of mentally ill death-row inmates. Quotes Principle VIII and Opinions 1.02 and 2.06. Lloyd, *Primum Non Nocere: Singleton v. Norris and the Ethical Dilemma of Medicating the Condemned,* 58 Ark. L. Rev. 225, 232, 233 (2005).

Journal 2005 Examines issues surrounding tort reform proposals. Concludes that more can be done to correct the current tort system before moving toward a "one size fits all" approach. Quotes Principles I, II, III, IV, V, VI, VII, VIII, and IX. Messerly & Warwick, *Nowhere to Turn: A Glance at the Facts Behind the Supposed Need for Tort "Reform,"* 28 Hamline L. Rev. 489, 506 (2005).

Journal 2005 Argues that in *Aetna v. Davila/Cigna v. Calad,* the Supreme Court missed an opportunity to overturn unjust ERISA policies. Concludes that the principle of complete ERISA preemption as articulated in these consolidated cases is unsatisfactory because it violates the separation of powers doctrine. Quotes Principle VIII. Cites Opinions 8.054, 8.13, 8.135, 9.123, 10.01, and 10.015. Nelson, *Aetna v. Davila/CIGNA v. Calad: A Missed Opportunity,* 31 Wm. Mitchell L. Rev. 843, 847, 849, 850, 880 (2005).

Journal 2004 Examines the requirements of the Privacy Rule regarding use and disclosure of a patient's identifiable health information in the context of research. Concludes that the Rule's burdensome administrative requirements may discourage research and thus outweigh any benefits for research subject autonomy. Quotes Principle VIII and Opinions 5.051, 8.031, and 10.015. Tovino, *The Use and Disclosure of Protected Health Information for Research Under the HIPAA Privacy Rule: Unrealized Patient Autonomy and Burdensome Government Regulation,* 49 S. D. L. Rev. 447, 496, 502 (2004).

Journal 2003 Examines social norms, using public choice theory, to determine how certain groups in society use these norms to benefit their members. Concludes that the benefits provided by social norms may dissipate depending on various considerations. Quotes Principles II and VIII. Miller, *Norms and Interests,* 32 Hofstra L. Rev. 637, 650, 670 (2003).

Journal 2002 Examines how managed care has adversely affected information disclosure in the physician-patient relationship. Concludes that, unless courts expand applicability of principles of informed consent, patient self-determination and autonomy will continue to be undermined. Quotes Principle VIII and Opinions 8.03, 8.053, 8.054, and 8.08. Morris, *Dissing Disclosure: Just What the Doctor Ordered,* 44 Ariz. L. Rev. 313, 344, 349, 362, 363, 366 (2002).

Journal 2002 Considers the dilemma of informed consent in the context of prescribing psychotropic medication to patients with mental illness and mental retardation. Recognizes the need for substituted decision-making in certain situations. Concludes that legislation would help address this issue. Quotes Preamble, Principles I, III, IV, VIII, and IX, and Opinion 8.08. O'Sullivan & Borcherding, *Informed Consent for Medication in Persons With Mental Retardation and Mental Illness*, 12 Health Matrix 63, 75, 86, 87, 88 (2002)

Journal 2002 Discusses legal and medical policies that protect confidentiality in the physician-patient relationship. Concludes that reducing the current level of privacy protection would jeopardize health care. Quotes Preamble and Opinions 2.136, 5.05, and 10.01. References Principles VIII and IX. Sciarrino, *Ferguson v. City of Charleston: "The Doctor Will See You Now, Be Sure to Bring Your Privacy Rights in With You!"* 12 Temp. Pol. & Civ. Rts. L. Rev. 197, 213, 215, 220, 221, 222 (2002).

Principle IX

Journal 2011 Argues the medical profession has no commitment to political advocacy because civic virtues are outside the professional realm, because civic participation is not necessary for civic virtue, and because the medical profession should not mandate any political stance for its members. Concludes the medical profession should be dedicated to competent and ethical professional work rather than require political advocacy. Quotes Principle IX. Huddle, *Medical Professionalism and Medical Education Should Not Involve Commitments to Political Advocacy*, 86 Acad. Med. 378, 379 (2011).

Journal 2010 Analyzes factors contributing to the emergence of medical repatriation and evaluates whether this practice comports with current legal and ethical standards. Proposes changes to federal regulations that govern hospitals and clarifications to medical ethical standards. Quotes the Preamble and Principles I, II, III, IV, V, VI, VII, VIII, and IX. Zoellner, *Medical Repatriation: Examining the Legal and Ethical Implications of an Emerging Practice*, 32 Wash. U. J. L. & Pol'y 515, 530-532 (2010).

Journal 2008 Examines the development of bioethics and environmental ethics, as well as laws promoting the role of bioethicists in decision making. Concludes environmental ethicists must convince legislatures of the role of environmental ethics in order to have a greater impact on decision making. Quotes Principles I, II, III, IV, V, VI, VII, VIII, and IX. Robertson, *Seeking a Seat at the Table: Has Law Left Environmental Ethics Behind as It Embraces Bioethics?* 32 Wm. & Mary Envtl. L. & Pol'y Rev. 273, 307 (2008).

Journal 2006 Examines ethical dilemmas physicians may face as providers of pay-for-performance medical care. Concludes that this strategy offers a benefit to patients as long as physicians uphold stringent ethical standards and work together to ensure optimum patient care. Cites Principles I, V, VIII, and IX and Opinions 2.035, 2.095, 6.01, 8.021, 8.03, 8.0501, 8.053, 8.054, and 8.121. Bostick, Sade, & McMahon, *Report of the Council on Ethical and Judicial Affairs: Physician Pay-For-Performance Programs*, 3 Ind. Health L. Rev. 429, 430, 431, 432-33, 434, 435, 436 (2006).

Journal 2006 Examines the legal and public health issues raised by increased rates of Hepatitis C in prison populations. Concludes that reform is needed to provide adequate health care to prisoners and that courts have the power to require such care under the Eighth Amendment. Quotes Preamble, Principles VII, VIII, and IX, and Opinion 10.015. Brunsden, *Hepatitis C in Prisons: Evolving Toward Decency Through Adequate Medical Care and Public Health Reform*, 54 UCLA L. Rev. 465, 500 (2006).

Journal 2006 Explores the legal and ethical issues surrounding concierge medicine. Concludes that concierge medicine is best restricted to a small class of wealthy individuals. Quotes Principle IX and Opinion 8.055. Cites Principle VI and Opinions 8.055, 8.11, 8.115, 9.065, and 10.05. Carnahan, *Law, Medicine, and Wealth: Does Concierge Medicine Promote Health Care Choice, or Is It a Barrier to Access?* 17 Stan. L. & Pol'y Rev. 121, 149-50, 151, 152, 153-54 (2006).

Journal 2006 Explores conscience clause legislation relating to the dispensing of oral contraceptives. Concludes that such legislation must balance the interests of the patient and the health care provider. Cites Principles I, II, III, IV, V, VI, VII, VIII, and IX. Collins, *Conscience Clauses and Oral Contraceptives: Conscientious Objection or Calculated Obstruction?* 15 Ann. Health L. 37, 54 (2006).

Journal 2006 Considers the interaction of laws, rules, and guidelines in the area of health law. Suggests that the legislature should revise current laws to reflect local variability in practice. Quotes Preamble and Principles VII and IX. Heimer, *Responsibility in Health Care: Spanning the Boundary Between Law and Medicine*, 41 Wake Forest L. Rev. 465, 498 (2006).

Journal 2006 Discusses the role of EMTALA in mandating care for the uninsured. Concludes EMTALA is inadequate and Congress should take steps toward establishing a program for universal health care. Quotes Principle IX and Ch. II, Art. V, Sec. 9 (May 1847) [now Opinion 9.065], and Ch. III, Art. I, Sec. 3 (May 1847) [now Opinion 9.065]. Hermer, *The Scapegoat: EMTALA and Emergency Department Overcrowding*, 14 J. L. & Pol'y 695, 713-14 (2006).

Journal 2005 Discusses legal and ethical problems associated with patient surcharges. Concludes that surcharges are necessary to combat rising malpractice insurance premiums and a declining payment environment. Cites Principle IX and Opinion 6.12. Landfair, *Transforming Physicians Into Business Savvy Entrepreneurs: Patient Surcharges Charge Onto the Scene of Physician Reimbursement*, 43 Duq. L. Rev. 257, 268, 269 (2005).

Journal 2005 Examines issues surrounding tort reform proposals. Concludes that more can be done to correct the current tort system before moving toward a "one size fits all" approach. Quotes Principles I, II, III, IV, V, VI, VII, VIII, and IX. Messerly & Warwick, *Nowhere to Turn: A Glance at the Facts Behind the Supposed Need for Tort "Reform,"* 28 Hamline L. Rev. 489, 506 (2005).

Journal 2005 Examines the practice of "boutique medicine" and considers legal and ethical implications. Concludes that boutique medical services would be ethical only if physicians used retainer money from their boutique clients to augment health care costs of the poor. Quotes Principles VII and IX and Opinion 8.055. Russano, *Is Boutique Medicine a New Threat to American Health Care or a Logical Way of Revitalizing the Doctor-Patient Relationship?* 17 Wash. U. J. L. & Pol'y 313, 331, 332 (2005).

Journal 2005 Discusses ethical, legal, and policy issues associated with treatment and research involving patients who are in a persistent vegetative or minimally conscious state. Concludes that patients in these states are at risk for therapeutic failures until physicians can more accurately determine which patients will benefit from treatment and accurately convey such information to families or surrogates. Quotes Principles VII and IX and Opinions 8.031, 8.0315, 9.065, 10.01, and 10.015. Tovino & Winslade, *A Primer on the Law and Ethics of Treatment, Research, and Public Policy in the Context of Severe Traumatic Brain Injury*, 14 Ann. Health L. 1, 18, 38, 39, 40, 41 (2005).

Journal 2002 Considers the dilemma of informed consent in the context of prescribing psychotropic medication to patients with mental illness and mental retardation. Recognizes the need for substituted decision-making in certain situations. Concludes that legislation would help address this issue. Quotes Preamble, Principles I, III, IV, VIII, and IX, and Opinion 8.08. O'Sullivan & Borcherding, *Informed Consent for Medication in Persons With Mental Retardation and Mental Illness*, 12 Health Matrix 63, 75, 86, 87, 88 (2002).

Journal 2002 Discusses legal and medical policies that protect confidentiality in the physician-patient relationship. Concludes that reducing the current level of privacy protection would jeopardize health care. Quotes Preamble and Opinions 2.136, 5.05, and 10.01. References Principles VIII and IX. Sciarrino, *Ferguson v. City of Charleston: "The Doctor Will See You Now, Be Sure to Bring Your Privacy Rights in With You!"* 12 Temp. Pol. & Civ. Rts. L. Rev. 197, 213, 215, 220, 221, 222 (2002).

Opinions of the Council on Ethical and Judicial Affairs

1 Patient-Physician Relationships

1.1.1 Patient-Physician Relationships

Minn. App. 2005 Minnesota Board of Medical Practice revoked the license of appellant, finding that appellant carried on an inappropriate sexual relationship with a patient. Quoting Opinion 10.015, the appeals court determined that the individual whom the appellant was treating fell within the definition of patient, and therefore, appellant's sexual relationship with the patient was a violation of the Minnesota Medical Practice Act, justifying the revocation of his license. *In re Woolley, 2005 WL 2077475, 6.*

Army Crim. App. 2004 Appellant, in a general court martial hearing, was found guilty of unpremeditated murder. The Court of Appeals for the Armed Forces set aside and remanded the judgment to the Army Court of Criminal Appeals to determine whether there was a conflict of interest in allowing mental health providers who had a prior psychotherapist-patient relationship with the appellant to serve on his sanity board. The court determined there was no conflict of interest. In making this determination, the court quoted Opinion 10.015 and cited Opinion 8.03 to analyze the aspects of the physician-patient relationship. *United States v. Best, 59 M.J. 886, 891 n. 8.*

Journal 2011 Reviews the issues surrounding the use of the Internet for medical consultations, as well as current guidelines and regulations. Concludes that, although online medical consultations may be cost-effective, the risks of liability outweigh the benefits. References Opinion 10.015. Bailey, *The Legal, Financial, and Ethical Implications of Online Medical Consultations, 16 J. Tech. L. & Pol'y 53, 95 (2011).*

Journal 2011 Describes off-label uses of prescription drugs and the associated risks and harms. Argues that such use should be restricted unless supported by high-quality evidence of efficacy and safety. Cites Opinions 10.01 and 10.015. Coleman & Rosoff, *The Case for Legal Regulation of Physicians' Off-Label Prescribing, 86 Notre Dame L. Rev. 649, 679 (2011).*

Journal 2011 Discusses the doctrine of informed consent and the influence of physician groups on the dissemination of information to patients. Concludes the doctrine of informed consent should be expanded by the courts, rather than continuing to allow professional societies to dictate provider guidelines for obtaining informed consent. Quotes Opinions 8.08, 10.01, and 10.015. References Opinion 2.065. Ginsberg, *Informed Consent: No Longer Just What the Doctor Ordered? The "Contributions" of Medical Associations and Courts to a More Patient Friendly Doctrine, 15 Mich. St. J. Med. & Law 17, 23, 24, 25, 26, 46 (2011).*

Journal 2011 Examines the Patient Protection and Affordable Care Act and its impact on patient access to physician services. Also considers the possibility that physicians might be required to provide services to all patients as a condition to practice. Concludes that regulations that try to conscript physician services would be practically ineffective, legally dubious, and unwise public policy. Quotes Opinions 9.06 and 10.015. Cites Opinion 2.09. Kapp, *Conscripted Physician Services and the Public's Health, 39 J. L. Med. & Ethics 414, 414, 418 (2011).*

Journal 2011 Discusses the far-reaching effects of 2005 Illinois medical liability reform legislation. Explains how the 2010 Illinois Supreme Court decision in *Lebron v. Gottlieb* invalidated many beneficial aspects of this legislation. Quotes Opinion 10.015. Cites Opinion 9.10. Nelson, Swanson, & Buckley, *Lebron v. Gottlieb Memorial Hospital: Capping Medical Practice Reform in Illinois, 20 Annals Health L. 1, 7, 11 (Winter 2011).*

Journal 2011 Reviews the use and current regulation of medical marijuana to alleviate pain in terminally ill patients. Focusing on patient autonomy, concludes that patients should have access to medical marijuana in controlled doses under controlled conditions. Quotes Principle III and Opinions 10.01, 10.015, and 10.02. References Principle VIII. Pfeifer, *Smoking Gun: The Moral and Legal Struggle for Medical Marijuana, 27 Touro L. Rev. 339, 340-41, 345-346 (2011).*

Journal 2010 Examines manufacturer-physician consulting arrangements and discusses the evolution of fair market valuation. Proposes a set of standards for calculating fair market value for physician services to ensure compliance with legal requirements. Quotes Opinion 8.061. Eaton & Reid, *Mirror, Mirror on the Wall: Evaluating Fair Market Value for Manufacturer-Physician Consulting Arrangements, 65 Food & Drug L. J. 141, 147 (2010).*

Journal 2010 Discusses issues arising from the enactment of legislation by North Dakota involving a minor's reproductive rights. Explores ethical principles that govern physician's actions within the context of reproductive health. Concludes that, while a patient's expectation of confidentiality with a physician is critical, competing values come into play when the patient is a minor and parental involvement may be important. Provides practical guidance to address issues in this context. Quotes Opinions 2.01, 2.015, 5.055, 8.08, 8.115, 9.12, 10.01, 10.015, and 10.05. Cites Opinions 5.05, 5.055, 8.08, 8.11, 8.115, 9.12, and 10.05. Haas, *"Doctor, I'm Pregnant and Fifteen—I Can't Tell My Parents—Please Help Me": Minor Consent, Reproductive Rights, and Ethical Principles for Physicians, 86 N.D. L. Rev. 63, 70, 73, 75-78, 82, 84, 86-88 (2010).*

Journal 2010 Argues that it is ethically improper for medical practitioners to use their position of influence arising from superior scientific knowledge to impose their moral preferences on patients. Concludes physicians need education about their professional and legal obligations so they may protect their ability to participate in, or refuse participation in, particular services while ensuring the patient is not harmed. Quotes Opinion 10.015. Morrison & Allokotte, *Duty First: Towards Patient-Centered Care and Limitations on the Right to Refuse for Moral, Religious or Ethical Reasons, 9 Ave Maria L. Rev. 141, 168 (2010).*

Journal 2010 Argues that physicians are more likely to avoid improperly prescribing controlled substances if put on notice of the additional criminal liability they face in the event of a patient's death. Concludes that physicians who have caused a patient's death by administering illegal and lethal doses should be charged under various sections of the Controlled Substances Act as well as with involuntary manslaughter. Quotes Opinion 10.015. Nunziato, *Preventing Prescription Drug Overdose in the Twenty-First Century: Is the Controlled Substances Act Enough? 38 Hofstra L. Rev. 1261, 1277 (2010).*

Journal 2010 Examines disciplinary functions of state medical licensing boards and identifies fundamental principles underlying their authority. Concludes that medical boards have lost sight of the primary goal of protecting patients and suggests that they renew their focus, prioritizing disciplinary actions taken on the basis of competence. Quotes Opinion 10.015. Sawicki, *Character, Competence, and the Principles of Medical Discipline, 13 J. Health Care L. & Pol'y 285, 291 (2010).*

Journal 2009 Considers a physician's role in educating patients about health care reform. Concludes that reform would be aided by educating patients on all aspects of the health care system. Quotes Opinion 10.015. Cites Opinion 9.012. Abemayor, *United We Stand, Divided We Fall, 135 Arch. Otolaryngol. Head Neck Surg. 432, 432, 433 (2009).*

Journal 2009 Explores the jurisprudential foundation of the fiduciary duty physicians owe their patients and discusses the failure of physicians to disclose to patients errors and other emergent medical risks. Concludes law should recognize the physician's duty to disclose such risks by enforcing a cause of action for breach of that duty. Quotes Principles III and VIII and Opinions 8.12, 10.015, and 10.02. References Opinion 8.12. Hafemeister, *Lean on Me: A Physician's Fiduciary Duty to Disclose an Emergent Medical Risk to the Patient, 86 Wash. U. L. Rev. 1167, 1172-1173, 1178, 1182, 1185, 1188, 1209 (2009).*

Journal 2009 Explores the nature of the physician-patient relationship and the impact of increased availability of medical information on patient autonomy and physician responsibility to exercise independent judgment. Concludes physicians must treat patients in accordance with their fiduciary obligation to use their own judgment when confronted with a patient demanding unnecessary medical services. Quotes Preamble, Principles I and VIII, and Opinions 2.035, 8.03, and 10.015. Hafemeister, *The Fiduciary Obligation of Physicians to "Just Say No" if an "Informed" Patient Demands Services That Are Not Medically Indicated, 39 Seton Hall L. Rev. 335, 372, 373, 374 (2009).*

Journal 2009 Discusses the judicial standard for reviewing physician noncompete covenants. Concludes courts should apply a strict standard to such covenants, rather than declare the covenants per se invalid. Quotes Principles IV and VII, Principles of Medical Ethics §5 (1957) [now Principle VI], Code of Medical Ethics Ch. II, Art. I §3 (1847) [now Opinion 5.02], Opinion 9.02, and Code of Medical Ethics Ch. II, Art. I §4 (1847) [now Opinion 9.09]. Cites Opinions 8.041, 8.115, 9.02, 9.06, 9.065, 9.067, 10.01, and 10.015. Koons, *Physician Employee Non-Compete Agreements on the Examining Table: The Need to Better Protect Patients' and the Public's Interests in Indiana, 6 Ind. Health L. Rev. 253, 272-77, 280-81 (2009).*

Journal 2008 Considers the utility of physician apologies for medical error and legal protection for physicians who apologize for mistakes. Concludes physicians must openly communicate with their patients and apologize for medical errors to strengthen the health care community. Quotes Opinions 8.08, 8.12, 10.01, and 10.015. References Opinion 8.12. Ebert, *Attorneys, Tell Your Clients to Say They're Sorry: Apologies in the Health Care Industry, 5 Ind. Health L. Rev. 337, 340-41, 344 (2008).*

Journal 2008 Studies the likelihood and causes of physicians discharging patients. Concludes that physicians should be educated about the ethical and legal consequences of discharging patients for reasons other than dangerous or illegal behavior. References Opinion 10.015. Farber, Jordan, Silverstein, Collier, Weiner, & Boyer, *Primary Care Physicians' Decisions About Discharging Patients From Their Practices, 23 J. of General Internal Med. 283, 283 (2008).*

Journal 2008 Discusses FDA advisory opinion preempting failure-to-warn claims brought against pharmaceutical companies and examines ethical problems throughout pharmaceutical industry. Concludes that litigation is an important check on the industry, encouraging quality research and safe medications. Quotes Opinion 10.015. Martin, *Hugs and Drugs: Research Ethics, Conflict of Interest, and Why the FDA's Attempt to Preempt Pharma Failure-to-Warn Claims Is a Dangerous Prescription, 6 Ave Maria L. Rev. 587, 621 (2008).*

Journal 2008 Examines the medical malpractice system and the reasons why patients sue. Argues that lack of effective communication between physician and patient is the underlying cause of litigation. Concludes voluntary mediation of claims may decrease medical malpractice litigation if attorneys, health professionals, and the federal government encourage use of mediation. Quotes Opinion 10.015. Meruelo, *The Need to Understand Why Patients Sue and a Proposal for a Specific Model of Mediation, 29 J. Legal Med. 285, 290 (2008).*

Journal 2008 Argues that as a matter of public health, physicians must control antibiotic administration to combat antibiotic resistance. Concludes that despite limited incentives for antibiotic conservation, physicians must acknowledge their important role in mitigating the public health threat of antibiotic resistance. Quotes Principles VII and VIII and Opinions 2.09 and 10.015. Cites Opinion 2.03. Saver, *In Tepid Defense of Population Health: Physicians and Antibiotic Resistance, 34 Am. J. L. & Med. 431, 457 (2008).*

Journal 2008 Explores the fiduciary relationship between physicians and patients, professional and ethical obligations of both physicians and lawyers, and the implications for conflict resolution in health care. Concludes physicians must put patient interests above their own and lawyers must work to discern clients' best interests and support client welfare. Quotes Principle VIII and Opinions 8.12 and 10.015. Cites Principles I and II and Opinions 10.01 and 10.015. Scott, *Doctors as Advocates, Lawyers as Healers, 29 Hamline J. Pub. L. Pol'y, 331, 340-41, 347, 371 (2008).*

Journal 2007 Addresses physician liability for an extramarital affair with a patient's spouse. Concludes that such an affair should be regarded as a breach of a fiduciary duty. Quotes Preamble, Principles I, II, and VIII, and Opinions 8.145, 9.04, 9.123, and 10.015. Demaine, *"Playing Doctor" With the Patient's Spouse: Alternative Conceptions of Health Professional Liability, 14 Va. J. Soc. Pol'y & L. 308, 325, 330-31, 331-32 (2007).*

Journal 2007 Examines the history and effectiveness of medical malpractice screening panels. Concludes that screening panels are ineffective, then proposes an alternative dispute resolution model. Quotes Opinion 10.015. Kaufman, *The Demise of Medical Malpractice Screening Panels and Alternative Solutions Based on Trust and Honesty, 28 J. Legal Med. 247, 250 (2007).*

Journal 2007 Discusses patients' right to refuse medical treatment and the corresponding duties of health care professionals. Concludes that detailed, carefully prepared advance directives are necessary to fulfill patients' wishes. Quotes Ch. II (1940) [now Opinions 8.08 and 8.082] and Opinions 2.035, 2.037, 2.20, 2.225, 8.081, and 10.015. Cites Opinions 9.11 and 9.115. Stamatakis, *Beyond Advance Directives: Personal Autonomy and the Right to Refuse Life-Sustaining Medical Treatment, 47 N. H. B. J. 20, 29-30 (2007).*

Journal 2006 Reviews the concept of therapeutic privilege. Concludes that the practice creates conflict between physician obligations under the concepts of autonomy and beneficence. Recommends that physicians maximize communication with patients by providing all pertinent information in the context of patient preferences. Cites Opinions 8.08, 8.081, 8.121, and 10.015. References Chap. I, Art. I, Sec. 4 (May 1847) [premise deleted from Code]. Bostick, Sade, McMahon, & Benjamin, *Report of the American Medical Association Council on Ethical and Judicial Affairs: Withholding Information From Patients: Rethinking the Propriety of "Therapeutic Privilege," 17 J. Clinical Ethics 302, 303 (Winter 2006).*

Journal 2006 Examines the efficacy of informed consent when a physician acts both as a researcher and care provider. Concludes that a patient cannot give truly informed consent in such cases. Cites Opinions 8.115 and 10.015. Lenrow, *The Treating Physician as Researcher: Is Assuming This Dual Role a Violation of the Nuremberg Code? 25 Temp. J. Sci. Tech. & Envtl. L. 15, 42-43 (2006).*

Journal 2006 Discusses tort liability for medical malpractice. Concludes that both physicians and attorneys should support a legal system which promotes patient safety. Quotes Opinions 8.12 and 10.015. Pegalis, *A Proposal to Use Common Ground That Exists Between the Medical and Legal Professions to Promote a Culture of Safety, 51 N. Y. L. Sch. L. Rev. 1057, 1070, 1073 (2006).*

Journal 2006 Examines the practice by physicians of billing a malpractice surcharge. Concludes that such practice is unethical and constitutes a breach of fiduciary duty. Quotes Opinions 10.015 and 10.018. Peterson, *The Malpractice Surcharge: A Simple Answer to Rising Malpractice Rates or a Greater Threat to Quality Patient Care? 27 J. Legal Med. 87, 96, 97-98 (2006).*

Journal 2006 Considers prisoners' rights to expression of sexuality and the state's legitimate interest in regulating that expression. Concludes that states should encourage healthy expressions of sexuality while protecting the goals of the Prison Rape Elimination Act. Cites Opinions 3.08, 8.14, 8.145, and 10.015. Smith, *Rethinking Prison Sex:*

Self-expression and Safety, 15 Colum. J. Gender & L. 185, 202 (2006).

Journal 2005 Discusses physician responses to the medical malpractice liability crisis. Concludes that certain responses may violate ethical obligations that physicians owe to their patients and to society as a whole. Cites Opinions 9.025 and 10.015. References Principle VIII. Kachalia, Choudhry, & Studdert, *Physician Responses to the Malpractice Crisis: From Defense to Offense, 33 J. L. Med. & Ethics 416, 419, 421, 424 (2005).*

Journal 2005 Argues that in *Aetna v. Davila/Cigna v. Calad*, the Supreme Court missed an opportunity to overturn unjust ERISA policies. Concludes that the principle of complete ERISA preemption as articulated in these consolidated cases is unsatisfactory because it violates the separation of powers doctrine. Quotes Principle VIII. Cites Opinions 8.054, 8.13, 8.135, 9.123, 10.01, and 10.015. Nelson, *AETNA v. DAVILA/CIGNA v. CALAD: A Missed Opportunity, 31 Wm. Mitchell L. Rev. 843, 847, 849, 850, 880 (2005).*

Journal 2005 Discusses ethical, legal, and policy issues associated with treatment and research involving patients who are in a persistent vegetative or minimally conscious state. Concludes that patients in these states are at risk for therapeutic failures until physicians can more accurately determine which patients will benefit from treatment and accurately convey such information to families or surrogates. Quotes Principles VII and IX and Opinions 8.031, 8.0315, 9.065, 10.01, and 10.015. Tovino & Winslade, *A Primer on the Law and Ethics of Treatment, Research, and Public Policy in the Context of Severe Traumatic Brain Injury, 14 Ann. Health L. 1, 18, 38, 39, 40, 41 (2005).*

Journal 2004 Analyzes various issues relating to the role of mental health professionals in capital punishment in light of Albert Bandura's model of "mechanisms of moral disengagement." Concludes that facilitating participation of mental health professionals in executions creates conflicts with the humanistic norms of the profession. Quotes Preamble and Opinions 1.01, 1.02, 2.06, 2.067, 2.20, 2.21, 2.211, and 8.14. Judges, *The Role of Mental Health Professionals in Capital Punishment: An Exercise in Moral Disengagement, 41 Hous. L. Rev. 515, 562, 568, 569, 570, 571-72, 581, 586, 588, 598 (2004).*

Journal 2004 Examines the requirements of the Privacy Rule regarding use and disclosure of a patient's identifiable health information in the context of research. Concludes that the Rule's burdensome administrative requirements may discourage research and thus outweigh any benefits for research subject autonomy. Quotes Principle VIII and Opinions 5.051, 8.031, and 10.015. Tovino, *The Use and Disclosure of Protected Health Information for Research Under the HIPAA Privacy Rule: Unrealized Patient Autonomy and Burdensome Government Regulation, 49 S. D. L. Rev. 447, 496, 502 (2004).*

Journal 2004 Addresses the problem of pediatric obesity and examines various treatment options, including gastric bypass. Concludes that, before surgery is undertaken, the best interests of the child must be prioritized, with consultative input from specialists who have no stake in the decision. Quotes 10.015. Wilde, *Bioethical and Legal Implications of Pediatric Gastric Bypass, 40 Willamette L. Rev. 575, 613 (2004).*

Journal 2003 Highlights the legal and ethical concerns surrounding use of noncompetition clauses. Concludes that physicians should carefully evaluate these clauses given their likely enforceability. Quotes Opinions 9.02, 9.06, 10.01, and 10.015. Loeser, *The Legal, Ethical, and Practical Implications of Noncompetition Clauses: What Physicians Should Know Before They Sign, 31 J. L. Med. & Ethics 283, 286, 287, 290 (2003).*

Journal 2002 Examines sports-related concussions among football players. Considers the responsibilities of team physicians. Concludes that litigation will increase without treatment guidelines for concussion management. References Opinion 10.015. Hecht, *Legal and Ethical Aspects of Sports-Related Concussions: The Merril Hoge Story, 12 Seton Hall J. Sport L. 17, 42-43 (2002).*

1.1.2 Prospective Patients

Journal 2011 Discusses advancements in modern reproductive technologies and the need for legislation to regulate these technologies. Concludes that regulating these technologies may violate modern views of personal autonomy and therefore should focus on the safety of the technologies and not be used to "protect" women from their ability to freely contract. Quotes Opinions 2.18 and 10.05. Neal, *Protecting Women: Preserving Autonomy in the Commodification of Motherhood, 17 Wm. & Mary J. Women & L. 611, 630, 635 (2011).*

Journal 2010 Discusses issues arising from the enactment of legislation by North Dakota involving a minor's reproductive rights. Explores ethical principles that govern physician's actions within the context of reproductive health. Concludes that, while a patient's expectation of confidentiality with a physician is critical, competing values come into play when the patient is a minor and parental involvement may be important. Provides practical guidance to address issues in this context. Quotes Opinions 2.01, 2.015, 5.055, 8.08, 8.115, 9.12, 10.01, 10.015, and 10.05. Cites Opinions 5.05, 5.055, 8.08, 8.11, 8.115, 9.12, and 10.05. Haas, *"Doctor, I'm Pregnant and Fifteen—I Can't Tell My Parents—Please Help Me": Minor Consent, Reproductive Rights, and Ethical Principles for Physicians, 86 N.D. L. Rev. 63, 70, 73, 75-78, 82, 84, 86-88 (2010).*

Journal 2009 Discusses the right of health care professionals to refuse to provide health care services to lesbian, gay, or bisexual (LGB) individuals, because of moral or religious objections, and its impact on access to health care services, including assisted reproduction and elder health care services, for such patients. Concludes physicians should adhere to professional ethical standards to promote LGB patients' autonomy and equal access to care. Quotes Preamble. Cites Opinion 10.05. Reibman, *The Patient Wanted the Doctor to Treat Her in the Closet, but the Janitor Wouldn't Open the Door: Healthcare Provider Rights of Refusal Versus LGB*

Rights to Reproductive and Elder Healthcare, 28 Temp. J. Sci. Tech. & Envtl. L. 65, 90-91 (2009).

Journal 2006 Explores the legal and ethical issues surrounding concierge medicine. Concludes that concierge medicine is best restricted to a small class of wealthy individuals. Quotes Principle IX and Opinion 8.055. Cites Principle VI and Opinions 8.055, 8.11, 8.115, 9.065, and 10.05. Carnahan, *Law, Medicine, and Wealth: Does Concierge Medicine Promote Health Care Choice, or Is It a Barrier to Access? 17 Stan. L. & Pol'y Rev. 121, 149-50, 151, 152, 153-54 (2006).*

1.1.3 Patient Rights

Colo. App. 1999 Physician filed suit seeking reinstatement, compensatory damages, and an opportunity to respond to the reasons for termination. The defendants claimed that the contract with the physician provided for termination without cause. The trial court granted the defendants' motion for summary judgment. The appellate court affirmed, holding that the termination clause allowed either party to terminate the contract without cause. In a separate dissenting opinion, judge stated that termination without cause significantly impacts the physician-patient relationship and referenced Fundamental Elements (5) [now Opinion 10.01], regarding the continuity of this relationship. *Grossman v. Columbine Medical Group, Inc., 1999 WL 1024015, 4-5.*

Ga. App. 2000 Plaintiff alleged failure on the part of a dentist to inform him of the risks of root canal in a malpractice action. The appeals court noted that state case law did not recognize the informed consent doctrine. In evaluating this precedent, the court quoted Opinion 8.08 and Fundamental Element (1) [now Opinion 10.01]. The court stated that the AMA Code of Medical Ethics should be understood to reflect the standard of care of the medical profession on the issue of informed consent. While the court ruled in favor of the dentist, it prospectively recognized the doctrine of informed consent. *Ketchup v. Howard, 247 Ga. App. 54, 543 S.E.2d 371, 376, 377.*

Ill. 2006 Physicians appealed a grant of preliminary injunction enforcing restrictive covenants in their employment contracts. Quoting Opinions 9.02, 9.06, and 10.01 and referencing Opinion 8.115, the Illinois Supreme Court gave thorough consideration to the AMA's position on restrictive covenants. While acknowledging the ethical problems associated with such contracts, the court found the covenants reasonable in scope. The decision to ban restrictive covenants, the court reasoned, was best left to the legislature. *Mohanty v. St. John Heart Clinic, S.C., 225 Ill.2d 52, 866 N.E.2d 85, 94, 106-07, 107-08.*

N.Y. Fam. 2006 During proceedings regarding a foster child, an issue was raised contesting the legality of the county department of human services' procedures for administering drugs to children. The mother's consent

for prescribing medication to the child was obtained by a caseworker, without direct consultation with a physician and with no explanation of side effects. The court cited Opinions 8.08, 8.081, 8.11, and 10.01 in determining the physician's duty to honor the decision of the parent/surrogate. The mother's consent was invalidated and she was given an opportunity to consult with a physician. *Matter of Lyle A., 14 Misc. 3d 842, 830 N.Y.S.2d 486, 492, 494.*

Tenn. App. 1998 Plaintiff challenged the constitutionality of various sections of state abortion statute. Among the provisions at issue was one requiring that a woman be "orally informed by her attending physician" as to specified information regarding the abortion. The court stated that the information requirement and physician counseling provision did not unduly burden a woman's right to an abortion. Physicians who supported this portion of the statute quoted Fundamental Element (1) [now Opinion 10.01], regarding a physician's duty to counsel a patient about the best treatments available. *Planned Parenthood of Middle Tennessee v. Sundquist, 1998 WL 467110, 33.*

Wis. App. 2007 Plaintiff brought action for medical abandonment against his physician. The physician had cancelled an elective surgery and terminated the relationship with the patient after the plaintiff sued the surgical center employing the physician. The circuit court granted summary judgment for the physician finding plaintiff's claim unsupported by expert testimony. With apparent reference to Opinions 8.115 and 10.01, the plaintiff argued that AMA ethics opinions supported his claim. The appeals court held, however, that expert testimony was required to prove the appropriate standard of care. *Casperson v. N.E. Wis. Ctr. for Surgery & Rehab of Hand, Ltd., 2007 WL 1191782, 3.*

Journal 2011 Describes off-label uses of prescription drugs and the associated risks and harms. Argues that such use should be restricted unless supported by high-quality evidence of efficacy and safety. Cites Opinions 10.01 and 10.015. Coleman & Rosoff, *The Case for Legal Regulation of Physicians' Off-Label Prescribing, 86 Notre Dame L. Rev. 649, 679 (2011).*

Journal 2011 Discusses the doctrine of informed consent and the influence of physician groups on the dissemination of information to patients. Concludes the doctrine of informed consent should be expanded by the courts, rather than continuing to allow professional societies to dictate provider guidelines for obtaining informed consent. Quotes Opinions 8.08, 10.01, and 10.015. References Opinion 2.065. Ginsberg, *Informed Consent: No Longer Just What the Doctor Ordered? The "Contributions" of Medical Associations and Courts to a More Patient Friendly Doctrine, 15 Mich. St. J. Med. & Law 17, 23, 24, 25, 26, 46 (2011).*

Journal 2011 Examines when constitutionally protected rights include a right to spend or give money to trigger them. Concludes that laws that restrict spending money on certain goods used to "speak," that are not distributed to the public via the market, are laws that protect the legislature's choice to remove that particular good from the market rather than laws that restrict speech. Cites Opinion 10.01. Hellman, *Money Talks But It Isn't Speech, 95 Minn. L. Rev. 953, 1002 (2011).*

Journal 2011 Examines the protection of a woman's autonomy in the context of reproductive choices including abortion. Argues that, when faced with such choices, women are not currently provided with balanced and comprehensive information necessary to promote autonomy. Concludes that the law should recognize the complexity involved in reproductive choices and provide an appropriate framework for women to make such choices in their own best interests. Cites Opinions 10.01 and 10.02. Laufer-Ukeles, *Reproductive Choices and Informed Consent: Fetal Interests, Women's Identity, and Relational Autonomy, 37 Am. J. L. & Med. 567, 575 (2011).*

Journal 2011 Examines the use of antibiotic prophylaxis for Lyme disease to prevent anaplasmosis from deer tick bites in patients in the upper Midwest. Concludes single-dose antibiotic prophylaxis is an appropriate response to bites, although an alternative recommendation of more aggressive antibiotic therapy following a bite may also be appropriate if patient is informed and such treatment is consistent with patient goals and values. References Opinions 10.01 and 10.02. Maloney, *The Management of Ixodes scapularis Bites in the Upper Midwest, 110 World Med. J. 78, 80 (2011).*

Journal 2011 Reviews the use and current regulation of medical marijuana to alleviate pain in terminally ill patients. Focusing on patient autonomy, concludes that patients should have access to medical marijuana in controlled doses under controlled conditions. Quotes Principle III and Opinions 10.01, 10.015, and 10.02. References Principle VIII. Pfeifer, *Smoking Gun: The Moral and Legal Struggle for Medical Marijuana, 27 Touro L. Rev. 339, 340-41, 345-346 (2011).*

Journal 2010 Assesses the legal environment underlying the identification, accommodation, response, and treatment of mental illnesses and behavioral conditions within the population during and after major emergencies. Concludes

that diagnostic and treatment protocols need to be altered by modifying laws regulating psychotropic medications, compelled treatment of nonadherent persons, and assisted therapies during such emergencies. Cites Opinion 10.01. Corcoran, Hodge, & Rutkow, *A Hidden Epidemic: Assessing the Legal Environment Underlying Mental and Behavioral Health Conditions in Emergencies, 4 St. Louis U. J. Health L. & Pol'y 33, 68 (2010).*

Journal 2010 Argues that a precise definition of death is needed to counteract the focus on reducing medical costs and increasing organ supplies for transplantations. Concludes that allowing dying patients more autonomy to determine conditions for organ donation will foster an atmosphere of trust in which more people will be willing to donate earlier in the dying process. Quotes Opinion 2.157. Cites Opinion 10.01. Fry-Revere, Ray, & Reher, *Death: A New Legal Perspective, 27 J. Contemp. Health L. & Pol'y 1, 11, 50, 53 (2010).*

Journal 2010 Discusses issues arising from the enactment of legislation by North Dakota involving a minor's reproductive rights. Explores ethical principles that govern physician's actions within the context of reproductive health. Concludes that, while a patient's expectation of confidentiality with a physician is critical, competing values come into play when the patient is a minor and parental involvement may be important. Provides practical guidance to address issues in this context. Quotes Opinions 2.01, 2.015, 5.055, 8.08, 8.115, 9.12, 10.01, 10.015, and 10.05. Cites Opinions 5.05, 5.055, 8.08, 8.11, 8.115, 9.12, and 10.05. Haas, *"Doctor, I'm Pregnant and Fifteen—I Can't Tell My Parents—Please Help Me": Minor Consent, Reproductive Rights, and Ethical Principles for Physicians, 86 N.D. L. Rev. 63, 70, 73, 75-78, 82, 84, 86-88 (2010).*

Journal 2009 Discusses the judicial standard for reviewing physician noncompete covenants. Concludes courts should apply a strict standard to such covenants, rather than declare the covenants per se invalid. Quotes Principles IV and VII, Principles of Medical Ethics §5 (1957) [now Principle VI], Code of Medical Ethics Ch. II, Art. I §3 (1847) [now Opinion 5.02], Opinion 9.02, and Code of Medical Ethics Ch. II, Art. I §4 (1847) [now Opinion 9.09]. Cites Opinions 8.041, 8.115, 9.02, 9.06, 9.065, 9.067, 10.01, and 10.015. Koons, *Physician Employee Non-Compete Agreements on the Examining Table: The Need to Better Protect Patients' and the Public's Interests in Indiana, 6 Ind. Health L. Rev. 253, 272-77, 280-81 (2009).*

Journal 2008 Discusses ex parte interviews with a treating physician in discovery before and after the HIPAA Privacy Rule and the issues facing physicians contacted for such interviews. Concludes courts and attorneys should work together to allow for efficient discovery while protecting physicians. Quotes Principles IV and VIII and Opinions 5.05 and 10.01. Burnette & Morning, *HIPAA and Ex Parte Interviews—The Beginning of the End? 1 J. Health & Life Sci. L. 73, 100-01 (2008).*

Journal 2008 Reviews the obligation of a physician to provide a referral for the termination of a pregnancy, when the treating physician objects to the procedure on ethical grounds. Concludes that the physician has an ethical duty to inform the patient of other providers who can offer competent care. Cites Opinion 10.01. Chervenak & McCullough, *The Ethics of Direct and Indirect Referral for Termination of Pregnancy*, 199 Am. J. Obstet. Gynecol. 232.e1, 232. e1 (2008).

Journal 2008 Considers the utility of physician apologies for medical error and legal protection for physicians who apologize for mistakes. Concludes physicians must openly communicate with their patients and apologize for medical errors to strengthen the health care community. Quotes Opinions 8.08, 8.12, 10.01, and 10.015. References Opinion 8.12. Ebert, *Attorneys, Tell Your Clients to Say They're Sorry: Apologies in the Health Care Industry*, 5 Ind. Health L. Rev. 337, 340-41, 344 (2008).

Journal 2008 Explores the fiduciary relationship between physicians and patients, professional and ethical obligations of both physicians and lawyers, and the implications for conflict resolution in health care. Concludes physicians must put patient interests above their own and lawyers must work to discern clients' best interests and support client welfare. Quotes Principle VIII and Opinions 8.12 and 10.015. Cites Principles I and II and Opinions 10.01 and 10.015. Scott, *Doctors as Advocates, Lawyers as Healers*, 29 Hamline J. Pub. L. Pol'y 331, 340-41, 347, 371 (2008).

Journal 2007 Reviews Deborah Rhode's analysis of pro bono obligations of lawyers from her book, *Pro Bono in Principle and in Practice: Public Service and the Professions*. Concludes that a mandatory pro bono requirement is a better solution than an incentive-based system. Quotes Opinion 10.01. References Opinion 9.065. Lininger, *From Park Place to Community Chest: Rethinking Lawyers' Monopoly*, 101 Nw. U. L. Rev. 1343, 1349 (2007).

Journal 2007 Considers relevant policy issues surrounding prenatal torts. Concludes that North Carolina should allow bringing of claims for prenatal, postconception malpractice. Quotes Opinion 10.01. McEntire, *Compensating Post-Conception Prenatal Medical Malpractice While Respecting Life: A Recommendation to North Carolina Legislators*, 29 Campbell L. Rev. 761, 763 (2007).

Journal 2006 Analyzes cases where a patient's right to refuse care conflicts with the physician's obligation to protect that patient's well-being. Concludes health care providers should seek a compromise that best promotes both patient autonomy and well-being. Quotes Principle IV and Ch. I, Art. II, Sec. 6 (May 1847) [now Opinion 10.01]. Carrese, *Refusal of Care: Patients' Well-being and Physicians' Ethical Obligations*, 296 JAMA 691, 692, 693 (2006).

Journal 2006 Reviews informed consent doctrine in the context of consumer-driven health care. Concludes that consumer-driven health care should not be undermined

by arguments about patient competence to make health care decisions. References Opinion 10.01. Kapp, *Patient Autonomy in the Age of Consumer-Driven Health Care: Informed Consent and Informed Choice*, 2 J. Health & Biomedical L. 1, 5 (2006).

Journal 2005 Discusses standard of care issues surrounding physicians using complementary and alternative medicine (CAM). Concludes that a prudent physician standard should apply to physicians practicing CAM. Quotes Opinion 10.01. Cites Opinion 10.02. Kallmyer, *A Chimera in Every Sense: Standard of Care for Physicians Practicing Complementary and Alternative Medicine*, 2 Ind. Health L. Rev. 225, 229, 231 (2005).

Journal 2005 Argues that in *Aetna v. Davila/Cigna v. Calad*, the Supreme Court missed an opportunity to overturn unjust ERISA policies. Concludes that the principle of complete ERISA preemption as articulated in these consolidated cases is unsatisfactory because it violates the separation of powers doctrine. Quotes Principle VIII. Cites Opinions 8.054, 8.13, 8.135, 9.123, 10.01, and 10.015. Nelson, *AETNA v. DAVILA/CIGNA v. CALAD: A Missed Opportunity*, 31 Wm. Mitchell L. Rev. 843, 847, 849, 850, 880 (2005).

Journal 2005 Discusses ethical, legal, and policy issues associated with treatment and research involving patients who are in a persistent vegetative or minimally conscious state. Concludes that patients in these states are at risk for therapeutic failures until physicians can more accurately determine which patients will benefit from treatment and accurately convey such information to families or surrogates. Quotes Principles VII and IX and Opinions 8.031, 8.0315, 9.065, 10.01, and 10.015. Tovino & Winslade, *A Primer on the Law and Ethics of Treatment, Research, and Public Policy in the Context of Severe Traumatic Brain Injury*, 14 Ann. Health L. 1, 18, 38, 39, 40, 41 (2005).

Journal 2004 Discusses medical errors in various health care settings and offers an ethical framework to support immediate implementation of proposed solutions. Concludes that federal and state legislators must place priority on developing policies that will help reduce the number of medical errors. Quotes Opinion 10.01. Clark, *Medication Errors in Family Practice, in Hospitals and After Discharge From the Hospital: An Ethical Analysis*, 32 J. L. Med & Ethics 349, 354 (2004).

Journal 2004 Analyzes Maryland's Drug Addiction at Birth Act, which was passed to help health care professionals deal with drug-exposed infants. Concludes that more effective legislation could be enacted to educate health care providers regarding treatment of infants with prenatal drug exposure. Quotes Opinion 10.01. Reese & Burry, *Evaluating Maryland's Response to Drug-Exposed Babies*, 10 Psychol. Pub. Pol'y & L. 343, 353 (2004).

Journal 2003 Reviews state laws designed to protect physicians acting as patient advocates in managed care organizations. Concludes that federal and state law must make it easier for physicians to challenge denials of or delays in patient care. Quotes Opinions 8.054, 8.13, and 10.01. Fentiman, *Patient Advocacy and Termination From Managed Care Organizations. Do State Laws Protecting Health Care Professional Advocacy Make Any Difference?* 82 Neb. L. Rev. 508, 515-16, 517-18 (2003).

Journal 2003 Highlights the legal and ethical concerns surrounding use of noncompetition clauses. Concludes that physicians should carefully evaluate these clauses given their likely enforceability. Quotes Opinions 9.02, 9.06, 10.01, and 10.015. Loeser, *The Legal, Ethical, and Practical Implications of Noncompetition Clauses: What Physicians Should Know Before They Sign, 31 J. L. Med. & Ethics 283, 286, 287, 290 (2003).*

Journal 2003 Considers the legal, medical, and ethical issues of physician-patient confidentiality in disclosure of paternity. Concludes that a balancing test should be applied to making determinations regarding disclosure of paternity. Quotes Principles I, IV, and V and Opinions 1.02, 5.055, and 10.01. Cites Principle II and Opinion 5.05. Richards & Wolf, *Medical Confidentiality and Disclosure of Paternity, 48 S. D. L. Rev. 409, 411, 412, 413 (2003).*

Journal 2003 Evaluates medical necessity decisions in managed care, with emphasis on therapeutic effectiveness. Concludes that, in order to be effective, review procedures and policies governing medical necessity determinations must be improved. Quotes Opinion 10.01. Sage, *Managed Care's Crimea: Medical Necessity, Therapeutic Benefit, and the Goals of Administrative Process in Health Insurance, 53 Duke L. J. 597, 634 (2003).*

Journal 2003 Argues that affirmative measures should be taken by the Air Force to ensure access to abortion services. Concludes that regulatory changes will reduce barriers to access. Quotes Opinion 10.01. Cites Opinion 8.08. Wilde, *Air Force Women's Access to Abortion Services and the Erosion of 10 USC § 1093, 9 Wm. & Mary J. Women & L. 351, 371 (2003).*

Journal 2003 Discusses potential liability of mental health care providers who administer court-ordered treatment to patients. Concludes that providers should treat these patients as much like voluntary patients as possible. References Opinion 10.01. Wilde, *The Liability of Alaska Mental Health Providers for Mandated Treatment, 20 Alaska L. Rev. 271, 276 (2003).*

Journal 2002 Argues for a more comprehensive approach in the management and treatment of intersex children. Emphasizes the importance of informed decision-making by parents and children. Quotes Opinion 10.01. Hermer, *Paradigms Revised: Intersex Children, Bioethics & the Law, 11 Annals Health L. 195, 221 (2002).*

Journal 2002 Discusses issues regarding regulation of elderly drivers. Concludes that mandating physicians to report unfit elderly patients will protect the public and help resolve ethical and legal dilemmas. Quotes Opinions 1.02, 2.24, 5.05, and 10.01. Kane, *Driving Into the Sunset:*

A Proposal for Mandatory Reporting to the DMV by Physicians Treating Unsafe Elderly Drivers, 25 U. Haw. L. Rev. 59, 59, 61, 62, 67, 69, 82, 83 (2002).

Journal 2002 Reviews how changes in the health care delivery system underscore the importance of information in patient empowerment. Concludes that patients should use information to take charge of their health care. Quotes Principle V and Opinion 10.02. Cites Opinion 10.01. Kane, *Information Is the Key to Patient Empowerment, 11 Annals Health L. 25, 29-30, 44 (2002).*

Journal 2002 Considers the ethical and legal issues regarding breach of confidentiality in situations where a patient is pregnant and uses teratogenic substances. Concludes that a breach of confidentiality causes damage to the physician-patient relationship. Quotes Principle IV and Opinion 10.01. Plambeck, *Divided Loyalties: Legal and Bioethical Considerations of Physician-Pregnant Patient Confidentiality and Prenatal Drug Abuse, 23 J. Legal Med. 1, 8, 25 (2002).*

Journal 2002 Analyzes the role of prognostication in physician-patient communication. Concludes that the patient-physician model of shared decision-making offers the best hope for reestablishing prognostication. Quotes Principles Ch. I, Art. I, Sec. 2 and 4 (1846) [now Principle IV and Opinions 8.12 and 10.01]. Cites Opinion 8.08. Rich, *Prognostication in Clinical Medicine: Prophecy or Professional Responsibility? 23 J. Legal Med. 297, 299, 318, 327 (2002).*

Journal 2002 Discusses legal and medical policies that protect confidentiality in the physician-patient relationship. Concludes that reducing the current level of privacy protection would jeopardize health care. Quotes Preamble and Opinions 2.136, 5.05, and 10.01. References Principles VIII and IX. Sciarrino, *Ferguson v. City of Charleston: "The Doctor Will See You Now, Be Sure to Bring Your Privacy Rights in With You!" 12 Temp. Pol. & Civ. Rts. L. Rev. 197, 213, 215, 220, 221, 222 (2002).*

Journal 2001 Explores the ethical and legal dilemmas associated with doctors and lawyers providing advice over the Internet. Concludes the law must ensure that cyberprofessionals comply with ethical and legal duties to their clients and their professions. Quotes Opinion 10.01. Deady, *Cyberadvice: The Ethical Implications of Giving Professional Advice Over the Internet, 14 Geo. J. Legal Ethics 891, 905 (2001).*

Journal 2001 Discusses whether the medical profession needs a policy on honesty. Reviews ethical codes and concludes they fail to offer physicians meaningful guidance about what constitutes "the truth" and when and how to disclose it. Quotes Principle II and Opinions 8.12 and 10.01. DeVita, *Honestly, Do We Need a Policy on Truth? 11 Kennedy Inst. Ethics J. 157, 158 (2001).*

Journal 2001 Discusses issues surrounding the privacy of genetic information. Considers the social, ethical, and legal responses to problems that arise in this context. Concludes with a unique view of privacy that would protect the right of individuals not to know genetic information about themselves. Quotes Principle IV and Opinion 10.01. Laurie, *Challenging Medical-Legal Norms: The Role of Autonomy, Confidentiality, and Privacy in Protecting Individual and Familial Group Rights in Genetic Information, 22 J. Legal Med. 1, 24 (2001).*

Journal 2001 Considers conflicts of interest in clinical research and other types of medical practice. Compares the way in which doctors and lawyers address conflicts of interest in professional practice. Concludes that physicians are unaware of the need to create a meaningful conflict-of-interest doctrine for medical practice. Quotes Preamble, Principle IV, and Opinions 2.07, 8.03, 8.031, and 10.01. Moore, *What Doctors Can Learn From Lawyers About Conflicts of Interest, 81 B. U. L. Rev. 445, 447, 449-50 (2001).*

Journal 2001 Compares ongoing efforts to control reproduction and to control drug abuse with a view toward finding more effective solutions in both areas. Concludes that a coherent approach will build stronger coalitions in support of drug policy reform and reproductive freedom. Quotes Opinion 10.01. Paltrow, *The War on Drugs and the War on Abortion: Some Initial Thoughts on the Connections, Intersections and the Effects, 28 S.U. L. Rev. 201, 219 (2001).*

Journal 2001 Considers how much information regarding the adverse effects of medication physicians should disclose to patients. Concludes that most patients want complete information. Quotes Opinion 10.01. Ziegler, Mosier, Buenaver, & Okuyemi, *How Much Information About Adverse Effects of Medication Do Patients Want From Physicians? 161 Arch. Intern. Med. 706, 710 (2001).*

Journal 2000 Introduces the debate surrounding the benefits and dangers of diagnosing and treating patients over the Internet and explores the issue of how cybermedicine will change the traditional physician-patient relationship. Concludes cybermedicine is the future of medical care, and the physician-patient relationship will have to change to accommodate the predicted online medical boom. Quotes Opinion 10.01. Gelein, *Are Online Consultations a Prescription for Trouble? The Uncharted Waters of Cybermedicine, 66 Brook. L. Rev. 209, 239 (2000).*

Journal 2000 Discusses patent law and policy. Examines whether those who practice medicine should be excused from patent laws because of the conflict that medical procedure patents create with respect to the practice of medicine. Concludes that Congress should repeal section 287(c) of the Patent Act. Quotes Principle V and Opinions 9.08 and 9.09. Cites Opinion 8.03. References Opinion 10.01. Ho, *Patents, Patients, and Public Policy: An Incomplete Intersection at 35 USC § 287(c), 33 U.C. Davis L. Rev. 601, 603, 623, 624, 625, 631 (2000).*

Journal 2000 Describes the fiduciary aspects of the physician-patient relationship. Explores the conflicts that

may occur between physicians and pregnant women in the health care setting. Proposes legal strategies to address these conflicts. Quotes Opinions 8.08 and 10.01. References Opinion 8.13. Oberman, *Mothers and Doctors' Orders: Unmasking the Doctor's Fiduciary Role in Maternal-Fetal Conflicts, 94 Nw. U. L. Rev. 451, 456, 462, 493 (2000).*

Journal 2000 Evaluates recent Texas legislation that affords immunity to health care professionals who provide free health care services to the poor. Concludes that such legislation creates a dual standard of care, requiring indigent patients to forfeit their legal rights in exchange for health care. Quotes Opinion 10.01. References Opinion 9.065. Pulido, *Immunity of Volunteer Health Care Providers in Texas: Bartering Legal Rights for Free Medical Care, 2 Scholar: St. Mary's L. Rev. Minority Issues 323, 330 (2000).*

Journal 2000 Considers the topic of physician liability for genetic malpractice. Explores how new genetic technologies may affect the medical and legal communities. Concludes by observing that the legal system is not prepared to address the wave of litigation that may grow out of emerging genetic technologies. Quotes Opinion 10.01. Reutenauer, *Medical Malpractice Liability in the Era of Genetic Susceptibility Testing, 19 QLR 539, 571 (2000).*

Journal 2000 Discusses managed care in terms of problems, responses, and accomplishments. Demonstrates how a physician union's collective bargaining process can benefit patients and physicians in addressing problems with managed care. Concludes that barriers preventing such unions should be removed. Quotes Principles VI and VII and Opinion 10.01. Rugg, *An Old Solution to a New Problem: Physician Unions Take the Edge Off Managed Care, 34 Colum. J. L. & Soc. Probs. 1, 41 (2000).*

Journal 2000 Examines ethical and legal issues regarding medical privacy. Discusses authorized and unauthorized uses of information contained in medical records and identifies who may access these records. Analyzes the ethical balance between patient privacy and societal benefits derived from sacrificing it. Concludes privacy is very important to maintaining a full and open physician-patient relationship. Quotes Opinion 10.01. Scott, *Is Too Much Privacy Bad for Your Health? An Introduction to the Law, Ethics, and HIPAA Rule on Medical Privacy, 17 Ga. St. U. L. Rev. 481, 494 (2000).*

Journal 2000 Discusses the development and history of the ethical doctrine of informed consent. Examines the current state of the law in Pennsylvania and concludes it does not adequately fulfill the goals of ethical and legal doctrines. Quotes Principle IV and Opinion 10.01. References Opinion 8.08. Warren, *Pennsylvania Medical Informed Consent Law: A Call to Protect Patient Autonomy Rights by Abandoning the Battery Approach, 38 Duq. L. Rev. 917, 925 (2000).*

Journal 1999 Examines reporting of AIDS and HIV under Texas law. Discusses limitations on a physician's ability to warn potentially at-risk third parties. Concludes that Texas law should be changed to place a duty upon physicians to notify at-risk third parties of a patient's HIV-positive status. Quotes Principle IV and Opinion 10.01. Acosta, *The Texas Communicable Disease Prevention and Control Act: Are We Offering Enough Protection to Those Who Need It Most? 36 Hous. L. Rev. 1819, 1822, 1830, 1831 (1999).*

Journal 1999 Discusses the need for physicians to advocate on behalf of patients' rights in the context of health care delivery. Evaluates the nature and scope of the physician's role as advocate, noting that physicians cannot be expected to engage in attorney-like advocacy. Quotes Principles IV and VI, Fundamental Elements (2), (4), and (6) [now Opinion 10.01], Patient Responsibilities 5 [now Opinion 10.02], and Opinions 2.03, 2.07, 2.09, 2.16, 2.19, 3.06, 4.01, 4.04, 6.01, 7.02, 8.02, 8.03, 8.13, 8.132, 9.06, 9.07, and 9.131. Cites Opinions 5.05, 5.09, 7.01, 8.135, and 9.02. Sage, *Physicians as Advocates, 35 Hous. L. Rev. 1529, 1537, 1541, 1542, 1552-53, 1554, 1556, 1557, 1559, 1561-62, 1564, 1571, 1574, 1576, 1580 (1999).*

Journal 1998 Discusses conflicts of interest in the physician-patient relationship arising out of use of financial incentives by managed care organizations. Considers how such conflicts are dealt with in the attorney-client relationship. Suggests that a financial incentive should be legally denounced if it unreasonably interferes with a physician's duty to properly care for and treat patients. Quotes Preamble, Fundamental Elements (1) [now Opinion 10.01], and Opinions 4.04, 5.01, 8.03, 8.13, and 9.06. Cites Fundamental Elements (4) [now Opinion 10.01] and Opinions 2.07, 2.08, and 2.132. Hall, *Third-Party Payor Conflicts of Interest in Managed Care: A Proposal for Regulation Based on the Model Rules of Professional Conduct, 29 Seton Hall L. Rev. 95, 96, 107, 108, 109, 110, 111, 112, 134, 135, 136 (1998).*

Journal 1997 Compares past ethical opinions to current opinions and notes the differences. Comments on the forces that have changed medical ethics through the years. Notes differing theories on the future course of medical ethics. Quotes Fundamental Elements (Preamble) and Opinions 5.05, 5.057, 7.01, 8.12, 9.12, and 9.131. Cites Fundamental Elements (5) [now Opinion 10.01] and Opinions 8.115 and 8.13. Buchanan, *Medical Ethics at the Millennium: A Brief Retrospective, 26 Colo. Law. 141, 142, 143, 144, 145 (1997).*

Journal 1997 Reviews ethical issues raised by genetic research. Explores the duty a physician may have to reveal the genetic diseases found in patients to their relatives. Considers case law and statutory law, and concludes that a limited duty to disclose exists. Quotes Fundamental Elements (4) [now Opinion 10.01]. Deftos, *Genomic Torts: The Law of the Future—The Duty of Physicians to Disclose the Presence of a Genetic Disease to the Relatives of Their Patients With the Disease, 32 USF. L. Rev. 105, 130 (1997).*

Journal 1997 Discusses physician frustration with managed care plans caused by gag clauses and cost-containment mechanisms. Reviews the development of managed care organizations and federal attempts at limiting the use of gag

clauses. Concludes that gag clauses are inherently flawed and compromise quality health care. Quotes Principles II and V, Fundamental Elements (1) [now Opinion 10.01], and Opinion 8.13. Note, *Physicians, Bound and Gagged: Federal Attempts to Combat Managed Care's Use of Gag Clauses, 21 Seton Hall Legis. J. 567, 601-02 (1997).*

Journal 1997 Considers the current approach to health care in the US. Examines financing mechanisms, and suggests that reform could be effected through a decentralized, community-based approach. Proposes use of volunteer systems in which medical personnel would care for certain patients free of charge or at reduced rates. Quotes Fundamental Elements (6) [now Opinion 10.01]. References Opinion 9.065. Solomon & Asaro, *Community-Based Health Care: A Legal and Policy Analysis, 24 Fordham Urb. L. J. 235, 276-77 (1997).*

Journal 1996 Describes the problem of lack of access to medical care by the indigent. Recognizes the commitment of the medical profession to providing care for indigent patients. Observes that state initiatives that provide physicians tort immunity in exchange for volunteer service can improve access to care by the indigent. Quotes Fundamental Elements (6) [now Opinion 10.01]. References Opinion 9.065. Comment, *Statutory Immunity for Volunteer Physicians: A Vehicle for Reaffirmation of the Doctor's Beneficent Duties—Absent the Rights Talk, 1 Widener L. Symp. J. 425, 448, 449 (1996).*

Journal 1996 Considers the ethical requirement for physicians to receive informed consent from patients before beginning treatment. Reviews the case of *Jacobson v. Massachusetts,* discussing its impact on informed consent and vaccination policy in the US. Quotes Fundamental Elements (2) [now Opinion 10.01]. References Opinion 8.08. Severyn, *Jacobson v. Massachusetts: Impact on Informed Consent and Vaccine Policy, 5 J. Pharmacy & L. 249, 253, 274 (1996).*

Journal 1996 Examines medically futile treatment in light of legislative enactments in Virginia and Maryland. Observes that the futility debate arises when requests for life-prolonging treatment are viewed as medically inappropriate by health care providers. Concludes that, while the ethical integrity of the medical profession justifies some legal recognition of futility, such recognition must be limited by respect for patient autonomy. References Fundamental Elements (5) [now Opinion 10.01]. Shiner, *Medical Futility: A Futile Concept? 53 Wash. & Lee L. Rev. 803, 834 (1996).*

Journal 1995 Examines the impact of health care reform on physician-patient relationships. Discusses how reform may threaten the physician's fiduciary duty of loyalty by forcing physicians to make rationing decisions and giving physicians financial incentives to limit use of health care resources. Quotes Fundamental Elements (5) [now Opinion 10.01]. Cites Opinion 5.05. Orentlicher, *Health Care Reform and the Patient-Physician Relationship, 5 Health Matrix 141, 143, 148 (1995).*

Journal 1994 Considers whether an exception should be made to physician-patient confidentiality that would allow a physician to reveal parental medical history to a child. Concludes that such an exception would not completely erode physician-patient confidentiality. Quotes Principles IV, Fundamental Elements (4) [now Opinion 10.01], and Opinion 5.05. Cites Principle I and Fundamental Elements (1). Friedland, physician-patient *Confidentiality: Time to Re-Examine a Venerable Concept in Light of Contemporary Society and Advances in Medicine, 15 J. Legal Med. 249, 257, 264, 276 (1994).*

Journal 1994 Explores the ethical issues involved in a multidisciplinary team working with children in legal proceedings. Focuses on the relationships between professionals and the conflicts that arise regarding disclosure of confidential information and forced disclosure of nonprivileged information. Quotes Principles III and IV, Fundamental Elements (4) [now Opinion 10.01], and Opinions 1.02 (1992) and 5.07 (1992) [now Opinion 5.05]. Cites Opinions 2.02. Glynn, *Multidisciplinary Representation of Children: Conflicts Over Disclosures of Client Communications, 27 J. Marshall L. Rev. 617, 625, 626, 630-32, 637, 639, 643 (1994).*

Journal 1994 Discusses physician-patient confidentiality and the exception that permits breach of a patient's confidence if required by law. Argues that this is always a legitimate exception to the confidentiality rule. Quotes Principle IV and Fundamental Elements (4) [now Opinion 10.01]. McConnell, *Confidentiality and the Law, 20 J. Med. Ethics 47, 47 (1994).*

Journal 1994 Reviews the evolution of the physician-patient relationship, with attention to the changing health care delivery environment. Quotes Preamble, Principles I, II, III, IV, V, and VI, Fundamental Elements (1) and (2) [now Opinion 10.01], and Opinions 1.02 and 8.07 (1981) [now Opinion 8.08]. Cites Opinion 1.01. Szczygiel, *Beyond Informed Consent, 21 Ohio N. U. L. Rev. 171, 217, 218, 220, 225, 226, 256 (1994).*

Journal 1994 Discusses the importance of confidentiality in the physician-patient relationship and under what circumstances patient information may be released. Examines unique considerations that apply when a physician provides medical care to a minor or an HIV-infected individual. Quotes Principle IV and Fundamental Elements (4) [now Opinion 10.01]. Weiner & Wettstein, *Confidentiality of Patient-Related Information, 112 Arch. Ophthalmology 1032, 1033 (1994).*

Journal 1993 Analyzes the implications of giving patients and their families an absolute right to control medical treatment. Argues that courts should refrain from ordering physicians to treat patients when physicians believe that treatment would be ineffective. Quotes Fundamental Elements (5) [now Opinion 10.01] and Opinions 2.11 (1982) [now Opinion 2.20] and 2.18 (1986) [now Opinion 2.20]. Comment, *Beyond Autonomy: Judicial Restraint and the Legal Limits Necessary to Uphold the Hippocratic Tradition and Preserve the Ethical Integrity of the Medical Profession, 9 J. Contemp. Health L. & Pol'y 451, 467, 468 (1993).*

1.1.4 Patient Responsibilities

Journal 2011 Examines the protection of a woman's autonomy in the context of reproductive choices including abortion. Argues that, when faced with such choices, women are not currently provided with balanced and comprehensive information necessary to promote autonomy. Concludes that the law should recognize the complexity involved in reproductive choices and provide an appropriate framework for women to make such choices in their own best interests. Cites Opinions 10.01 and 10.02. Laufer-Ukeles, *Reproductive Choices and Informed Consent: Fetal Interests, Women's Identity, and Relational Autonomy, 37 Am. J. L. & Med. 567, 575 (2011).*

Journal 2011 Examines the use of antibiotic prophylaxis for Lyme disease to prevent anaplasmosis from deer tick bites in patients in the upper Midwest. Concludes single-dose antibiotic prophylaxis is an appropriate response to bites, although an alternative recommendation of more aggressive antibiotic therapy following a bite may also be appropriate if patient is informed and such treatment is consistent with patient goals and values. References Opinions 10.01 and 10.02. Maloney, *The Management of Ixodes scapularis Bites in the Upper Midwest, 110 World Med. J. 78, 80 (2011).*

Journal 2011 Reviews the use and current regulation of medical marijuana to alleviate pain in terminally ill patients. Focusing on patient autonomy, concludes that patients should have access to medical marijuana in controlled doses under controlled conditions. Quotes Principle III and Opinions 10.01, 10.015, and 10.02. References Principle VIII. Pfeifer, *Smoking Gun: The Moral and Legal Struggle for Medical Marijuana, 27 Touro L. Rev. 339, 340-41, 345-346 (2011).*

Journal 2009 Explores the jurisprudential foundation of the fiduciary duty physicians owe their patients and discusses the failure of physicians to disclose to patients errors and other emergent medical risks. Concludes law should recognize the physician's duty to disclose such risks by enforcing a cause of action for breach of that duty. Quotes Principles III and VIII and Opinions 8.12, 10.015, and 10.02. References Opinion 8.12. Hafemeister, *Lean on Me: A Physician's Fiduciary Duty to Disclose an Emergent Medical Risk to the Patient, 86 Wash. U. L. Rev. 1167, 1172-1173, 1178, 1182, 1185, 1188, 1209 (2009).*

Journal 2002 Reviews how changes in the health care delivery system underscore the importance of information in patient empowerment. Concludes that patients should use information to take charge of their health care. Quotes Principle V and Opinion 10.02. Cites Opinion 10.01. Kane, *Information Is the Key to Patient Empowerment, 11 Annals Health L. 25, 29-30, 44 (2002).*

Journal 2002 Discusses state regulation of health information and the Federal Health Privacy Rule, noting that it provides inadequate protection. Concludes state laws can bridge gaps in protection. Quotes Opinion 10.02. Pritts, *Altered States: State Health Privacy Laws and the Impact of the Federal Health Privacy Rules, 2 Yale J. Health Pol'y, L. & Ethics 327, 351 (2002).*

Journal 1999 Discusses the need for physicians to advocate on behalf of patients' rights in the context of health care delivery. Evaluates the nature and scope of the physician's role as advocate, noting that physicians cannot be expected to engage in attorney-like advocacy. Quotes Principles IV and VI, Fundamental Elements (2), (4), and (6) [now Opinion 10.01], Patient Responsibilities 5 [now Opinion 10.02], and Opinions 2.03, 2.07, 2.09, 2.16, 2.19, 3.06, 4.01, 4.04, 6.01, 7.02, 8.02, 8.03, 8.13, 8.132, 9.06, 9.07, and 9.131. Cites Opinions 5.05, 5.09, 7.01, 8.135, and 9.02. Sage, *Physicians as Advocates, 35 Hous. L. Rev. 1529, 1537, 1541, 1542, 1552-53, 1554, 1556, 1557, 1559, 1561-62, 1564, 1571, 1574, 1576, 1580 (1999).*

Journal 1994 Discusses notions of quality in health care, asking who is responsible to define quality, who is responsible to deliver it, and who is responsible for quality of care when it is unsatisfactory. Concludes that significant economic changes will require a reallocation of these responsibilities among patients, providers, and payers. References Patient Responsibilities (1), (4), and (5) [now Opinion 10.02]. Morreim, *Redefining Quality by Reassigning Responsibility, 20 Am. J. Law & Med. 79, 103 (1994).*

1.1.5 Terminating a Patient-Physician Relationship

Ill. 2006 Physicians appealed a grant of preliminary injunction enforcing restrictive covenants in their employment contracts. Quoting Opinions 9.02, 9.06, and 10.01 and referencing Opinion 8.115, the Illinois Supreme Court gave thorough consideration to the AMA's position on restrictive covenants. While acknowledging the ethical problems associated with such contracts, the court found the covenants reasonable in scope. The decision to ban restrictive covenants, the court reasoned, was best left to the legislature. *Mohanty v. St. John Heart Clinic, S.C., 225 Ill.2d 52, 866 N.E.2d 85, 94, 106-07, 107-08.*

Mass. Super. 1993 Plaintiff sought to enjoin defendant-physician from contacting patients that defendant treated while employed with plaintiff. The court denied the injunction, noting that under Opinion 8.11 [now Opinion 8.115] defendant has a duty to notify his patients before withdrawing from a case and an injunction would force defendant to choose between violating professional ethics and violating a court order. *Plastic Surgical Servs. of New England, P.C. v. Hall, 1993 WL 818637.*

Wis. App. 2007 Plaintiff brought action for medical abandonment against his physician. The physician had cancelled an elective surgery and terminated the relationship with the patient after the plaintiff sued the surgical center employing the physician. The circuit court granted summary judgment for the physician finding plaintiff's claim unsupported by expert testimony. With apparent reference to Opinions 8.115 and 10.01, the plaintiff argued that AMA ethics opinions supported his claim. The appeals court held, however, that expert testimony was required to prove the appropriate standard of care. *Casperson v. N.E. Wis. Ctr. for Surgery & Rehab of Hand, Ltd., 2007 WL 1191782, 3.*

Journal 2010 Examines instances where physicians assert a right to refuse to participate in certain activities deemed immoral based upon claims of conscience. Concludes that this right may be limited by various factors, such as the risk of patient harm. Further concludes that through the informed consent process and other means, physicians can properly accommodate patient care needs and their right of conscience. Cites Opinion 8.115. Antommaria, *Conscientious Objection in Clinical Practice: Notice, Informed Consent, Referral, and Emergency Treatment, 9 Ave Maria L. Rev. 81, 98 (2010).*

Journal 2010 Discusses issues arising from the enactment of legislation by North Dakota involving a minor's reproductive rights. Explores ethical principles that govern physician's actions within the context of reproductive health. Concludes that, while a patient's expectation of confidentiality with a physician is critical, competing values come into play when the patient is a minor and parental involvement may be important. Provides practical guidance to address issues in this context. Quotes Opinions 2.01, 2.015, 5.055, 8.08, 8.115, 9.12, 10.01, 10.015, and 10.05. Cites Opinions 5.05, 5.055, 8.08, 8.11, 8.115, 9.12, and 10.05. Haas, *"Doctor, I'm Pregnant and Fifteen—I Can't Tell My Parents—Please Help Me": Minor Consent, Reproductive Rights, and Ethical Principles for Physicians, 86 N.D. L. Rev. 63, 70, 73, 75-78, 82, 84, 86-88 (2010).*

Journal 2009 Discusses the judicial standard for reviewing physician noncompete covenants. Concludes courts should apply a strict standard to such covenants, rather than declare the covenants per se invalid. Quotes Principles IV and VII, Principles of Medical Ethics §5 (1957) [now Principle VI], Code of Medical Ethics Ch. II, Art. I §3 (1847) [now Opinion 5.02], Opinion 9.02, and Code of Medical Ethics

Ch. II, Art. I §4 (1847) [now Opinion 9.09]. Cites Opinions 8.041, 8.115, 9.02, 9.06, 9.065, 9.067, 10.01, and 10.015. Koons, *Physician Employee Non-Compete Agreements on the Examining Table: The Need to Better Protect Patients' and the Public's Interests in Indiana, 6 Ind. Health L. Rev. 253, 272-77, 280-81 (2009).*

Journal 2008 Examines patient-provider conflicts in end-of-life care and the use of dispute resolution mechanisms. Concludes dispute resolution processes are needed to aid interaction among the various participants in the health care system to prevent injustice to patients. Cites Opinion 8.115. Antommaria, *How Can I Give Her IV Antibiotics at Home When I Have Three Other Children to Care For? Using Dispute System Design to Address Patient Provider Conflicts in Health Care, 29 Hamline J. Pub. L. & Pol'y 273, 275 (2008).*

Journal 2008 Explores the ethical issues associated with writing prescriptions for family members and acquaintances. Concludes that informal treatment often compromises the quality of care, and that a referral to an objective provider is the best choice. Quotes Opinion 8.19. Cites Opinion 8.115. Ares, *An Uncommon Skin Condition Illustrates the Need for Caution When Prescribing for Friends, 20 J. Am. Acad. of Nurse Prac. 389, 390 (2008).*

Journal 2007 Reviews the legal and ethical problems surrounding concierge medical practice. Concludes that concierge medicine should remain restricted to a small class of wealthy individuals. Cites Opinions 8.05, 8.055, 8.115, 9.06, and 9.065. Carnahan, *Concierge Medicine: Legal and Ethical Issues, 35 J. L. Med. & Ethics 211, 212-13 (2007).*

Journal 2007 Compares laws of client abandonment with those of patient abandonment by physicians. Concludes that physicians should be required to show good cause to justify abandonment. Quotes Ch. II, Art. I, Sec. 5 (1903) [now Preamble]. References Opinion 8.115. LeBlanc, *Abandoning Patients and Clients: Where Medicine Can Learn From Law, 1 Charleston L. Rev. 237, 237-38, 256 (2007).*

Journal 2006 Explores the legal and ethical issues surrounding concierge medicine. Concludes that concierge medicine is best restricted to a small class of wealthy individuals. Quotes Principle IX and Opinion 8.055. Cites Principle VI and Opinions 8.055, 8.11, 8.115, 9.065, and 10.05. Carnahan, *Law, Medicine, and Wealth: Does Concierge Medicine Promote Health Care Choice, or Is It a Barrier to Access? 17 Stan. L. & Pol'y Rev. 121, 149-50, 151, 152, 153-54 (2006).*

Journal 2006 Discusses the evolution of health law in Virginia. Concludes that the area of health law continues to expand, develop, and be refined. Cites Opinions 3.03, 3.08, 5.01, 5.015, 5.02, 5.04, 5.055, 6.02, 6.021, 6.03, 6.04, 7.03, 7.04, 7.05, 8.054, 8.08, 8.081, 8.085, 8.115, 8.12, 8.14, 8.145, 8.19, and 9.045. Guanzon, *Health Care Law, 41 U. Rich. L. Rev. 179, 199 (2006).*

Journal 2006 Examines the efficacy of informed consent when a physician acts both as a researcher and care provider. Concludes that a patient cannot give truly informed consent in such cases. Cites Opinions 8.115 and 10.015. Lenrow, *The Treating Physician as Researcher: Is Assuming This Dual Role a Violation of the Nuremberg Code? 25 Temp. J. Sci. Tech. & Envtl. L. 15, 42-43 (2006).*

Journal 2006 Examines physician restrictive covenants. Concludes that under the current balancing test, courts should give considerable weight to the public interest in preserving the physician-patient relationship. Quotes Opinions 9.02 and 9.06. Cites Opinions 6.11, 8.11, 8.115, and 9.06. Malloy, *Physician Restrictive Covenants: The Neglect of Incumbent Patient Interests, 41 Wake Forest L. Rev. 189, 207-08, 217, 218 (2006).*

Journal 2004 Discusses the law in Tennessee regarding surrogate decision-making. Concludes that recent legislation passed in Tennessee will assist those who care for incapacitated patients. Cites Opinions 2.035, 8.081, and 8.115. Wampler, *To Be or Not to Be in Tennessee: Deciding Surrogate Issues, 34 U. Mem. L. Rev. 333, 365 (2004).*

Journal 1998 Explains the connection and differences between bioethics and the law. States that the distinction between ethics and law is that ethics places additional emphasis on moral ideals. References Opinions 8.08 and 8.115. Sullivan & Reynolds, *Where Law and Bioethics Meet . . . and Where They Don't, 75 U. Det. Mercy L. Rev. 607, 612 (1998).*

Journal 1997 Compares past ethical opinions to current opinions and notes the differences. Comments on the forces that have changed medical ethics through the years. Notes differing theories on the future course of medical ethics. Quotes Fundamental Elements (Preamble) and Opinions 5.05, 5.057, 7.01, 8.12, 9.12, and 9.131. Cites Fundamental Elements (5) and Opinions 8.115 and 8.13. Buchanan, *Medical Ethics at the Millennium: A Brief Retrospective, 26 Colo. Law. 141, 142, 143, 144, 145 (1997).*

1.2.1 Treating Self or Family

Journal 2008 Explores the ethical issues associated with writing prescriptions for family members and acquaintances. Concludes that informal treatment often compromises the quality of care, and that a referral to an objective provider is the best choice. Quotes Opinion 8.19. Cites Opinion 8.115. Ares, *An Uncommon Skin Condition Illustrates the Need for Caution When Prescribing for Friends, 20 J. Am. Acad. of Nurse Prac. 389, 390 (2008).*

Journal 2008 Explores the role of an attorney and the attorney's obligation to provide dispassionate counsel and to avoid emotional conflicts. Concludes the American Bar Association Model Rules of Professional Conduct should be amended to prohibit attorney representation of persons with whom the attorney has a significant emotional relationship. Quotes Opinion 8.19. Buhai, *Emotional Conflicts: Impaired Dispassionate Representation of Family Members, 21 Geo. J. Legal Ethics 1159, 1191-92 (2008).*

Journal 2007 Questions whether it is ethical for a physician to provide medical care to a family member. Concludes that providing such care becomes increasingly problematic as

the likelihood of complications increases. Quotes Principle VI and Opinion 8.19. Oberheu, Jones, & Sade, *A Surgeon Operates on His Son: Wisdom or Hubris? 84 Ann. Thorac. Surg. 723, 725, 726 (2007).*

Journal 2006 Discusses the evolution of health law in Virginia. Concludes that the area of health law continues to expand, develop, and be refined. Cites Opinions 3.03, 3.08, 5.01, 5.015, 5.02, 5.04, 5.055, 6.02, 6.021, 6.03, 6.04, 7.03, 7.04, 7.05, 8.054, 8.08, 8.081, 8.085, 8.115, 8.12, 8.14, 8.145, 8.19, and 9.045. Guanzon, *Health Care Law, 41 U. Rich. L. Rev. 179, 199 (2006).*

1.2.2 Disruptive Behavior by Patients

Journal 2010 Explores how participation in online social networks may blur boundaries between personal and professional relationships for health care professionals and how such risks may be mitigated by use of network privacy and security settings. Suggests that health care institutions are likely to institute online social-networking policies for employees. Quotes Opinions 5.026, 5.027, 5.045, 5.046, 5.05, 5.059, 5.0591, 8.14, 9.08, and 9.123. Cites Opinions 5.026, 9.031, and 9.12. Terry, *Physicians and Patients Who "Friend" or "Tweet": Constructing a Legal Framework for Social Networking in a Highly Regulated Domain, 43 Ind. L. Rev. 285, 314-16, 319, 334-36, 338 (2010).*

Journal 2007 Addresses physician liability for an extra-marital affair with a patient's spouse. Concludes that such an affair should be regarded as a breach of a fiduciary duty.

Quotes Preamble, Principles I, II, and VIII, and Opinions 8.145, 9.04, 9.123, and 10.015. Demaine, *"Playing Doctor" With the Patient's Spouse: Alternative Conceptions of Health Professional Liability, 14 Va. J. Soc. Pol'y & L. 308, 325, 330-31, 331-32 (2007).*

Journal 2005 Argues that in *Aetna v. Davila/Cigna v. Calad,* the Supreme Court missed an opportunity to over-turn unjust ERISA policies. Concludes that the principle of complete ERISA preemption as articulated in these consolidated cases is unsatisfactory because it violates the separation of powers doctrine. Quotes Principle VIII. Cites Opinions 8.054, 8.13, 8.135, 9.123, 10.01, and 10.015. Nelson, *AETNA v. DAVILA/CIGNA v. CALAD: A Missed Opportunity, 31 Wm. Mitchell L. Rev. 843, 847, 849, 850, 880 (2005).*

1.2.3 Consultation, Referral, and Second Opinions

6th Cir. 1989 Plaintiff, a chiropractic association, alleged that the AMA and several other professional associations violated antitrust law by conspiring to contain and ultimately eliminate the practice of chiropractic. The court provided an historical overview of the AMA's gradual, but incomplete, recognition of chiropractors and limited licensed practitioners referring specifically to Principle 3 (1957) as well as to the Opinions and Reports of the Judicial Council Sec. 3, Para. 8 (1969) and to the Opinions and Reports 3.60 and 3.70 (1977) [now Principle VI and Opinions 3.01 and 3.04]. Based on its reading of these Principles and Opinions, the court reversed the trial court's grant of summary judgment to the AMA because there remained a material issue of fact of whether it had continued to illegally boycott chiropractic. *Chiropractic Coop. Ass'n v. AMA, 867 F.2d 270, 272-75.*

E.D. Mich. 1986 Plaintiff-chiropractors claimed violation of the Sherman Antitrust Act alleging that the AMA conspired with others to injure them professionally and financially. In support of their claim, plaintiffs cited Principle 3 (1957) and the Opinions and Reports of the Judicial Council Sec.

3, Para. 8 (1969) [now Principles VI and Opinions 3.01 and 3.04]. The court, noting the 1977 change in the AMA's position regarding chiropractic reflected in the Opinions and Reports of the Judicial Council 3.60 and 3.70 (1977) [now Opinion 3.04] held that plaintiffs failed to demonstrate evidence of an overt act by the AMA within the statutory limitations period. Summary judgment entered for AMA. *Chiropractic Coop. Ass'n v. AMA, 1986-2 Trade Cas. (CCH) & 67,294, aff'd in part and rev'd in part, 867 F.2d 270 (6th Cir. 1989).*

E.D. Mich. 1985 In an antitrust case brought by plaintiff-chiropractic association against the AMA, plaintiffs presented the court with a motion in limine asking that the court strike defendant's affirmative defense of a good faith concern with public health and patient care. Plaintiffs argued that the defense was unprecedented, in conflict with existing law, and dramatically wrong. Plaintiffs referred to Principle 3 (1957) [now Principle VI and Opinions 3.01 and 3.04] as the source of the AMA's antitrust violations. The court denied plaintiffs' motion to strike, stating that under the rule of reason test, the AMA had the right to present evidence that its actions furthered the public interest and patient care. *Chiropractic Coop. Ass'n v. AMA, 617 F. Supp. 264, 266, aff'd in part and rev'd in part, 867 F.2d 270 (6th Cir. 1989).*

D.N.M. 1987 In an antitrust action against major health insurance provider and state medical society, group of chiropractors alleged that a conspiracy existed in which the insurer refused to provide health cost reimbursement coverage for chiropractic services. Plaintiffs urged court to apply a per se analysis, rather than the rule of reason analysis to determine the legality of defendants' restrictive practices. The court declined to apply the per se test. In part, court's conclusion was based on view that concerns of defendant-physicians about relationship with chiropractors because of ethical restrictions imposed by Principle 3 (1957) [now Principle VI and Opinions 3.01 and 3.04] deserved more consideration than the per se test would afford. *Johnson v. Blue Cross/Blue Shield, 677 F. Supp. 1112, 1118.*

S.D. Ohio 1995 Physician accused of soliciting bribes in return for referring patients to Medicaid provider moved to dismiss the indictment which alleged mail fraud and violations of Medicaid antikickback statute. In denying physician's motion to dismiss indictment, the court noted that physician's fiduciary duty under Opinion 3.04 supported an intangible rights mail fraud charge. *United States v. Neufeld, 908 F. Supp. 491, 500.*

Journal 1994 Focuses on physicians' legal and ethical duties to pregnant women to provide medical information relevant to patient choice regarding abortion and to make referrals for services that physicians are unable or unwilling to perform. Concludes that medical educators, professional associations, women's groups, and state legislatures should address these issues. Cites Opinions 3.04 and 8.04. Law, *Silent No More: Physicians' Legal and Ethical Obligations to Patients Seeking Abortions, 21 N. Y. U. Rev. L. & Soc. Change 279, 289, 290, 300 (1994).*

Journal 1993 Focuses on how antitrust laws might be used to prevent exclusion of chiropractors by health maintenance organizations (HMOs) by discussing two theories under which it might be illegal. Concludes that chiropractors challenging their exclusion from HMOs may establish an antitrust claim under the theories of "structural conspiracy" and "tacit collusion" if certain criteria are met. Quotes Opinion 3.04. Note, *HMO Exclusion of Chiropractors, 66 So. Cal. L. Rev. 807, 823 (1993).*

D.S.C. 1968 Military dependent sued government physicians under Federal Tort Claims Act where child with acute abdominal pain was twice referred to naval hospital with diagnosis of possible appendicitis and twice sent home without treatment, eventually suffering ruptured appendix and serious complications. In finding for the plaintiff, the court quoted Principle 8 (1957) [now Principle V and Opinion 8.04] in considering whether the physicians had a duty to seek consultation in such a situation. *Steeves v. United States, 294 F. Supp. 446, 454.*

Wash. 1951 Plaintiff, a charitable, not-for-profit medical corporation, offered prepaid health care services to members and their families. Suit was filed against county medical society and others for damages and injunction for defendants' alleged efforts to monopolize prepaid medical care in area and unlawfully restrain competition by plaintiff and its physicians. Defendants alleged as affirmative defense that their efforts were designed to curb unethical prepaid contract practice by plaintiff. Court examined at length AMA's position regarding contract practice including Principles Ch. III, Art. VI, Secs. 3 and 4 (1947) [now Principle VI and Opinions 8.05 and 9.06] concluding nothing in plaintiff's practice violated the AMA's ethical guidelines. Further, quoting Principles Ch. III, Art. III, Sec.1 (1947) [now Opinion 8.04] dealing with consultations, court noted that defendants' efforts impeded plaintiff's physicians from obtaining consultations. Court concluded defendants' actions constituted unlawful, monopolistic behavior and issued an injunction, although it declined to award damages. *Group Health Coop. v. King County Medical Soc'y, 39 Wash. 2d 586, 237 P.2d 737, 744, 750-51, 759-60.*

Journal 1998 Examines mechanisms of oversight for expert witness testimony by medical, legal, legislative, and regulatory agencies. Points out that the amount of malpractice litigation will increase the need for medical expert witnesses. Concludes that improvements in this context must uphold principles of due process and be acceptable to the medical and legal communities. Cites Opinions 6.01, 8.04, and 9.07. McAbee, *Improper Expert Medical Testimony: Existing and Proposed Mechanisms of Oversight, 19 J. Legal Med. 257, 265 (1998).*

Journal 2009 Discusses the judicial standard for reviewing physician noncompete covenants. Concludes courts should apply a strict standard to such covenants, rather than declare the covenants per se invalid. Quotes Principles IV and VII, Principles of Medical Ethics §5 (1957) [now Principle VI], Code of Medical Ethics Ch. II, Art. I §3 (1847) [now Opinion 5.02], Opinion 9.02, and Code of Medical Ethics Ch. II, Art. I §4 (1847) [now Opinion 9.09]. Cites Opinions 8.041, 8.115, 9.02, 9.06, 9.065, 9.067, 10.01, and 10.015. Koons, *Physician Employee Non-Compete Agreements on the Examining Table: The Need to Better Protect Patients' and the Public's Interests in Indiana, 6 Ind. Health L. Rev. 253, 272-77, 280-81 (2009).*

Journal 2010 Reviews a book with case studies of controversial issues of bioethics, health law, and human rights. Concludes that, while in many areas bioethics relates to human rights issues, human rights issues not directly involving the conduct of health professionals or human health are not within the scope of expertise of bioethicist. Quotes Opinion 8.02. Rothstein, *Worst Case Bioethics: Death, Disaster, and Public Health, 31 J. Legal Med. 331, 333 (2010).*

Journal 2001 Examines issues relating to health care cost containment. Concludes that, if physicians are to meet the goals assigned to them in a cost-constrained health care system, then professional standards must be reevaluated and modified to afford meaningful guidance for clinical decision-making in the face of health care spending controls. Quotes Opinions 2.03, 2.09, 2.095, 8.032, and 9.04. Cites Opinions 8.02, 8.021, 8.051, and 8.13. Agrawal, *Resuscitating Professionalism: Self-regulation in the Medical Marketplace, 66 Mo. L. Rev. 341, 354, 355, 360, 361, 378, 388 (2001).*

Journal 2001 Discusses the prohibition on nonlawyer ownership of legal service providers. Considers how ethical rules and standards governing physicians have been directed toward preserving independent judgment. Concludes that ethical conflicts created by abandoning the prohibition on nonlawyer ownership of legal service providers may be managed by following the medical ethics model. Quotes Principle VI and Opinions 2.03, 2.09, 8.02, 8.021, 8.03, 8.05, 8.051, 8.054, 8.13, and 8.132. Harris & Foran, *The Ethics of Middle-Class Access to Legal Services and What We Can Learn From the Medical Profession's Shift to a Corporate Paradigm, 70 Fordham L. Rev. 775, 817, 821, 822, 823, 824 (2001).*

Journal 1999 Discusses the need for physicians to advocate on behalf of patients' rights in the context of health care delivery. Evaluates the nature and scope of the physician's role as advocate, noting that physicians cannot be expected to engage in attorney-like advocacy. Quotes Principles IV and VI, Fundamental Elements (2), (4), and (6) [now Opinion 10.01], Patient Responsibilities 5 [now Opinion 10.02], and Opinions 2.03, 2.07, 2.09, 2.16, 2.19, 3.06, 4.01, 4.04, 6.01, 7.02, 8.02, 8.03, 8.13, 8.132, 9.06, 9.07, and 9.131. Cites Opinions 5.05, 5.09, 7.01, 8.135, and 9.02. Sage, *Physicians as Advocates, 35 Hous. L. Rev. 1529, 1537, 1541, 1542, 1552-53, 1554, 1556, 1557, 1559, 1561-62, 1564, 1571, 1574, 1576, 1580 (1999).*

Journal 1997 Discusses the practice of ex parte communications between treating physicians and their patients' legal adversaries without informing the patient or obtaining consent. Examines harms that may occur in these situations. Argues that Oklahoma needs to prohibit treating physicians from communicating ex parte with their patients' legal adversaries. Quotes Opinions 5.05, 5.07, 5.08, 8.02, 8.03, and 9.07. Cites Opinion 7.02. McNaughton & McNaughton, *Divided Loyalty: The Dilemma of the Treating Physician Advocate, 22 Okla. City U. L. Rev. 1051, 1052, 1054, 1056, 1058, 1059, 1062 (1997).*

Journal 2007 Examines the ethical obligations of a corporate health lawyer. Concludes that the ethical health lawyer must balance obligations to the client with obligations to patients and the public. Quotes Opinion 8.09. Weeks, *Loopholes: Opportunity, Responsibility, or Liability? 35 J. L. Med. & Ethics 320, 322 (2007).*

1.2.5 Sports Medicine

Journal 2008 Discusses medical and legal issues facing the National Football League stemming from concussions sustained by players. Argues steps must be taken to minimize the impact of concussions on active players and increase assistance for former injured players. Quotes Opinion 3.06. Lipsky, *Dealing With the NFL's Concussion Problems of Yesterday, Today, and Tomorrow, 18 Fordham Intell. Prop. Media & Ent. L. J. 959, 988 (2008).*

Journal 2007 Examines ethical issues that arise when physicians are employed by sports teams. Concludes that for team physicians, special guidelines apply to informed consent, advertising, confidentiality, and third-party influences. Quotes Opinion 3.06. Dunn, George, Churchill, & Spindler, *Ethics in Sports Medicine, 35 The Am. J. of Sports Med. 840, 841, 842 (2007).*

Journal 1999 Describes conflicts of interest faced by professional sports team physicians. Examines cases where athletes have sued team physicians for failing to follow the proper standard of care. Provides a clear standard of care and suggests ways team physicians can reduce conflicts of interest. Quotes Opinion 3.06. Keim, *Physicians for Professional Sports Teams: Health Care Under the Pressure of Economic and Commercial Interests, 9 Seton Hall. J. Sport L. 196, 218-19 (1999).*

Journal 1999 Discusses the need for physicians to advocate on behalf of patients' rights in the context of health care delivery. Evaluates the nature and scope of the physician's role as advocate, noting that physicians cannot be expected to engage in attorney-like advocacy. Quotes Principles IV and VI, Fundamental Elements (2), (4), and (6) [now Opinion 10.01], Patient Responsibilities 5 [now Opinion 10.02], and Opinions 2.03, 2.07, 2.09, 2.16, 2.19, 3.06, 4.01, 4.04, 6.01, 7.02, 8.02, 8.03, 8.13, 8.132, 9.06, 9.07, and 9.131. Cites Opinions 5.05, 5.09, 7.01, 8.135, and 9.02. Sage, *Physicians as Advocates, 35 Hous. L. Rev. 1529, 1537, 1541, 1542, 1552-53, 1554, 1556, 1557, 1559, 1561-62, 1564, 1571, 1574, 1576, 1580 (1999).*

Journal 1993 Discusses an athlete's rights to assume serious health risks by playing a sport, despite a physical abnormality or medical condition. Considers the team physician's conflicting duties toward the patient/player and the team. Concludes that physicians or athletes should bear legal responsibility if either violates their obligations in this context. Cites Opinion 3.06. Mitten, *Team Physicians and Competitive Athletes: Allocating Legal Responsibility for Athletic Injuries, 55 U. Pitt. L. Rev. 129, 140 (1993).*

1.2.6 Work-Related and Independent Medical Examinations

Alaska 2010 Workers' compensation claimant appealed summary judgment in medical malpractice action against physician who performed independent medical examination. The court quoted Opinion 10.03 in holding that the claimant did not present any evidence the physician failed to abide by ethical standards. The court concluded in part that the claims were dependent upon claimant establishing a physician-patient relationship with the physician and affirmed the lower court's ruling. *Smith v. Radecki, 238 P.3d 111, 116.*

Ariz. 2003 Employee appealed summary judgment and dismissal in malpractice action against a radiologist and x-ray company for failure to inform her of medical results that could have led to an earlier diagnosis of lung cancer. Employee was referred by her employer to the radiologist for a chest x-ray. The radiologist did not inform the employee of abnormalities noted in his report. Quoting Opinion 10.03, the appellate court held the physician had a duty to directly inform the employee of the results. The x-ray company was not liable, however, since the radiologist was an independent contractor. *Stanley v. McCarver, 204 Ariz. 339, 63 P.3d 1076, 1081.*

N.J. 2001 Deceased patient's wife filed a medical malpractice action against a physician who conducted pre-employment screening. The physician failed to inform the deceased about a condition he discovered during the physical. The New Jersey Supreme Court reversed the lower courts and held that a physician under contract with a third party to perform pre-employment physicals has a nondelegable duty to inform the patient of any potentially serious medical conditions. The court quoted Opinion 10.03, expressing the view that, although this may not be a traditional physician-patient relationship, the physician still has a responsibility to inform the patient. *Reed v. Bojarski, 166 N.J.89, 764 A.2d 433, 444.*

N.Y. 2009 Plaintiff in a personal injury action sued the physician designated by the defendant in that action to conduct an independent medical examination of plaintiff. Plaintiff claimed he was injured during the examination by the physician. The court relied on Opinion 10.03 in distinguishing the relationship between a physician performing an independent medical examination on a person and an examination undertaken in a traditional physician-patient relationship. The court held that the duty owed to the examinee is to perform the examination in a manner so as not to cause physical harm to the examinee. The court found that plaintiff's claim was governed by the statute of limitations for professional malpractice actions. *Bazakos v. Lewis, 12 N.Y.3d 631, 911 N.E.2d 847, 850, 883 N.Y.S.2d 785.*

N.Y. App. 2008 Plaintiff in personal injury action brought suit against physician hired by alleged tortfeasor to conduct statutory medical examination to recover for injuries sustained during examination. The court quoted Opinion 10.03 in determining that a limited patient-physician relationship exists between the physician and the examinee in such a case. The court held that, despite precedent dictating otherwise, there was no physician-patient relationship in this case and that the statute of limitations for negligence should apply, rather than the statute of limitations for medical malpractice actions. *Bazakos v. Lewis, 56 A.D.3d 15, 864 N.Y.S.2d 505, 512, n. 3, rev'd, 12 N.Y.3d 631, 911 N.E.2d 847, 883 N.Y.S.2d 785.*

1.2.8 Gifts from Patients

Journal 2008 Argues that organ donation from a patient to his or her physician is unethical. Concludes that this practice would be exploitative to the patient and undermine public trust in the medical profession. Cites Opinions 8.14, 10.017, and 10.018. Steinberg & Pomfret, *A Novel Boundary Issue: Should a Patient Be an Organ Donor for Their Physician? 34 J. Med. Ethics 772, 772 (2008).*

1.2.10 Political Action by Physicians

Journal 2006 Examines medical resident labor rights. Concludes that hospitals should allow residents to unionize. References Opinion 9.025. Geiger, *The Ailing Labor Rights of Medical Residents: Curable Ill or a Lost Cause? 8 U. Pa. J. Lab. & Emp. L. 523, 538 (2006)*

Journal 2005 Discusses physician responses to the medical malpractice liability crisis. Concludes that certain responses may violate ethical obligations that physicians owe to their patients and to society as a whole. Cites Opinions 9.025 and 10.015. References Principle VIII. Kachalia, Choudhry, & Studdert, *Physician Responses to the Malpractice Crisis: From Defense to Offense, 33 J. L. Med. & Ethics 416, 419, 421, 424 (2005).*

Journal 2004 Examines whether unionization is a feasible solution to the commodification of the professional work force. Concludes that unionization is a tool used to protect the class status and livelihood of professional employees and that the law should support such efforts. References Opinion 9.025. Crain, *The Transformation of the Professional Workforce, 79 Chi.-Kent L. Rev. 543, 582 (2004).*

Journal 1999 Considers the growing interest on the part of physicians to unionize and engage in collective bargaining. Discusses how legislatures and the courts may affect the evolution of physician unions. Analyzes potential benefits and detriments of unionization. References Opinion 9.025. Phan, *Physician Unionization: The Impact on the Medical Profession, 20 J. Legal Med. 115, 136, 137 (1999).*

2 Consent, Communication, and Decision Making

2.1.1 Informed Consent

7th Cir. 2002 Prosecutors appealed order enjoining enforcement of informed consent provisions of Indiana abortion statute on the grounds that they unconstitutionally created an undue burden. Court of Appeals reversed and held injunction was an abuse of discretion. The court found the statute was substantively identical to a law upheld in previous decisions. Further, the court held that the state was entitled to have the law evaluated on the basis of actual experience. Dissenting judge quoted Opinion 8.08 regarding need for patient to be capable of giving informed consent. *A Woman's Choice-East Side Women's Clinic v. Newman, 305 F.3d 684, 716.*

Alaska 2002 Patient brought malpractice and informed consent claims against physician. In part, patient alleged physician's failure to appropriately advise her regarding her abdominal pain after surgery led to permanent injuries. Trial court entered judgment for physician. On appeal, Alaska Supreme Court remanded the informed consent claim, holding that the jury instruction should have reflected a "reasonable patient" standard. Quotes Opinion 8.08. *Marsingill v. O'Malley, 58 P.3d 495, 499, 504-05.*

Ga. App. 2000 Plaintiff alleged failure on the part of a dentist to inform him of the risks of root canal in a malpractice action. The appeals court noted that state case law did not recognize the informed consent doctrine. In evaluating this precedent, the court quoted Opinion 8.08 and Fundamental Element (1) [now Opinion 10.01]. The court stated that the *AMA Code of Medical Ethics* should be understood to reflect the standard of care of the medical profession on the issue of informed consent. While the court ruled in favor of the dentist, it prospectively recognized the doctrine of informed consent. *Ketchup v. Howard, 247 Ga. App. 54, 543 S.E.2d 371, 376, 377.*

Ind. 1992 Plaintiffs filed suit against physician after medical review panel found no evidence that physician committed malpractice in performing a bladder suspension and cryosurgery that resulted in plaintiff's cervix adhering to wall of her vagina. The trial court granted summary judgment for the defendant but appellate court reversed in part holding that the informed consent claim did not require expert medical testimony. The state Supreme Court affirmed the summary judgment, determining that the reasonably prudent physician standard applied in informed consent cases. In support of its decision, the court quoted Opinion 8.08, regarding informed consent. The court also held that expert medical testimony was required for plaintiff's informed consent claim because the standard of care for the procedure performed was not common knowledge for lay persons. *Culbertson v. Mernitz, 602 N.E.2d 98, 103, 106.*

Ind. App. 1999 Patient brought malpractice suit against surgeon, claiming that he would not have consented to surgery if the surgeon had disclosed that he would perform only a fusion for the patient's back, rather than the recommended procedure. The trial court granted summary judgment. The appellate court reversed, and held that a plaintiff is not required to introduce expert testimony to establish the standard of care or the causation elements in an informed consent action when lay people can understand that a failure to meet the standard of care occurred. The court cited *Culbertson v. Mernitz*, 602 N.E.2d 98 (Ind. 1992), where the Indiana Supreme Court quoted Opinion 8.08, regarding informed consent. *Bowman v. Beghin, 713 N.E.2d 913, 916.*

N.J. 2007 After consultation with her physician, plaintiff signed a consent form and had an abortion. Plaintiff was later diagnosed with an incomplete abortion which, she alleged, alerted her to the fact that the procedure resulted in the death of a human being. She sued her physician for negligent infliction of emotional distress and failure to obtain informed consent. Summary judgment was granted for the physician and plaintiff appealed. The Supreme Court of New Jersey, quoting Opinion 8.08, considered whether a reasonable patient would find the information regarding whether a human being was killed material in giving consent. Finding that there is no consensus that a "human being" is killed during an abortion, that a fetus has not been deemed to be a person under the Constitution, and that the question is a value judgment, the court found no duty for a physician to provide such information. *Acuna v. Turkish, 192 N.J. 399, 930 A.2d 416, 425.*

N.J. 1999 Patient sued surgeon for lack of informed consent and malpractice on grounds that the surgeon decided to treat patient's hip fracture with bed rest rather than utilizing other alternatives. The trial court held that the patient could not sustain a claim for lack of informed consent. The New Jersey Supreme Court held that the informed consent requirement extends to noninvasive procedures. The court quoted Opinion 8.08 regarding a patient's right to be fully informed of medically reasonable treatments. *Matthies v. Mastromonaco, 160 N.J. 26, 733 A.2d 456, 463.*

N.Y. Fam. 2006 During proceedings regarding a foster child, an issue was raised contesting the legality of the County Department of Human Services' procedures for administering drugs to children. The mother's consent for prescribing medication to the child was obtained by a caseworker, without direct consultation with a physician and with no explanation of side effects. The court cited Opinions 8.08, 8.081, 8.11, and 10.01 in determining the physician's duty to honor the decision of the parent/surrogate. The mother's consent was invalidated and she was given an opportunity to consult with a physician. *Matter of Lyle A., 14 Misc. 3d 842, 830 N.Y.S.2d 486, 492, 494.*

W. Va. 1995 West Virginia Board of Medicine received a complaint from patient that physician was using depossession treatment. The hearing examiner in part found that there had been a lack of informed consent for such treatment. The Board changed the examiner's report and added sanctions. In doing so, it quoted Opinion 8.08. On appeal, the circuit court reversed, finding the Board's order arbitrary and an abuse of discretion. The appellate court agreed that the Board abused its discretion, but remanded the case for consideration of the issue of informed consent for depossession treatment. *Modi v. West Virginia Board of Medicine, 465 S.E.2d230,236.*

Journal 2011 Discusses the doctrine of informed consent and the influence of physician groups on the dissemination of information to patients. Concludes the doctrine of informed consent should be expanded by the courts, rather than continuing to allow professional professional societies to dictate provider guidelines for obtaining informed consent. Quotes Opinions 8.08, 10.01, and 10.015. References Opinion 2.065. Ginsberg, *Informed Consent: No Longer Just What the Doctor Ordered? The "Contributions" of Medical Associations and Courts to a More Patient Friendly Doctrine, 15 Mich. St. J. Med. & Law 17, 23, 24, 25, 26, 46 (2011).*

Journal 2011 Argues that autonomy should be compromised for the welfare of certain research subjects who would benefit from the particular medical research. Concludes that although autonomy is sometimes sacrificed for welfare, it should go even further to prefer subject groups with the greatest risk/benefit ratio. Quotes Opinion 8.08. Stein & Savulescu, *Welfare Versus Autonomy in Human Subjects Research, 38 Fla. St. U. L. Rev. 303, 332 (2011).*

Journal 2010 Examines a prisoner's substantive due process right under the Fourteenth Amendment to receive sufficient information to make an informed decision on whether to consent to or refuse medical treatment. Concludes that the doctrinal grounds for this claimed right are weak and that public policy considerations counsel against it. Quotes Opinion 8.08. Gatter, *A Prisoner's Constitutional Right to Medical Information: Doctrinally Flawed and a Threat to State Informed Consent Law, 45 Wake Forest L. Rev. 1025, 1062 (2010).*

Journal 2010 Discusses issues arising from the enactment of legislation by North Dakota involving a minor's reproductive rights. Explores ethical principles that govern physician's actions within the context of reproductive health. Concludes that, while a patient's expectation of confidentiality with a physician is critical, competing values come into play when the patient is a minor and parental involvement may be important. Provides practical guidance to address issues in this context. Quotes Opinions 2.01, 2.015, 5.055, 8.08, 8.115, 9.12, 10.01, 10.015, and 10.05. Cites Opinions 5.05, 5.055, 8.08, 8.11, 8.115, 9.12, and 10.05. Haas, *"Doctor, I'm Pregnant and Fifteen—I Can't Tell My Parents—Please Help Me": Minor Consent, Reproductive Rights, and Ethical Principles for Physicians, 86 N.D. L. Rev. 63, 70, 73, 75-78, 82, 84, 86-88 (2010).*

Journal 2010 Analyzes the practice of coerced sterilization of HIV-positive women to prevent transmission of the virus to offspring and discusses current litigation challenging such sterilization as a rights violation. Concludes forced sterilization is a major problem in Latin America and Africa, and the human rights community must work closely with the medical community to ensure patients are making informed medical decisions. Cites Opinion 8.08. Nair, *Litigating Against the Forced Sterilization of HIV-Positive Women: Recent Developments in Chile and Nambia, 23 Harv. Hum. Rts. J. 223, 226 (2010).*

Journal 2009 Discusses the availability and scope of the doctrine of informed consent in Georgia, citing *Doreika v. Blotner* as an important pending case in which the Georgia Supreme Court will review the doctrine. Concludes *Doreika* should be affirmed to provide full recognition of a patient's rights to self-determination and bodily integrity in Georgia. Cites Opinions 8.08 and 8.15. Leppert, *Doreika v. Blotner: Affirming Ketchup Against Judicial Mustard, 60 Mercer L. Rev. 807, 817, 820 (2009).*

Journal 2009 Argues race-based genetic biomedical research is necessary because of the significant impact of race and ethnicity on various aspects of life. Concludes law and policy should promote socially responsible race-based genetic research to gain more meaningful and applicable scientific knowledge. Quotes Opinion 8.08. Malinowski, *Dealing With the Realities of Race and Ethnicity: A Bioethics-Centered Argument in Favor of Race-Based Genetics Research, 45 Hous. L. Rev. 1415, 1463 (2009).*

Journal 2009 Compares the tort law doctrine of informed consent to abortion law's approach to informed consent. Discusses woman-protective reasoning as the cause of divergence between the two bodies of law. Concludes abortion law lacks confidence in women's decision-making capabilities and that lawmakers should recognize abortion law's approach to informed consent is contrary to other patient health care decision-making and denies women equal treatment. References Opinion 8.08. Manian, *The Irrational Woman: Informed Consent and Abortion Decision-Making, 16 Duke J. Gender L. & Pol'y 223, 241 (2009).*

Journal 2009 Argues First Amendment rights of physicians are being violated by government control and imposition of ideology through statutes, using South Dakota's informed consent to abortion statute as an example. Concludes statutes endorsing a particular ideology damage the physician-patient relationship and infringe upon physician First Amendment rights. References Code of Ethics Art. I(4) (1847) [now Opinion 8.08]. Robbins, *Open Your Mouth and Say "Ideology": Physicians and the First Amendment, 12 U. Pa. J. Const. L. 155, 159 (2009).*

Journal 2009 Discusses potential liability of a medical device or pharmaceutical company due to its representative's presence in the treatment room, including privacy claims and claims based on the representative's acts or omissions. Concludes companies must be aware of such liability risks and train their representatives accordingly. Quotes Opinion 8.08. Summerhill & Chandler, *Company Representatives in the Operating & Treatment Room: How to Navigate the Ever-Expanding Theories of Liability for Medical Device & Pharmaceutical Companies, 12 DePaul J. Health Care L. 253, 258-259 (2009).*

Journal 2008 Reviews procedural guidelines for fine-needle aspiration of the thyroid gland. Concludes, in part, that particular attention must be paid to the informed consent process to ensure patients undergoing such procedures appropriately understand procedure risks and benefits. References Opinion 8.08. Cibas, Alexander, Benson, Patricio de Agustín, Doherty, Faquin, Middleton, Miller, Raab, White, & Mandel, *Indications for Thyroid FNA and Pre-FNA Requirements: A Synopsis of the National Cancer Institute Thyroid Fine-Needle Aspiration State of the Science Conference, 36 Diagnostic Cytopathology 390, 394 (2008).*

Journal 2008 Considers the utility of physician apologies for medical error and legal protection for physicians who apologize for mistakes. Concludes physicians must openly communicate with their patients and apologize for medical errors to strengthen the health care community. Quotes Opinions 8.08, 8.12, 10.01, and 10.015. References Opinion 8.12. Ebert, *Attorneys, Tell Your Clients to Say They're Sorry: Apologies in the Health Care Industry, 5 Ind. Health L. Rev. 337, 340-41, 344 (2008).*

Journal 2008 Argues the Alaska Supreme Court erroneously extended the physician's informed consent duty to disclose to situations in which the physician had no opportunity to evaluate the patient. Concludes *Marsingill v. O'Malley* requires physicians to inconvenience patients or bear unreasonable risk. Quotes Opinion 8.08. Hutchinson, *Marsingill v. O'Malley: The Duty to Disclose Becomes the Duty to Divine, 25 Alaska L. Rev. 241, 252 (2008).*

Journal 2008 Explores issues regarding treatment decisions for incapacitated patients. Concludes patient decision-making capacity should be tested in many situations to ensure the treatment decisions made are those the patient would make if competent. Cites Opinion 8.08. Vars, *Illusory Consent: When an Incapacitated Patient Agrees to Treatment, 87 Or. L. Rev. 353, 359 (2008).*

Journal 2007 Discusses the evolution of informed consent doctrine. Concludes that, in context of research, informed consent exceptions should be substantially narrowed. Quotes Ch. I, Art. I, Sec. 4 (May 1847) [now Opinion 8.082] and Ch. I, Art. I, Sec. 1 (May 1847) [now Principles I and VIII]. References Opinions 2.08 and 8.08. Grimm, *Informed Consent for All! No Exceptions, 37 N. M. L. Rev. 39, 39, 61 (2007).*

Journal 2007 Discusses patients' right to refuse medical treatment and the corresponding duties of health care professionals. Concludes that detailed, carefully prepared advance directives are necessary to fulfill patients' wishes. Quotes Ch. II (1940) [now Opinions 8.08 and 8.082] and Opinions 2.035, 2.037, 2.20, 2.225, 8.081, and 10.015. Cites Opinions 9.11 and 9.115. Stamatakis, *Beyond Advance Directives: Personal Autonomy and the Right to Refuse Life-Sustaining Medical Treatment, 47 N. H. B. J. 20, 29-30 (2007).*

Journal 2007 Examines statutes giving pharmacists the right to refuse dispensing of emergency contraceptives. Concludes that a woman should be allowed to bring a wrongful conception claim against a pharmacist who refuses her medication. References Opinion 8.08. Weisser, *Abolishing the Pharmacist's Veto: An Argument in Support of a Wrongful Conception Cause of Action Against Pharmacists Who Refuse to Provide Emergency Contraception, 80 S. Cal. L. Rev. 865, 881-81 (2007).*

Journal 2006 Reviews the concept of therapeutic privilege. Concludes that the practice creates conflict between physician obligations under the concepts of autonomy and beneficence. Recommends that physicians maximize communication with patients by providing all pertinent information in the context of patient preferences. Cites Opinions 8.08, 8.081, 8.121, and 10.015. References Chap. I, Art. I, Sec. 4 (May 1847) [premise deleted from Code]. Bostick, Sade, McMahon, & Benjamin, *Report of the American Medical Association Council on Ethical and Judicial Affairs: Withholding Information From Patients: Rethinking the Propriety of "Therapeutic Privilege," 17 J. Clinical Ethics 302, 303 (Winter 2006).*

Journal 2006 Discusses the evolution of health law in Virginia. Concludes that the area of health law continues to expand, develop, and be refined. Cites Opinions 3.03, 3.08, 5.01, 5.015, 5.02, 5.04, 5.055, 6.02, 6.021, 6.03, 6.04, 7.03, 7.04, 7.05, 8.054, 8.08, 8.081, 8.085, 8.115, 8.12, 8.14, 8.145, 8.19, and 9.045. Guanzon, *Health Care Law, 41 U. Rich. L. Rev. 179, 199 (2006).*

Journal 2005 Speculates on the issues raised if the US government were to force drug addicts to take pharmaceuticals designed to prevent reaction to illegal drug. Concludes that such a policy violates multiple constitutional rights as well as the ethical principles underlying informed consent. Quotes Opinion 8.08. Boire, *Neurocops: The Politics of Prohibition and the Future of Enforcing Social Policy From Inside the Body*, 19 J. L. & Health 215, 237 (2005)

Journal 2005 Evaluates informed consent in the practice of teaching medical students by having them perform unnecessary procedures on hospital patients. Concludes that consent must be obtained in all cases. Cites Opinion 8.08. Oberman, *Panel Discussion American Association of Law Schools Panel: Panel on the Use of Patients for Teaching Purposes Without Their Knowledge or Consent*, 8 J. Health Care L. & Pol'y 210, 210 (2005).

Journal 2004 Examines whether performing genital reconstruction surgery on intersexed children to prevent psychological harm is necessary. Concludes that courts around the world should prohibit medically unnecessary genital reconstruction surgery during childhood. Quotes Opinion 8.08. Haas, *Who Will Make Room for the Intersexed?* 30 Am. J. L. & Med. 41, 63 (2004).

Journal 2003 Discusses whether, and how, legal rights may be waived. Concludes that, in addressing these questions, emphasis should be placed on concepts of autonomy and voluntariness. Cites Opinion 8.08. Berg, *Understanding Waiver*, 40 Hous. L. Rev. 281, 329 (2003).

Journal 2003 Examines the manner in which psychiatrists participate in the criminal justice system. Concludes that, in some situations, this participation may violate principles of medical ethics. Cites Opinions 2.06 and 8.08. Dolin, *A Healer or an Executioner? The Proper Role of a Psychiatrist in a Criminal Justice System*, 17 J. L. & Health 169, 206, 213-14 (2003).

Journal 2003 Evaluates patient autonomy in the physician-patient relationship. Concludes that it may be time to reject its dominance in favor of requiring physicians to provide patients with the maximum benefit of their expertise without imposing authority in areas beyond that expertise. Quotes Opinion 8.08. Dworkin, *Getting What We Should From Doctors: Rethinking Patient Autonomy and the Doctor-Patient Relationship*, 13 Health Matrix 235, 240 (2003).

Journal 2003 Argues that affirmative measures should be taken by the Air Force to ensure access to abortion services. Concludes that regulatory changes will reduce barriers to access. Quotes Opinion 10.01. Cites Opinion 8.08. Wilde, *Air Force Women's Access to Abortion Services and the Erosion of 10 USC § 1093*, 9 Wm. & Mary J. Women & L. 351, 371 (2003).

Journal 2002 Examines how managed care has adversely affected information disclosure in the physician-patient relationship. Concludes that, unless courts expand applicability of principles of informed consent, patient self-determination

and autonomy will continue to be undermined. Quotes Principle VIII and Opinions 8.03, 8.053, 8.054, and 8.08. Morris, *Dissing Disclosure: Just What the Doctor Ordered*, 44 Ariz. L. Rev. 313, 344, 349, 362, 363, 366 (2002).

Journal 2002 Considers the dilemma of informed consent in the context of prescribing psychotropic medication to patients with mental illness and mental retardation. Recognizes the need for substituted decision-making in certain situations. Concludes that legislation would help address this issue. Quotes Preamble, Principles I, III, IV, VIII, and IX, and Opinion 8.08. O'Sullivan & Borcherding, *Informed Consent for Medication in Persons With Mental Retardation and Mental Illness*, 12 Health Matrix 63, 75, 86, 87, 88 (2002).

Journal 2002 Analyzes the role of prognostication in physician-patient communication. Concludes that the patient-physician model of shared decision-making offers the best hope for reestablishing prognostication. Quotes Principles Ch. I, Art. I, Sec. 2 and 4 (1846) [now Principle IV and Opinions 8.12 and 10.01]. Cites Opinion 8.08. Rich, *Prognostication in Clinical Medicine: Prophecy or Professional Responsibility?* 23 J. Legal Med. 297, 299, 318, 327 (2002).

Journal 2000 Examines physician value neutrality (PVN). Defines PVN as providing a foundation to suggest physicians must keep their values—religious, political, or otherwise—out of the patient-physician relationship. Concludes it is not clear how values can be removed from the patient-physician relationship without removing the very thing PVN supporters are trying to protect, the intrinsic value of persons. References Opinions 2.01, 2.02, 8.032, 8.05, 8.08, and 8.132. Beckwith & Peppin, *Physician Value Neutrality: A Critique*, 28 J. L. Med. & Ethics 67, 72-73 (2000).

Journal 2000 Explores the US Supreme Court's use of the First Amendment's viewpoint neutrality mandate. Concludes that viewpoint discrimination should be applied to limit government censorship of private speech in nonpublic forums and selective subsidy programs. Quotes Opinion 8.08. Casarez, *Public Forums, Selective Subsidies, and Shifting Standards of Viewpoint Discrimination*, 64 Alb. L. Rev. 501, 558 (2000).

Journal 2000 Considers the objective of the informed consent doctrine. Concludes that, in practice, the doctrine falls short of its intended purpose. Quotes Opinion 8.08. Kurtz, *The Law of Informed Consent: From "Doctor Is Right" to "Patient Has Rights,"* 50 Syracuse L. Rev. 1243, 1245 (2000).

Journal 2000 Describes the fiduciary aspects of the physician-patient relationship. Explores the conflicts that may occur between physicians and pregnant women in the health care setting. Proposes legal strategies to address these conflicts. Quotes Opinions 8.08 and 10.01. References Opinion 8.13. Oberman, *Mothers and Doctors' Orders: Unmasking the Doctor's Fiduciary Role in Maternal-Fetal Conflicts*, 94 Nw. U. L. Rev. 451, 456, 462, 493 (2000).

Journal 2000 Examines issues relating to parental consent to circumcision. Identifies legal and ethical requirements for consent when medical professionals are treating adult patients. Analyzes the implications of those requirements for routine circumcision of infant males. Concludes that only when the male is an adult and capable of making decisions can circumcision be ethically and legally performed. Quotes Opinion 8.08. References Opinions 8.03 and 9.011. Svoboda, Van Howe, & Dwyer, *Informed Consent for Neonatal Circumcision: An Ethical and Legal Conundrum, 17 J. Contemp. Health L. & Pol'y 61, 67, 73, 82 (2000)*.

Journal 2000 Discusses traditional medical ethics and the physician's duty to benefit patients. Concludes that, in the 21st century, physicians will no longer be expected to determine on their own what will benefit their patients. Quotes Principle II and Opinion 8.08. Veatch, *Doctor Does Not Know Best: Why in the New Century Physicians Must Stop Trying to Benefit Patients, 25 J. Med. & Phil. 701, 710, 711 (2000)*.

Journal 2000 Discusses the development and history of the ethical doctrine of informed consent. Examines the current state of the law in Pennsylvania and concludes it does not adequately fulfill the goals of ethical and legal doctrines. Quotes Principle IV and Opinion 10.01. References Opinion 8.08. Warren, *Pennsylvania Medical Informed Consent Law: A Call to Protect Patient Autonomy Rights by Abandoning the Battery Approach, 38 Duq. L. Rev. 917, 925 (2000)*.

Journal 1999 Observes that, under statute and common law, the doctrine of informed consent in Pennsylvania does not apply in situations involving nonsurgical procedures. Argues that state law should be expanded to include a duty to obtain informed consent in these situations. Quotes Opinion 8.08. Durst, *Cutting Through Pennsylvania's Medical Informed Consent Statute: A Reasonable Interpretation Abolishing the Surgical Requirement, 104 Dick. L. Rev. 197, 225 (1999)*.

Journal 1998 Discusses legal aspects of physician-assisted suicide. Identifies acceptable end-of-life choices and compares them to physician-assisted suicide. Points out that physician-assisted suicide has the potential for abuse and that safeguards have not been implemented to protect people from that risk. Quotes Opinion 2.211. Cites Opinions 2.20 and 8.08. Mitchell, *Physician-Assisted Suicide: A Survey of the Issues Surrounding Legalization, 74 N. D. L. Rev. 341, 349 (1998)*.

Journal 1998 Discusses current abortion malpractice claims. Describes three general types of malpractice causes of action. Argues that specialized procreative torts should be implemented to adequately protect a woman's procreative autonomy. Quotes Opinion 8.08. Northern, *Procreative Torts: Enhancing the Common-Law Protection for Reproductive Autonomy, 1998 U. Ill. L. Rev. 489, 525 (1998)*.

Journal 1998 Explains the connection and differences between bioethics and the law. States that the distinction between ethics and law is that ethics places additional emphasis on moral ideals. References Opinions 8.08 and 8.115. Sullivan & Reynolds, *Where Law and Bioethics Meet . . . and Where They Don't, 75 U. Det. Mercy L. Rev. 607, 612 (1998)*.

Journal 1997 Examines the evolution of the Indiana health care system. Discusses developments in Indiana jurisprudence regarding the physician-patient relationship. Explores various challenges facing the relationship and recognizes the need for legal rules to help address these challenges. Quotes Opinion 8.08. Cites Opinions 2.20, 9.06, and 9.12. Kinney & Selby, *History and Jurisprudence of the physician-patient Relationship in Indiana, 30 Ind. L. Rev. 263, 269, 272, 276 (1997)*.

Journal 1997 Explores the meaning of cardiopulmonary resuscitation and legal issues involving do-not-resuscitate (DNR) orders. Considers problems created by DNR orders in operating rooms in light of patients' rights. Concludes that hospitals must adopt clear policies for their surgical teams to follow. Quotes Opinion 8.08. References Opinion 2.22. Lonchyna, *To Resuscitate or Not . . . In the Operating Room: The Need for Hospital Policies for Surgeons Regarding DNR Orders, 6 Annals Health L. 209, 215, 217 (1997)*.

Journal 1996 Examines the constitutional implications of government-subsidized speech. Proposes two key characterization questions that should be answered when undertaking legal analysis. Observes, among other things, that potential ethical conflicts may exist when governmental subsidies are utilized to control the discourse between physicians and their patients. Quotes Opinion 8.08. Post, *Subsidized Speech, 106 Yale L. J. 151, 173 (1996)*.

Journal 1996 Discusses new abortion legislation in Utah. Notes that patient consent must be obtained in accordance with AMA ethical standards, requiring physicians to provide all relevant data. Concludes that new laws require more detailed and comprehensive information be given to women. Quotes Opinion 8.08. Schnibbe, *Recent Legislative Developments in Utah Law: Family Law, 1996 Utah L. Rev. 1335, 1394 (1996)*.

Journal 1996 Considers the ethical requirement for physicians to receive informed consent from patients before beginning treatment. Reviews the case of *Jacobson v. Massachusetts*, discussing its impact on informed consent and vaccination policy in the US. Quotes Fundamental Elements (2). References Opinion 8.08. Severyn, *Jacobson v. Massachusetts: Impact on Informed Consent and Vaccine Policy, 5 J. Pharmacy & L. 249, 253, 274 (1996)*.

Journal 1995 Observes that physicians are unable to obtain informed consent because they cannot guess which treatment alternatives will best serve an individual patient's interests. Suggests that this situation would be improved if patients were paired with physicians who share their personal values. Quotes Opinion 8.08. Veatch, *Abandoning*

Informed Consent, 25 Hastings Center Rep. 5, 6 (March/April 1995).

Journal 1994 Discusses how physicians historically have taken too much license with patients' bodies and placed greater value on longevity than on quality of life. Suggests that greater emphasis should be given to physician disclosure obligations in order to improve the quality of patient consent. Quotes Opinion 8.07 (1981) [now Opinion 8.08]. Katz, *Informed Consent: Must It Remain a Fairy Tale? 10 J. Contemp. Health L. & Pol'y 69, 80 (1994).*

Journal 1994 Reviews the evolution of the physician-patient relationship, with attention to patient autonomy. Examines the changing health care delivery environment. Quotes Preamble, Principles I, II, III, IV, V, and VI, Fundamental Elements (1) and (2), and Opinions 1.02 and 8.07 (1981) [now Opinion 8.08]. Cites Opinion 1.01. Szczygiel, *Beyond Informed Consent, 21 Ohio N. U. L. Rev. 171, 217, 218, 220, 225, 226, 256 (1994).*

Journal 1993 Considers how patient self-determination may be affected by cardiopulmonary resuscitation and do-not-resuscitate policies. Opposes a "futility" exception to informed consent as being violative of a physician's fiduciary duties to patients. Cites Opinion 8.07 (1986) [now Opinion 8.08]. References Opinion 2.22. Boozang, *Death Wish: Resuscitating Self-determination for the Critically Ill, 35 Ariz. L. Rev. 23, 24, 28, 52 (1993).*

Journal 1993 Discusses physicians' duty to disclose medical treatment alternatives to patients that are not readily available. Proposes that based on the historical development and legal requirements of the informed consent doctrine, physicians should be required to inform patients of non–readily available alternatives or face liability for breach of such obligation. Quotes Principles I, II, III, IV, and V and Opinion 8.08. Note, *Informed Choice: Physicians' Duty to Disclose Nonreadily Available Alternatives, 43 Case W. Res. L. Rev. 491, 491, 498-499, 508, 509 (1993).*

Journal 1993 Examines the case of *Rust v. Sullivan*, in which the Supreme Court sustained regulations barring abortion counseling and referral at federally funded clinics. Criticizes the Court's deference to the executive branch and its failure to classify the regulations as violative of constitutional rights to free speech. Quotes Opinion 8.08. Note, *Rust on the Constitution: Politics and Gag Rules, 37 How. L. J. 83, 96 (1993).*

Journal 1993 Critiques the Supreme Court's decision in *Rust v. Sullivan*, which upheld regulations prohibiting employees of Title X–funded clinics from discussing abortions with patients. Advocates an affirmative government obligation to provide abortion counseling to Title X patients. Cites Opinion 8.08. Roberts, *Rust v. Sullivan and the Control of Knowledge, 61 Geo. Wash. L. Rev. 587, 641 (1993).*

Journal 1993 Discusses legal attempts to control reproduction by HIV-positive women. Suggests that controls will not achieve the goal of lessening children's suffering, but will discourage HIV-positive women from seeking health care services. Quotes Opinion 8.08. Sangree, *Control of Childbearing by HIV-Positive Women: Some Responses to Emerging Legal Policies, 41 Buff. L. Rev. 309, 362 (1993).*

Journal 1992 Examines the constitutionality of certain restrictions on speech in federally funded programs. Advocates greater First Amendment protections in these situations. Quotes Opinion 8.08. Cole, *Beyond Unconstitutional Conditions: Charting Spheres of Neutrality in Government-Funded Speech, 67 N. Y. U. L. Rev. 675, 744 (1992).*

Journal 1992 Discusses the problem of protecting the privacy and confidentiality of public figures in light of contemporary tabloid journalism. Argues that current tort law does not adequately address this problem and advocates a new cause of action based on breach of confidentiality. Quotes Opinion 8.08. Harvey, *Confidentiality: A Measured Response to the Failure of Privacy, 140 Univ. Pa. L. Rev. 2385, 2454 (1992).*

Journal 1992 Analyzes the case of *Rust v. Sullivan* in which the US Supreme Court let stand regulations restricting abortion counseling in federally funded clinics. Concludes that *Rust* limits this right by expanding government powers. Cites Opinion 8.08. Note, *Constitutional Law—Judicial Deference—Supreme Court Will Defer to "Reasonable" Abortion Restrictions, 14 Univ. Ark. Little Rock 557, 573 (1992).*

Journal 1992 Discusses limitations on abortion counseling in federally funded clinics in light of the US Supreme Court decision in *Rust v. Sullivan*. Concludes that the *Rust* decision improperly limits freedom of speech. Cites Opinion 8.08. Note, *The Policy Against Federal Funding for Abortions Extends Into the Realm of Free Speech After Rust v. Sullivan, 19 Pepperdine L. Rev. 637, 681 (1992).*

Journal 1991 Discusses the manner in which a changing economy and an evolving health care system require society to expand its understanding of the physician-patient relationship. Concludes that open patient-physician discussion about available medical services and costs may become part of the standard of care. References Opinions 8.08 and 8.12. Morreim, *Economic Disclosure and Economic Advocacy: New Duties in the Medical Standard of Care, 12 J. Legal Med. 275, 306 (1991).*

Journal 1991 Considers how administrative restrictions on abortion counseling in Title X–funded clinics were affected by the Supreme Court's decision in *Rust v. Sullivan*. Concludes that *Rust* expands the powers of administrative agencies and narrows First Amendment free speech rights and Fifth Amendment due process rights. Cites Opinion 8.08. Note, *Administrative Agencies Get Their Way Over Constitutional Rights in Rust v. Sullivan, 28 Willamette L. Rev. 173, 193 (1991).*

Journal 1991 Examines legal, ethical, and economic concerns surrounding pharmaceutical company promotions. Concludes that pharmaceutical freebies can serve a positive role in health care if adequately regulated. Quotes Opinions 8.061 and 8.08. Note, *The Economic Wisdom of Regulating Pharmaceutical "Freebies," 1991 Duke L. J. 206, 216, 233, 234 (1991).*

Journal 1990 Examines Minnesota's "Crack Baby" law as a response to the increasing problem of drug abuse. Concludes that Minnesota's "Crack Baby" law endangers basic constitutional rights of women. Quotes Opinion 8.07 (1986) [now Opinion 8.08]. Johnson, *Minnesota's "Crack Baby" Law: Weapon of War or Link in a Chain? 8 Law & Ineq. 485, 494, 495, 496 (1990).*

Journal 1983 Discusses both moral and legal dilemmas in the use of placebos in treating patients. Concludes that, while arguments against placebo therapy are noble, a complete ban of placebo therapy is impractical and undesirable. Quotes Opinions 8.07 (1982) [now Opinion 8.08] and 8.11 (1982) [now Opinion 8.12]. Kapp, *Placebo Therapy and the Law: Prescribe With Care, 8 Am. J. Law & Med. 371, 391 (1983).*

2.1.2 Decisions for Adult Patients Who Lack Capacity

N.Y. Fam. 2006 During proceedings regarding a foster child, an issue was raised contesting the legality of the County Department of Human Services' procedures for administering drugs to children. The mother's consent for prescribing medication to the child was obtained by a caseworker, without direct consultation with a physician and with no explanation of side effects. The court cited Opinions 8.08, 8.081, 8.11, and 10.01 in determining the physician's duty to honor the decision of the parent/surrogate. The mother's consent was invalidated and she was given an opportunity to consult with a physician. *Matter of Lyle A., 14 Misc. 3d 842, 830 N.Y.S.2d 486, 492, 494.*

Journal 2010 Discusses conflicts between surrogates and health care professionals in the context of "futile" care for patients. Further, discusses how "surrogate selection" laws may be used to replace a surrogate demanding inappropriately aggressive end-of-life treatment. Concludes that while surrogate selection has resolved some futility issues, an increase in independent ethics committees would be beneficial in dispelling other major issues. Quotes and cites Opinions 2.20 and 8.081. Pope, *Surrogate Selection: An Increasingly Viable, but Limited, Solution to Intractable Futility Disputes, 3 St. Louis U. J. Health L. & Pol'y 183, 207, 208, 211-214, 224, 228 (2010).*

Journal 2009 Examines the question of when a physician should seek a court order to override a surrogate decision maker's authority. Concludes that such an order should be sought only if the surrogate choices do not accurately reflect the wishes of the patient. Quotes Opinion 8.081. D'Amico, Krasna, Krasna, & Sade, *No Heroic Measures: How Soon Is Too Soon to Stop? 87 Ann. Thorac. Surg. 11, 17 (2009).*

Journal 2007 Discusses patients' right to refuse medical treatment and the corresponding duties of health care professionals. Concludes that detailed, carefully prepared advance directives are necessary to fulfill patients' wishes. Quotes Ch. II (1940) [now Opinions 8.08 and 8.082] and Opinions 2.035, 2.037, 2.20, 2.225, 8.081, and 10.015. Cites Opinions 9.11 and 9.115. Stamatakis, *Beyond Advance Directives: Personal Autonomy and the Right to Refuse Life-Sustaining Medical Treatment, 47 N. H. B. J. 20, 29-30 (2007).*

Journal 2006 Reviews the concept of therapeutic privilege. Concludes that the practice creates conflict between physician obligations under the concepts of autonomy and beneficence. Recommends that physicians maximize communication with patients by providing all pertinent information in the context of patient preferences. Cites Opinions 8.08, 8.081, 8.121, and 10.015. References Chap. I, Art. I, Sec. 4 (May 1847) [premise deleted from Code]. Bostick, Sade, McMahon, & Benjamin, *Report of the American Medical Association Council on Ethical and Judicial Affairs: Withholding Information From Patients: Rethinking the Propriety of "Therapeutic Privilege," 17 J. Clinical Ethics 302, 303 (Winter 2006).*

Journal 2006 Discusses the evolution of health law in Virginia. Concludes that the area of health law continues to expand, develop, and be refined. Cites Opinions 3.03, 3.08, 5.01, 5.015, 5.02, 5.04, 5.055, 6.02, 6.021, 6.03, 6.04, 7.03, 7.04, 7.05, 8.054, 8.08, 8.081, 8.085, 8.115, 8.12, 8.14, 8.145, 8.19, and 9.045. Guanzon, *Health Care Law, 41 U. Rich. L. Rev. 179, 199 (2006).*

Journal 2004 Discusses the law in Tennessee regarding surrogate decision-making. Concludes that recent legislation passed in Tennessee will assist those who care for incapacitated patients. Cites Opinions 2.035, 8.081, and 8.115. Wampler, *To Be or Not to Be in Tennessee: Deciding Surrogate Issues, 34 U. Mem. L. Rev. 333, 365 (2004).*

2.1.3 Withholding Information from Patients

Journal 2007 Analyzes problems with the current medical malpractice system. Concludes that Hillary Clinton's proposed National Medical Error and Compensation (MEDiC) Act of 2005 would be effective in facilitating physician apologies, reducing incidence of medical errors, and improving resolution of malpractice disputes. Quotes Opinion 8.12. References Opinion 8.082. Geckeler, *The Clinton-Obama Approach to Medical Malpractice Reform: Reviving the Most Meaningful Features of Alternative Dispute Resolution,* 8 Pepp. Disp. Resol. L. J. 171, 193 (2007).

Journal 2007 Discusses the evolution of informed consent doctrine. Concludes that, in context of research, informed consent exceptions should be substantially narrowed. Quotes Ch. I, Art. I, Sec. 4 (May 1847) [now Opinion 8.082] and Ch. I, Art. I, Sec. 1 (May 1847) [now Principles I and VIII]. References Opinions 2.08 and 8.08. Grimm, *Informed Consent for All! No Exceptions,* 37 N. M. L. Rev. 39, 39, 61 (2007).

Journal 2007 Discusses patients' right to refuse medical treatment and the corresponding duties of health care professionals. Concludes that detailed, carefully prepared advance directives are necessary to fulfill patients' wishes. Quotes Ch. II (1940) [now Opinions 8.08 and 8.082] and Opinions 2.035, 2.037, 2.20, 2.225, 8.081, and 10.015. Cites Opinions 9.11 and 9.115. Stamatakis, *Beyond Advance Directives: Personal Autonomy and the Right to Refuse Life-Sustaining Medical Treatment,* 47 N. H. B. J. 20, 29-30 (2007).

Journal 2007 Argues for informed consent in the process of child adoption. Concludes that prospective parents have a right to be informed of any general increases in prevalence of learning or developmental problems among adopted children. Cites Opinion 8.082. Wertheimer, *Of Apples and Trees: Adoption and Informed Consent,* 25 QLR 601, 618 (2007).

Journal 2006 Explores the possibility of "Medicare-led malpractice reform." Concludes that such reform may be successful if beneficiaries are given the proper incentives and the option of opting out. References Opinion 8.082. Kinney & Sage, *Resolving Medical Malpractice Claims in the Medicare Program: Can It Be Done?* 12 Conn. Ins. L. J. 77, 105 (2006).

2.1.4 Use of Placebo in Clinical Practice

Journal 2011 Compares academic psychiatrist patterns of placebo use with those of physicians in other specialties to evaluate physician attitudes and beliefs toward placebos. Concludes psychiatrists are less likely to report that placebos have no clinical benefit and suggests greater discussion is needed to optimally incorporate placebos into medical practice. Quotes Opinion 8.083. Raz, Campbell, Guindi, Holcraft, Déry, & Cukier, *Placebos in Clinical Practice: Comparing Attitudes, Beliefs, and Patterns of Use Between Academic Psychiatrists and Nonpsychiatrists,* 56 Can. J. Psychiatry 199 (2011).

Journal 2009 Proposes an ethical approach for the administration of opioid therapy in treatment of chronic nonmalignant pain. Concludes that bioethical principles can guide a treatment plan, but that widespread consensus is still needed on rules for ethical treatment. Cites Opinion 8.083. Novy, Ritter, & McNeill, *A Primer of Ethical Issues Involving Opioid Therapy for Chronic Nonmalignant Pain in a Multidisciplinary Setting,* 10 Pain Med. 356, 360 (2009).

2.1.6 Substitution of Surgeon

Ala. 1985 Patient sued physicians alleging fraud and conspiracy to commit fraud. The court clarified its previous holding in the case (461 So. 2d 775) that a new trial was ordered only on fraud and conspiracy to commit fraud theories. The court also noted that the trier of fact would need to decide whether the Current Opinions of the Judicial Council of the AMA pamphlet was properly excluded under the learned treatise doctrine and whether, if properly authenticated, it might be admissible at a new trial as to the issue of whether ghost surgery, condemned by Opinion 8.12 (1984) [now Opinion 8.16], constitutes fraud. *McMurray v. Johnson,* 481 So. 2d 887, 889.

Md. 2000 Plaintiff scheduled surgery with the defendant physician. During surgery, a resident mistakenly dissected the common bile duct. Plaintiff sued for negligence and breach of contract, alleging that defendant had agreed personally to perform all incisions. The circuit court dismissed the contract claim as subsumed by the negligence claim. While the Court of Appeals of Maryland found a contractual relationship does exist between a physician and patient, citing Opinions 8.12 (1982) [now Opinion 8.16] and 8.16, the court nonetheless held for the physician because the jury had found he never made the alleged promise. *Dingle v. Belin,* 358 Md. 354, 749 A.2d 157, 168.

Md. App. 1999 Patient sued hospital and the surgeon named in consent form for negligence and breach of contract. The plaintiff claimed that the defendants breached their contract when a resident performed surgery, rather than the surgeon authorized by the plaintiff. The trial court dismissed the breach of contract claim and entered judgment upon the jury verdict for the defendants. The appeals court cited Opinion 8.12 (1982) [now Opinion 8.16], stating that it is unethical and deceitful for another surgeon to perform an operation without the patient's knowledge or consent. *Belin v. Dingle, 127 Md. App. 68, 732 A.2d 301, 302-03, 307.*

N.J. 1983 Patient who consented to surgery by one surgeon, but was actually operated on by another, sued both surgeons. Pursuant to state law, patient submitted case to malpractice panel, which found no basis to patient's claims, and jury returned verdict for defendant surgeons. In holding that failure to permit plaintiff to show possible bias of panel doctor and to impeach the testimony constituted reversible error, the court quoted Opinion 8.12 (1982) [now Opinion 8.16] indicating that substitution of one surgeon for another without patient consent is a deceit and deviates from standard medical care, constituting the violation of a legal obligation as well as a tenet of the medical profession. *Perna v. Pirozzi, 92 N.J. 446, 457 A.2d 431, 434, 440, n.3.*

N.J. Super. 1991 Two physicians were sued by a patient claiming that one of the physician-surgeons had committed "ghost surgery" battery. The court acknowledged the rule in *Perna v. Pirozzi*, 92 N.J. 446, 457 A.2d 431 (1983). The court there, taking judicial notice of the standard of care set out by Opinion 8.12 (1982) [now Opinion 8.16], held that an intent to injure is not required to establish battery when a medical procedure is performed by a "substitute" physician. However, the court here held that the plaintiff had failed to establish by competent medical opinion that one of the physicians was an unauthorized operating surgeon. Furthermore, the court stated that to hold otherwise would create a punitive damage claim based on a patient's lay opinion concerning the proper role of an authorized surgeon in team surgery. *Monturi v. Englewood Hosp., 246 N.J. Super. 547, 552, 588 A.2d 408, 410, 411.*

N.J. Super. 1982 In a medical malpractice suit against a surgeon for negligence and for allowing a different surgeon to operate on plaintiff without plaintiff's express consent, the court noted Opinions and Reports of the Judicial Council Sec. 1, Para. 5 (1969) [now Opinion 8.16] as quoted in 209 *JAMA* 947-48 (1969) that it is fraudulent and deceitful for a surgeon to allow another surgeon to operate on a patient without that patient's consent. The court ultimately concluded that the doctrine of informed consent is a theory of professional liability independent from malpractice, and thus was not relevant to the case at bar. *Perna v. Pirozzi, 182 N.J. Super. 510, 442 A.2d 1016, 1019, rev'd, 92 N.J. 446, 457 A.2d 431 (1983).*

Okla. App. 1974 Owner of a bull sued veterinarian for malpractice and failure to disclose possible adverse reactions to penicillin. The appellate court held that the veterinarian was liable for damages to the plaintiff resulting from the death of the bull. In so holding, the court noted Opinions and Reports of the Judicial Council Sec. 1, Para. 5 (1969) [now Opinion 8.16] which, inter alia, requires a surgeon to make a complete disclosure of all facts relevant to the operation to be performed. *Hull v. Tate, No. 46443 (Okla. Ct. App. April 16, 1974) (LEXIS, States library, Okla. file), rev'd, No. 46443 (Okla. Sup. Ct. Oct. 29, 1974) (LEXIS, States library, Okla. file).*

Pa. Super. 1998 Parents of child who died during a catheterization procedure sued the pediatrician, cardiologist, and the hospital on various theories including battery. In referring to an earlier decision, the court quoted Opinion 8.12 (1982) [now Opinion 8.16], in support of a patient's right to consent to a specific physician to perform a medical procedure. The court held that the jury should have decided whether the parents consented for the pediatrician, instead of the cardiologist, to perform the procedure. *Taylor v. Albert Einstein Medical Ctr., 723 A.2d 1027, 1036.*

Pa. Super. 1996 Physician told patient he would perform necessary surgery. As a result of the surgery, patient developed a drop foot which would drag whenever he walked. The patient later discovered that his treating physician did not appear for or participate in his surgery. When the hospital was unable to reach the physician, it contacted his office where another physician instructed the hospital to perform the surgery with a third physician. All of this was done without patient's consent and was not disclosed after recovery. Patient sued the physician for failure to perform the surgery and for directing or permitting a third party to perform the surgery. The court quoted from Opinion 8.12 (1982) [now Opinion 8.16] which provides that the patient is entitled to choose his or her physician and should be permitted to acquiesce in or refuse to accept any substitutions. *Grabowski v. Quigley, 454 Pa. Super. 27, 684 A.2d 610, 617.*

Journal 2006 Evaluates standard of care rules for medical residents. Proposes a minimum standard equivalent to that of a general practitioner and an appropriate standard of care for residents who fully disclose their status. Quotes Opinions 8.12 (1982) [now Opinion 8.16] and Opinion 8.16. King, *The Standard of Care for Residents and Other Medical School Graduates in Training,* 55 Am. U. L. Rev. 683, 727 (2006).

Journal 2006 Reviews informed consent law. Concludes that physicians in certain jurisdictions may be required to disclose their level of experience. Quotes Opinion 8.12 (1982) [now Opinion 8.16]. Wiltbank, *Informed Consent and Physician Inexperience: A Prescription for Liability?* 42 Willamette L. Rev. 563, 570 (2006).

Journal 1996 Considers how practice guidelines may be used in malpractice litigation as inculpatory or exculpatory evidence. Concludes that use of guidelines as inculpatory evidence should not be eliminated until there is evidence of undesirable effects. Quotes Opinion 8.16. Hyams, Shapiro, & Brennan, *Medical Practice Guidelines in Malpractice Litigation: An Early Retrospective,* 21 J. Health Pol. Pol'y & L. 289, 298 (1996).

Journal 1996 Discusses tort liability in cases of substitution of surgeons without patient consent. Explores whether substitutions are a battery thereby allowing recovery, regardless of outcome. Concludes that ghost surgery should not automatically constitute a battery but that courts should allow recovery for infliction of emotional distress stemming from the substitution. Quotes Opinion 8.12 (1982) [now Opinion 8.16]. Lundmark, *Surgery by an Unauthorized Surgeon as a Battery*, 10 J. L. & Health 287, 293 (1996).

2.2.2 Confidential Health Care for Minors

Journal 2010 Discusses issues arising from the enactment of legislation by North Dakota involving a minor's reproductive rights. Explores ethical principles that govern physician's actions within the context of reproductive health. Concludes that, while a patient's expectation of confidentiality with a physician is critical, competing values come into play when the patient is a minor and parental involvement may be important. Provides practical guidance to address issues in this context. Quotes Opinions 2.01, 2.015, 5.055, 8.08, 8.115, 9.12, 10.01, 10.015, and 10.05. Cites Opinions 5.05, 5.055, 8.08, 8.11, 8.115, 9.12, and 10.05. Haas, *"Doctor, I'm Pregnant and Fifteen—I Can't Tell My Parents—Please Help Me": Minor Consent, Reproductive Rights, and Ethical Principles for Physicians*, 86 N.D. L. Rev. 63, 70, 73, 75-78, 82, 84, 86-88 (2010).

Journal 2010 Discusses the importance of adolescent consent and confidentiality in providing quality health care to youth. Summarizes the relevant legal and ethical principles related to adolescent consent and confidentiality. Concludes the confidential care of minors is an integral component of routine adolescent care. Quotes Opinion 5.055. Berlan & Bravender, *Confidentiality, Consent and Caring for the Adolescent Patient*, 21 Current Opinion Pediatrics 450, 455 (2009).

Journal 2008 Discusses confidentiality rights of pediatric patients and the ethical considerations of physicians when establishing policies for managing patient confidentiality. Concludes that physicians must exercise discretion to protect the health interests of pediatric patients. Quotes Opinion 5.055. McGuire & Bruce, *Keeping Children's Secrets: Confidentiality in the* physician-patient *Relationship, 8 Hous. J. Health L. & Pol'y 315, 332 (2008)*.

Journal 2006 Discusses the evolution of health law in Virginia. Concludes that the area of health law continues to expand, develop, and be refined. Cites Opinions 3.03, 3.08, 5.01, 5.015, 5.02, 5.04, 5.055, 6.02, 6.021, 6.03, 6.04, 7.03, 7.04, 7.05, 8.054, 8.08, 8.081, 8.085, 8.115, 8.12, 8.14, 8.145, 8.19, and 9.045. Guanzon, *Health Care Law, 41 U. Rich. L. Rev. 179, 199 (2006)*.

Journal 2003 Highlights HIPAA privacy issues that need to be monitored and have yet to be resolved. Concludes that HIPAA poses many challenges and it remains unclear whether HIPAA will increase privacy protection. Cites Opinions 5.05, 5.055, 5.057, 5.06, 5.07, 5.075, 5.08, and 5.09. Kutzko, Boyer, Thoman, & Scott, *HIPAA in Real Time: Practical Implications of the Federal Privacy Rule, 51 Drake L. Rev. 403, 408 (2003)*.

Journal 2003 Considers the legal, medical, and ethical issues of physician-patient confidentiality in disclosure of paternity. Concludes that a balancing test should be applied to making determinations regarding disclosure of paternity. Quotes Principles I, IV, and V and Opinions 1.02, 5.055, and 10.01. Cites Principle II and Opinion 5.05. Richards & Wolf, *Medical Confidentiality and Disclosure of Paternity, 48 S. D. L. Rev. 409, 411, 412, 413 (2003)*.

2.2.3 Mandatory Parental Consent to Abortion

6th Cir. 1999 Plaintiff challenged state law requiring minors to appeal, within 24 hours, a denied petition to bypass parental consent to obtain an abortion. The court stated that the 24-hour appeal requirement did not unduly burden the minor's ability to obtain an abortion. The dissent cited Opinion 2.015, to support its view that the 24-hour appeal requirement imposed an undue burden by jeopardizing the minor's ability to obtain an abortion. *Memphis Planned Parenthood v. Sundquist, 175 F.3d 456, 473*.

8th Cir. 1995 Court held several provisions of the South Dakota abortion law unconstitutional, including parental notice provision. In ruling that parental notice requirement, which lacked a bypass provision, unduly burdened liberty interests of some minors, the court cited AMA Council on Ethical and Judicial Affairs, Mandatory Parental Consent to Abortion, 269 *JAMA* 82 (1993) [now Opinion 2.015]. *Planned Parenthood v. Miller, 63 F.3d 1452, 1462*.

Mass. 1997 Plaintiffs brought suit seeking a declaration that statute prohibiting, with certain exceptions, a pregnant unmarried minor from obtaining an abortion unless either both parents consent or a judge authorizes the procedure, is unconstitutional. The court concluded that the statute did not facially violate due process or equal protection and was thus constitutional. However, the court struck down the provision requiring both parents' consent as lacking sufficient justification to overcome the minor's constitutional right to choose. The court cited AMA Council on Ethical and Judicial Affairs, Mandatory Parental Consent to Abortion, 269

JAMA 82 (1993) [now Opinion 2.015]. *Planned Parenthood League of Massachusetts, Inc. v. Attorney General, 424 Mass. 586, 596, 608, 677 N.E.2d 101, 107, 114.*

N.J. 2000 Prior to the effective date of the Parental Notification for Abortion Act, the plaintiffs sought a declaratory judgment and preliminary injunction precluding the enforcement of the Act. The trial court dismissed the challenge, but the state Supreme Court struck down the statute. The state, in support of the Act, argued that it was passed to facilitate and foster familial communications. The court rejected this as a legitimate governmental interest, noting that the Act applies to many young women who are justified in not telling their parents about their abortion decisions. The court quoted AMA Council on Ethics and Judicial Affairs, Mandatory Parental Consent to Abortion, 269 *JAMA* 82 (1983) [now Opinion 2.015] in support of this argument. *Planned Parenthood of Central New Jersey v. Farmer, 165 N.J. 609, 762 A.2d 620, 640.*

Journal 2010 Discusses issues arising from the enactment of legislation by North Dakota involving a minor's reproductive rights. Explores ethical principles that govern physician's actions within the context of reproductive health. Concludes that, while a patient's expectation of confidentiality with a physician is critical, competing values come into play when the patient is a minor and parental involvement may be important. Provides practical guidance to address issues in this context. Quotes Opinions 2.01, 2.015, 5.055, 8.08, 8.115, 9.12, 10.01, 10.015, and 10.05. Cites Opinions 5.05, 5.055, 8.08, 8.11, 8.115, 9.12, and 10.05. Haas, *"Doctor, I'm Pregnant and Fifteen—I Can't Tell My Parents—Please Help Me": Minor Consent, Reproductive Rights, and Ethical Principles for Physicians, 86 N.D. L. Rev. 63, 70, 73, 75-78, 82, 84, 86-88 (2010).*

Journal 2003 Uses the medical self-consent rights of minors to challenge the legal assumption that teens lack decisional capacity for abortions. Concludes with discussion of an empirical study that supports this challenge. References Opinion 2.015. Ehrlich, *Grounded in the Reality of Their Lives: Listening to Teens Who Make the Abortion Decision Without Involving Their Parents, 18 Berkeley Women's L. J. 61, 72, 84-85, 175-76 (2003).*

Journal 2003 Explores conflict in the legal treatment of minors in situations involving reproductive decision-making and the commission of crimes. Concludes that different approaches are justified. References Opinion 2.015. Ehrlich, *Shifting Boundaries: Abortion, Criminal Culpability and the Indeterminate Legal Status of Adolescents, 18 Wis. Women's L. J. 77, 105 (2003).*

Journal 2002 Argues attorneys should be appointed to represent minors in judicial bypass proceedings. Concludes that appointing a guardian ad litem raises ethical and constitutional problems. References Opinion 2.015. Graybill, *Assisting Minors Seeking Abortions in Judicial Bypass Proceedings: A Guardian Ad Litem Is No Substitute for an Attorney, 55 Vand. L. Rev. 581, 583 (2002).*

Journal 2002 Examines how Alabama juvenile courts are handling petitions for waiver of parental consent for abortion. Concludes the courts are not correctly handling these matters, thus adversely affecting the rights of pregnant minors. References Opinion 2.015. Silverstein & Speitel, *"Honey, I Have No Idea": Court Readiness to Handle Petitions to Waive Parental Consent for Abortion, 88 Iowa L. Rev. 75, 116, 117 (2002).*

Journal 2001 Considers proposed state legislation requiring a minor to notify a parent when she intends to obtain an abortion. Concludes that notification serves the minor's best interests. References Opinion 2.015. Collett, *Protecting Our Daughters: The Need for the Vermont Parental Notification Law, 26 Vt. L. Rev. 101, 106-07 (2001).*

Journal 2000 Explores issues associated with mandatory parental consent to abortion laws. Examines the failure of the US Supreme Court to consider medical decision-making by minors when evaluating the constitutionality of such laws. References Opinion 2.015. Ehrlich, *Minors as Medical Decision Makers: The Pretextual Reasoning of the Court in the Abortion Cases, 7 Mich. J. Gender & L. 65, 91 (2000).*

Journal 1999 Discusses minors' rights to an abortion. Examines parental notification requirements and procedures to bypass parental notification laws. Argues that minors should be afforded the same rights in seeking an abortion as adult women. References Opinion 2.015. Katz, *The Pregnant Child's Right to Self-determination, 62 Alb. L. Rev. 1119, 1142 (1999).*

Journal 1998 Discusses parental consent laws pertaining to minors seeking abortions. Examines *Roe v. Wade* and the federal constitutional challenge to the Massachusetts parental consent law. States that the purpose of parental involvement laws is to limit abortion rights, rather than to promote family discourse. References Opinion 2.015. Ehrlich, *Journey Through the Courts: Minors, Abortion and the Quest for Reproductive Fairness, 10 Yale J. L. & Feminism 1, 19 (1998).*

Journal 1997 Addresses the issue of teenage pregnancy. Examines governmental actions that have made it more difficult for teenagers to receive abortions. Suggests that parental consent and judicial bypass provisions are an infringement on their reproductive freedom. Advocates lawyer participation in abortion reform. References Opinion 2.015. Schiff, *The Lawyer's Role in Restoring Adolescents' Abortion Rights, 44 Fed. Law. 60, 62 (May 1997).*

Journal 1996 Reviews Supreme Court decisions that address parental involvement in the abortion decisions of mature minors. Suggests that the Court's position on parental involvement should be reevaluated. Posits that many young women are mature enough to make their own pregnancy decisions. References Opinion 2.015. O'Shaughnessy, *The Worst of Both Worlds? Parental Involvement Requirements and the Privacy Rights of Mature Minors, 57 Ohio St. L. J. 1731, 1764-65 (1996).*

2.2.4 Treatment Decisions for Seriously Ill Newborns

N.Y. Sup. 2003 Mother petitioned court to remove her daughter from a respirator. Hospital policy denied mother the authorization to withdraw care. Court granted petition and held parents have a right to refuse medical treatment for their children. Applying the best interest test, the court held that the burdens of prolonging life exceeded the benefits and that, absent extraordinary circumstances or disagreement between parents, judicial intervention is not required to withhold medical treatment from a minor in a vegetative state. Quotes Opinion 2.215. References Opinion 2.20. *In re AB, 196 Misc. 2d 940, 768 N.Y.S. 2d 256, 268-69.*

Journal 2004 Discusses the lack of a rational basis for a distinction between physician-assisted suicide and a physician's cooperation with a patient's refusal of life-sustaining treatment. Concludes that once legally permissible means of hastening death are widely known by physicians, restrictions on physician-assisted death may become anomalous. Cites Opinion 2.215. Cantor, *On Kamisar, Killing, and the Future of Physician-Assisted Death, 102 Mich. L. Rev. 1793, 1825 (2004).*

Journal 2002 Explores the implications of withholding medical treatment when abortion results in a live birth. Concludes that, in these situations, abortive parents and physicians should not solely decide the child's best interest. Quotes Preamble, Principles I and III, and Opinions 2.035, 2.20, and 2.215. Casagrande, *Children Not Meant to Be: Protecting the Interests of the Child When Abortion Results in Live Birth, 6 Quinnipiac Health L. J. 19, 44, 45, 47-48 (2002).*

Journal 2001 Examines end-of-life care given to infants under the age of one. Concludes that palliative care consultations may improve the end-of-life care that terminally ill infants and their families currently receive. References Opinion 2.215. Pierucci, Kirby, & Leuthner, *End-of-Life Care for Neonates and Infants: The Experience and Effects of a Palliative Care Consultation Service, 108 Pediatrics 653, 659 (2001).*

Journal 2001 Discusses neonatal euthanasia and the related moral dilemmas. Explores the background and current legal status of neonatal euthanasia in the US. Concludes that the moral and legal status of passive neonatal euthanasia is unclear and should be reviewed and clarified. Quotes Opinion 2.215. Sklansky, *Neonatal Euthanasia: Moral Considerations and Criminal Liability, 27 J. Med. Ethics 5, 8, 9 (2001).*

2.2.5 Genetic Testing of Children

Journal 2007 Explores the impact of genetic testing on disability insurance. Concludes that predictive genetic tests should not act to limit access to disability insurance. Cites Opinion 2.138. Wolf & Kahn, *Genetic Testing and the Future of Disability Insurance: Ethics, Law & Policy, 35 J. L. Med. & Ethics 6, 23 (2007).*

Journal 1999 Discusses regulatory concerns regarding genetic technology. Provides ideas on how society might regulate genetic enhancements. Argues that a variety of means of regulation need to be utilized to govern genetic technology. Quotes Opinion 2.11. Cites Opinion 9.065. References Opinion 2.138. Mehlman, *How Will We Regulate Genetic Enhancement? 34 Wake Forest L. Rev. 671, 693-94, 695 (1999).*

Journal 1998 Discusses ramifications of genetic research. Points out that genetic information affects not only the tested individual, but the person's family as well. Suggests that a greater awareness of potential risk will reduce possible hazards stemming from genetic research. Cites Opinion 2.138. Green & Thomas, *DNA: Five Distinguishing Features for Policy Analysis, 11 Harv. J. L. & Tech. 571, 582-83 (1998).*

Journal 1997 Discusses the National Human Genome Research Institute and the activities of the Office of Genome Ethics. Offers an overview and evaluation, with emphasis on bioethical education and counsel that was provided to genetic researchers. References Opinion 2.138. Green, *NHGRI's Intramural Ethics Experiment, 7 Kennedy Inst. of Ethics J. 181, 185, 188 (1997).*

2.3.1 Health Information Sites and Services Outside an Existing Patient-Physician Relationship

Wash. App. 2007 The defendant-physician resided in New Jersey and was licensed to practice medicine in Washington. Complaints were filed alleging he had prescribed pharmaceuticals over the Internet without any direct contact with patients. His license was revoked by the State Department of Health for unprofessional conduct. Defendant appealed, challenging the sufficiency of the evidence proving he created an unreasonable risk of harm to patients. With apparent reference to Opinions 5.026 and 5.027, the court found that defendant violated the AMA's ethical guidelines. The court reasoned that the Opinions are incorporated into state guidelines and are highly persuasive. The court found ample evidence to show defendant created an unreasonable risk to patients. *Ancier v. State Dept. of Health, 140 Wash. App 564, 166 P.3d 829, 833, 836, 837.*

Journal 2010 Explores how participation in online social networks may blur boundaries between personal and professional relationships for health care professionals and how such risks may be mitigated by use of network privacy and security settings. Suggests that health care institutions are likely to institute online social-networking policies for employees. Quotes Opinions 5.026, 5.027, 5.045, 5.046, 5.05, 5.059, 5.0591, 8.14, 9.08, and 9.123. Cites Opinions 5.026, 9.031, and 9.12. Terry, *Physicians and Patients Who "Friend" or "Tweet": Constructing a Legal Framework for Social Networking in a Highly Regulated Domain, 43 Ind. L. Rev. 285, 314-16, 319, 334-36, 338 (2010).*

Journal 2004 Explores whether treatment of patients over the Internet without a prior physician-patient relationship is

a violation of conventional standards of care. Concludes that the Federation of State Medical Boards must address this concern and that uniform online medicine guidelines must be adopted by the states. References Opinion 5.027. Reed, *Cybermedicine: Defying and Redefining Patient Standards of Care, 37 Ind. L. Rev. 845, 850, 859, 862 (2004).*

Journal 2004 Discusses legal and policy issues surrounding Internet drug prescribing and dispensing. Concludes that the current regulatory scheme may impede development of innovative and efficient online prescription models. Quotes Opinion 5.026. References 5.027. Terry, *Prescriptions sans Frontières (or How I Stopped Worrying About Viagra on the Web but Grew Concerned About the Future of Healthcare Delivery), 4 Yale J. Health Pol'y L. & Ethics 183, 240, 244, 251 (2004).*

2.3.2 Electronic Communication with Patients

Wash. App. 2007 The defendant-physician resided in New Jersey and was licensed to practice medicine in Washington. Complaints were filed alleging he had prescribed pharmaceuticals over the Internet without any direct contact with patients. His license was revoked by the State Department of Health for unprofessional conduct. Defendant appealed, challenging the sufficiency of the evidence proving he created an unreasonable risk of harm to patients. With apparent reference to Opinions 5.026 and 5.027, the court found that defendant violated the AMA's ethical guidelines. The court reasoned that the Opinions are incorporated into state guidelines and are highly persuasive. The court found ample evidence to show defendant created an unreasonable risk to patients. *Ancier v. State Dept. of Health, 140 Wash. App 564, 166 P.3d 829, 833, 836, 837.*

Journal 2010 Explores how participation in online social networks may blur boundaries between personal and professional relationships for health care professionals and how such risks may be mitigated by use of network privacy and security settings. Suggests that health care institutions are likely to institute online social-networking policies for employees. Quotes Opinions 5.026, 5.027, 5.045, 5.046, 5.05, 5.059, 5.0591, 8.14, 9.08, and 9.123. Cites Opinions 5.026, 9.031, and 9.12. Terry, *Physicians and Patients Who "Friend" or "Tweet": Constructing a Legal Framework for*

Social Networking in a Highly Regulated Domain, 43 Ind. L. Rev. 285, 314-16, 319, 334-36, 338 (2010).

Journal 2006 Argues that state and federal law enforcement agencies are unable to regulate online sale of pharmaceuticals. Concludes that alternative tactics must be used, such as controlling the price of pharmaceuticals. Quotes Opinion 5.026 (incorrectly cited as 5.06). Castronova, *Operation Cyber Chase and Other Agency Efforts to Control Internet Drug Trafficking, 27 J. Legal Med. 207, 219 (2006).*

Journal 2006 Argues that states have authority to regulate Internet pharmacies within the constraints of the Dormant Commerce Clause. Concludes that the federal government does not have sole authority to regulate Internet pharmacies. References Opinion 5.026. Vanderstappen, *Internet Pharmacies and the Specter of the Dormant Commerce Clause, 22 Wash. U. J. L. & Pol'y 619, 628 (2006).*

Journal 2004 Discusses legal and policy issues surrounding Internet drug prescribing and dispensing. Concludes that the current regulatory scheme may impede development of innovative and efficient online prescription models. Quotes Opinion 5.026. References 5.027. Terry, *Prescriptions sans Frontières (or How I Stopped Worrying About Viagra on the Web but Grew Concerned About the Future of Healthcare Delivery), 4 Yale J. Health Pol'y L. & Ethics 183, 240, 244, 251 (2004).*

2.3.4 Informing Families of a Patient's Death

Journal 1995 Examines four essential principles of bioethics—patient autonomy, nonmaleficence, beneficence, and justice—and describes the application of these in clinical settings according to bioethical norms and AMA opinions. Concludes that such an approach promotes compassionate

medical caregiving and that laws should reflect these values. Quotes Opinions 2.01 and 8.18. References Opinion 2.211. Cohen, *Toward a Bioethics of Compassion, 28 Ind. L. Rev. 667, 673, 681-82, 683 (1995).*

2.3.5 Political Communications

Journal 2009 Considers a physician's role in educating patients about health care reform. Concludes that reform would be aided by educating patients on all aspects of the health care system. Quotes Opinion 10.015. Cites Opinion 9.012. Abemayor, *United We Stand, Divided We Fall, 135 Arch. Otolaryngol. Head Neck Surg. 432, 432, 433 (2009).*

2.3.6 Soliciting Charitable Contributions from Patients

Journal 2008 Argues that organ donation from a patient to his or her physician is unethical. Concludes that this practice would be exploitative to the patient and undermine public trust in the medical profession. Cites Opinions 8.14, 10.017, and 10.018. Steinberg & Pomfret, *A Novel Boundary Issue: Should a Patient Be an Organ Donor for Their Physician? 34 J. Med. Ethics 772, 772 (2008).*

Journal 2006 Examines the practice by physicians of billing a malpractice surcharge. Concludes that such practice is unethical and constitutes a breach of fiduciary duty. Quotes Opinions 10.015 and 10.018. Peterson, *The Malpractice Surcharge: A Simple Answer to Rising Malpractice Rates or a Greater Threat to Quality Patient Care? 27 J. Legal Med. 87, 96, 97-98 (2006).*

3 Privacy, Confidentiality and Medical Records

3.1.3 Privacy in Health Care

Utah App. 2006 Following an automobile accident, plaintiff filed a personal injury suit against the driver. Plaintiff discovered that his treating physician had been subpoenaed by the driver's lawyer, had agreed to testify against plaintiff, and had engaged in ex parte communications with defense counsel. Plaintiff sued the physician. With apparent reference to Opinions 5.05 and 5.059 plaintiff relied in part on the AMA ethical principles to establish the standard of care. The court of appeals held that the physician could be liable for breach of the fiduciary duty of confidentiality as well as for intentional infliction of emotional distress. *Sorensen v. Barbuto, 143 P.3d 295, 299.*

Journal 2010 Explores how participation in online social networks may blur boundaries between personal and professional relationships for health care professionals and how such risks may be mitigated by use of network privacy and security settings. Suggests that health care institutions are likely to institute online social-networking policies for employees. Quotes Opinions 5.026, 5.027, 5.045, 5.046, 5.05, 5.059, 5.0591, 8.14, 9.08, and 9.123. Cites Opinions 5.026, 9.031, and 9.12. Terry, *Physicians and Patients Who "Friend" or "Tweet": Constructing a Legal Framework for Social Networking in a Highly Regulated Domain, 43 Ind. L. Rev. 285, 314-16, 319, 334-36, 338 (2010).*

Journal 2007 Explores solutions to the growing need for palliative care of prison inmates. Concludes that a partnership between community and correctional physicians is the optimal solution. References Opinion 5.059. Linder & Meyers, *"Don't Let Me Die in Prison"—Palliative Care for Prison Inmates, 298 JAMA 894, 898 (2007).*

3.1.2 Patient Privacy and Outside Observers of the Clinical Encounter

Journal 2010 Explores how participation in online social networks may blur boundaries between personal and professional relationships for health care professionals and how such risks may be mitigated by use of network privacy and security settings. Suggests that health care institutions are likely to institute online social-networking policies for employees. Quotes Opinions 5.026, 5.027, 5.045, 5.046, 5.05, 5.059, 5.0591, 8.14, 9.08, and 9.123. Cites Opinions 5.026, 9.031, and 9.12. Terry, *Physicians and Patients Who "Friend" or "Tweet": Constructing a Legal Framework for Social Networking in a Highly Regulated Domain, 43 Ind. L. Rev. 285, 314-16, 319, 334-36, 338 (2010).*

3.1.3 Audio or Visual Recording of Patients for Education in Health Care

Journal 2010 Explores how participation in online social networks may blur boundaries between personal and professional relationships for health care professionals and how such risks may be mitigated by use of network privacy and security settings. Suggests that health care institutions are likely to institute online social-networking policies for employees. Quotes Opinions 5.026, 5.027, 5.045, 5.046, 5.05, 5.059, 5.0591, 8.14, 9.08, and 9.123. Cites Opinions 5.026, 9.031, and 9.12. Terry, *Physicians and Patients Who "Friend" or "Tweet": Constructing a Legal Framework for Social Networking in a Highly Regulated Domain, 43 Ind. L. Rev. 285, 314-16, 319, 334-36, 338 (2010).*

3.1.4 Audio or Visual Recording of Patients for Public Education

Journal 2010 Explores how participation in online social networks may blur boundaries between personal and professional relationships for health care professionals and how such risks may be mitigated by use of network privacy and security settings. Suggests that health care institutions are likely to institute online social-networking policies for employees. Quotes Opinions 5.026, 5.027, 5.045, 5.046, 5.05, 5.059, 5.0591, 8.14, 9.08, and 9.123. Cites Opinions 5.026, 9.031, and 9.12. Terry, *Physicians and Patients Who "Friend" or "Tweet": Constructing a Legal Framework for Social Networking in a Highly Regulated Domain, 43 Ind. L. Rev. 285, 314-16, 319, 334-36, 338 (2010).*

3.1.5 Professionalism in Relationships with Media

Journal 2006 Discusses the evolution of health law in Virginia. Concludes that the area of health law continues to expand, develop, and be refined. Cites Opinions 3.03, 3.08, 5.01, 5.015, 5.02, 5.04, 5.055, 6.02, 6.021, 6.03, 6.04, 7.03, 7.04, 7.05, 8.054, 8.08, 8.081, 8.085, 8.115, 8.12, 8.14, 8.145, 8.19, and 9.045. Guanzon, *Health Care Law, 41 U. Rich. L. Rev. 179, 199 (2006).*

Journal 1999 Explores the increased use of physician-patient communication through e-mail. Analyzes current laws regarding medical privacy. Suggests that patients' communications to their physicians are part of their medical record and should be given the same protections. Quotes Opinions 5.05 and 5.07. Cites Opinions 5.04 and 5.06. Spielberg, *Online Without a Net: physician-patient Communication by Electronic Mail, 25 Am. J. Law & Med. 267, 284-85 (1999).*

Journal 1998 Examines the use of e-mail in the physician-patient relationship. Focuses on privacy concerns stemming from the use of e-mail in the medical context. Suggests that physicians should discuss the implications of communicating through e-mail with their patients and should obtain informed consent prior to communicating in this manner. Cites Opinions 5.04, 5.05, 5.057, 5.07, 5.075, and 5.08.

Spielberg, *On Call and Online: Sociohistorical, Legal, and Ethical Implications of E-mail for the Patient-Physician Relationship, 280 JAMA 1353, 1356 (1998).*

Journal 1995 Addresses presidential disability, its past impact on American government, and possible solutions to potential problems. Proposes enhancement of the role of the President's physician. Quotes Opinion 8.03. Cites Opinions 5.04 and 5.05. Abrams, *The Vulnerable President and the Twenty-Fifth Amendment, With Observations on Guidelines, a Health Commission, and the Role of the President's Physician, 30 Wake Forest L. Rev. 453, 466, 471 (1995).*

Journal 1984 Observes that available ethical and legal guidelines are insufficient to aid physicians in addressing issues of patient privacy and confidentiality. Concludes that there is need for legislation in order to provide suitable guidance to physicians who fulfill an important role in protecting patient privacy. Cites 1982 Opinions 5.03 [now Opinion 5.04], 5.04, 5.05 [now Opinion 5.06], 5.06 [now Opinion 5.07], 5.07 [now Opinion 5.08], and 5.08 [now Opinion 5.09]. Gellman, *Prescribing Privacy: The Uncertain Role of the Physician in the Protection of Patient Privacy, 62 No. Carolina L. Rev. 255, 271 (1984).*

3.2.1 Confidentiality

US 2001 Obstetrical patients at a state university hospital who were arrested after testing positive for cocaine filed suit challenging the nonconsensual drug tests given to them by the hospital and later used for law enforcement purposes. The lower courts found for the respondents. The Supreme Court reversed, finding the searches unconstitutional and not within the "special needs" category of constitutional, nonconsensual searches. The Court quoted Opinion 5.05, noting that this was not a case where the physicians were required to report to law enforcement the threat of harm by a patient. *Ferguson v. City of Charleston, 532 US 67, 121 S. Ct. 1281, 1290.*

E.D. Ark. 1992 Plaintiff sought an injunction to prevent defendant's attorneys from contacting patient's nonparty treating physicians and interviewing them privately without the patient's consent. Quoting Opinion 5.05, the court stated that patients have a right not to have privileged information disclosed by their physician without express authorization. While the privilege may be partially waived where the patient's medical condition is put in issue by the filing of a lawsuit, patients still retain the right to insist that disclosure be made pursuant to formal discovery methods, absent express consent to ex parte contact. *Harlan v. Lewis, 141 F.R.D. 107, 109 n.5.*

D. Kan. 1991 With apparent reliance on Principle IV and Opinion 5.05, plaintiff claimed that other than in discovery or judicial proceedings, the physician-patient privilege is absolute and precludes ex parte communications with defense counsel. While recognizing the confidential nature of the physician-patient relationship, the court held that the ethical standards promulgated by the AMA are not binding law and that, where a litigant-patient has placed his or her medical status in issue, the physician is released from the constraints imposed by the physician-patient relationship for the purposes of the litigation. *Bryant v. Hilst, 136 F.R.D. 487, 490.*

E.D. La. 2005 Plaintiff filed a motion to modify the district court's order requiring five days' notice to opposing counsel before interviewing plaintiff's prescribing physician. The court quoted Opinion 5.05 and cited Principle IV when discussing the physician-patient relationship and the physician's duty to protect confidences revealed by a patient. The court granted the plaintiff's motion and modified the order to ensure that defendants were faced with the same restrictions as the plaintiff and that plaintiff could conduct ex parte interviews with physicians not named as defendants. *In re Vioxx Products Liability Litigation, 230 F.R.D. 473, 476 n. 17.*

E.D. Pa. 1992 Patient sued state mental institution and psychiatrist for violation of her right to privacy under the Fourteenth Amendment. Defendants had disclosed to law enforcement personnel and to plaintiff's supervisor threats made by plaintiff during the course of her treatment. While recognizing a strong public policy against breaches of confidentiality, the court held that the state's interest in protecting its citizens from serious bodily harm was overriding. The court noted that the limits placed on patient-therapist confidentiality by Opinion 5.05 (1989) are in accordance with the judicially recognized duty that a mental health professional take reasonable steps to prevent harm to others threatened by his or her patient. *Ms. B. v. Montgomery County Emergency Service, Inc., 799 F. Supp. 534, 539 cert denied, 114 S.Ct. 174 (1993).*

M.D. Pa. 1987 Plaintiff in a medical malpractice action sought to preclude his treating physicians from serving as defendant's expert witnesses at trial. The court held that

defense counsel's failure to provide prior notice of ex parte communication with plaintiff's treating physicians barred their use as defense experts. Referring to *Petrillo v. Syntex Laboratories, Inc.*, 148 Ill. App. 3d 581, 499 N.E.2d 952 (1986), the court noted that the court there favorably cited Principle IV and Opinions 5.05, 5.06, and 5.07 (1984) in support of a public policy protecting confidentiality between physician and patient and against ex parte discussion. *Manion v. N.P.W. Medical Center of N.E. Pa., Inc., 676 F. Supp. 585, 591.*

Ala. 1973 Physician revealed patient information to the patient's employer, contrary to instructions of patient. Patient sued for breach of fiduciary duty. Citing Principle 9 (1957) [now Principle IV and Opinion 5.05] as well as cases from other states, the court held that even in the absence of a testimonial privilege statute, as a matter of public policy, a physician has a fiduciary duty not to make extrajudicial disclosures of patient information acquired in the course of treatment unless the public interest or the private interest of the patient demands otherwise. In holding that the physician had breached his contract with patient, the court found the Principles together with state licensing requirements sufficient to establish the public policy of confidentiality. *Horne v. Patton, 291 Ala. 701, 287 So. 2d 824, 829, 832.*

Alaska 1977 Physician–school board member failed to fully comply with state's conflict of interest law by refusing to reveal the names of patients from whom he had received over $100 in income. The physician claimed a legal privilege or ethical duty not to disclose the information under Principle 9 (1957) [now Principle IV and Opinion 5.05] and, alternatively, that the conflict of interest law unconstitutionally invaded a patient's right to privacy. The court held that disclosure was not barred by a legal privilege or ethical mandate, but that the conflict of interest law unconstitutionally invaded patient privacy due to the absence of protective regulations. In ruling on the ethical duty issue, the court noted that under Alaska law, a physician's license may be revoked for violating the Principles. However, the court found this licensing provision irrelevant to the privileged relationship exception in the conflict of interest law. The court found that otherwise the privilege exception in the statute could be changed by the AMA, a private organization, simply by amending the Principles. *Falcon v. Alaska Pub. Offices Comm'n, 570 P.2d 469, 474 n.13.*

Ariz. App. 1989 In a medical malpractice action, defense counsel interviewed several of plaintiff's treating physicians ex parte and notified plaintiff of this in preparation for a medical liability review panel hearing. Plaintiff moved to bar all testimony by those physicians and to disqualify defense counsel from representing defendants. The appellate court noted a physician's obligation of confidentiality pursuant to Principle IV and Opinion 5.05 and held that defense counsel in a medical malpractice action may not engage in nonconsensual ex parte communications with plaintiff's treating physicians. *Duquette v. Superior Court, 161 Ariz. 269, 778 P.2d 634, 641.*

Cal. 1994 Plaintiff alleged that treating physician and medical group violated her statutory and constitutional right to privacy by engaging in ex parte communications with original physician's insurance company during discovery in a medical malpractice action against her original physician. The court concluded that state law clearly exempts the defendants from liability and that plaintiff failed to allege a sufficiently serious invasion of privacy to warrant relief. The dissent quoted Opinion 5.05 to emphasize the fiduciary nature of the physician-patient relationship. *Heller v. Norcal Mutual Ins. Co., 8 Cal. 4th 30, 876 P.2d 999, 32 Cal. Rptr. 2d 200, 220, cert. denied, 115 S. Ct. 669, 130 L. Ed. 2d 602 (1994).*

Cal. 1976 Parents sued psychotherapists to recover for murder of daughter by psychiatric patient, alleging that failure to warn victim of patient's violent threat was a proximate cause of her death. In considering whether such a revelation would have been a violation of professional ethics, the court noted that Principle 9 (1957) [now Principle IV and Opinion 5.05] recognized that the confidential nature of a physician-patient communication must yield when disclosure is necessary to protect an individual or community as a whole. The court concluded that, in the circumstances of this case, disclosure would not have violated medical ethics and held that psychotherapists are under a duty to warn when they determine or should determine that a patient poses a serious danger of violence to someone else. *Tarasoff v. Regents of Univ. of Cal., 17 Cal. 3d 425, 551 P.2d 334, 347, 131 Cal. Rptr. 14, 27.*

Cal. 1970 Psychiatrist-witness in civil assault case applied for writ of habeas corpus after being held in contempt of court for refusing to produce patient's psychiatric records. Patient, plaintiff in the assault action, neither expressly claimed nor waived the statutory psychotherapist-patient privilege. The court held that the litigant-patient exception to the statutory psychotherapist-patient privilege does not unconstitutionally infringe rights of privacy of either psychotherapists or their patients. The court noted that in such a context a psychiatrist does not violate Principle 9 (1957) [now Principle IV and Opinion 5.05] since the Principle allows for legally compelled disclosure. *In re Lifschutz, 2 Cal. 3d 415, 467 P.2d 557, 565-66 n.9, 85 Cal. Rptr. 829, 837-38 n.9.*

Cal. App. 1982 Defendant was convicted of lewd act with a child and child molestation or annoyance, after licensed clinical psychologist reported defendant's admission of sexual conduct to authorities. The court held that the psychologist's testimony was properly admitted since a statute requiring the reporting of actual or suspected child abuse expressly made the psychotherapist-patient privilege inapplicable. The court quoted Principle 9 (1957) [now Principle IV and Opinions 2.02 and 5.05] in concluding the disclosure was not a breach of professional ethics. *People v. Stritzinger, 126 Cal. App. 3d 135, 186 Cal. Rptr. 750, 752 rev'd, 34 Cal. 3d 505, 668 P.2d 738, 194 Cal. Rptr. 431 (1983).*

Cal. App. 1968 Plaintiff-physician sought dissolution of a medical partnership with defendant's decedent, and also sought a larger percentage of the partnership receipts based upon an alleged oral agreement. Defendant cross-claimed to enjoin plaintiff from taking physical control of the partnership offices and patient records. The trial court enjoined plaintiff from treating previous patients, requiring that he return all medical records and pay defendant all fees received from patients he had treated during the time of dispute. The appellate court reversed insofar as the injunction prohibited the plaintiff from treating the patient who desired to continue to receive his services or prevented access to medical records essential for this purpose, citing Opinions and Reports of the Judicial Council Sec. 7, Para. 16, Sec. 5, Para. 21, and Sec. 9 (1966) [now Opinions 6.08, 5.02, and 5.05] to support view that patients may not be regarded as the subject of ownership. *Jones v. Fakehany, 261 Cal. App. 2d 298, 67 Cal. Rptr. 810, 815, 816 n.1.*

Colo. 1989 Spouse of police officer killed by released psychiatric patient sued state mental hospital and psychiatrist for negligence. Patient had blamed police for his misfortunes during repeated involuntary commitments for paranoid schizophrenia, and psychiatrist knew that patient would have access to a gun after release. The court held that a psychiatrist owed a duty of care in determining whether patient had propensity for violence and posed unreasonable risk of serious bodily harm to others. In so holding, the court cited Principle 9 (1957) [now Principle IV and Opinion 5.05], in support of the view that there are situations in which the need to protect an individual or the community from the threat of harm from a patient may outweigh the strong policy in favor of nondisclosure of patient confidences. *Perreira v. State, 768 P.2d 1198, 1210 n.7.*

D.C. App. 1985 Patient sued plastic surgeon for breach of confidential physician-patient relationship following surgeon's use of before and after photographs of her plastic surgery in a department store presentation. In considering whether such a breach was an actionable tort, the court made reference to an earlier case quoting Principles Ch. II, Sec. 2 (1947) [erroneously cited in the earlier case as Ch. II, Sec. 1 (1943)] [now Principle IV and Opinion 5.05], as evidence of the strong public policy which exists in favor of maintaining a patient's confidences. *Vassiliades v. Garfinckel's, Brooks Bros., 492 A.2d 580, 590, 591.*

Fla. App. 1995 The court considered the issue of the effect of § 455.241(2) of the Florida Statutes on right of defense in a medical malpractice action to engage in ex parte communications with plaintiff's nonparty treating physician. The court held that a 1988 amendment to § 455.241(2) negated the applicability of the statute to medical malpractice cases. The dissent, citing *Petrillo v. Syntex Laboratories, Inc.,* 148 Ill. App. 3d 581, 499 N.E.2d 952 (1986), quoted Principles II and IV and Opinions 5.05, 5.06, and 5.08 as strong public policy support for its position that ex parte communications should be barred altogether. *Castillo-Plaza v. Green, 655 So. 2d 197, 206 n.4.*

Ill. 1997 Trial court held various statutory sections, including those permitting unlimited disclosure of a patient's medical records, unconstitutional. On appeal, state Supreme Court affirmed. Regarding provisions mandating consent to the disclosure of medical records, the court noted, with reference to Principle IV and Opinion 5.05, the crucial importance of confidentiality in the physician-patient relationship. *Best v. Taylor Machine Works, 179 Ill. 2d 367, 689 N.E. 2d 1057, 1099.*

Ill. App. 1987 In appeal of malpractice action, an issue was whether expert testimony of plaintiff's treating physician, based upon discussions with the defense counsel without patient's consent, was admissible. The court held that ex parte communications between a plaintiff's treating physician and legal adversary violated public policy. In determining the existence of such a policy favoring the sanctity of the doctor-patient relationship, the court noted *Petrillo v. Syntex Laboratories, Inc.,* 148 Ill. App. 3d 581, 499 N.E.2d 952 (1st Dist. 1986) and its reference to the Principles and Opinions, namely Principle IV and Opinion 5.05 (1984), which establish an ethical obligation to keep physician-patient communications confidential, generally requiring a patient's consent before information is released. *Yates v. El-Deiry, 160 Ill. App. 3d 198, 513 N.E.2d 519, 522.*

Ill. App. 1986 Defense attorney in product liability suit was held in contempt of court for conducting ex parte discussions with plaintiff-patient's treating physician without patient's consent and contrary to authorized methods of discovery. The court held that the strong public policy favoring physician-patient confidentiality articulated in Principles II and IV and Opinions 5.05, 5.06, 5.07, and 5.08 (1984) justified a rule against such ex parte discussions. Further, the court held that the public has the right to rely on physicians to faithfully execute their ethical obligations. *Petrillo v. Syntex Laboratories, Inc., 148 Ill. App. 3d 581, 499 N.E.2d 952, 957, 958, 959, cert. denied, 483 US 1007 (1987).*

Ill. App. 1979 Patient filed suit against physician for breach of contract and breach of confidential relationship after physician's employee disclosed patient's name to police. Patient alleged that implied contract arose out of a statutory physician-patient privilege, and provisions of the Canons of Medical Ethics, with apparent reference to Principle 9 (1957) [now Principle IV and Opinion 5.05]. The court held that disclosure of patient's name alone by a physician or the physician's agents is insufficient to state a cause of action in contract and does not violate the physician-patient privilege. *Geisberger v. Willuhn, 72 Ill. App. 3d 435, 390 N.E.2d 945, 946, 948.*

Ind. App. 1996 A patient filed suit against a mental health counseling center for disclosing to a third party death threats made by the patient during therapy. The patient claimed this was a breach of the standard of care owed to her. The trial court found that the counseling center was not statutorily prohibited from disclosing death threats the patient made. On appeal, the court affirmed the decision. It noted, with apparent reference to Principle IV and Opinion 5.05, that

physicians may disclose confidential information to ensure the safety of the public or of individuals. In clarifying its holding, the court observed that while free and frank communication should be promoted to aid proper diagnosis and treatment, public policy supports disclosure of confidential information when appropriate. *Rocca v. Southern Hills Counseling Center, Inc., 671 N.E. 2d 913, 916.*

La. App. 2009 Accused criminal sued emergency room physician for defamation and false arrest and imprisonment after he was charged with second-degree murder based on physician's report to police that accused's deceased girlfriend had been shot. The court, quoting Opinion 5.05, noted that while a physician has a duty of confidentiality to a patient, because state law required report of gunshot wounds to local law enforcement, and because the physician did not fabricate the report, the physician was immune from liability. *Mitchell v. Villien, 19 So. 3d 557, 567, n. 14.*

Md. App. 2007 In an espionage case, a psychiatrist was engaged to evaluate defendant's competency. Defendant disclosed confidential information, which the psychiatrist later disclosed to defendant's wife and the media. Defendant and his wife filed a complaint for breach of confidentiality with the State Board of Physicians, which revoked the psychiatrist's medical license. On appeal, the psychiatrist denied any unprofessional conduct. The court, quoting Principle IV, found the psychiatrist's behavior was unethical and unprofessional. With apparent reference to Opinion 5.05, the psychiatrist argued there was an exception to the duty of confidentiality when disclosure would protect the "community interest." The court found no such "community interest" exception. *Salerian v. Maryland State Board of Physicians, 176 Md. App. 231, 932 A.2d 1225, 1235-36, 1241-42.*

Ky. 2002 Patient appealed denial of writ to prevent release to grand jury of psychiatric treatment records. Records were requested to demonstrate that patient had visited multiple physicians to obtain the same prescription drugs. Trial judge reviewed the records in camera and denied writ. The Supreme Court of Kentucky reversed, holding that the evidence reviewed in camera was inadmissible. The court found that a sufficient evidentiary basis must be shown to permit in camera review of privileged records. Concurring judge quotes Opinion 5.05. *Stidham v. Clark, 74 S.W.3d 719, 729, 730.*

Md. Att'y Gen. 1977 Opinion addresses the obligation of a psychiatrist to report child abuse information obtained from a parent-patient. Referring to state statutes and to Principle 9 (1957) [now Principle IV and Opinions 2.02 and 5.05] the opinion concludes that the question of whether to disclose suspected child abuse is a matter left to the individual psychiatrist's professional and moral judgment. *Maryland Att'y Gen. Opinion, 62 Op. Att'y Gen. Md. 157, 160.*

Mass. 1984 Employee sued employer for libel and invasion of privacy following disclosure of medical facts about employee to other employees. In part, claim involved disclosure of opinion about employee's mental state to his supervisor by physician retained by employer. Citing Principle 9 (1957) [now Principle IV and Opinions 5.05 and 5.09], the court held that a physician retained by an employer may disclose to the employer information concerning an employee if receipt of the information is reasonably necessary to serve a substantial and valid business interest of the employer. *Bratt v. Int'l Business Mach. Corp., 392 Mass. 508, 467 N.E.2d 126, 137 n.23.*

Minn. 1976 Plaintiff-patient in malpractice action appealed trial court's order to provide authorization for private, informal interview between defense counsel and patient's treating physician. In holding that formal pretrial discovery provided the exclusive procedure by which defendant could obtain medical testimony, the court noted, without deciding the issue, that a physician who discloses confidential patient information in a private interview may be subject to tort liability for breach of patient's right to privacy or professional discipline for unprofessional conduct, citing Principle 9 (1957) [now Principle IV and Opinion 5.05]. *Wenninger v. Muesing, 240 N.W.2d 333, 337 n.3.*

Mo. 1993 Patient sued physicians alleging a breach of fiduciary duty of confidentiality for participating in an unauthorized ex parte discussion with defendant's attorney. While recognizing this duty, the court held that, where the plaintiff's medical condition is in issue, this constitutes a waiver of both the testimonial privilege and the physician's fiduciary duty insofar as the information is related to the medical issues. Quoting Opinion 5.05 and citing Principle IV, the court stated that courts may apply ethical principles to frame the specific limits of the legal duty of confidentiality. *Brandt v. Medical Defense Assoc., 856 S.W.2d 667, 671 n.1.*

Mo. 1989 In a personal injury suit, plaintiff challenged trial court's authority to compel plaintiff to authorize ex parte meetings between defendant insurance company and plaintiff's treating physician. Applying a balancing test between preserving the physician-patient confidential and fiduciary relationship, the physician-patient testimonal privilege, and the quest for truth in civil litigation, the court held that such information could be obtained through the methods of formal discovery. The court quoted Principle IV and Opinion 5.05 (1984) as statements of the policy underlying medical confidentiality and a basis for a patient's affirmative right to rely on the confidential nature of disclosures to a treating physician. *State ex. rel. Woytus v. Ryan, 776 S.W.2d 389, 392-93.*

Mo. App. 1985 In a prohibition proceeding arising from a medical malpractice action, defense attorneys sought order compelling plaintiff to authorize a private interview between defense attorneys and physician who treated plaintiff for injuries allegedly caused by defendant-physician. The appellate court, after discussing Principle IV and Opinion 5.05 (1984), held that the defense attorneys had the right to seek an ex parte interview with the treating physician, subject to the willingness of the physician to grant the interview. Furthermore, the court noted that Opinion 5.05 prevents a

physician from revealing a patient's confidences only where there is a lack of consent from the patient and found that consent did exist here in the form of a medical authorization executed by plaintiff during pendency of the malpractice action. *State ex rel. Stufflebam v. Appelquist, 694 S.W.2d 882, 886, 888 n.7, overruled by State ex. rel. Woytus v. Ryan, 776 S.W.2d 389 (Mo. 1989).*

N.J. 1985 Plaintiff provided authorization for release of decedent's medical records from former treating physicians but refused to consent to depositions or interviews between defense counsel and physicians. The court noted physicians' ethical duty to avoid unauthorized disclosure, as stated in Principle 9 (1957) [now Principle IV and Opinion 5.05], but recognized that a patient's right to confidentiality was not absolute. After balancing the competing interests involved, the court held that defense counsel had a right to seek ex parte interviews of decedent's other treating physicians regarding litigation matters, provided procedural safeguards were met including clear statements that participation in such an interview is voluntary on the part of a physician. *Stempler v. Speidell, 100 N.J. 368, 495 A.2d 857, 860, cert. denied, 483 US 1007 (1987).*

N.J. 1979 In wrongful death action against a psychiatrist whose patient murdered plaintiff's decedent, the court concluded, in accord with Principle 9 (1957) [now Principle IV], that a psychiatrist may owe a duty to warn potential victims of possible danger from psychiatrist's patient despite the general emphasis on confidentiality. The court also noted the Preamble and Principles 1 and 3 (1957) [now revised Preamble, Principle I, and Opinion 5.05] in discussing the psychiatrist-patient relationship. *McIntosh v. Milano, 168 N.J. Super. 466, 403 A.2d 500, 510, 512-13.*

N.J. 1962 Parents sued pediatrician for unauthorized disclosure to life insurer of deceased infant's congenital heart defect. The court quoted Principle 9 (1957) [now Principle IV and Opinion 5.05] as an articulation of a physician's legal duty to his or her patient subject to exceptions of compelling social or patient interests. The court held that the parents had lost their limited right to nondisclosure by filing an insurance claim. *Hague v. Williams, 37 N.J. 328, 181 A.2d 345, 347.*

N.J. Super. 1991 Physician's estate sued hospital alleging that it violated state law against discrimination by restricting the physician's surgery privileges and requiring him to inform patients of his HIV-infected status before performing invasive procedures. The defendant hospital was also alleged to have breached its duty to maintain confidentiality of his seropositive diagnosis. The court held that the hospital had not discriminated against the physician since the hospital had relied on ethical and professional standards, including a report of the Council on Ethical and Judicial Affairs of the AMA dealing with the issue of AIDS [now Opinions 9.13 and 9.131]. However, the hospital was held to have breached its fiduciary duty to maintain the confidentiality of the physician's medical records. Referring to *McIntosh v. Milano, 168 N.J. Super. 466, 403 A.2d 500 (1979),* which had quoted AMA Principles of Medical Ethics sec. 9 (1957) [now Principle IV and Opinion 5.05] in applying the "duty to warn" exception, the court noted that the disclosure in this case went far beyond the medical personnel directly involved in the treatment of the physician and those patients entitled to informed consent. *Estate of Behringer v. Medical Ctr., 249 N.J. Super. 597, 614, 633, 592 A.2d 1251, 1259, 1268.*

N.J. Super. 1988 Several portions of state department of corrections regulations concerning exceptions to privileged communications between psychologist and inmates were invalidated by appellate court because they permitted disclosure of confidences that did not present clear and imminent danger to the inmate or others, or failed to identify any intended victim. Court made general reference (with erroneous quotation) to Principle 9 (1957) [now Principle IV and Opinion 5.05]. *In re Rules Adoption, 224 N.J. Super. 252, 540 A.2d 212, 215.*

N.J. Super. 1987 Defendant in a personal injury suit sought to offer testimony from plaintiff's treating physician regarding plaintiff's prognosis. The court denied plaintiff's motion to exclude that evidence, despite the ethical obligation of physicians to uphold patients' communications as confidential under Principle 9 (1957) [now Principle IV and Opinion 5.05]. The court's decision was based on New Jersey case law permitting disclosure of a patient's medical condition to someone having a legitimate interest where the physical condition of the patient is made an element of a claim. *Kurdek v. West Orange Bd. of Educ., 222 N.J. Super. 218, 536 A.2d 332, 335.*

N.J. Super. 1967 In a suit for separate maintenance, communications between plaintiff-wife and her psychiatrist were not protected from disclosure during depositions, despite Principle 9 (1957) [now Principle IV and Opinion 5.05], which prohibited physicians from disclosing patient confidences except where necessary to protect the welfare of the individual or of the community. The court concluded that the patient had only a limited right of nondisclosure, subject to exceptions created by supervening interest of society and that the institution of litigation by the patient constituted a vitiation of that right. *Ritt v. Ritt, 98 N.J. Super. 590, 238 A.2d 196, 199, rev'd, 52 N.J. 177, 244 A.2d 497 (1968).*

N.Y. Sup. 2000 Physician brought wrongful discharge claim against corporate employer. The physician alleged she was discharged because she refused to reveal confidential medical information regarding employees. With apparent reference to Principle IV and Opinions 5.05 and 5.09, the affidavit filed by the physician claimed she had an ethical and legal duty to protect patient confidentiality. The court found termination of an employee at will based upon such grounds is sufficient to state a cause of action for breach of contract. The court ruled that obligations of good faith and fair dealing may be implied in a contract for the employment of a physician and that no physician should be placed in the position of choosing between retaining employment and violating ethical standards. *Horn v. New York Times, 186 Misc. 2d 469, 719 N.Y.S. 2d 471, 474.*

N.Y. Sup. 1977 Plaintiff, a psychiatric patient, sued her psychiatrist and the psychiatrist's spouse for violating several state statutes and her privacy rights by publishing a book about the intimate details of plaintiff's psychotherapy. The court found for plaintiff, basing its decision in part upon Principle 9 (1957) [now Principle IV and Opinion 5.05], which requires a physician to uphold the confidences of a patient. *Doe v. Roe, 93 Misc. 2d 201, 400 N.Y.S.2d 668, 674.*

N.Y. Surr. 1977 In a discovery proceeding, respondent-psychiatrist, who had treated some patients of deceased psychiatrist subsequent to his death, allegedly misappropriated decedent's patient records. Estate petitioned court for return of records and damages for injury to value of decedent's practice. Respondent sought dismissal of claim arguing that estate could not sell patient records. The court rejected respondent's request. In so ruling, the court noted that under Principle 9 (1957) [now Principle IV and Opinion 5.05] prohibiting physicians from revealing patient confidences, various guidelines had been issued regarding sale of a medical practice [now Opinion 7.04]. Whether respondent's actions had interfered with the estate's efforts to dispose of decedent's practice in keeping with these guidelines presented the court with factual issues for later resolution. *Estate of Finkle, 90 Misc. 2d 550, 395 N.Y.S.2d 343, 346.*

N.C. 1990 Plaintiff in a malpractice case was granted an order prohibiting ex parte conferences between defendant's attorney and nonparty treating physicians. The court noted that both the Principles of Medical Ethics and Current Opinions affirm the physician's duty to protect patient confidentiality, in apparent reference to Principle IV and Opinion 5.05. In consideration of (1) the patient's right to privacy, (2) physician-patient confidentiality, (3) the adequacy of formal discovery procedures, and (4) the dilemma in which nonparty treating physicians are placed by ex parte conferences, the court held that an attorney may not interview a patient's nonparty treating physicians privately without express authorization. *Crist v. Moffatt, 326 N.C. 326, 333, 389 S.E.2d 41, 46.*

N.C. App. 1999 Plaintiff appealed industrial commission's finding for the plaintiff's employer on the grounds that there was insufficient medical evidence to find that the plaintiff's absence from work was attributed to injury. The plaintiff in part alleged that his employer engaged in ex parte communications with the plaintiff's treating physician. The court held that the commission erroneously placed on the plaintiff the burden of proving that the medical treatment he sought related to his injury. The court quoted Opinion 5.05, noting that it is improper for a physician to engage in ex parte communications with a defendant. The court stated, however, that the plaintiff failed to present evidence of such ex parte communications. *Reininger v. Prestige Fabricators, Inc., 523 S.E.2d 720, 724.*

Ohio 1999 Patients brought a class action suit against hospital on grounds that the hospital disclosed patients' confidential medical information to the hospital's law firm, in order to determine whether the patients were eligible for government benefits to pay for unpaid hospital bills. The trial court granted defendants' motion for summary judgment. On appeal, the court held that a physician or a hospital can be held liable for unauthorized out-of-court disclosure of patients' confidential information. Additionally, the court found that an independent tort exists for unauthorized, unprivileged disclosure of patients' private medical information to a third party. The court cited Principle 9 (1957) [now Principle IV and Opinion 5.05], noting that courts have looked to such sources in providing a cause of action for breach of patient confidentiality. *Biddle v. Warren General Hospital, 86 Ohio St. 3d 395, 715 N.E.2d 518, 523.*

Ohio 1997 Estates of victims who were killed by their mentally ill son brought suit against son's psychotherapist for failing to disclose potential for violence. Son had been institutionalized and treated for schizophrenia. After release, he continued to take medication and see a psychotherapist. Despite parents' objections and attempts to have him involuntarily recommitted, psychotherapist reduced his medication and continued to recommend outpatient treatment. The court held that the psychotherapist had a duty to exercise reasonable care to control the son so as to prevent him from causing harm to his family. The court expressed concern for safeguarding the confidentiality of psychotherapeutic communications but noted that Principle 9 (1957) [now Principle IV and Opinion 5.05] has long allowed breaches of confidence when it becomes necessary to protect the welfare of the individual or the community. *Estates of Morgan v. Fairfield Family Counseling Center, 77 Ohio St. 3d 284, 303, 673 N.E.2d 1311, 1326.*

Ohio 1988 Administrator sued psychiatrist for wrongful death after recently discharged patient killed her infant daughter. In determining whether a professional judgment rule should be adopted in the malpractice standard of care where the prediction of violent behavior is involved, the court referred favorably to Principle 9 (1957) [now Principle IV and Opinion 5.05], which allows breaches of patient confidences when necessary to protect potential victims. *Littleton v. Good Samaritan Hospital, 39 Ohio St. 3d 86, 529 N.E.2d 449, 459 n.19.*

Okla. 1988 In response to a police request, physician reported patient treated for a penile bite. Patient sued physician for negligence after information furnished by physician led to patient's arrest and conviction for rape. Patient alleged a tortious breach of the physician-patient confidential relationship, breach of contract, violation of licensing statute, and breach of Principle 9 (1957) [now Principle IV and Opinion 5.05]. The court reasoned that the benefit of the divulgence inured to the public at large and thus fell within the public policy exception to the testimonial privilege, created no liability in tort or contract, and was not a breach of medical ethics under the licensing statute or the Principles. *Bryson v. Tillinghast, 749 P.2d 110, 113, 114.*

Pa. 1999 Administratrix of estate of victim murdered by a mental patient filed suit against the mental health center and

member of professional staff. The trial court found in favor of the defendants. The Pennsylvania Supreme Court held that mental health professionals have a duty to warn a third party who is the subject of patient's threats when there is a immediate risk of serious bodily harm. The court quoted Opinion 5.05, noting that the AMA allows an exception to the duty of confidentiality when safety is a reasonable concern. The court found that the defendants had the duty to warn the victim and had fulfilled that duty when the victim was warned not to go to the patient's apartment. *Emerich v. Philadelphia Center for Human Development, Inc., 554 Pa. 209, 720 A.2d 1032, 1043.*

Pa. 1973 Plaintiff in personal injury suit resulting from auto accident claimed that trial court should have allowed showing on cross-examination that defendant's expert medical witness, who had treated plaintiff, violated Principle 9 (1957) [now Principle IV and Opinion 5.05] by ex parte communications with defense counsel, in order to impeach his medical testimony. The court held that any connection between an alleged breach of medical ethics and the credibility of a physician on the witness stand was tenuous. Therefore, the trial court's decision barring further inquiry in this regard was proper. *Downey v. Weston, 451 Pa. 259, 301 A.2d 635, 638.*

Pa. Super. 1998 The court denied a social worker's motion to quash a subpoena compelling her to testify before a grand jury regarding a client's murder. The court explained that the duty of confidentiality should be waived because the deceased client was not a crime suspect and because the information was necessary to solve a crime. The court further reasoned that disclosure of the confidential information was in the client's best interest because it would aid in solving the client's murder. The court, citing an earlier case, referenced Opinion 5.05, in support of the notion that confidentiality may be waived under special circumstances such as overriding public safety concerns. *In re Subpoena No. 22., Appeal of A.B., 709 A.2d 385, 391.*

Pa. Super. 1988 Plaintiff-patient sued her physician for breach of confidentiality when physician conferred with defense counsel in plaintiff's malpractice suit against the hospital (physician's employer). In its majority opinion, the court cited Principle IV, commenting that it gave very little guidance to physicians but nonetheless was not violated by the physician. The court also noted Opinion 5.07 (1986) finding that the plaintiff's suit minimized her expectations of confidentiality. The dissent, however, interpreted these same provisions, along with Opinion 5.05 (1986), as protecting plaintiff's expectations of confidentiality. *Moses v. McWilliams, 379 Pa. Super. 150, 549 A.2d 950, 956, 962 (dissent), appeal denied, 521 Pa. 630, 558 A.2d 532 (1989).*

Tenn. App. 1994 Plaintiff sought damages for wrongful death from defendant-surgeon. Defendant requested that the court require plaintiff to sign a form authorizing release of medical records and information to defense counsel. Trial court denied defendant's motion noting, with apparent reference to Principle IV and Opinion 5.05, that confidential relationship exists between physician and patient. Appellate court affirmed although it did not reach the ethical issue of the propriety of disclosures by a physician. *Wright v. Wasudev, 1994 Tenn. App. LEXIS 657.*

Utah App. 2006 Following an automobile accident, plaintiff filed a personal injury suit against the driver. Plaintiff discovered that his treating physician had been subpoenaed by the driver's lawyer, had agreed to testify against plaintiff, and had engaged in ex parte communications with defense counsel. Plaintiff sued the physician. With apparent reference to Opinions 5.05 and 5.059 plaintiff relied in part on the AMA ethical principles to establish the standard of care. The court of appeals held that the physician could be liable for breach of the fiduciary duty of confidentiality as well as for intentional infliction of emotional distress. *Sorensen v. Barbuto, 143 P.3d 295, 299.*

Utah Att'y Gen. 1978 A physician who, acting in good faith, discloses confidential information to proper authorities concerning a patient's unfitness to drive is not liable for doing so. Reference is made to Principle 9 (1957) [now Principle IV and Opinion 5.05] to support propriety of such disclosure where the public interest is involved. *Utah Att'y Gen. Op. No. 77-294.*

Wash. 1988 Personal representative brought wrongful death action against decedent's physicians. At issue was whether defense counsel in a personal injury action may communicate ex parte with plaintiff's treating physician where plaintiff has waived the physician-patient relationship. In holding that defense counsel may not engage in ex parte communication, and is limited to formal discovery methods, the court cited Principle IV and Opinion 5.05 (1986) with approval, reasoning that the mere threat of disclosure of private conversations between a physician and defense counsel would chill the physician-patient relationship and hinder further treatment. *Loudon v. Mhyre, 110 Wash. 2d 675, 756 P.2d 138, 141, 141 n.3.*

W. Va. 1993 Plaintiff, in a malpractice action, sought a writ of prohibition to prevent the enforcement of a trial court order allowing ex parte interviews. The court, in granting the writ, held that any benefit from ex parte interviews that occurs is minimal compared to the danger that they will undermine the confidential nature of the physician-patient relationship. Quoting Principles of Medical Ethics Ch. II, sec. 1 (1943) [now Principle IV and Opinion 5.05], the court noted that the medical profession is well aware of the importance of patient confidentiality. *State ex. rel. Kitzmiller v. Henning, 437 S.E.2d 452, 454.*

Wis. 1995 In medical malpractice suit, the court held that (1) subject to restrictions, defense counsel may engage in ex parte communications with plaintiff's treating physician if the communications do not involve disclosure of confidential information; (2) outside a judicial proceeding, defendant-physician may communicate ex parte with plaintiff's treating physician subject to a physician's duty of confidentiality; and (3) if defense counsel elicits confidential information from a treating physician during ex parte communications, the

appropriate sanction is within the discretion of the court. The court expressly overruled *State ex rel. Klieger v. Alby*, 125 Wis. 2d 468, 373 N.W.2d 57 (Ct. App. 1985), and the cases applying it. The majority and concurring opinions referred to Principle IV and Opinion 5.05. *Steinberg v. Jensen, 194 Wis. 2d 440, 534 N.W.2d 361, 370, 377.*

Wis. App. 1999 Defendant who pled guilty to carrying a concealed weapon appealed on grounds that the police officer's search of the defendant was based on information obtained from the defendant's psychotherapist. The appellate court held that the defendant's statements made to his psychotherapist could be considered in evaluating the reasonableness of the search because the defendant posed a threat of danger. The court quoted Opinion 5.05, regarding confidentiality and noted the exception where safety is a concern. *State v. Agacki, 226 Wis. 2d 349, 595 N.W.2d 31, 37.*

Wis. App. 1994 In medical malpractice suit, defense counsel engaged in ex parte communications with plaintiff's consulting physicians. Plaintiff amended her complaint seeking punitive damages for breach of confidentiality. The court concluded that the rule of *State ex rel. Klieger v. Alby*, 125 Wis. 2d 468, 373 N.W.2d 57 (Ct. App. 1985), which prohibits ex parte communications that have the potential to breach physician-patient confidentiality, was violated and sanctions were required. The court referred to *Petrillo v. Syntax Labs., Inc.*, 148 Ill. App. 3d 581, 499 N.E.2d 952 (1986), and its use of Principle IV and Opinion 5.05. *Steinberg v. Jensen, 186 Wis. 2d 237, 519 N.W.2d 753, 761 n.9, rev'd, 194 Wis. 2d 440, 534 N.W.2d 361 (1995).*

Wis. Att'y Gen. 1987 Physicians may report cases of suspected child abuse or neglect when a patient discloses that he or she has abused a child in some manner. Where report is made in good faith, physicians are immune from any civil or criminal liability. Passing reference is made to Principle 9 (1957) [now Principle IV and Opinions 2.02 and 5.05] in support of this position. *Wisconsin Att'y Gen. Op. 10-87 (March 16, 1987) (LEXIS, States library, Wis. file).*

Journal 2011 Explores intimate partner violence (IPV) and various attempts to address it, such as mandatory reporting laws. Emphasizes the importance of distinguishing types of IPV and developing a multifaceted approach for responding to the needs of IPV victims. Cites Opinion 5.05. Hafemeister, *If All You Have Is a Hammer: Society's Ineffective Response to Intimate Partner Violence, 60 Cath. U. L. Rev. 919, 962 (2011).*

Journal 2011 Addresses why private Internet activity should always be protected by the warrant and probable cause requirements of the Fourth Amendment. Concludes that private Internet activity is exactly the type of activity that the courts and Congress have sought to protect from unreasonable searches and seizures by law enforcement. References Opinion 5.05. Mitter, *Deputizing Internet Service Providers: How the Government Avoids Fourth Amendment Protections, 67 N.Y.U. Ann. Surv. Am. L. 235, 273 (2011).*

Journal 2011 Considers the role of empirical evidence and moral principles in relation to the controversy surrounding attorney/client confidentiality. Concludes that rules of confidentiality should be revised to accommodate extreme situations where the lawyer has good reason to think that maintaining silence will cause serious undeserved harm to others. Further concludes that lawyers should not fear censure for coming forward in such situations. Cites Opinion 5.05. Morawetz, *Confidentiality and Common Sense: Insights From Philosophy*, 48 San Diego L. Rev. 357, 373 (2011).

Journal 2010 Discusses issues arising from the enactment of legislation by North Dakota involving a minor's reproductive rights. Explores ethical principles that govern physician's actions within the context of reproductive health. Concludes that, while a patient's expectation of confidentiality with a physician is critical, competing values come into play when the patient is a minor and parental involvement may be important. Provides practical guidance to address issues in this context. Quotes Opinions 2.01, 2.015, 5.055, 8.08, 8.115, 9.12, 10.01, 10.015, and 10.05. Cites Opinions 5.05, 5.055, 8.08, 8.11, 8.115, 9.12, and 10.05. Haas, *"Doctor, I'm Pregnant and Fifteen—I Can't Tell My Parents—Please Help Me": Minor Consent, Reproductive Rights, and Ethical Principles for Physicians*, 86 N.D. L. Rev. 63, 70, 73, 75-78, 82, 84, 86-88 (2010).

Journal 2010 Examines published resources within the medical and legal fields that focus on confidentiality and evaluates those resources to determine if they help clarify confidentiality issues. Further, discusses differences between these professions that may be hindrances when serving the same patient or client. Concludes that, while both professions guard against disclosure of patient/client communications, they also allow for disclosure in certain instances such as imminent death, harm, or injury. References Principle IV and cites Opinions 2.02, 2.23, 2.24, and 5.05. Johns, *Multidisciplinary Practice and Ethics Part II—Lawyers, Doctors, and Confidentiality*, 6 NAELA J. 55, 57-65, 68 (2010).

Journal 2010 Discusses the effects of using deidentified health information on privacy and considers the dangers of nonconsensual use of health information. Concludes deidentification of health information is a necessary though insufficient protection of privacy, and further research and regulations should be developed to demonstrate respect for individuals without unduly burdening research. Quotes Principle IV and Opinions 5.05 and 7.025. Rothstein, *Is Deidentification Sufficient to Protect Health Privacy in Research?* 10 Am. J. Bioethics 3, 5 (Sept. 2010).

Journal 2010 Explores how participation in online social networks may blur boundaries between personal and professional relationships for health care professionals and how such risks may be mitigated by use of network privacy and security settings. Suggests that health care institutions are likely to institute online social-networking policies for employees. Quotes Opinions 5.026, 5.027, 5.045, 5.046, 5.05, 5.059, 5.0591, 8.14, 9.08, and 9.123. Cites Opinions 5.026, 9.031, and 9.12. Terry, *Physicians and Patients Who "Friend" or "Tweet": Constructing a Legal Framework for Social Networking in a Highly Regulated Domain*, 43 Ind. L. Rev. 285, 314-16, 319, 334-36, 338 (2010).

Journal 2010 Examines legislative and judicial efforts to address hazards posed by drivers' use of cell phones and other communication technology with distracted driver laws. Concludes that the scope of a phone search under the automobile exception to verify suspected violations of such laws is limited to verifying when a message was sent or received. Cites Opinion 5.05. Williams, *The Trouble With Texting: The Future of Searches Under the Automobile Exception After Arizona v. Gant*, 4 Charleston L. Rev. 919, 929 (2010).

Journal 2009 Explains that, while the Restatement (Third) of Torts recognizes a mental health therapist's duty to warn foreseeable victims of risks posed by a patient, it takes no position regarding such a duty for physicians in other settings (eg, infectious diseases). Concludes while there is a basis to question this distinction, the issue is sufficiently complex and the considerations sufficiently balanced that the Restatement's position is justifiable. Cites Principles of Medical Ethics § 9 (1957) [now Opinion 5.05]. Cardi, *A Pluralistic Analysis of the Therapist/Physician Duty to Warn Third Parties*, 44 Wake Forest L. Rev. 877, 881 (2009).

Journal 2009 Discusses state open records statutes and the treatment of concealed carry permit records. Concludes concealed carry permit records should be disclosed to the public in order to achieve greater consistency in open records laws and to increase public safety. Quotes Opinion 5.05. Swanson, *The Right to Know: An Approach to Gun Licenses and Public Access to Government Records*, 56 UCLA L. Rev. 1579, 1594 (2009).

Journal 2009 Discusses the tension between duties of confidentiality and to protect third parties owed by mental health professionals to their patients and the public. Analyzes current Illinois law regarding these duties. Argues because Illinois law causes confusion regarding a professional's duty to disclose, inappropriately restricts the protected class, and leads to unnecessary breaches of confidentiality, clarification is necessary. Quotes Preamble and Opinion 5.05. Wood, *Protective Privilege Versus Public Peril: How Illinois Has Failed to Balance Patient Confidentiality With the Mental Health Professional's Duty to Protect the Public*, 29 N. Ill. U. L. Rev. 571, 581, 598 (2009).

Journal 2008 Discusses ex parte interviews with a treating physician in discovery before and after the HIPAA Privacy Rule and the issues facing physicians contacted for such interviews. Concludes courts and attorneys should work together to allow for efficient discovery while protecting physicians. Quotes Principles IV and VIII and Opinions 5.05 and 10.01. Burnette & Morning, *HIPAA and Ex Parte Interviews—the Beginning of the End?* 1 J. Health & Life Sci. L. 73, 100-01 (2008).

Journal 2008 Examines law governing the duty to warn a threatened individual. Proposes new criteria by which to evaluate whether a statement triggers a duty to warn, incorporating linguistic imperatives and professional standards. Quotes Opinion 5.05. Harmon, *Back from Wonderland: A Linguistic Approach to Duties Arising From Threats of Physical Violence, 37 Cap. U. L. Rev. 27, 33 (2008).*

Journal 2008 Argues a general physician-patient privilege is needed in West Virginia and outlines the manner in which the privilege could be adopted. Concludes that the privilege will allow physicians to maintain their fiduciary role, foster open communication between patient and physician, and encourage patients to freely seek medical treatment. Quotes Principle IV and Opinion 5.05. Johnson, *"I Will Not Divulge": How to Resolve the "Mass of Legal Confusion" Surrounding the* physician-patient *Relationship in West Virginia, 110 W. Va. L. Rev. 1231, 1247 (2008).*

Journal 2008 Examines prescription privacy and the sale of deidentified medical records. Suggests HIPAA must modernize its deidentification requirements to protect patient privacy amid technological advances in data mining. Quotes Opinion 5.05. Klocke, *Prescription Records for Sale: Privacy and Free Speech Issues Arising From the Sale of De-identified Medical Data, 44 Idaho L. Rev. 511, 518 (2008).*

Journal 2008 Examines the practicability and constitutionality of restrictions on drivers' licensing for the elderly. Concludes there are high-risk drivers in all age groups and licensing restrictions must not unfairly limit autonomy for the elderly. Cites Opinion 5.05. Mikel, *Drivers' Licenses and Age Limits: Imposition of Driving Restrictions on Elderly Drivers, 9 Marq. Elder's Advisor 359, 379 (2008).*

Journal 2008 Discusses privacy and disability laws concerning the mental health of college students. Concludes law and policy should be changed to promote student well-being while limiting liability for institutions. References Opinion 5.05. Pena, *Reevaluating Privacy and Disability Laws in the Wake of the Virginia Tech Tragedy: Considerations for Administrators and Lawmakers, 87 N. C. L. Rev. 305, 334 (2008).*

Journal 2008 Discusses student privacy and campus safety with respect to Family Education Rights and Privacy Act (FERPA) obligations and HIPAA regulations. Argues campus professionals should work together to effectively communicate pertinent student information to promote campus safety. Quotes Opinion 5.05 as it read before 2007 revision. Tribbensee, *Privacy and Confidentiality: Balancing Student Rights and Campus Safety, 34 J. C. & U. L. 393, 406-07 (2008).*

Journal 2007 Analyzes scientific, ethical, and legal issues raised in the exhumation and genetic analysis of historical figures. Concludes that biohistorical review boards should be created to generate guidelines for such research. Quotes Preamble and Opinion 2.08. Cites Opinions 2.079, 2.105, 5.05, 5.051, 5.075, 8.03, 8.031, 9.095, and 9.10. Paradise & Andrews, *Tales From the Crypt: Scientific, Ethical, and Legal Considerations for Biohistorical Analysis of Deceased Historical Figures, 26 Temp. J. Sci. Tech. & Envtl. L. 223, 287-88 (2007).*

Journal 2007 Examines relative vs absolute rights to confidentiality for military detainees considering the utilitarian need to protect the public at large. Concludes that evolving standards may favor individual rights to confidentiality, even from a utilitarian perspective. Quotes Opinions 1.02 and 5.05. References Principle III. Wynia, *Breaching Confidentiality to Protect the Public: Evolving Standards of Medical Confidentiality for Military Detainees, 7 Am. J. Bioethics, 1, 2 (Aug. 2007).*

Journal 2006 Analyzes the ethical and legal problems of confidentiality which arise in the context of genetic testing. Concludes that the disclosure of a patient's genetic disease to others is only allowable when the patient is a minor and the family has a right to know. Quotes Principle IV and References Principle 9 (1957) [now Principle IV and Opinion 5.05]. Denbo, *What Your Genes Know Affects Them: Should Patient Confidentiality Prevent Disclosure of Genetic Test Results to a Patient's Biological Relatives? 43 Am. Bus. L. J. 561, 572, 577 (2006).*

Journal 2006 Evaluates the influence that Justice Blackmun's experience at the Mayo Clinic had on his opinions related to medicine. Concludes that Blackmun's experience had less of an impact on his opinions than is traditionally assumed. Quotes Principle 9 (1957) [now Principle IV and Opinion 5.05]. Hunter, *Justice Blackmun, Abortion, and the Myth of Medical Independence, 72 Brooklyn L. Rev. 147, 190-91 (2006).*

Journal 2006 Examines a mental health professional's competing duties of confidentiality and reporting a patient's threats of violence. Suggests new legislation should clarify duty to report a threat. Quotes Preamble and Principles III, IV, and VIII. Cites Opinion 5.05. Mossman, *Critique of Pure Risk Assessment or, Kant Meets Tarasoff, 75 U. Cin. L. Rev. 523, 579 (2006).*

Journal 2006 Analyzes the privacy risks associated with introducing a system of electronic medical records. Concludes that cost and confidentiality concerns mandate that security must be built into the initial system. Cites Ch. I, Art. I, Sec. 2 (May 1847) [now Principle IV and Opinion 5.05]. Rothstein & Talbott, *Compelled Disclosure of Health Information: Protecting Against the Greatest Potential Threat to Privacy, 295 JAMA 2882, 2883 (2006).*

Journal 2006 Examines situations where physician-patient confidentiality may be breached to prevent violations of human rights. Suggests that new laws should be enacted to specify when a physician may testify about a violation of human rights. Quotes Principle IV and Opinion 5.05. Weissbrodt & Wilson, *Piercing the Confidentiality Veil: Physician Testimony in International Criminal Trials Against Perpetrators of Torture, 15 Minn. J. Int'l L. 43, 68, 68-69 (2006).*

Journal 2005 Reviews the lack of confidentiality in peer-run self-help programs. Concludes that new laws need to be enacted to protect participant confidentiality in such programs. References Opinion 5.05. Coleman, *Privilege and Confidentiality in 12-Step Self-Help Programs*, 26 J. Legal Med. 435, 441 (2005).

Journal 2005 Examines the argument that data privacy regulations violate the First Amendment. Concludes that neither privacy rights nor First Amendment free speech rights must be sacrificed in protecting data, and that balancing the two is a policy rather than a constitutional concern. Quotes Opinion 5.05. Richards, *Reconciling Data Privacy and the First Amendment*, 52 UCLA L. Rev. 1149, 1195 (2005).

Journal 2004 Argues that the intent of Congress to protect health information is clearly signaled in the language of HIPAA. Concludes that, despite this fact, a federal physician-patient privilege should be recognized, to ensure that gaps in the scope of available protection may be addressed. Quotes Opinion 5.05. Ruebner & Reis, *Hippocrates to HIPAA: A Foundation for a Federal physician-patient Privilege*, 77 Temp. L. Rev. 505, 572 (2004).

Journal 2004 Discusses the need for a greater understanding of and openness to religious values by the professions. Concludes that, although such openness is important, problems may arise when professional values and religious values clash. Quotes Opinion 5.05. References Principle v. Sullivan, *Naked Fitzies and Iron Cages: Individual Values, Professional Virtues, and the Struggle for Public Space*, 78 Tul. L. Rev. 1687, 1702, 1703 (2004).

Journal 2004 Argues that the privacy model rather than the property model is the most appropriate way to protect an individual's interest in genetic information. Concludes that privacy interests must nevertheless be balanced against other societal factors. References Principle IV and Opinion 5.05. Suter, *Disentangling Privacy From Property: Toward a Deeper Understanding of Genetic Privacy*, 72 Geo. Wash. L. Rev. 737, 787 (2004).

Journal 2003 Argues the legal profession must become meaningfully involved in efforts to address the causes and effects of domestic violence. Concludes that lawyers must do more in an effort to protect the interests of clients. Quotes Opinion 5.05. Burman, *Lawyers and Domestic Violence: Raising the Standard of Practice*, 9 Mich. J. Gender & L. 207, 254 (2003).

Journal 2003 Highlights HIPAA privacy issues that need to be monitored and have yet to be resolved. Concludes that HIPAA poses many challenges and it remains unclear whether HIPAA will increase privacy protection. Cites Opinions 5.05, 5.055, 5.057, 5.06, 5.07, 5.075, 5.08, and 5.09. Kutzko, Boyer, Thoman, & Scott, *HIPAA in Real Time: Practical Implications of the Federal Privacy Rule*, 51 Drake L. Rev. 403, 408 (2003).

Journal 2003 Considers the legal, medical, and ethical issues of physician-patient confidentiality in disclosure of

paternity. Concludes that a balancing test should be applied to making determinations regarding disclosure of paternity. Quotes Principles I, IV, and V and Opinions 1.02, 5.055, and 10.01. Cites Principle II and Opinion 5.05. Richards & Wolf, *Medical Confidentiality and Disclosure of Paternity*, 48 S. D. L. Rev. 409, 411, 412, 413 (2003).

Journal 2003 Discusses legal principles governing electronic personal information and other digital media. Concludes that biometric security methods will become the standard for protecting private information. Quotes Opinion 5.05. Yang & Gorman, *What's Yours Is Mine: Protection and Security in a Digital World*, 36 Md. B. J. 24, 28-29 (Nov./Dec. 2003).

Journal 2002 Discusses issues regarding regulation of elderly drivers. Concludes that mandating physicians to report unfit elderly patients will protect the public and help resolve ethical and legal dilemmas. Quotes Opinions 1.02, 2.24, 5.05, and 10.01. Kane, *Driving Into the Sunset: A Proposal for Mandatory Reporting to the DMV by Physicians Treating Unsafe Elderly Drivers*, 25 U. Haw. L. Rev. 59, 59, 61, 62, 67, 69, 82, 83 (2002).

Journal 2002 Discusses legal and medical policies that protect confidentiality in the physician-patient relationship. Concludes that reducing the current level of privacy protection would jeopardize health care. Quotes Preamble and Opinions 2.136, 5.05, and 10.01. References Principles VIII and IX. Sciarrino, *Ferguson v. City of Charleston: "The Doctor Will See You Now, Be Sure to Bring Your Privacy Rights in With You!"* 12 Temp. Pol. & Civ. Rts. L. Rev. 197, 213, 215, 220, 221, 222 (2002).

Journal 2002 Discusses the lapse of Fourth Amendment protection in the collection of third-party records by the government. Concludes that a new paradigm is needed for regulating government collection of third-party information. Quotes Opinion 5.05. Solove, *Digital Dossiers and the Dissipation of Fourth Amendment Privacy*, 75 S. Cal. L. Rev. 1083, 1155 (2002).

Journal 2002 Considers issues of health information privacy in the electronic age. Concludes that protections afforded by the HIPAA privacy rules and common law will be increasingly important. Quotes Opinion 5.05. Winn, *Confidentiality in Cyberspace: The HIPAA Privacy Rules and the Common Law*, 33 Rutgers L. J. 617, 622 (2002).

Journal 2001 Examines ethical issues surrounding physician disclosure of information to attorneys. Observes that attorneys do not have an absolute right to interfere with the physician-patient relationship. Concludes that attorneys' efforts to obtain information may give rise to lawsuits for aiding and abetting the physician's breach of a fiduciary duty to preserve confidentiality. Quotes Opinion 5.05. Freeman, *Dealing With Doctors*, 13 S. C. Law 11, 11 (July/Aug. 2001).

Journal 2001 Explores the Uniform Mediation Act (UMA). Describes how certain exceptions to confidentiality in mediation arise from an inability to balance the means of confidentiality and the ends of self-determination. Concludes that, under the UMA, confidentiality does not promote self-determination. Quotes Opinion 5.05. Hughes, *The Uniform Mediation Act: To the Spoiled Go the Privileges*, 85 Marq. L. Rev. 9, 26 (2001).

Journal 2001 Compares the American system of patient confidentiality to the Austrian system. Discusses the debate between patients' rights and public safety. Concludes that the duty to warn third parties of dangerous patients should be discretionary instead of mandatory, except in cases of HIV seropositivity, which should involve mandatory disclosure to public health officials. Quotes Opinions 2.23, 5.05, and 5.06. Kenworthy, *The Austrian Psychotherapy Act: No Legal Duty to Warn*, 11 Ind. Int'l & Comp. L. Rev. 469, 480-81, 485, 490, 496 (2001).

Journal 2001 Considers whether it is ethical for physicians to prescribe, and pharmacists to dispense, syringes for use by injection drug users. Concludes that ethical considerations suggest such actions are permissible but not obligatory. Quotes Principle III and Opinion 1.02. References Opinion 5.05. Lazzarini, *An Analysis of Ethical Issues in Prescribing and Dispensing Syringes to Injection Drug Users*, 11 Health Matrix 85, 107, 119 (2001).

Journal 2001 Focuses on the case of *Weld v. CVS Pharmacy, Inc.* Examines whether an individual's privacy is invaded when pharmacies disclose prescription information about customers to aid other private organizations with implementation of marketing activities. Quotes Opinion 5.05. Schawbel, *Are You Taking Any Prescription Medication? A Case Comment on Weld v. CVS Pharmacy, Inc.*, 35 New Eng. L. Rev. 909, 957 (2001).

Journal 2001 Evaluates current forms of cybermedicine and Internet resources that support it. Explores patient and regulatory concerns, including privacy issues, insurance reimbursement problems, licensure, and liability, which may thwart the growth of cybermedicine. Concludes that cybermedicine may facilitate delivery of cost-effective, quality medical care. Quotes Opinions 5.05, 6.02, and 6.03. Scott, *Cybermedicine and Virtual Pharmacies*, 103 W. Va. L. Rev. 407, 441, 451 (2001).

Journal 2001 Discusses the history of fetal abuse prosecution and the Medical University of South Carolina's Interagency Policy of Management of Substance Abuse During Pregnancy. Concludes that, although the *Ferguson v. City of Charleston* decision will continue to allow pregnant drug users to access prenatal care, it leaves open questions regarding the future of fetal abuse prosecutions. Quotes Opinion 5.05. Toll, *For My Doctor's Eyes Only: Ferguson v. City of Charleston*, 33 Loy. U. Chi. L. J. 267, 305 (2001).

Journal 2000 Explores confidentiality and discusses the legal standards pertaining to attorneys, physicians, and social workers. Concludes that the concept of confidentiality is the backbone of each profession and without privileged communications such professions would fail the American public. Quotes Opinion 5.05. Clark, *Confidential Communications in a Professional Context: Attorney,*

Physician, and Social Worker, 24 J. Legal Prof. 79, 92 (2000).

Journal 2000 Describes possible solutions designed to improve postapproval regulation of prescription drugs so that fewer patients will suffer from adverse drug reactions. Concludes that the FDA along with physicians and clinical researchers should rethink the existing approach to monitoring of unexpected side effects. Quotes Principle V and Opinion 9.032. Cites Opinion 5.05. Noah, *Adverse Drug Reactions: Harnessing Experimental Data to Promote Patient Welfare*, 49 Cath. U. L. Rev. 449, 477, 497-98 (2000).

Journal 2000 Addresses the philosophical conflict between free speech and privacy. Examines the commercial speech doctrine and discusses the constitutional and human rights implications of use of private sector data. Cites Opinion 5.05. Singleton, *Privacy Versus the First Amendment: A Skeptical Approach*, 11 Fordham Intell. Prop. Media & Ent. L. J. 97, 122 (2000).

Journal 2000 Defines and explores current and future applications of telemedicine. Considers issues of cost, quality, access, and regulation. Concludes that telemedicine holds tremendous promise for improving the US health care system. Quotes Opinions 5.05 and 5.07. Volkert, *Telemedicine: Rx for the Future of Health Care*, 6 Mich. Telecomm. & Tech. L. Rev. 147, 214, 225 (2000).

Journal 1999 Explores changes in technology and the resulting impact on privacy of medical information. Observes that current federal and state laws inadequately protect medical information privacy and suggests that Congress needs to enact legislation addressing this issue. Quotes Opinion 5.05. References Opinions 7.02 and 7.05. Carter, *Health Information Privacy: Can Congress Protect Confidential Medical Information in the "Information Age"?* 25 Wm. Mitchell L. Rev. 223, 236, 273 (1999).

Journal 1999 Discusses the "ever-expanding" disclosure of confidential medical record information regarding patients. Emphasizes organizational problems relating to access and security in medical record systems. Argues in favor of stronger regulations limiting access to and use of information. Quotes Opinion 5.05. Hall, *Confidentiality as an Organizational Ethics Issue*, 10 J. Clinical Ethics 230, 232 (1999).

Journal 1999 Discusses the need for physicians to advocate on behalf of patients' rights in the context of health care delivery. Evaluates the nature and scope of the physician's role as advocate, noting that physicians cannot be expected to engage in attorney-like advocacy. Quotes Principles IV and VI, Fundamental Elements (2), (4), and (6) [now Opinion 10.01], Patient Responsibilities 5 [now Opinion 10.02], and Opinions 2.03, 2.07, 2.09, 2.16, 2.19, 3.06, 4.01, 4.04, 6.01, 7.02, 8.02, 8.03, 8.13, 8.132, 9.06, 9.07, and 9.131. Cites Opinions 5.05, 5.09, 7.01, 8.135, and 9.02. Sage, *Physicians as Advocates*, 35 Hous. L. Rev. 1529, 1537, 1541, 1542,

1552-53, 1554, 1556, 1557, 1559, 1561-62, 1564, 1571, 1574, 1576, 1580 (1999).

Journal 1999 Explores the increased use of physician-patient communication through e-mail. Analyzes current laws regarding medical privacy. Suggests that patients' communications to their physicians are part of their medical record and should be given the same protections. Quotes Opinions 5.05 and 5.07. Cites Opinions 5.04 and 5.06. Spielberg, *Online Without a Net:* physician-patient *Communication by Electronic Mail,* 25 Am. J. Law & Med. 267, 284-85 (1999).

Journal 1999 Explores Model Rules of Professional Conduct focusing on the attorney-client relationship. Compares confidentiality provisions in the Model Rules with the rules of confidentiality governing the medical profession. Observes that existing confidentiality rules are incomplete and ambiguous. Concludes that one remedy is to embrace a discretionary confidentiality rule. Quotes Opinion 5.05. Cites Principle IV and Opinion 5.07. Zer-Gutman, *Revising the Ethical Rules of Attorney-Client Confidentiality: Towards a New Discretionary Rule,* 45 Loy. L. Rev. 669, 683-84, 699, 709, 718 (1999).

Journal 1998 Describes the special nature of confidentiality in the relationship between the psychotherapist and patient. States that not many breach of confidentiality cases involve psychotherapists. Concludes that patients and psychotherapists must better understand their rights and responsibilities in this context. Quotes Opinion 5.05. Cites Opinions 5.06, 5.07, 5.08, and 5.09. Grabois, *The Liability of Psychotherapists for Breach of Confidentiality,* 12 J. Law & Health 39, 53-54 (1998).

Journal 1998 Explains risks involved with the use of electronic medical records. States that patients need to be aware of who has access to their medical records. Concludes that health care providers should equalize the risks and benefits related to the use of electronic medical records. Cites Opinion 5.05. References Opinion 5.07. Jurevic, *When Technology and Health Care Collide: Issues With Electronic Medical Records and Electronic Mail,* 66 UMKC L. Rev. 809, 819-20 (1998).

Journal 1998 Discusses issues of patient consent regarding disclosure of medical information. Points out that recent changes in the health care system have presented medical record privacy concerns. Discloses findings of a study regarding hospital consent forms and calls for more research to be conducted. Cites Principle IV and Opinion 5.05. Merz, Sankar, & Yoo, *Hospital Consent for Disclosure of Medical Records,* 26 J. Law Med. & Ethics 241, 248 (1998).

Journal 1998 Points out that most victims of elder abuse are socially isolated and thus few incidents of elder abuse are reported to authorities. Argues that current protections against elder abuse are inadequate. Suggests that the legal system and health professionals can make a difference in reducing elder abuse. Quotes Opinion 5.05. References Opinion 2.02. Moskowitz, *Saving Granny From the Wolf:*

Elder Abuse and Neglect—The Legal Framework, 31 Conn. L. Rev. 77, 116, 120, 121, 122 (1998).

Journal 1998 Discusses issues of privacy concerning the collection and use of computerized pharmacy records by pharmaceutical companies. Concludes that federal legislation is needed to protect the privacy of prescription information. Quotes Opinion 5.05. Mowery, *A Patient's Right of Privacy in Computerized Pharmacy Records,* 66 U. Cin. L. Rev. 697, 717 (1998).

Journal 1998 Discusses the ramifications of physician license revocation for failing to pay child support. Points out that patients stand to lose access to trusted physicians and confidence in the health care system. Concludes that children need the most protection and that patients will have an easier time finding another physician than children will have finding another means for support. Quotes Opinion 5.05. Cites Opinions 9.02 and 9.06. Noyes, *Higher Penalties for Failing to Pay Child Support: A Look at Medical License Revocation,* 19 J. Legal Med. 127, 138 (1998).

Journal 1998 Explores the role of pharmacy benefits managers. Discusses the impact of pharmacy benefits managers on patients, consumers, and the medical field. Analyzes potential privacy problems stemming from pharmacy benefits managers. Cites Opinion 5.05. Rosoff, *The Changing Face of Pharmacy Benefits Management: Information Technology Pursues a Grand Mission,* 42 St. Louis U. L. J. 1, 25-26 (1998).

Journal 1998 Examines the use of e-mail in the physician-patient relationship. Focuses on privacy concerns stemming from the use of e-mail in the medical context. Suggests that physicians should discuss the implications of communicating through e-mail with their patients and should obtain informed consent prior to communicating in this manner. Cites Opinions 5.04, 5.05, 5.057, 5.07, 5.075, and 5.08. Spielberg, *On Call and Online: Sociohistorical, Legal, and Ethical Implications of E-mail for the Patient-Physician Relationship,* 280 JAMA 1353, 1356 (1998).

Journal 1998 Explores the increased use and benefits of telemedicine. Points out that there is inadequate protection of privacy rights regarding electronic medical information. Concludes that federal law does not uniformly address medical record privacy and that Missouri law lacks adequate specificity. Quotes Principle IV. References Opinion 5.05. Young, *Telemedicine: Patient Privacy Rights of Electronic Medical Records,* 66 UMKC L. Rev. 921, 926 (1998).

Journal 1997 Compares past ethical opinions to current opinions and notes the differences. Comments on the forces that have changed medical ethics through the years. Notes differing theories on the future course of medical ethics. Quotes Fundamental Elements (Preamble) and Opinions 5.05, 5.057, 7.01, 8.12, 9.12, and 9.131. Cites Fundamental Elements (5) and Opinions 8.115 and 8.13. Buchanan, *Medical Ethics at the Millennium: A Brief Retrospective,* 26 Colo. Law. 141, 142, 143, 144, 145 (1997).

Journal 1997 Describes the DNA profile and its use in the scientific community. Examines common misconceptions about the DNA profile. Considers implication of the DNA profile as a unique identifier in the context of community health information networks. Quotes Principle 9 (1957) [now Opinion 5.05]. Dahm, *Using DNA Profile as the Unique Patient Identifier in the Community Health Information Network: Legal Implications, 15 J. Marshall J. Computer & Info. L. 227, 266, 275 (1997).*

Journal 1997 Considers how breast cancer has given rise to numerous medical malpractice lawsuits. Discusses trial techniques and strategies for litigating these types of claims. Quotes Opinions 5.05 and 5.06. Hillerich, Ellerin, & Frieder, *Selecting and Presenting a Failure to Diagnose Breast Cancer Case, 20 Am. J. Trial Advoc. 253, 271 (1996-97).*

Journal 1997 Considers principles of confidentiality in the physician-patient relationship. Notes the current trend emphasizing public reporting obligations of physicians to protect members of society. Emphasizes need for balance between patient rights and societal interests. Quotes Principle IV and Opinion 5.05. References Preamble. Jozefowicz, *The Case Against Having Professional Privilege in the* physician-patient *Relationship, 16 Med. & L. 385, 386-87, 391 (1997).*

Journal 1997 Suggests that ex parte conferences between treating physicians and opposing counsel undermine the physician-patient relationship. Notes that there are no significant benefits within the fact-finding process that justify the conflicts of interest created. Concludes that ex parte conferences are unnecessary. Quotes Principle IV and Opinion 5.05. Kassel, *Counterpoint . . . Defense Counsel's Ex Parte Communication With Plaintiff's Doctors: A Bad One-Sided Deal, 9 S. C. Law. 42, 43 (Sept./Oct. 1997).*

Journal 1997 Discusses the practice of ex parte communications between treating physicians and their patients' legal adversaries without informing the patient or obtaining consent. Examines harms that may occur in these situations. Argues that Oklahoma needs to prohibit treating physicians from communicating ex parte with their patients' legal adversaries. Quotes Opinions 5.05, 5.07, 5.08, 8.02, 8.03, and 9.07. Cites Opinion 7.02. McNaughton & McNaughton, *Divided Loyalty: The Dilemma of the Treating Physician Advocate, 22 Okla. City U. L. Rev. 1051, 1052, 1054, 1056, 1058, 1059, 1062 (1997).*

Journal 1997 Considers Connecticut AIDS statute, which relates to testing and confidentiality of patient medical information. Discusses statutory construction of provisions of this law by the Connecticut Supreme Court in *Doe v. Marselle.* Quotes Opinion 5.05. Note, *A Case Study of New Textualism in State Courts: Doe v. Marselle and the Confidentiality of HIV-Related Information, 30 Conn. L. Rev. 295, 297 (1997).*

Journal 1997 Considers whether the physician-patient privilege should be extended to protect communications to alternative health practitioners. Suggests that these practitioners treat and diagnose patients within the meaning of the

privilege. Advocates an extension of the privilege to recognize the importance of confidentiality. Quotes Opinion 5.05. Note, *Healer-Patient Privilege: Extending the* physician-patient *Privilege to Alternative Health Practitioners in California, 48 Hastings L. J. 633, 657 (1997).*

Journal 1996 Explains the benefits of high-tech access to patient information by pharmacists. Considers related issues of patient confidentiality. Advocates a pharmacist-patient privilege. Quotes Opinion 5.05. Berger, *Patient Confidentiality in a High Tech World, 5 J. Pharmacy & L., 139, 141 (1996).*

Journal 1996 Suggests that attorneys representing HIV-infected and sexually active adolescents face an ethical conflict between their duty of client confidentiality and the duty to protect third parties. Notes that attorneys failing to warn third parties may face liability. Concludes that clients should be informed of potential limitations on the right to confidentiality. Quotes Opinion 5.05. Katner, *The Ethical Dilemma Awaiting Counsel Who Represent Adolescents With HIV/AIDS: Criminal Law and Tort Suits Pressure Counsel to Breach the Confidentiality of the Clients' Medical Status, 70 Tul. L. Rev. 2311, 2341 (1996).*

Journal 1996 Discusses sexual abuse litigation in which accusers have recovered memories of molestation in psychotherapy sessions. Observes that, to successfully defend against such claims, it is necessary for the accused to have access to the clinical record. Posits that confidentiality problems can be eliminated with in camera record inspections. References Principle IV and Opinion 5.05. Loftus, Paddock, & Guernsey, *Patient-Psychotherapist Privilege: Access to Clinical Records in the Tangled Web of Repressed Memory Litigation, 30 U. Rich L. Rev. 109, 127 (1996).*

Journal 1996 Reviews two Washington State Supreme Court decisions in which subsequent treating physicians testified against their patients and on behalf of defendant physicians in malpractice litigation. Observes that these decisions erode the physician-patient privilege. Posits that the decisions are inconsistent with current medical ethics and proposes a statutory enactment as a solution. Quotes Opinion 5.05. Cites Principle 9 (1957) [now Principle IV]. Oppenheim, *Physicians as Experts Against Their Own Patients? What Happened to the Privilege? 63 Def. Couns. J. 254, 257, 261 (1996).*

Journal 1996 Considers prearraignment forensic evaluations. Notes the prohibition against use of such evaluations. Examines underlying ethical precepts. Observes that principles of beneficence are misapplied to forensic psychiatry in this context. Advocates a new ethical framework. Quotes Preamble. References Principle IV and Opinion 5.05. Ornish, Mills, & Ornish, *Prearraignment Forensic Evaluations: Toward a New Policy, 24 Bull. Am. Acad. Psychiatry Law 453, 454, 469 (1996).*

Journal 1996 Examines the psychiatrist-patient duty of confidentiality. Notes that Principles of Medical Ethics prohibit the disclosure of patient confidences and medical records. Observes that exceptions to this prohibition exist when required by law or to protect the community. Quotes Principle 9 (1957) [now Principle IV and Opinion 5.05]. Sadoff, *Ethical Obligations for the Psychiatrist: Confidentiality, Privilege, and Privacy in Psychiatric Treatment,* 29 Loy. L. A. L. Rev. 1709, 1710, 1711 (1996).

Journal 1995 Addresses presidential disability, its past impact on American government, and possible solutions to potential problems. Proposes enhancement of the role of the President's physician. Quotes Opinion 8.03. Cites Opinions 5.04 and 5.05. Abrams, *The Vulnerable President and the Twenty-Fifth Amendment, With Observations on Guidelines, a Health Commission, and the Role of the President's Physician,* 30 Wake Forest L. Rev. 453, 466, 471 (1995).

Journal 1995 Discusses the belief of health care providers that they have an ethical obligation to warn the partners of HIV-positive patients. Examines both the scope of a Massachusetts statute that prevents providers from releasing HIV test results of patients and possible defenses that providers may assert. Quotes Principle IV and Opinion 5.05. Friedland, *HIV Confidentiality and the Right to Warn—The Health Care Provider's Dilemma,* 80 Mass. L. Rev. 3, 4 (March 1995).

Journal 1995 Considers how the use of health care identification cards and medical record databases would threaten privacy rights. Concludes that federal legislation should be enacted to protect health care record privacy and prevent misuse of health care identification cards. Quotes Opinion 5.05. Minor, *Identity Cards and Databases in Health Care: The Need for Federal Privacy Protections,* 28 Colum. J. L. & Soc. Probs. 253, 279 (1995).

Journal 1995 Examines the impact of health care reform on physician-patient relationships. Discusses how reform may threaten the physician's fiduciary duty of loyalty by forcing physicians to make rationing decisions and giving physicians financial incentives to limit use of health care resources. Quotes Fundamental Elements (5) [now Opinion 10.0]. Cites Opinion 5.05. Orentlicher, *Health Care Reform and the Patient-Physician Relationship,* 5 Health Matrix 141, 143, 148 (1995).

Journal 1995 Analyzes the secular approach to the duty to treat HIV-infected individuals and the duty to warn those who are sexual partners of, or who share needles with, people infected with HIV. Observes that the secular approach leaves these issues unresolved but indicates that Jewish law compels physicians both to treat and to warn. Quotes Opinions 5.05 and 9.131. Shorr, *AIDS, Judaism, and the Limits of the Secular Society,* 20 Second Opinion 23, 24, 27 (1995).

Journal 1994 Considers whether an exception should be made to physician-patient confidentiality that would allow a physician to reveal parental medical history to a child. Concludes that such an exception would not completely erode physician-patient confidentiality. Quotes Principle IV, Fundamental Elements (4), and Opinion 5.05. Cites Principle I and Fundamental Elements (1). Friedland, physician-patient *Confidentiality: Time to Re-Examine a Venerable Concept in Light of Contemporary Society and Advances in Medicine,* 15 J. Legal Med. 249, 257, 264, 276 (1994).

Journal 1994 Explores the ethical issues involved in a multidisciplinary team working with children in legal proceedings. Focuses on the relationships between professionals and the conflicts that arise regarding disclosure of confidential information and forced disclosure of nonprivileged information. Quotes Principles III and IV, Fundamental Elements (4), and Opinions 1.02 (1992) and 5.07 (1992) [now Opinion 5.05]. Cites Opinions 2.02. Glynn, *Multidisciplinary Representation of Children: Conflicts Over Disclosures of Client Communications,* 27 J. Marshall L. Rev. 617, 625, 626, 630-32, 637, 639, 643 (1994).

Journal 1994 Compares Texas law with Illinois law on the issue of ex parte communications between defense counsel and the patient/plaintiff's physician in civil litigation. Argues that preservation of the physician-patient relationship requires prohibition of such contact. Quotes Principles II and IV and Opinion 5.05. Comment, *From the Land of Lincoln a Healing Rule: Proposed Texas Rule of Civil Procedure Prohibiting Ex Parte Contact Between Defense Counsel and a Plaintiff's Treating Physician,* 25 Tex. Tech L. Rev. 1081, 1081, 1082 (1994).

Journal 1994 Considers how computerized medical records might threaten patient confidentiality. Explores proposed legislation for computerized records and the potential need for new legal standards in this area. Cites Opinion 5.05. Field, *Overview: Computerized Medical Records Create New Legal and Business Confidentiality Problems,* 11 HealthSpan 3, 4 (1994).

Journal 1993 Discusses family privacy rights and considers the meaning of justice, self-respect, and the fundamental principles of physician ethics. Concludes that physicians have an ethical duty to intervene in domestic violence so long as such intervention does not breach confidentiality or violate patient autonomy. Quotes Principle IV and Opinion 5.05. References Opinions 8.14 and 9.131. Jecker, *Privacy Beliefs and the Violent Family: Extending the Ethical Argument for Physician Intervention,* 269 JAMA 776, 778, 779 (1993).

Journal 1993 Evaluates the legal issues surrounding AIDS and HIV. Examines various aspects of the law that would be relevant to a medical or health care lawyer. Quotes Opinion 5.05. Skiver & Hickey, *AIDS: Legal Issues 1992,* 19 Ohio No. Univ. L. Rev. 839, 860 (1993).

Journal 1991 Discusses current law protecting confidential genetic information obtained in the workplace and presents several safeguard mechanisms. Analyzes the legal grounds upon which various parties may access this information. References Opinion 5.05. Andrews & Jaeger, *Confidentiality of Genetic Information in the Workplace,* XVII Am. J. Law & Med. 75, 78 (1991).

Journal 1991 Examines the problem of AIDS in this country and the risk of HIV transmission via sexual assault. Concludes that state laws requiring HIV testing for sex offenders are necessary to preserve the rights of victims of sexual assault. Quotes Opinion 5.05. McGuire, *AIDS and the Sexual Offender: The Epidemic Now Poses New Threats to the Victim and the Criminal Justice System, 96 Dickinson L. Rev. 95, 109, 110 (1991).*

Journal 1991 Focuses on the case *Crist v. Moffatt*, where a court permitted ex parte interview of a plaintiff's physician only after the plaintiff signed a written authorization. Concludes that Crist was correctly decided, but warns against expanding the decision to the point of unduly restricting discovery. Quotes Opinion 5.05. Note, *Restricting Ex Parte Interviews With Nonparty Treating Physicians: Crist v. Moffatt, 69 No. Carolina L. Rev. 1381, 1391, 1392 (1991).*

Journal 1991 Discusses confidentiality with respect to a patient's HIV status. Notes how confidentiality may be lost in the hospital setting and emphasizes importance of heightened attention to this issue by institutional health care providers. Quotes Opinion 5.05. Obade, *Whisper Down the Lane: AIDS, Privacy, and the Hospital Grapevine, 2 J. Clinical Ethics 133, 133 (1991).*

Journal 1990 Discusses the legal and ethical considerations associated with genetic research, including recombinant DNA technology. Offers case examples illustrating issues raised by the application of this technology in the clinical setting. Quotes Opinion 5.05. Elsas, *A Clinical Approach to Legal and Ethical Problems in Human Genetics, 39 Emory L. J. 811, 816, 820 (1990).*

Journal 1990 Advocates physician liability for failure to warn third parties of the potential risk of being infected with HIV from the physician's patient. Concludes that there should be no liability for disclosure because public health concerns outweigh an individual patient's right to confidentiality. References Opinion 5.05. Note, *AIDS: Establishing a Physician's Duty to Warn, 21 Rutgers L. J. 645, 652 (1990).*

Journal 1989 Discusses the history of the physician-patient privilege up through changes implemented under the Ohio Tort Reform Act of 1987. Aspects of the physician-patient privilege that are most significantly affected by this Tort Reform Act are highlighted, with recommendations for further refinement of the privilege in Ohio. Quotes Principles II and IV and Opinion 5.05. Note, *The Ohio physician-patient Privilege: Modified, Revised, and Defined, 49 Ohio St. L. J. 1147, 1167 (1989).*

3.2.2 Confidentiality Postmortem

Journal 2011 Examines current legal and ethical frameworks governing the return of a deceased research participant's individual research results to related family members, including Canadian, American, and French legislation. Concludes that there is a lack of international consensus and that additional ethical and professional guidelines are necessary. Quotes Opinion 5.051. Tasse, *The Return of Results of Deceased Research Participants, 39 J. L. Med. & Ethics 621, 624-625 (2011).*

Journal 2007 Analyzes scientific, ethical, and legal issues raised in the exhumation and genetic analysis of historical figures. Concludes that biohistorical review boards should be created to generate guidelines for such research. Quotes Preamble and Opinion 2.08. Cites Opinions 2.079, 2.105, 5.05, 5.051, 5.075, 8.03, 8.031, 9.095, and 9.10. Paradise & Andrews, *Tales From the Crypt: Scientific, Ethical, and Legal Considerations for Biohistorical Analysis of Deceased Historical Figures, 26 Temp. J. Sci. Tech. & Envtl. L. 223, 287-88 (2007).*

Journal 2004 Examines the requirements of the Privacy Rule regarding use and disclosure of a patient's identifiable health information in the context of research. Concludes that the Rule's burdensome administrative requirements may discourage research and thus outweigh any benefits for research subject autonomy. Quotes Principle VIII and Opinions 5.051, 8.031, and 10.015. Tovino, *The Use and Disclosure of Protected Health Information for Research Under the HIPAA Privacy Rule: Unrealized Patient Autonomy and Burdensome Government Regulation, 49 S. D. L. Rev. 447, 496, 502 (2004).*

Journal 2001 Analyzes postmortem patient confidentiality and proposes a framework for appropriate information disclosure. Concludes that, following death, decisions regarding disclosure of confidential information should be made on a case-by-case basis. Quotes Opinions 5.051 and 7.02. Berg, *Grave Secrets: Legal and Ethical Analysis of Postmortem Confidentiality, 34 Conn. L. Rev. 81, 87, 117 (2001).*

3.2.3 Industry-Employed Physicians and Independent Medical Examiners

Mass. 1984 Employee sued employer for libel and invasion of privacy following disclosure of medical facts about employee to other employees. In part, claim involved disclosure of opinion about employee's mental state to

his supervisor by physician retained by employer. Citing Principle 9 (1957) [now Principle IV and Opinions 5.05 and 5.09], the court held that a physician retained by an employer may disclose to the employer information concerning an employee if receipt of the information is reasonably necessary to serve a substantial and valid business interest of the employer. *Bratt v. International Business Mach. Corp., 392 Mass. 508, 467 N.E.2d 126, 137 n.23.*

N.Y. Sup. 2000 Physician brought wrongful discharge claim against corporate employer. The physician alleged she was discharged because she refused to reveal confidential medical information regarding employees. With apparent reference to Principle IV and Opinions 5.05 and 5.09, the affidavit filed by the physician claimed she had an ethical and legal duty to protect patient confidentiality. The court found termination of an employee at will based upon such grounds is sufficient to state a cause of action for breach of contract. The court ruled that obligations of good faith and fair dealing may be implied in a contract for the employment of a physician and that no physician should be placed in the position of choosing between retaining employment and violating ethical standards. *Horn v. New York Times, 186 Misc. 2d 469, 719 N.Y.S. 2d 471, 474.*

Journal 2003 Highlights HIPAA privacy issues that need to be monitored and have yet to be resolved. Concludes that HIPAA poses many challenges and it remains unclear whether HIPAA will increase privacy protection. Cites Opinions 5.05, 5.055, 5.057, 5.06, 5.07, 5.075, 5.08, and 5.09. Kutzko, Boyer, Thoman, & Scott, *HIPAA in Real Time: Practical Implications of the Federal Privacy Rule, 51 Drake L. Rev. 403, 408 (2003).*

Journal 2001 Discusses same-sex marriages in the transgender community. Explores Defense of Marriage Act statutes. Considers whether same-sex transgender marriages can prevail against attacks brought under such statutes. Cites Opinions 2.132, 2.135, 2.137, 5.08, and 5.09. Frye & Meiselman, *Same-Sex Marriages Have Existed Legally in the United States for a Long Time Now, 64 Alb. L. Rev. 1031, 1053 (2001).*

Journal 2000 Evaluates transgender legal and political activity in the US. Discusses the International Bill of Gender Rights against the background of the Texas case, *Littleton v. Prange.* Cites Opinions 2.132, 2.135, 2.137, 5.08, and 5.09. Frye, *The International Bill of Gender Rights vs. the Cider House Rules: Transgenders Struggle With the Courts Over What Clothing They Are Allowed to Wear on the Job, Which Restroom They Are Allowed to Use on the Job, Their Right to Marry, and the Very Definition of Their Sex, 7 Wm. & Mary J. Women & L. 133, 149 (2000).*

Journal 1999 Discusses the need for physicians to advocate on behalf of patients' rights in the context of health care

delivery. Evaluates the nature and scope of the physician's role as advocate, noting that physicians cannot be expected to engage in attorney-like advocacy. Quotes Principles IV and VI, Fundamental Elements (2), (4), and (6) [now Opinion 10.01], Patient Responsibilities 5 [now Opinion 10.02], and Opinions 2.03, 2.07, 2.09, 2.16, 2.19, 3.06, 4.01, 4.04, 6.01, 7.02, 8.02, 8.03, 8.13, 8.132, 9.06, 9.07, and 9.131. Cites Opinions 5.05, 5.09, 7.01, 8.135, and 9.02. Sage, *Physicians as Advocates, 35 Hous. L. Rev. 1529, 1537, 1541, 1542, 1552-53, 1554, 1556, 1557, 1559, 1561-62, 1564, 1571, 1574, 1576, 1580 (1999).*

Journal 1998 Analyzes the decision in *Spaulding v. Zimmerman.* Discusses the issue of an attorney's obligation to disclose information to protect a third-party's health or safety. Includes in this discussion consideration of the duty of an "examining" physician to disclose such information to an examinee. Cites Opinion 5.09. Cramton & Knowles, *Professional Secrecy and Its Exceptions: Spaulding v. Zimmerman Revisited, 83 Minn. L. Rev. 63, 98 (1998).*

Journal 1998 Describes the special nature of confidentiality in the relationship between the psychotherapist and patient. States that not many breach of confidentiality cases involve psychotherapists. Concludes that patients and psychotherapists must better understand their rights and responsibilities in this context. Quotes Opinion 5.05. Cites Opinions 5.06, 5.07, 5.08, and 5.09. Grabois, *The Liability of Psychotherapists for Breach of Confidentiality, 12 J. Law & Health 39, 53-54 (1998).*

Journal 1991 Explores ethical problems unique to the field of forensic psychiatry. Presents the results of a survey of members of the American Academy of Psychiatry and the Law (AAPL), asking their opinions regarding proposed ethical guidelines. Quotes Opinions 1.02 and 5.09. Weinstock, Leong, & Silva, *Opinions by AAPL Forensic Psychiatrists on Controversial Ethical Guidelines: A Survey, 19 Bull. Am. Acad. Psychiatry Law 237, 238 (1991).*

Journal 1984 Observes that available ethical and legal guidelines are insufficient to aid physicians in addressing issues of patient privacy and confidentiality. Concludes that there is need for legislation in order to provide suitable guidance to physicians who fulfill an important role in protecting patient privacy. Cites 1982 Opinions 5.03 [now Opinion 5.04], 5.04, 5.05 [now Opinion 5.06], 5.06 [now Opinion 5.07], 5.07 [now Opinion 5.08], and 5.08 [now Opinion 5.09]. Gellman, *Prescribing Privacy: The Uncertain Role of the Physician in the Protection of Patient Privacy, 62 No. Carolina L. Rev. 255, 271 (1984).*

3.2.4 Access to Medical Records by Data Collection Companies

Journal 2007 Analyzes scientific, ethical, and legal issues raised in the exhumation and genetic analysis of historical figures. Concludes that biohistorical review boards should be created to generate guidelines for such research. Quotes

Preamble and Opinion 2.08. Cites Opinions 2.079, 2.105, 5.05, 5.051, 5.075, 8.03, 8.031, 9.095, and 9.10. Paradise & Andrews, *Tales From the Crypt: Scientific, Ethical, and Legal Considerations for Biohistorical Analysis of*

Deceased Historical Figures, 26 Temp. J. Sci. Tech. & Envtl. L. 223, 287-88 (2007).

Journal 2003 Highlights HIPAA privacy issues that need to be monitored and have yet to be resolved. Concludes that HIPAA poses many challenges and it remains unclear whether HIPAA will increase privacy protection. Cites Opinions 5.05, 5.055, 5.057, 5.06, 5.07, 5.075, 5.08, and 5.09. Kutzko, Boyer, Thoman, & Scott, *HIPAA in Real Time: Practical Implications of the Federal Privacy Rule, 51 Drake L. Rev. 403, 408 (2003).*

Journal 1998 Examines the use of e-mail in the physician-patient relationship. Focuses on privacy concerns stemming from the use of e-mail in the medical context. Suggests that physicians should discuss the implications of communicating through e-mail with their patients and should obtain informed consent prior to communicating in this manner. Cites Opinions 5.04, 5.05, 5.057, 5.07, 5.075, and 5.08. Spielberg, *On Call and Online: Sociohistorical, Legal, and Ethical Implications of E-mail for the Patient-Physician Relationship, 280 JAMA 1353, 1356 (1998).*

Journal 1998 Examines the transition from paper medical records to electronic medical records. Identifies issues of confidentiality and privacy that arise as a result of the move to electronic medical records. Concludes that federal protection is needed to safeguard personal medical information. Quotes Principle IV and Opinions 5.07 and 5.075. Cites Opinion 8.061. Tsai, *Cheaper and Better: The Congressional Administrative Simplification Mandate Facilitates the Transition to Electronic Medical Records, 19 J. Legal Med. 549, 570, 581 (1998).*

3.3.1 Management of Medical Records

D. Colo. 2007 Plaintiff-inmate sued prison medical staff members claiming insufficient care and improper denial of outside care following an assault. The district court considered whether the plaintiff's Eighth Amendment right to receive adequate medical care had been violated. In support of his allegations, plaintiff attempted to show that in one instance a physician's recommendation for a second opinion was intentionally ignored. The court, quoting Opinion 7.01, found that the physician had merely transferred plaintiff's medical records to another physician upon request, consistent with his ethical obligation. The court held that plaintiff failed to show the required intent to disregard a substantial risk to his health. *Schaal v. Fender, 2007 WL 2461642, 7.*

N.D. Ill. 2010 Sister of deceased patient brought adversary proceeding against bankrupt physician to except from discharge debt stemming from physician's alleged breach of fiduciary duties. The bankruptcy court quotes Opinions 7.01 and 8.03 in finding that a fiduciary duty was established by nature of the physician-patient relationship that continued after patient's death. *In re Odeh, 431 B.R. 807, 814.*

Del. Super. 2002 Medical group sued physician for misappropriation of trade secrets and solicitation of patients while still employed with group. Group authorized physician to notify his patients of his departure. The physician used group's records and insurance data to send a mass-mail letter to about 900 patients. Appeals court held that the letter sent went beyond a notification and was instead a solicitation and that the group had not authorized him to use trade secrets to solicit patients. In so ruling the court quoted Opinions 7.01 and 7.03. *Total Care Physicians v. O'Hara, 2002 Del. Super. LEXIS 493, *19.*

Me. 1999 Physician appealed decision of the Board of Licensure in Medicine imposing a civil penalty for his failure to release medical records to patient's physicians. Physician argued that the board did not specify the ethical standards that his conduct violated. The court vacated the board's decision on the grounds that the physician was denied the opportunity to refute evidence of a violation of professional standards or to develop a defense predicated on those standards. The board, in defense of its decision, presented Opinions 7.01 and 7.02 to the court. The court, in vacating the decision, pointed out that the hearing record did not demonstrate which Opinions the board applied. Furthermore, the court, quoting Principle IV, stated that the physician had a responsibility to protect the patient's medical records. *Balian v. Board of Licensure in Medicine, 722 A.2d 364, 368.*

N.Y. Surr. 1968 Patients of a deceased physician filed an action seeking to obtain or copy records maintained by the decedent during his lifetime regarding them. The executor had refused to deliver the records by reason of a provision in the decedent's will directing that his "office records" be destroyed. Quoting Opinions and Reports of the Judicial Council, Sec. 9 Paras. 3, 4, 5, 6, and 7 (1966) [now Opinions 7.01, 7.02, 7.03, and 7.05], the court ruled that, while patient records are the property of the physician, it would be against public policy to permit their destruction. As a result, the court ordered the executor to make the records available to the patients' succeeding physicians at their request. *In re Culbertson's Will, 57 Misc. 2d 391, 292 N.Y.S.2d 806, 808-10.*

S.C. Att'y Gen. 1978 Citing Opinions 5.61, 5.62, and 5.63 (1977) [now Opinions 7.01, 7.02, and 7.03], state attorney general found that patient medical records are the property of the physician or hospital which compiled them and that patients have no ownership rights in them. Further, the opinion concludes that patients have a right to information contained in their records and the right to have records sent to another physician. Patients do not, however, have the right to unlimited direct access to their medical records. *South Carolina Att'y Gen. Op., 1978 S.C. AG LEXIS 806.*

Journal 1999 Discusses the need for physicians to advocate on behalf of patients' rights in the context of health care delivery. Evaluates the nature and scope of the physician's role as advocate, noting that physicians cannot be expected to engage in attorney-like advocacy. Quotes Principles IV and VI, Fundamental Elements (2), (4), and (6) [now Opinion 10.01], Patient Responsibilities 5 [now Opinion 10.02], and Opinions 2.03, 2.07, 2.09, 2.16, 2.19, 3.06, 4.01, 4.04, 6.01, 7.02, 8.02, 8.03, 8.13, 8.132, 9.06, 9.07, and 9.131. Cites Opinions 5.05, 5.09, 7.01, 8.135, and 9.02. Sage, *Physicians as Advocates, 35 Hous. L. Rev. 1529, 1537, 1541, 1542, 1552-53, 1554, 1556, 1557, 1559, 1561-62, 1564, 1571, 1574, 1576, 1580 (1999).*

Journal 1997 Compares past ethical opinions to current opinions and notes the differences. Comments on the forces that have changed medical ethics through the years. Notes differing theories on the future course of medical ethics. Quotes Fundamental Elements (Preamble) and Opinions 5.05, 5.057, 7.01, 8.12, 9.12, and 9.131. Cites Fundamental Elements (5) and Opinions 8.115 and 8.13. Buchanan, *Medical Ethics at the Millennium: A Brief Retrospective, 26 Colo. Law. 141, 142, 143, 144, 145 (1997).*

Tenn. App. 2007 Pursuant to a state statute, the Tennessee Board of Medical Examiners sought patient records from a physician. The physician refused the request. The court of appeals found that while patient privacy and a physician's right to practice were protected by substantive due process, these interests are balanced against the interest of the state in protecting the public health and welfare. Citing Opinion 7.02, the court found that the right to practice medicine freely was not infringed here because the statutory obligations were analogous to existing professional obligations. *McNiel v. Cooper, 241 S.W.3d 886, 897.*

Journal 2001 Analyzes postmortem patient confidentiality and proposes a framework for appropriate information disclosure. Concludes that, following death, decisions regarding disclosure of confidential information should be made on a case-by-case basis. Quotes Opinions 5.051 and 7.02. Berg, *Grave Secrets: Legal and Ethical Analysis of Postmortem Confidentiality, 34 Conn. L. Rev. 81, 87, 117 (2001).*

Journal 1999 Explores changes in technology and the resulting impact on privacy of medical information. Observes that current federal and state laws inadequately protect medical information privacy and suggests that Congress needs to enact legislation addressing this issue. Quotes Opinion 5.05. References Opinions 7.02 and 7.05. Carter, *Health Information Privacy: Can Congress Protect Confidential Medical Information in the "Information Age"? 25 Wm. Mitchell L. Rev. 223, 236, 273 (1999).*

Journal 1997 Discusses the practice of ex parte communications between treating physicians and their patients' legal adversaries without informing the patient or obtaining consent. Examines harms that may occur in these situations. Argues that Oklahoma needs to prohibit treating physicians from communicating ex parte with their patients' legal

adversaries. Quotes Opinions 5.05, 5.07, 5.08, 8.02, 8.03, and 9.07. Cites Opinion 7.02. McNaughton & McNaughton, *Divided Loyalty: The Dilemma of the Treating Physician Advocate, 22 Okla. City U. L. Rev. 1051, 1052, 1054, 1056, 1058, 1059, 1062 (1997).*

Journal 2010 Discusses the effects of using deidentified health information on privacy and considers the dangers of nonconsensual use of health information. Concludes deidentification of health information is a necessary though insufficient protection of privacy, and further research and regulations should be developed to demonstrate respect for individuals without unduly burdening research. Quotes Principle IV and Opinions 5.05 and 7.025. Rothstein, *Is Deidentification Sufficient to Protect Health Privacy in Research? 10 Am. J. Bioethics 3, 5 (Sept. 2010).*

Journal 2003 Addresses the importance of medical record privacy for patients with HIV/AIDS. Concludes that US privacy laws afford patients less protection than privacy laws in the European Union. References Opinion 7.025. Gilbert, *Emerging Issues in Global AIDS Policy: Preserving Privacy, 25 Whittier L. Rev. 273, 276 (2003).*

N.D. Ill. 1996 A corporation which provided hair transplants brought suit against a physician group under contract to provide medical services to the corporation. The complaint alleged that the defendants had breached the contract in bad faith by attempting to start their own company, by hiring staff members away, and by threatening to enforce noncompetition covenants in their contracts should any physicians attempt to remain with the corporation. The court referred to Opinion 9.02 as explicitly discouraging the use of restrictive covenants in contracts with physicians. Additionally, with apparent reference to Opinion 7.03, the court noted that defendants had not sent notices advising patients of the departure of physicians from the corporation, or of the departing physicians' new practice locations. *Cleveland Hair Clinic, Inc. v. Puig, 968 F. Supp. 1227, 1246.*

Ark. App. 2003 Clinic appealed summary judgment for a medical group that hired two physicians previously practicing in the clinic. Clinic did not pay the physicians and had no noncompetition agreement with them. Physicians notified their patients of their departure. Clinic alleged the medical group solicited its patients by employing the physicians and using patient lists. Appeals court found the clinic failed to establish an employment relationship or rights to the records. The court held the physicians had a right to terminate their association with the clinic and that their patients had a right to follow them. Cites Opinion 7.03. *Springdale Diagnostic Clinic v. Northwest Physicians, 2003 Ark. App. LEXIS 697, *13, n.1.*

N.Y. Sup. 2006 Following termination from a medical group, a physician sought possession of her patients' original medical records. Her employment contract specified that the group would retain all original records and that the physician was entitled to copies. Plaintiff cited a state statute, as well as Opinions 7.03 and 7.04, arguing that a physician has a duty to personally maintain patient records. The court, while acknowledging the physician's duty in this regard, held there was no violation of the statute. There was no reason to believe the group would not safeguard the original records and comply with all statutory requirements. *Pullman v. Gormley, 13 Misc.3d 1234(A), 831 N.Y.S.2d 356, 2006 WL 3232182, 3.*

Journal 2006 Discusses the evolution of health law in Virginia. Concludes that the area of health law continues to expand, develop, and be refined. Cites Opinions 3.03, 3.08, 5.01, 5.015, 5.02, 5.04, 5.055, 6.02, 6.021, 6.03, 6.04, 7.03, 7.04, 7.05, 8.054, 8.08, 8.081, 8.085, 8.115, 8.12, 8.14, 8.145, 8.19, and 9.045. Guanzon, *Health Care Law, 41 U. Rich. L. Rev. 179, 199 (2006).*

N.Y. Surr. 1977 In a discovery proceeding, respondent-psychiatrist, who had treated some patients of deceased psychiatrist subsequent to his death, allegedly misappropriated decedent's patient records. Estate petitioned court for return of records and damages for injury to value of decedent's practice. Respondent sought dismissal of claim arguing that estate could not sell patient records. The court rejected respondent's request. In so ruling, the court noted that under Principle 9 (1957) [now Principle IV and Opinion 5.05] prohibiting physicians from revealing patient confidences, various guidelines had been issued regarding sale of a medical practice [now Opinion 7.04]. Whether respondent's actions had interfered with the estate's efforts to dispose of decedent's practice in keeping with these guidelines presented the court with factual issues for later resolution. *Estate of Finkle, 90 Misc. 2d 550, 395 N.Y.S.2d 343, 346.*

Journal 2004 Discusses the practice of using an attorney retaining lien over a client's papers and argues that the practice should be abolished. Concludes that this practice is coercive and inconsistent with a lawyer's role as a fiduciary. Quotes Opinion 7.02. References Opinion 8.10. Leubsdorf, *Against Lawyer Retaining Liens, 72 Fordham L. Rev. 849, 864, 865 (2004).*

Tex. 1998 Plaintiff, whose daughter was injured at birth, sued physician for intentional spoliation of medical records pertinent to lawsuit against hospital. The Texas Supreme Court refused to recognize a separate cause of action for intentional or negligent spoliation of evidence by parties to litigation. The court stated that creating a new cause of action for spoliation would result in duplicative litigation. Concurring judge explained other remedies available to the plaintiff. Quoting Opinion 7.05, judge stated that the ethical duty to retain medical records could be treated as a legal duty. *Trevino v. Ortega, 41 Tex. Sup. Ct. J. 907, 969 S.W.2d 950, 955.*

Journal 2007 Highlights inconsistencies in applying judicial deference to medical ethics. Concludes that courts should afford greater deference to established medical ethics standards. Quotes Principle I and Opinions 2.06 and Ch. II, Art. I, Sec. 3 (May 1847) [now Opinion 5.02]. Cites Opinions 4.01 and 7.05. Lerman, *Second Opinion: Inconsistent Deference to Medical Ethics in Death Penalty Jurisprudence, 95 Geo. L. J. 1941, 1945, 1974-75, 1976, 1977 (2007).*

Journal 2007 Examines regulation of medical tourism and the outsourcing of medical goods and services. Concludes that little regulation currently exists, and that patient privacy is a foremost concern. Quotes Opinion 7.05. Terry, *Under-Regulated Health Care Phenomena in a Flat World: Medical Tourism and Outsourcing, 29 W. New Eng. L. Rev. 421, 441 (2007).*

Journal 1999 Explores changes in technology and the resulting impact on privacy of medical information. Observes that current federal and state laws inadequately protect medical information privacy and suggests that Congress needs to enact legislation addressing this issue. Quotes Opinion 5.05. References Opinions 7.02 and 7.05. Carter, *Health Information Privacy: Can Congress Protect Confidential Medical Information in the "Information Age"? 25 Wm. Mitchell L. Rev. 223, 236, 273(1999).*

3.3.2 Confidentiality and Electronic Medical Records

M.D. Pa. 1987 Plaintiff in a medical malpractice action sought to preclude his treating physicians from serving as defendant's expert witnesses at trial. The court held that defense counsel's failure to provide prior notice of ex parte communication with plaintiff's treating physicians barred their use as defense experts. Referring to *Petrillo v. Syntex Laboratories, Inc.*, 148 Ill. App. 3d 581, 499 N.E.2d 952 (1986), the court noted that the court there favorably cited Principle IV and Opinions 5.05, 5.06, and 5.07 (1984) in support of a public policy protecting confidentiality between physician and patient and against ex parte discussion. *Manion v. N.P.W. Medical Center of N.E. Pa., Inc., 676 F.Supp. 585, 591.*

Ill. App. 1986 Defense attorney in product liability suit was held in contempt of court for conducting ex parte discussions with plaintiff-patient's treating physician without patient's consent and contrary to authorized methods of discovery. The court held that the strong public policy favoring physician-patient confidentiality articulated in Principles II and IV and Opinions 5.05, 5.06, 5.07, and 5.08 (1984) justified a rule against such ex parte discussions. Further, the court held that the public has the right to rely on physicians to faithfully execute their ethical obligations. *Petrillo v. Syntex Laboratories, Inc., 148 Ill. App. 3d 581, 499 N.E.2d 952, 957, 958, 959, cert. denied 483 US 1007 (1987).*

Pa. Super. 1988 Plaintiff-patient sued her physician for breach of confidentiality when physician conferred with defense counsel in plaintiff's malpractice suit against the hospital (physician's employer). In its majority opinion, the court cited Principle IV, commenting that it gave very little guidance to physicians but nonetheless was not violated by the physician. The court also noted Opinion 5.07 (1986) finding that the plaintiff's suit minimized her expectations of confidentiality. The dissent, however, interpreted these same provisions, along with Opinion 5.05 (1986), as protecting plaintiff's expectations of confidentiality. *Moses v. McWilliams, 379 Pa. Super. 150, 549 A.2d 950, 956, 962 (dissent) appeal denied 521 Pa. 630, 558 A.2d 532 (1989).*

Journal 2006 Examines the benefits and privacy concerns associated with the adoption of electronic medical records. Suggests the federal government should embrace HIPAA to simultaneously protect privacy and facilitate transition to the new system. Cites Opinion 5.07. McLaughlin, *Pandora's Box: Can HIPAA Still Protect Patient Privacy Under a National Health Care Information Network? 42 Gonz. L. Rev. 29, 42 (2006).*

Journal 2003 Highlights HIPAA privacy issues that need to be monitored and have yet to be resolved. Concludes that HIPAA poses many challenges and it remains unclear whether HIPAA will increase privacy protection. Cites Opinions 5.05, 5.055, 5.057, 5.06, 5.07, 5.075, 5.08, and 5.09. Kutzko, Boyer, Thoman, & Scott, *HIPAA in Real Time: Practical Implications of the Federal Privacy Rule, 51 Drake L. Rev. 403, 408 (2003).*

Journal 2000 Defines and explores current and future applications of telemedicine. Considers issues of cost, quality, access, and regulation. Concludes that telemedicine holds tremendous promise for improving the US health care system. Quotes Opinions 5.05 and 5.07. Volkert, *Telemedicine: Rx for the Future of Health Care, 6 Mich. Telecomm. & Tech. L. Rev. 147, 214, 225 (2000).*

Journal 1999 Explores the increased use of physician-patient communication through e-mail. Analyzes current laws regarding medical privacy. Suggests that patients' communications to their physicians are part of their medical record and should be given the same protections. Quotes Opinions 5.05 and 5.07. Cites Opinions 5.04 and 5.06. Spielberg, *Online Without a Net: physician-patient Communication by Electronic Mail, 25 Am. J. Law & Med. 267, 284-85 (1999).*

Journal 1999 Explores Model Rules of Professional Conduct focusing on the attorney-client relationship. Compares confidentiality provisions in the Model Rules with the rules of confidentiality governing the medical profession. Observes that existing confidentiality rules are incomplete and ambiguous. Concludes that one remedy is to embrace a discretionary confidentiality rule. Quotes Opinion 5.05. Cites Principle IV and Opinion 5.07. Zer-Gutman, *Revising the Ethical Rules of Attorney-Client Confidentiality: Towards a New Discretionary Rule, 45 Loy. L. Rev. 669, 683-84, 699, 709, 718 (1999).*

Journal 1998 Describes the special nature of confidentiality in the relationship between the psychotherapist and patient. States that not many breach of confidentiality cases involve psychotherapists. Concludes that patients and psychotherapists must better understand their rights and responsibilities in this context. Quotes Opinion 5.05. Cites Opinions 5.06, 5.07, 5.08, and 5.09. Grabois, *The Liability of Psychotherapists for Breach of Confidentiality, 12 J. Law & Health 39, 53-54 (1998).*

Journal 1998 Explains risks involved with the use of electronic medical records. States that patients need to be aware of who has access to their medical records. Concludes that health care providers should equalize the risks and benefits related to the use of electronic medical records. Cites Opinion 5.05. References Opinion 5.07. Jurevic, *When Technology and Health Care Collide: Issues With Electronic Medical Records and Electronic Mail, 66 UMKC L. Rev. 809, 819-20 (1998).*

Journal 1998 Examines the use of e-mail in the physician-patient relationship. Focuses on privacy concerns stemming from the use of e-mail in the medical context. Suggests that physicians should discuss the implications of communicating through e-mail with their patients and should obtain informed consent prior to communicating in this manner. Cites Opinions 5.04, 5.05, 5.057, 5.07, 5.075, and 5.08. Spielberg, *On Call and Online: Sociohistorical, Legal, and Ethical Implications of E-mail for the Patient-Physician Relationship, 280 JAMA 1353, 1356 (1998).*

Journal 1998 Examines the transition from paper medical records to electronic medical records. Identifies issues of confidentiality and privacy that arise as a result of the move to electronic medical records. Concludes that federal protection is needed to safeguard personal medical information. Quotes Principle IV and Opinions 5.07 and 5.075. Cites Opinion 8.061. Tsai, *Cheaper and Better: The Congressional Administrative Simplification Mandate Facilitates the Transition to Electronic Medical Records, 19 J. Legal Med. 549, 570, 581 (1998).*

Journal 1997 Discusses the practice of ex parte communications between treating physicians and their patients' legal adversaries without informing the patient or obtaining consent. Examines harms that may occur in these situations. Argues that Oklahoma needs to prohibit treating physicians from communicating ex parte with their patients' legal adversaries. Quotes Opinions 5.05, 5.07, 5.08, 8.02, 8.03, and 9.07. Cites Opinion 7.02. McNaughton & McNaughton, *Divided Loyalty: The Dilemma of the Treating Physician Advocate, 22 Okla. City U. L. Rev. 1051, 1052, 1054, 1056, 1058, 1059, 1062 (1997).*

Journal 1997 Examines the benefits of unconstrained access to personal medical information. Discusses drawbacks to full disclosure and absolute confidentiality of medical information. Advocates increased awareness of how medical data are used. Proposes guidelines for the best approach to regulation of health care data. Cites Opinion 5.07. Schwartz, *Privacy and the Economics of Personal Health Care Information, 76 Tex. L. Rev. 1, 59 (1997).*

Journal 1997 Considers new data-collection technology enabling collection, storage, and dissemination of data, including medical records information. Discusses the confidentiality problems triggered by increased utilization of computers in health care delivery. Quotes Opinion 5.07. Woodward, *Medical Record Confidentiality and Data Collection: Current Dilemmas, 25 J. Law Med. & Ethics 88, 90, 95 (1997).*

Journal 1995 Examines federal legislative proposals intended to protect confidentiality of computerized medical records. Concludes that proposed legislation will significantly undermine confidentiality. Cites Opinion 5.07. References Principle IV. Hoge, *Proposed Federal Legislation Jeopardizes Patient Privacy, 23 Bull. Am. Acad. Psychiatry Law 495, 498, 500 (1995).*

Journal 1993 Discusses the issues surrounding the confidentiality of electronic and computerized medical records.

Concludes that any legal standard addressing this problem should balance the need to protect patient confidentiality with the practical constraints limiting ideal security. References Principle IV and Opinion 5.07. Waller & Fulton, *The Electronic Chart: Keeping It Confidential and Secure, 26 J. Health & Hosp. L. 104, 105 (April 1993).*

Journal 1984 Observes that available ethical and legal guidelines are insufficient to aid physicians in addressing issues of patient privacy and confidentiality. Concludes that there is need for legislation in order to provide suitable guidance to physicians who fulfill an important role in protecting patient privacy. Cites 1982 Opinions 5.03 [now Opinion 5.04], 5.04, 5.05 [now Opinion 5.06], 5.06 [now Opinion 5.07], 5.07 [now Opinion 5.08], and 5.08 [now Opinion 5.09]. Gellman, *Prescribing Privacy: The Uncertain Role of the Physician in the Protection of Patient Privacy, 62 No. Carolina L. Rev. 255, 271 (1984).*

4 Genetics and Reproductive Medicine

4.1.1 Genetic Testing and Counseling

Journal 2006 Evaluates policies regarding regulation of preimplantation genetic diagnosis. Concludes the US should require a separate license for health care professionals to perform the procedure. Cites Opinion 2.12. Fahrenkrog, *A Comparison of International Regulation of Preimplantation Genetic Diagnosis and a Regulatory Suggestion for the United States, 15 Transnat'l L. & Contemp. Probs. 757, 759 (2006).*

Journal 2006 Discusses the ethical issues surrounding preimplantation genetic diagnosis (PGD) for cancer syndromes. Concludes that patients must be afforded psychosocial support for participation in PGD and that there is ongoing need for professional guidance to physicians on this topic. Quotes Opinion 2.12. Offit, Sagi, & Hurley, *Preimplantation Genetic Diagnosis for Cancer Syndromes: A New Challenge for Preventive Medicine, 296 JAMA 2727, 2727 (2006).*

Journal 2003 Applies professional standards to determine the technology that practitioners should utilize in prenatal diagnosis. Concludes that appropriate uses of prenatal diagnostic methodologies must be articulated by society. Quotes Opinion 2.12. Botkin, *Prenatal Diagnosis and the Selection of Children, 30 Fla. St. U. L. Rev. 265, 289 (2003).*

Journal 2003 Proposes a method to distinguish between good and bad eugenics. Concludes that prenatal testing for Down syndrome, followed by termination of pregnancy, characterizes bad eugenics. References Opinion 2.12. Mahowald, *Aren't We All Eugenicists? Commentary on Paul Lombardo's "Taking Eugenics Seriously," 30 Fla. St. U. L. Rev. 219, 234 (2003).*

Journal 2003 Considers the medical, ethical, and legal issues associated with using preimplantation genetic diagnosis (PGD) to create a stem cell donor. Concludes by offering important guidelines and limitations in connection with use of PGD. Quotes Opinion 2.12. Wolf, Kahn, & Wagner, *Using Preimplantation Genetic Diagnosis to Create a Stem Cell Donor: Issues, Guidelines & Limits, 31 J. L. Med. & Ethics 327, 329, 339 (2003).*

Journal 2000 Defines and describes human genetic enhancement. Explores the legal implications of this emerging technology as well as related societal concerns. Quotes Opinion 2.11. References Opinion 2.12. Mehlman, *The Law of Above Averages: Leveling the New Genetic Enhancement Playing Field, 85 Iowa L. Rev. 517, 527-28, 559 (2000).*

Journal 1998 Discusses genetic testing to determine hereditary hearing impairment. Explains ways in which genetic counselors can assist people. Points out how presymptomatic diagnosis can help parents and children. References Opinion 2.12. Chen, Mueller, Prasad, Greinwald, Manaligod, Muilenburg, Verhoeven, Van Camp, & Smith, *Presymptomatic Diagnosis of Nonsyndromic Hearing Loss by Genotyping, 124 Arch. Otolaryngol. Head Neck Surg. 20, 23 (1998).*

Journal 1997 Discusses techniques and possibilities for genetic testing. Presents a series of problems designed as a starting point for understanding the conflicts surrounding genetic testing. Reviews the applications of state-of-the-art genetic research. Suggests potential difficulties that testing may cause in society. References Opinion 2.12. Underwood

& Cadle, *Genetics, Genetic Testing, and the Specter of Discrimination: A Discussion Using Hypothetical Cases*, 85 Ky. L. J. 665, 684 (1996-97).

Journal 2007 Examines the legal and ethical considerations surrounding disclosure of *BRCA1/2* genetic testing results to family members. Concludes that genetic providers play a valuable role in facilitating the communication process between family members. Cites Opinion 2.131. DeMarco & McKinnon, *Life After BRCA1/2 Testing: Family Communication and Support Issues*, 27 Breast Disease 127, 127 (2007).

Journal 2004 Discusses the conflict between a physician's duty to keep genetic information private and potential liability for failure to inform at-risk relatives of the possibility of genetic disorders. Concludes that physicians should encourage patients to share genetic information with at-risk relatives, while abiding by legal and ethical principles. Quotes Opinion 2.131. Offit, Groeger, Turner, Wadsworth, & Weiser, *The "Duty to Warn" a Patient's Family Members About Hereditary Disease Risks*, 292 JAMA 1469, 1471 (2004).

Journal 2001 Examines the distinction between preplacement and postplacement examinations in the workplace. Analyzes the possible dangers that might result if preplacement medical testing is not restricted. Concludes that any such testing must relate to the potential employee's ability to perform assigned job duties. References Opinions 2.132 and 2.139. Hoffman, *Preplacement Examinations and Job-Relatedness: How to Enhance Privacy and Diminish Discrimination in the Workplace*, 49 U. Kan. L. Rev. 517, 534, 535, 556, 565 (2001).

Journal 2000 Explores issues relating to genetic privacy and considers how the law should evolve in this context. Identifies contrasting ideological viewpoints regarding the role government should play in regulating public use of personal genetic data. Concludes that because of unregulated information markets, people may be afraid to use genetic technologies. References Opinion 2.139. Fedder, *To Know or Not to Know: Legal Perspectives on Genetic Privacy and Disclosure of an Individual's Genetic Profile*, 21 J. Legal Med. 557, 563 (2000).

Journal 2000 Explores the legal, ethical, social, and economic considerations associated with use of new genetic techniques in the prediction and diagnosis of Alzheimer disease. Outlines the potential responsibilities and liabilities of physicians in connection with use of these techniques. References Opinions 2.132, 2.139, and 8.032. Kapp, *Physicians' Legal Duties Regarding the Use of Genetic Tests to Predict and Diagnose Alzheimer Disease*, 21 J. Legal Med. 445, 456-57, 465-66 (2000).

4.1.2 Genetic Testing for Reproductive Decision Making

Journal 2006 Evaluates policies regarding regulation of preimplantation genetic diagnosis. Concludes the US should require a separate license for health care professionals to perform the procedure. Cites Opinion 2.12. Fahrenkrog, *A Comparison of International Regulation of Preimplantation Genetic Diagnosis and a Regulatory Suggestion for the United States*, 15 Transnat'l L. & Contemp. Probs. 757, 759 (2006).

Journal 2006 Discusses the ethical issues surrounding preimplantation genetic diagnosis (PGD) for cancer syndromes. Concludes that patients must be afforded psychosocial support for participation in PGD and that there is ongoing need for professional guidance to physicians on this topic. Quotes Opinion 2.12. Offit, Sagi, & Hurley, *Preimplantation Genetic Diagnosis for Cancer Syndromes: A New Challenge for Preventive Medicine*, 296 JAMA 2727, 2727 (2006).

Journal 2003 Applies professional standards to determine the technology that practitioners should utilize in prenatal diagnosis. Concludes that appropriate uses of prenatal diagnostic methodologies must be articulated by society. Quotes Opinion 2.12. Botkin, *Prenatal Diagnosis and the Selection of Children*, 30 Fla. St. U. L. Rev. 265, 289 (2003).

Journal 2003 Proposes a method to distinguish between good and bad eugenics. Concludes that prenatal testing for Down syndrome, followed by termination of pregnancy, characterizes bad eugenics. References Opinion 2.12. Mahowald, *Aren't We All Eugenicists? Commentary on Paul Lombardo's "Taking Eugenics Seriously,"* 30 Fla. St. U. L. Rev. 219, 234 (2003).

Journal 2003 Considers the medical, ethical, and legal issues associated with using preimplantation genetic diagnosis (PGD) to create a stem cell donor. Concludes by offering important guidelines and limitations in connection with use of PGD. Quotes Opinion 2.12. Wolf, Kahn, & Wagner, *Using Preimplantation Genetic Diagnosis to Create a Stem Cell Donor: Issues, Guidelines & Limits*, 31 J. L. Med. & Ethics 327, 329, 339 (2003).

Journal 2000 Defines and describes human genetic enhancement. Explores the legal implications of this emerging technology as well as related societal concerns. Quotes Opinion 2.11. References Opinion 2.12. Mehlman, *The Law of Above Averages: Leveling the New Genetic Enhancement Playing Field*, 85 Iowa L. Rev. 517, 527-28, 559 (2000).

Journal 1998 Discusses genetic testing to determine hereditary hearing impairment. Explains ways in which genetic counselors can assist people. Points out how presymptomatic diagnosis can help parents and children. References Opinion 2.12. Chen, Mueller, Prasad, Greinwald, Manaligod, Muilenburg, Verhoeven, Van Camp, & Smith, *Presymptomatic Diagnosis of Nonsyndromic Hearing Loss* *by Genotyping, 124 Arch. Otolaryngol. Head Neck Surg. 20, 23 (1998).*

Journal 1997 Discusses techniques and possibilities for genetic testing. Presents a series of problems designed as a starting point for understanding the conflicts surrounding

genetic testing. Reviews the applications of state-of-the-art genetic research. Suggests potential difficulties that testing may cause in society. References Opinion 2.12. Underwood & Cadle, *Genetics, Genetic Testing, and the Specter of Discrimination: A Discussion Using Hypothetical Cases, 85 Ky. L. J. 665, 684 (1996-97).*

4.1.3 Third-Party Access to Genetic Information

Journal 2007 Evaluates the ethical issues surrounding "neoeugenics." Concludes that, in formulating future policy, societal concerns must be balanced with individual rights to reproductive autonomy. References Opinion 2.137. Suter, *A Brave New World of Designer Babies? 22 Berkeley Tech. L. J. 897, 936-37 (2007).*

Journal 2003 Focuses on the controversial use of genetic information in employment and insurance. Concludes that reformers must reexamine the ethical and legal duties of professionals regarding protection of genetic information. References Opinion 2.132. Partlett, *Misuse of Genetic Information: The Common Law and Professionals' Liability, 42 Washburn L. J. 489, 503 (2003).*

Journal 2001 Discusses same-sex marriages in the transgender community. Explores Defense of Marriage Act statutes. Considers whether same-sex transgender marriages can prevail against attacks brought under such statutes. Cites Opinions 2.132, 2.135, 2.137, 5.08, and 5.09. Frye & Meiselman, *Same-Sex Marriages Have Existed Legally in the United States for a Long Time Now, 64 Alb. L. Rev. 1031, 1053 (2001).*

Journal 2001 Examines the distinction between preplacement and postplacement examinations in the workplace. Analyzes the possible dangers that might result if preplacement medical testing is not restricted. Concludes that any such testing must relate to the potential employee's ability to perform assigned job duties. References Opinions 2.132 and 2.139. Hoffman, *Preplacement Examinations and Job-Relatedness: How to Enhance Privacy and Diminish Discrimination in the Workplace, 49 U. Kan. L. Rev. 517, 534, 535, 556, 565 (2001).*

Journal 2000 Explores the benefits and harms of the new era of genomic medicine. Discusses the needs of tissue donors, noting they should be carefully balanced with the needs of the medical research community. Concludes that a multifaceted effort is essential to ensuring trust in the medical community as the benefits of genomic medicine are realized. References Opinion 2.132. Ashburn, Wilson, & Eisenstein, *Human Tissue Research in the Genomic Era of Medicine, 160 Arch. Intern. Med. 3377, 3378 (2000).*

Journal 2000 Examines the effects of genetic information on medical care. Concludes that the existing rules and regulations, which try to protect a patient's absolute control over personal genetic data, should be modified. Suggests that a statutory board might better decide when personal genetic

information may be divulged to others. References Opinion 2.132. Bruns & Wolman, *Morality of the Privacy of Genetic Information: Possible Improvements of Procedures, 19 Med. Law 127, 129 (2000).*

Journal 2000 Evaluates transgender legal and political activity in the US. Discusses the International Bill of Gender Rights against the background of the Texas case, *Littleton v. Prange.* Cites Opinions 2.132, 2.135, 2.137, 5.08, and 5.09. Frye, *The International Bill of Gender Rights vs. the Cider House Rules: Transgenders Struggle With the Courts Over What Clothing They Are Allowed to Wear on the Job, Which Restroom They Are Allowed to Use on the Job, Their Right to Marry, and the Very Definition of Their Sex, 7 Wm. & Mary J. Women & L. 133, 149 (2000).*

Journal 2000 Explores the legal, ethical, social, and economic considerations associated with use of new genetic techniques in the prediction and diagnosis of Alzheimer disease. Outlines the potential responsibilities and liabilities of physicians in connection with use of these techniques. References Opinions 2.132, 2.139, and 8.032. Kapp, *Physicians' Legal Duties Regarding the Use of Genetic Tests to Predict and Diagnose Alzheimer Disease, 21 J. Legal Med. 445, 456-57, 465-66 (2000).*

Journal 2000 Discusses the adverse effects of predisposition genetic testing on personal and familial relationships as well as insurability and employment opportunities. Concludes that health care providers and policy makers must ensure that individuals who undergo genetic testing have access to proper counseling, appropriate medical resources, and protection from genetic discrimination. References Opinion 2.132. Schneider, *Adverse Impact of Predisposition Testing on Major Life Activities: Lessons From BRCA1/2 Testing, 3 J. Health Care L. & Pol'y 365, 380 (2000).*

Journal 1999 Explains physicians' potential liability as corporate professionals and how that reinforces professional standards. Discusses physicians' pursuit of preventive health and its impact on reducing company liability. References Opinion 2.132. Draper, *Preventive Law by Corporate Professional Team Players: Liability and Responsibility in the Work of Company Doctors, 15 J. Contemp. Health L. & Pol'y. 525, 564 (1999).*

Journal 1999 Argues that current Fourth Amendment jurisprudence needs to be changed. Describes two different theories—an antidiscrimination model and an individual rights model—and applies them to different situations.

States that the Fourth Amendment needs to protect personal sovereignty for the sake of the individual and society. References Opinion 2.132. Luna, *Sovereignty and Suspicion, 48 Duke L. J. 787, 884 (1999).*

Journal 1998 Discusses conflicts of interest in the physician-patient relationship arising out of use of financial incentives by managed care organizations. Considers how such conflicts are dealt with in the attorney-client relationship. Suggests that a financial incentive should be legally denounced if it unreasonably interferes with a physician's duty to properly care for and treat patients. Quotes Preamble, Fundamental Elements (1) [now Opinion 10.01], and Opinions 4.04, 5.01, 8.03, 8.13, and 9.06. Cites Fundamental Elements (4) [now Opinion 10.01] and Opinions 2.07, 2.08, and 2.132. Hall, *Third-Party Payor Conflicts of Interest in Managed Care: A Proposal for Regulation Based on the Model Rules of Professional Conduct, 29 Seton Hall L. Rev. 95, 96, 107, 108, 109, 110, 111, 112, 134, 135, 136 (1998).*

Journal 1998 Discusses the use of genetic information by employers. Argues that people may forgo genetic testing for fear that the results will be used by their employers in a discriminatory manner. Concludes that the Minnesota statute prohibiting employers from performing medical tests or obtaining medical information, which is not job-related, is better than other approaches. References Opinion 2.132. Rothstein, Gelb, & Craig, *Protecting Genetic Privacy by Permitting Employer Access Only to Job-Related Employee Medical Information: Analysis of a Unique Minnesota Law, 24 Am. J. Law & Med. 399, 400 (1998).*

Journal 1997 Explores the legality of pre-employment screening techniques. Considers legal reforms that would balance the interests of employers and job applicants. Offers suggestions that would enhance fairness and consistency in this screening process. References Opinion 2.132. Befort, *Pre-Employment Screening and Investigation: Navigating Between a Rock and a Hard Place, 14 Hofstra Lab. L. J. 365, 391 (1997).*

Journal 1997 Explores parents' legal rights to subject their children to genetic testing for untreatable, late-onset disorders or for carrier status. Examines potential negative aspects of genetic testing. Proposes that parents should not have the right to subject their children to such testing. References Opinion 2.132. Holland, *Should Parents Be Permitted to Authorize Genetic Testing for Their Children? 31 Fam. L. Q. 321, 346-47 (1997).*

Journal 1997 Discusses the collection and storage of human tissues. Notes the use of genetic testing by employers. Examines whether those with biomedical experience perceive genetic research as dangerous. Considers problems of privacy and confidentiality raised by genetic technology and the storage of tissues. References Opinion 2.132. Merz, *Psychosocial Risks of Storing and Using Human Tissues in Research, 8 Risk Health Safety & Env't. 235, 236 (1997).*

Journal 1993 Examines how genetic tests to diagnose disease may be useful to private insurance companies in identifying persons for whom coverage will be provided. Concludes that this issue should be considered as part of the national health care reform debate. References Opinion 2.132. Jecker, *Genetic Testing and the Social Responsibility of Private Health Insurance Companies, 21 J. Law Med. & Ethics 109, 112 (1993).*

4.1.4 Forensic Genetics

Journal 2002 Discusses legal and medical policies that protect confidentiality in the physician-patient relationship. Concludes that reducing the current level of privacy protection would jeopardize health care. Quotes Preamble and Opinions 2.136, 5.05, and 10.01. References Principles VIII and IX. Sciarrino, *Ferguson v. City of Charleston: "The Doctor Will See You Now, Be Sure to Bring Your Privacy Rights in With You!" 12 Temp. Pol. & Civ. Rts. L. Rev. 197, 213, 215, 220, 221, 222 (2002).*

4.2.1 Assisted Reproductive Technology

Journal 2010 Describes how physicians act as bankers in financing fertility treatments for patients and how this significantly contributes to medical debt and bankruptcies. Proposes regulations which would address these issues within fertility markets. Quotes Opinion 6.08. Cites Opinion 2.055. Hawkins, *Doctors as Bankers: Evidence From Fertility Markets, 84 Tul. L. Rev. 841, 848, 874 (2010).*

Journal 2009 Discusses the costs parents, children, and society incur as a result of multiple gestation pregnancies. Concludes the US should adopt increased regulation similar to that prevalent in European countries to address these costs. Quotes Opinion 2.055. Velikonja, *The Costs of Multiple Gestation Pregnancies in Assisted Reproduction, 32 Harv. J. L. & Gender 463, 484 (2009).*

Journal 2005 Examines legal controversies triggered by advances in technology, using in vitro fertilization as an example. Concludes that no single legislative solution is capable of dealing with the many problems associated with changes in technology. Cites Opinions 2.055 and 2.141. Moses, *Understanding Legal Responses to Technological Change: The Example of In Vitro Fertilization*, 6 Minn. J. L. Sci. & Tech. 505, 543, 615 (2005).

Journal 2005 Discusses legal and ethical issues in conducting embryonic research in the US. Concludes that failure to pursue such research may be viewed as unethical and that the British experience might offer a model for moving forward in this regard. Cites Opinion 2.14. Clemmens, *Creating Human Embryos for Research: A Scientist's Perspective on Managing the Legal and Ethical Issues*, 2 Ind. Health L. Rev. 95, 99 (2005).

Journal 1991 Considers how the use of in vitro fertilization (IVF) has blurred the distinction between medical practice and research. Argues that medical-professional responsibility standards should be used to curtail the creation of life in vitro. Quotes Opinions 2.10 and 2.14. Comment, *Dangerous*

Relations: Doctors and Extracorporeal Embryos, The Need for New Limits to Medical Inquiry, 7 J. Contemp. Health L. & Pol'y 307, 309 (1991).

Journal 1987 Examines various ethical issues surrounding surrogate motherhood, artificial insemination, in vitro fertilization, and embryonic/fetal research. Reports on the positions of four ethics groups: the Warnock Committee of Inquiry Into Human Fertilization and Embryology; the AMA's Council on Ethical and Judicial Affairs; the Ethics Committee of the American Fertility Society; and the Ethics Committee of the American College of Obstetricians and Gynecologists. References Opinions 2.04, 2.05, and 2.13 (1986) [now Opinion 2.14]. Quotes Opinion 2.18. Rosner, Cassell, Friedland, Landolt, Loeb, Numann, Ora, Risemberg, & Sordillo, *Ethical Considerations of Reproductive Technologies*, 87 N. Y. State J. Med. 398, 399-400 (1987).

4.2.2 Gamete Donation

Colo. 1989 State statute prohibiting a sperm donor from asserting his parental status was held to be inapplicable where known donor and unmarried recipient agreed that the donor would have parental rights. Concurring opinion argued that the statute bars any nonhusband donor, regardless of relationship to the recipient, from asserting parental rights. However, the concurring opinion found the statute inapplicable because its provision requiring "supervision" by a physician had not been met. In apparent reference to the standards set out under Opinions 2.04 and 2.05, the concurring opinion said that "supervision" should at the least require an examination to determine whether there are any health risks to the recipient as a result of the procedure and to protect the child from hereditary disease. *In re R.C.*, 775 P.2d 27, 37 n.3.

Journal 2010 Addresses issues involving posthumous conception. Concludes that an estate fiduciary does not have absolute discretion to make decisions regarding the disposition of a decedent's reproductive matter. Cites Opinion 2.04. Cooper & Harper, *Life After Death: The Authority of Estate Fiduciaries to Dispose of Decedents' Reproductive Matter*, 26 Touro L. Rev. 649, 658 (2010).

Journal 2009 Discusses advancements in assisted reproductive technology and the law concerning posthumous conception. Concludes the Model Act Concerning Assisted Reproductive Technology should be used as a basis for legislation to regulate the use of assisted reproductive technology for posthumous conception. Cites Opinion 2.04. O'Brien, *The Momentum of Posthumous Conception: A Model Act*, 25 J. Contemp. Health L. & Pol'y 332, 363 (2009).

Journal 2006 Examines protection and regulation of sperm donor genetic information. Concludes that children born as a result of artificial insemination should have a legal right to both medical and genetic information about the donor. References 2.05. D'Orazio, *Half of the Family Tree: A Call For Access to a Full Genetic History for Children Born by Artificial Insemination*, 2 J. Health & Biomedical L. 249, 256 (2006).

Journal 2004 Explores whether a child born through postmortem conception (PMC) can claim an inheritance from a deceased father. Concludes that, under common law rules, a PMC child generally will not be able to inherit; however, the final outcome may be affected by available extrinsic evidence. Quotes Opinion 2.04. Knaplund, *Postmortem Conception and a Father's Last Will*, 46 Ariz. L. Rev. 91, 96 (2004).

Journal 1987 Examines various ethical issues surrounding surrogate motherhood, artificial insemination, in vitro fertilization, and embryonic/fetal research. Reports on the positions of four ethics groups: the Warnock Committee of Inquiry into Human Fertilization and Embryology; the AMA's Council on Ethical and Judicial Affairs; the Ethics Committee of the American Fertility Society; and the Ethics Committee of the American College of Obstetricians and Gynecologists. References Opinions 2.04, 2.05, and 2.13 (1986) [now Opinion 2.14]. Quotes Opinion 2.18. Rosner, Cassell, Friedland, Landolt, Loeb, Numann, Ora, Risemberg, & Sordillo, *Ethical Considerations of Reproductive Technologies*, 87 N. Y. State J. Med. 398, 399-400 (1987).

4.2.3 Therapeutic Donor Insemination

Colo. 1989 State statute prohibiting a sperm donor from asserting his parental status was held to be inapplicable where known donor and unmarried recipient agreed that the donor would have parental rights. Concurring opinion argued that the statute bars any nonhusband donor, regardless of relationship to the recipient, from asserting parental rights. However, the concurring opinion found the statute inapplicable because its provision requiring "supervision" by a physician had not been met. In apparent reference to the standards set out under Opinions 2.04 and 2.05, the concurring opinion said that "supervision" should at the least require an examination to determine whether there are any health risks to the recipient as a result of the procedure and to protect the child from hereditary disease. *In re R.C.,* 775 *P.2d 27, 37 n.3.*

Journal 2010 Addresses issues involving posthumous conception. Concludes that an estate fiduciary does not have absolute discretion to make decisions regarding the disposition of a decedent's reproductive matter. Cites Opinion 2.04. Cooper & Harper, *Life After Death: The Authority of Estate Fiduciaries to Dispose of Decedents' Reproductive Matter,* 26 Touro L. Rev. 649, 658 (2010).

Journal 2009 Discusses advancements in assisted reproductive technology and the law concerning posthumous conception. Concludes the Model Act Concerning Assisted Reproductive Technology should be used as a basis for legislation to regulate the use of assisted reproductive technology for posthumous conception. Cites Opinion 2.04. O'Brien, *The Momentum of Posthumous Conception: A Model Act,* 25 J. Contemp. Health L. & Pol'y 332, 363 (2009).

Journal 2006 Examines protection and regulation of sperm donor genetic information. Concludes that children born as a result of artificial insemination should have a legal right to both medical and genetic information about the donor. References 2.05. D'Orazio, *Half of the Family Tree: A Call For Access to a Full Genetic History for Children Born by Artificial Insemination,* 2 J. Health & Biomedical L. 249, 256 (2006).

Journal 2004 Explores whether a child born through postmortem conception (PMC) can claim an inheritance from a deceased father. Concludes that, under common law rules, a PMC child generally will not be able to inherit; however, the final outcome may be affected by available extrinsic evidence. Quotes Opinion 2.04. Knaplund, *Postmortem Conception and a Father's Last Will,* 46 Ariz. L. Rev. 91, 96 (2004).

Journal 1987 Examines various ethical issues surrounding surrogate motherhood, artificial insemination, in vitro fertilization, and embryonic/fetal research. Reports on the positions of four ethics groups: the Warnock Committee of Inquiry into Human Fertilization and Embryology; the AMA's Council on Ethical and Judicial Affairs; the Ethics Committee of the American Fertility Society; and the Ethics Committee of the American College of Obstetricians and Gynecologists. References Opinions 2.04, 2.05, and 2.13 (1986) [now Opinion 2.14]. Quotes Opinion 2.18. Rosner, Cassell, Friedland, Landolt, Loeb, Numann, Ora, Risemberg, & Sordillo, *Ethical Considerations of Reproductive Technologies,* 87 N. Y. State J. Med. 398, 399-400 (1987).

4.2.4 Third-Party Reproduction

Journal 2011 Discusses advancements in modern reproductive technologies and the need for legislation to regulate these technologies. Concludes that regulating these technologies may violate modern views of personal autonomy and therefore should focus on the safety of the technologies and not be used to "protect" women from their ability to freely contract. Quotes Opinions 2.18 and 10.05. Neal, *Protecting Women: Preserving Autonomy in the Commodification of Motherhood,* 17 Wm. & Mary J. Women & L. 611, 630, 635 (2011).

Journal 2000 Examines questions regarding the legality of such practices as voluntary stopping of eating and drinking (VSED), use of risky analgesics, and terminal sedation. Explores the distinctions between physician-assisted suicide and other palliative interventions. Concludes VSED, risky analgesics, and certain types of terminal sedation are lawful and should be made available to dying patients who make informed decisions to accept the risks involved. Quotes

Opinions 2.21 and 2.211. Cites Opinions 2.18 and 2.20. Cantor & Thomas, *The Legal Bounds of Physician Conduct Hastening Death,* 48 Buff. L. Rev. 83, 110, 131, 158 (2000).

Journal 1990 Argues that gestational surrogacy, because of its inherent medical, ethical, and legal complications, is not an acceptable reproductive alternative. Discusses the California Superior Court case of *Johnson v. Calvert* in which a gestational surrogacy contract was held valid and the genetic parents were found to have exclusive custody and parental rights. Quotes Opinion 2.18 (1988). Rothenberg, *Gestational Surrogacy and the Health Care Provider: Put Part of the IVF Genie Back Into the Bottle,* 18 Law Med. & Health Care 345, 346 (1990).

Journal 1987 Examines various ethical issues surrounding surrogate motherhood, artificial insemination, in vitro fertilization, and embryonic/fetal research. Reports on the positions of four ethics groups: the Warnock Committee of Inquiry Into Human Fertilization and Embryology;

the AMA's Council on Ethical and Judicial Affairs; the Ethics Committee of the American Fertility Society; and the Ethics Committee of the American College of Obstetricians and Gynecologists. References Opinions 2.04, 2.05, and 2.13 (1986) [now Opinion 2.14]. Quotes Opinion

2.18. Rosner, Cassell, Friedland, Landolt, Loeb, Numann, Ora, Risemberg, & Sordillo, *Ethical Considerations of Reproductive Technologies*, 87 N. Y. State J. Med. 398, 399-400 (1987).

4.2.5 Storage and Use of Human Embryos

Journal 2006 Discusses the ethical issues surrounding embryonic stem cell research, gamete donation, and embryo adoption. Concludes that conflation of these concepts does not advance solutions in the current climate of abortion politics. Cites Opinion 2.141. Conde, *Embryo Donation: The Government Adopts a Cause*, 13 Wm. & Mary J. Women & L. 273, 288 (2006).

Journal 2005 Examines legal controversies triggered by advances in technology, using in vitro fertilization as an example. Concludes that no single legislative solution is capable of dealing with the many problems associated with changes in technology. Cites Opinions 2.055 and 2.141. Moses, *Understanding Legal Responses to Technological Change: The Example of In Vitro Fertilization*, 6 Minn. J. L. Sci. & Tech. 505, 543, 615 (2005).

Journal 2003 Reviews legal methods for resolving disputes involving disposition of cryopreserved pre-embryos. Concludes that federal legislation is needed to address existing problems. Cites Opinion 2.141. Windsor, *Disposition of Cryopreserved Preembryos After Divorce*, 88 Iowa L. Rev. 1001, 1026 (2003).

Journal 2001 Examines the ethical and legal dilemmas associated with stem cell and fetal tissue research. Discusses current federal law. Concludes that Congress should allow researchers to obtain stem cells from discarded human embryos provided by in vitro fertilization clinics. Cites Opinion 2.141. Casell, *Lengthening the Stem: Allowing Federally Funded Researchers to Derive Human Pluripotent Stem Cells From Embryos*, 34 U. Mich. J. L. Ref. 547, 563 (2001).

Journal 1999 Describes cryopreservation and in vitro fertilization (IVF) procedures. Examines statutory and case law regarding the use of IVF and discusses theories about how frozen pre-embryos should be discarded. Concludes by suggesting that, in legal disputes, the party opposing implantation ordinarily should prevail. Quotes Opinion 2.141. Fiestal, *A Solomonic Decision: What Will Be the Fate of Frozen Preembryos?* 6 Cardozo Women's L. J. 103, 110 (1999).

Journal 1999 Describes the approaches various courts have taken toward disposition of cryopreserved embryos after dissolution of marriage. Concludes that, while a prior

agreement should be binding, various contract defenses may apply where circumstances have substantially changed. References Opinion 2.141. Haut, *Divorce and the Disposition of Frozen Embryos*, 28 Hofstra L. Rev. 493, 519 (1999).

Journal 1998 Addresses the ethical and legal issues regarding storage and disposition of frozen human embryos. Suggests that courts should seek to honor the donors' wishes. Proposes that future legislation should mandate embryo disposition after a certain length of time. Quotes Opinion 2.141. Forster, *The Legal and Ethical Debate Surrounding the Storage and Destruction of Frozen Human Embryos: A Reaction to the Mass Disposal in Britain and the Lack of Law in the United States*, 76 Wash. U. L. Q. 759, 766-67, 770 (1998).

Journal 1998 Discusses legal issues regarding reproductive biotechnology, with emphasis on freezing of eggs and embryos, research involving frozen embryos, and cloning. Argues that legislation should protect society from unacceptable uses of reproductive technology but, at the same time, ensure advancement of technology for the benefit of society. References Opinion 2.141. Godoy, *Where Is Biotechnology Taking the Law? An Overview of Assisted Reproductive Technology, Research on Frozen Embryos and Human Cloning*, 19 J. Juv. L. 357, 363 (1998).

Journal 1990 Considers ways in which the frozen pre-embryo can be legally described and argues that it should not be considered either person or property. Concludes that in vitro fertilization research is valuable to society and proposes research guidelines. References Opinion 2.141. Martin & Lagod, *The Human Preembryo, the Progenitors, and the State: Toward a Dynamic Theory of Status, Rights, and Research Policy*, 5 High Tech. L. J. 257, 304 (1990).

Journal 1990 Considers problems created by frozen pre-embryos that result from in vitro fertilization therapy. Explores problems with disposing of these pre-embryos and how prior agreements between couples have surfaced as a potential solution. References Opinion 2.141. Robertson, *Prior Agreements for Disposition of Frozen Embryos*, 51 Ohio St. L. J. 407, 419 (1990).

4.2.6 Cloning for Reproduction

Journal 2009 Explores ethical concerns surrounding organ donation from anencephalic infants. Concludes that, by viewing anencephalic infants as having been born into a state of death, an infant's organs may be donated without violating the dead donor rule. Cites Opinion 2.147. References Opinion 2.162. Khan & Lea, *Paging King Solomon: Towards Allowing Organ Donation From Anencephalic Infants, 6 Ind. Health L. Rev. 17, 38 (2009).*

Journal 1999 Discusses arguments against cloning. Points out that, as medical knowledge advances, and physicians can safely undertake this procedure, increasing emphasis will be placed on ethical concerns. Concludes that cloning may benefit infertile couples and single people who want to have children without involving a third party in their procreational activities. References Opinion 2.147. Orentlicher, *Cloning and the Preservation of Family Integrity, 59 La. L. Rev. 1019, 1022 (1999).*

4.2.7 Abortion

U.S. 1973 Pregnant woman and physician sought declaratory relief and injunction against Texas criminal abortion statute. In holding that the constitutional right of privacy includes a woman's decision whether to terminate a pregnancy prior to viability, the Court reviewed the medical and legal history of abortion, including the AMA's lobbying efforts in support of criminal abortion statutes (1859, 1871), its opposition to induced abortion except when threat to life or health of mother exists (1967), its statement that lobbying efforts were consistent with the Principles of Medical Ethics (1957), and the Preamble, Sec. 10 (1971) [now Opinion 2.01], which stated that a physician was not prohibited from performing an abortion in accordance with good medical practice and consistent with local law. *Roe v. Wade, 410 U.S. 113, 144 n.39.*

Journal 2010 Discusses issues arising from the enactment of legislation by North Dakota involving a minor's reproductive rights. Explores ethical principles that govern physician's actions within the context of reproductive health. Concludes that, while a patient's expectation of confidentiality with a physician is critical, competing values come into play when the patient is a minor and parental involvement may be important. Provides practical guidance to address issues in this context. Quotes Opinions 2.01, 2.015, 5.055, 8.08, 8.115, 9.12, 10.01, 10.015, and 10.05. Cites Opinions 5.05, 5.055, 8.08, 8.11, 8.115, 9.12, and 10.05. Haas, *"Doctor, I'm Pregnant and Fifteen—I Can't Tell My Parents—Please Help Me": Minor Consent, Reproductive Rights, and Ethical Principles for Physicians, 86 N.D. L. Rev. 63, 70, 73, 75-78, 82, 84, 86-88 (2010).*

Journal 2005 Discusses Wisconsin Act 110. Concludes the Act was unnecessary, and that if an infant does survive an abortion, the decision of whether treatment should be administered must be left to the physician. Quotes Opinion 2.01. Frishman, *Wisconsin Act 110: When an Infant Survives an Abortion, 20 Wis. Women's L. J. 101, 117 (2005).*

Journal 2005 Examines the legal and ethical aspects of physician participation in capital punishment. Concludes that federal and state laws addressing this practice must be amended to harmonize the law with applicable principles of medical ethics. Quotes Opinion 2.06. Cites Opinion 2.21. References Opinion 2.01. Levy, *Conflict of Duty: Capital Punishment Regulations and AMA Medical Ethics, 26 J. Legal Med. 261, 268, 269, 270, 273 (2005).*

Journal 2004 Asks whether pharmacists should be protected from civil liability when they refuse to dispense birth control medication based on their moral convictions. Concludes that moral beliefs of health care providers should not get in the way of patient care. Cites Opinion 2.01. Cantor & Baum, *The Limits of Conscientious Objection—May Pharmacists Refuse to Fill Prescriptions for Emergency Contraception? 351 New Eng. J. Med. 2008, 2012 (2004).*

Journal 2000 Examines physician value neutrality (PVN). Defines PVN as providing a foundation to suggest physicians must keep their values—religious, political, or otherwise—out of the patient-physician relationship. Concludes it is not clear how values can be removed from the patient-physician relationship without removing the very thing PVN supporters are trying to protect, the intrinsic value of persons. References Opinions 2.01, 2.02, 8.032, 8.05, 8.08, and 8.132. Beckwith & Peppin, *Physician Value Neutrality: A Critique, 28 J. L. Med. & Ethics 67, 72-73 (2000).*

Journal 1995 Examines four essential principles of bioethics—patient autonomy, nonmaleficence, beneficence, and justice—and describes their application in clinical settings according to bioethical norms and AMA opinions. Concludes that such an approach promotes compassionate medical caregiving and that laws should reflect these values. Quotes Opinions 2.01 and 8.18. References Opinion 2.211. Cohen, *Toward a Bioethics of Compassion, 28 Ind. L. Rev. 667, 673, 681-82, 683 (1995).*

5 Caring for Patients at the End of Life

5.2 Advance Directives

Journal 2009 Argues new physician orders for life-sustaining treatment (POLST) legislation should be enacted in Florida because the POLST form can more effectively achieve the purposes of advance directives. Concludes the POLST form will reduce problems with advance directives by creating a system to translate a patient's wishes into standardized physician's orders. Quotes Opinion 2.225. Sonderling, *POLST: A Cure for the Common Advance Directive—It's Just What the Doctor Ordered*, 33 Nova L. Rev. 451, 470, 478 (2009).

Journal 2007 Discusses patients' right to refuse medical treatment and the corresponding duties of health care professionals. Concludes that detailed, carefully prepared advance directives are necessary to fulfill patients' wishes. Quotes Ch. II (1940) [now Opinions 8.08 and 8.082] and Opinions 2.035, 2.037, 2.20, 2.225, 8.081, and 10.015. Cites Opinions 9.11 and 9.115. Stamatakis, *Beyond Advance Directives: Personal Autonomy and the Right to Refuse Life-Sustaining Medical Treatment*, 47 N. H. B. J. 20, 29-30 (2007).

Journal 2000 Discusses the process of advance care planning. Identifies five steps for success: appropriate introduction of the topic; structured discussions covering specific situations; documentation of patient preferences; updating of directives; and application of directives when indicated. References Opinion 2.225. Emanuel, von Gunten, & Ferris, *Advance Care Planning, 9 Arch. Fam. Med. 1181, 1181 (2000)*.

Journal 1999 States that a distrust of the medical profession arose from changes in the health care system and federal law. Explains how legislation may help alleviate some of the distrust. Suggests that people need more access to information about their health plans. References Opinions 2.20 and 2.225. Cerminara, *Protecting Participants in and Beneficiaries of ERISA-Governed Managed Health Care Plans*, 29 U. Mem. L. Rev. 317, 324 (1999).

5.3 Withholding or Withdrawing Life-Sustaining Treatment

U.S. 1997 Several physicians and terminally ill patients sued the state seeking a declaration that its prohibition against physician-assisted suicide violates the Fourteenth Amendment's Equal Protection Clause. The trial court disagreed, but the Second Circuit reversed, holding that the state accords different treatment to those terminally ill patients who wish to hasten their death by self-administering prescribed drugs and to those patients who wish to do so by directing the removal of life support systems. The Supreme Court reversed holding that the prohibition against assisting suicide does not violate the Equal Protection Clause. The Court concluded that there is a distinction between assisting suicide and withdrawing treatment, quoting reports of the AMA Council on Ethical and Judicial Affairs [now Opinions 2.20 and 2.211]. *Vacco v. Quill, 117 S. Ct. 2293, 2298, 138 L. Ed. 2d 834.*

U.S. 1990 Parents of patient in persistent vegetative state appealed denial of request to discontinue gastrotomy feeding tube. The Supreme Court held that the federal constitution did not forbid the state's requirement of clear and convincing evidence of an incompetent patient's wishes regarding the withdrawal of life-prolonging treatment. The Court acknowledged that a competent person has a liberty interest under the due process clause in refusing unwanted medical care; however, the Court assumed the existence of a constitutionally protected right to refuse artificial hydration

and nutrition only for purposes of the case. In a concurring opinion, Justice O'Connor cited Opinion 2.20 for the proposition that artificial feeding cannot be distinguished from other forms of medical treatment. In his dissent, Justice Brennan likewise cited Opinion 2.20 for this point. *Cruzan v. Director, Missouri Department of Health, 497 U.S. 261.*

9th Cir. 1996 Suit was brought by several physicians and a not-for-profit corporation which provides information, assistance, and counseling to competent terminally ill adult patients contemplating suicide, asserting that a state statute making it a crime to aid anyone in attempting to commit suicide unconstitutionally prevents terminally ill patients from exercising their protected liberty interests. Appeals court, en banc, held that the choice of how and when to die is a liberty interest and that the statute violates the due process rights of competent, terminally ill adults who wish to hasten their deaths by obtaining medication prescribed by their physicians. Stating that physician-assisted suicide runs counter to medical ethics, the dissent cited Opinions 2.20, 2.21, and 2.211 and quoted Opinion 2.211. *Compassion in Dying v. Washington, 79 F.3d 790, 840, 855, replacing 49 F.3d 586 (9th Cir. 1995).*

E.D.N.Y. 2011 The court confronted the question of how to sentence young defendants whose drug addiction led to violations of criminal drug laws. In finding an ethical obligation of physicians to treat chronic pain, the court quotes Opinion

2.20. The court holds that where the defendant's drug addiction is causatively intertwined with a violation of criminal law, every effort should be made to minimize incarceration in favor of closely supervised, intensive medical treatment outside of prison. *United States v. Ilayayev, 800 F. Supp. 2d 417, 435.*

Ariz. 1987 Guardian of nursing home patient in persistent vegetative state sought removal of nasogastric tube and retention of do-not-resuscitate and do-not-hospitalize orders. Patient had not communicated desires regarding life-sustaining procedures while competent. In assessing whether safeguarding the integrity of the medical profession might be a state interest that outweighed the patient's right to refuse medical treatment, the court noted Opinion 2.18 (1986) [now Opinion 2.20] to support the view that the medical profession itself now recognizes that it is no longer obligated to provide medical treatment in all situations. Since the Opinion would allow the disputed orders for a patient suffering from an irreversible coma, the court concluded that the same action would be allowed in a case of irreversible chronic vegetative state and thus concluded that the case did not bring into disrepute the ethical integrity of the medical profession. *Rasmussen v. Fleming, 154 Ariz. 207, 741 P.2d 674, 684, 685.*

Ariz. App. 1986 Guardian of nursing home patient in persistent vegetative state sought removal of nasogastric tube and retention of do-not-resuscitate and do-not-hospitalize orders. Patient had not communicated her desires regarding life-sustaining procedures while competent. The court quoted Opinion 2.18 (1986) [now Opinion 2.20] in holding that competing state interests, including the ethical integrity of the medical profession, did not outweigh patient's constitutional right to privacy and held that rights of incompetent patient could be asserted vicariously. *Rasmussen v. Fleming, 154 Ariz. 200, 741 P.2d 667, 671, 672, 673 n.4, aff'd in part and rev'd in part, 154 Ariz. 207, 741 P.2d 674 (1987).*

Cal. App. 1988 Conservator sought an injunction requiring physician to remove nasogastric feeding tube from a patient who was in a persistent vegetative state. The court held that while a conservator may authorize withdrawal or withholding of medical treatment, he may not force a physician to do so against the physician's personal moral objections if the patient can be transferred to the care of a physician who will follow the directive. Citing Opinion 2.18 (1986) [now Opinion 2.20], the court noted that the physician's compliance with the conservator's decision would not have violated the ethical code of the medical profession. *Morrison v. Abramovice, 206 Cal. App. 3d 304, 309, 253 Cal. Rptr. 530, 533.*

Cal. App. 1988 Conservator of patient in persistent vegetative state sought permission for removal of nasogastric feeding tube claiming such relief would serve the patient's best interests. Patient had expressed a desire never to be kept alive through artificial means. The court held that a conservator is authorized to order that artificial life support be withdrawn after considering medical advice and the patient's

best interests. In so holding, the court quoted Opinion 2.18 (1986) [now Opinion 2.20] showing support within the medical community for its analysis. *In re Drabick, 200 Cal. App. 3d 185, 245 Cal. Rptr. 840, 845 n.8.*

Cal. App. 1986 Mentally competent, physically debilitated patient sought authorization to discontinue forced feedings through nasogastric tube. Patient had dictated instructions to her lawyers and signed them with an x by means of a pen held in her mouth. In holding that a competent adult patient has the legal right to refuse medical treatment even though such refusal will hasten her death, the court quoted Opinion 2.18 (1986) [now Opinion 2.20]. *Bouvia v. Superior Court, 179 Cal. App. 3d 1127, 225 Cal. Rptr. 297, 303-04.*

Conn. 1989 Family of comatose, terminal patient in nursing home sought injunction to discontinue life support services. In holding that removal of a gastrostomy tube was authorized by statute and no compelling state interests outweighed the patient's rights, the court cited Opinion 2.18 (1986) [now Opinion 2.20] for its view that the provision of nutrition and hydration is a form of life-prolonging medical treatment. *McConnell v. Beverly Enterprises-Connecticut, Inc., 209 Conn. 692, 553 A.2d 596, 603 n.13.*

Fla. App. 1986 Husband of terminally ill patient in persistent vegetative state sought declaratory judgment to permit removal of nasogastric feeding tube. In recognizing a right to allow the natural consequence of removal of artificial life-sustaining measures, the court quoted Opinion 2.18 (1986) [now Opinion 2.20]. *Corbett v. D'Alessandro, 487 So. 2d 368, 371 n.1.*

Ill. 1989 Daughter of permanently unconscious patient petitioned to withdraw life-prolonging gastrotomy feeding tube. The court cited with approval Opinion 2.18 (1986) [now Opinion 2.20] that the AMA considers artificial hydration and nutrition to be medical treatments which may be withdrawn under certain circumstances. The court based the right to refuse life-prolonging procedures upon the state's common law of informed consent, probate law, and power of attorney for health care statute. The court established guidelines for a guardian's exercise of this right. The patient must be terminally ill, in a persistent vegetative state, and the guardian must exercise the substituted judgment of the patient as shown through clear and convincing evidence in a judicial proceeding. *In re Longeway, 133 Ill. 2d 33, 549 N.E.2d 292, 295-96.*

Ill. App. 1988 Guardian of patient in persistent vegetative state petitioned to withdraw artificial feeding tube. Prior to her incompetence, the patient had stated in writing and in conversations with friends that she desired no artificial means of treatment if there was no hope for her recovery, and had completed a living will form, but had failed to obtain the requisite number of witness signatures. The trial court dismissed the case upon the patient's death. On appeal, the court held that the guardian, using the doctrine of substituted judgment, could consent to the removal of a feeding tube from a patient in a persistent vegetative state. In so holding, the court quoted Opinion 2.18 [now Opinion 2.20], noting that it was within a physician's ethical parameters to discontinue such treatment. *In re Prange, 166 Ill. App. 3d 1091, 520 N.E.2d 946, vacated, 121 Ill. 2d 570, 527 N.E.2d 303 (1988).*

Ind. 1991 State statute provided procedures by which parents of an incompetent patient, in consultation with the patient's physician, could withhold or withdraw life-prolonging medical treatment. The court held that barring any challenge from the treating physician or interested parties, the family could make these decisions without a court proceeding. Quoting Opinion 2.20 (1989), the court concluded that medical treatment includes artificial nutrition and hydration. *In re Lawrance, 579 N.E.2d 32, 40.*

Kan. App. 1998 Physician was convicted of attempted murder of a terminally ill patient, and intentional and malicious second-degree murder of another terminally ill patient. The court quoted Opinion 2.22, to exemplify a physician's duty to provide cardiopulmonary resuscitation unless the physician believes that such action would be futile. Additionally, the court referenced Opinion 2.20, in support of a physician's duty to provide a terminally ill patient adequate pain relief. The court reversed the physician's convictions, stating that the jury could not disregard the testimony of several physicians who concurred with the defendant-physician's treatment of the deceased patients. *State v. Naramore, 25 Kan. App. 2d 302, 965 P.2d 211, 214, 216.*

Ky. 2004 Plaintiff challenged the constitutionality of a provision of the Kentucky Living Will Directive Act which allows a judicially appointed guardian or surrogate to decide to withhold or withdraw life-sustaining medical treatment from a patient in a persistent vegetative state or who is permanently unconscious. The Kentucky Supreme Court quoted Opinion 2.20 in determining that the challenged provision does not violate any modern legal, moral, or ethical standards. The court found the statute constitutional, but stated that if the family and the guardian disagree as to whether to withhold or withdraw life-sustaining treatment, those attempting to withhold or withdraw treatment must show by clear and convincing evidence that the patient is in a permanently unconscious or persistent vegetative state or that death is imminent and that withholding or withdrawing life-sustaining treatment is in the patient's best interest. *Woods v. Commonwealth, 142 S.W.3d 24, 46, 47.*

Ky. 1993 In a declaratory judgment action, the court was asked to allow a surrogate to exercise the right to withdraw life-prolonging treatment for a patient who had orally expressed her wishes not to be sustained artificially. Since common law recognizes a patient's right to withdraw or withhold medical treatment, the court held that a surrogate could rely on the patient's statement of choice made before patient became incompetent to exercise "substituted judgment." The court quoted from guidelines for state courts deciding life-sustaining medical treatment cases issued by the National Center for State Courts. Citing Opinion 2.20 and other sources, the Guidelines stated that a consensus had

already been reached on the primary ethical issues relating to life-prolonging treatment. *DeGrella v. Elston, 858 S.W.2d 698, 707 n.5.*

Me. 1987 Guardian sought to have nasogastric feeding tube withdrawn from patient in persistent vegetative state. Investigation by a state agency corroborated evidence of patient's prior statements that he desired no life-sustaining procedures if in a persistent vegetative state. The court noted that under state's common law an individual has a personal right to refuse medical treatment, including life-sustaining procedures. The court held that where the patient had clearly and convincingly expressed his desire not to be maintained by life-sustaining procedures if in a persistent vegetative state, health professionals had a duty to respect that decision. The court cited Opinion 2.18 (1986) [now Opinion 2.20] for the concept that artificial hydration and nutrition should be equated with other life-sustaining treatments in delineating the patient's right to reject such treatment. *In re Gardner, 534 A.2d 947, 954.*

Md. Att'y Gen. 1988 Attorney general was asked whether persons with capacity to decide about medical care have a right to instruct that artificially administered sustenance not be provided if they become terminally ill or permanently comatose. An opinion was also requested regarding decision-making for incompetent persons who have given no prior instructions about artificial feeding. In response, Opinion 2.18 (1986) [now Opinion 2.20] is cited to support the view that no distinction should be drawn between artificial feeding and other forms of life-prolonging treatment. Further, in delineating procedures for deciding to forgo treatment for an incompetent, terminally ill patient who has given no prior instructions, Opinion 2.18 (1986) [now Opinion 2.20] is also cited in terms of the physician's role in advising whether withdrawal is medically proper. Finally, while disallowing family members, without court approval, to terminate tube feeding for a nonterminal, permanently comatose patient, it is recognized that under this Opinion it is not unethical to discontinue life-sustaining treatment for such a patient. *Maryland Att'y Gen. Op. No. 88-046, 73 Op. Att'y Gen. 162.*

Mass. 1992 Request of parents of a patient in a persistent vegetative state to employ "substituted judgment" in order to withdraw medical treatment was granted. Citing Opinion 2.18 (1986) [now Opinion 2.20], the court noted that medical treatment includes artificial hydration and nutrition. *In re Doe, 411 Mass. 512, 517 n.11, 583 N.E.2d 1263, 1267 n.11.*

Mass. 1986 Guardian of patient in persistent vegetative state who, according to trial court, would have declined food and water, sued for declaratory judgment requesting authority to have artificial hydration and nutrition discontinued. The court held that while the hospital had a right to refuse to participate in the removal of the gastrostomy tube, the guardian was authorized to transfer the patient to other physicians who would honor the guardian's request. The court cited Opinion 2.18 (1986) [now Opinion 2.20] in finding that the patient's right to refuse medical treatment did not violate the state's interest in the maintenance of the ethical integrity of the medical profession as long as the hospital was not forced to participate in the removal or clamping of the gastronomy tube. *Brophy v. New England Sinai Hosp., Inc., 398 Mass. 417, 497 N.E.2d 626, 638-39 n.38.*

Mich. App. 2001 State brought criminal action against physician for the murder of a patient by lethal injection. The trial court convicted the physician of second-degree murder and delivering a controlled substance. On appeal, the trial court decision was affirmed. The physician asked the appellate court to conclude that euthanasia is legal and to reverse his conviction on constitutional grounds. The appellate court relied on *Washington v. Glucksberg*, 521 U.S. 702 (1997) in determining there is no constitutional right to commit euthanasia, so that an individual can be free from intolerable and irremediable suffering. In discussing Glucksberg, the court observed that a state has a legitimate interest in protecting the integrity and ethics of the medical profession. The court noted Glucksberg's reference to Opinions 2.20, 2.21, and 2.211 in this regard. *People v. Kevorkian, 248 Mich. App. 373, 639 N.W.2d 291, 305 n. 42.*

Mo. 1988 Parents-guardians of a nonterminal patient in a persistent vegetative state sought a declaratory judgment after a state hospital refused to terminate artificial hydration and nutrition. The court found that the patient's burden in being fed through gastronomy tube did not outweigh the state's interest in preserving life and that guardians could not order withdrawal of hydration and nutrition. The court, in refusing to classify artificial hydration and nutrition as medical treatment, rejected Opinion 2.18 (1986) [now Opinion 2.20], which expresses a contrary view. *Cruzan v. Harmon, 760 S.W.2d 408, 423 n.18, aff'd, 497 U.S. 261.*

N.J. 1987 Husband applied to court for authorization to discontinue wife's hydration and nutrition after nursing home refused his request to do so. The court held that the right of a patient in an irreversible vegetative state to refuse life-sustaining procedures may be exercised by the patient's family or close friend after two independent neurologists have confirmed the diagnosis and prognosis. The court further stated that the processes of surrogate decision-making should be substantially the same regardless of type of medical facility. In so holding, the court cited Opinion 2.18 (1986) [now Opinion 2.20] with approval. *In re Jobes, 108 N.J. 394, 529 A.2d 434, 446.*

N.J. 1987 Elderly nursing home patient was comatose in a persistent vegetative state. Patient's designee, under power of attorney for health care decisions, sought appointment as guardian and authorization for removal of patient's artificial nutrition and hydration. The court held that where there is clear and convincing proof that patient would refuse such treatment if competent, a surrogate may effect that decision regardless of the patient's life expectancy. The court quoted with approval Opinion 2.18 (1986) [now Opinion 2.20] stating that artificial hydration and nutrition is a form of medical treatment. *In re Peter, 108 N.J. 365, 529 A.2d 419, 427-28.*

N.J. 1987 Husband of competent, terminally ill patient applied to be special medical guardian to effectuate patient's desire to remove respirator. In holding that the right of a competent, terminally ill patient to decline medical treatment outweighed the state's interests in preserving life, preventing suicide, protecting innocent third parties, and safeguarding the integrity of the medical profession, the court cited as reflective of the views of the medical profession the Judicial Council's report at 253 *JAMA* 2424 (1985) [now Opinion 2.20]. *In re Farrell, 108 N.J. 335, 529 A.2d 404, 412.*

N.J. Super. 1983 Guardian of elderly nursing home patient suffering from severe organic brain syndrome sought to remove nasogastric tube from patient. Trial court granted guardian's petition, and patient's guardian ad litem appealed. Appellate court reversed, in part based upon Opinions 2.11 (1981) and 5.17 (1979) [now Opinions 2.17 and 2.20], and held that it is improper and would violate medical ethics to allow dehydration and starvation in a noncomatose, non–brain-dead patient not facing imminent death, not maintained by any life-support machine, and not able to speak for herself. *In re Conroy, 190 N.J. Super. 453, 464 A.2d 303, 313-15, rev'd, 98 N.J. 321, 486 A.2d 1209 (1985).*

N.Y. 1990 Jehovah's Witness was given blood transfusion against her express wishes. The court held that the lower court erred in ordering the transfusions without giving the patient or her family notice and a hearing. Barring any superior interest of the state, the patient had a right to determine the course of her own treatment. Concurring opinion argued that the majority rule created an absolute right to refuse treatment. Quoting from Opinion 2.21 (1989) [now Opinion 2.20], the concurring opinion held that a physician had a corresponding ethical duty to render treatment which, in his judgment, benefits the patient. Note that Opinion 2.20 does not retain the specific language of former Opinion 2.21 relied on by concurring judge. *Fosmire v. Nicoleau, 75 N.Y.2d 218, 236 n.2, 551 N.E.2d 77, 87 n.2, 551 N.Y.S.2d 876, 886 n.2.*

N.Y. Sup. 2003 Mother petitioned court to remove her daughter from a respirator. Hospital policy denied mother the authorization to withdraw care. Court granted petition and held parents have a right to refuse medical treatment for their children. Applying the best interest test, the court held that the burdens of prolonging life exceeded the benefits and that, absent extraordinary circumstances or disagreement between parents, judicial intervention is not required to withhold medical treatment from a minor in a vegetative state. Quotes Opinion 2.215. References Opinion 2.20. *In re AB, 196 Misc. 2d 940, 768 N.Y.S. 2d 256, 268-69.*

N.Y. Sup. 1986 Plaintiff petitioned for judicial authorization to remove feeding tube from her 33-year-old husband, a patient in a permanent chronic vegetative state. In denying the petition, the court noted the AMA's position set out in 245 *JAMA* 819 (1981), later included as Opinion 2.11 (1981) [now Opinion 2.20] that, in such cases, members of the family and physicians should decide whether to continue treatment. However, the court concluded that the legislature must resolve the issue and denied the petition. *Delio v. Westchester County Medical Center, 134 Misc. 2d 206, 510 N.Y.S.2d 415, 419, rev'd, 129 A.D. 2d 1, 516 N.Y.S. 2d 677 (1987).*

Ohio App. 1989 The divorced parents of a patient in a persistent vegetative state each petitioned to be appointed guardian of their son. The mother was initially appointed guardian and testified that it would be in the best interests of her son, and consistent with his wishes, to terminate nutrition and hydration. Over the father's objections, the probate court granted the mother, as guardian, the right to make decisions regarding her son's treatment and care. On appeal, the appellate court modified the lower court's order, pursuant to a state statute enacted after that order was entered. Although recognizing that the lower court's decision was consistent with the position of the AMA as articulated in Opinion 2.20, the appellate court held that to allow termination of nutrition and hydration in this case would violate the public policy as expressed in recent legislation. *Couture v. Couture, 48 Ohio App. 3d 208, 549 N.E.2d 571, 574.*

Pa. Super. 1995 Parent of nursing home patient in persistent vegetative state sought removal of gastrostomy tube. Nursing home refused to comply with request without court order. Trial court, applying best interests test, authorized removal of tube. On appeal, court held that consent of close family member, with approval of two qualified physicians, is sufficient without court order to terminate life-sustaining treatment for patient in a long-term persistent vegetative state. Court referred to *In re Grant*, 109 Wash. 2d 545, 747 P.2d 445 (1987) citing Opinion 2.18 [now Opinion 2.20] for proposition that medical ethical principles permit withdrawal of nutrition and hydration for patient in persistent vegetative state. *In re Fiori, 438 Pa. Super. 610, 652 A.2d 1350, 1354, app. granted, 655 A.2d 989 (Pa. 1995).*

Phila. Co. 1987 In a declaratory judgment action, the court held that a patient has a right to withhold or withdraw medical treatment. This right is subject to the state's interest in (1) the preservation of life, (2) protection of innocent third parties, (3) prevention of suicide, and (4) protecting the ethical integrity of the medical profession. The court held that the withholding or withdrawal of life support by a physician or hospital or their agents did not constitute a criminal act or give rise to any civil liability. Citing Opinion 2.18 (1986) [now Opinion 2.20]), the court noted that respect for a patient's autonomy and decision to withdraw life support was consistent with medical ethics. *In re Doe, 16 Phila. 229, 1987 Phila. Cty. Rptr. LEXIS 30 (1987).*

Tenn. App. 2002 Patient was in a vegetative state and had metastasized breast cancer. Her family sought to terminate nutrition and hydration. Trial court found clear and convincing evidence showed patient did not want to live by artificial nutrition. However, court also ruled that state statute required a valid written document in order for an incompetent person to refuse nutrition and hydration. Appellate court reversed, holding that lower court misinterpreted the statute.

The court held that patient had an inherent fundamental right to refuse medical treatment. Quotes Opinion 2.18 [now Opinion 2.20]. *San Juan-Torregosa v. Garcia, 80 S.W.3d 539, 543.*

Va. Att'y Gen. 1990 Attorney general answered in the affirmative when asked whether a competent adult could create a document authorizing a surrogate to consent to the withholding or withdrawal of medical treatment if the person later enters a persistent vegetative state but is not terminally ill. Quoting Opinion 2.18 (1986) [now Opinion 2.20], the attorney general concluded that medical treatment includes artificial hydration and nutrition. *Va. Att'y Gen. Op., 1990 Va. AG LEXIS 63.*

Wash. 1987 Court authorization sought by guardian to withhold mechanical or artificial life-sustaining procedures from incompetent patient with terminal disorder. Trial court denied request as premature because patient was not yet comatose or vegetative, and did not yet need intrusive medical procedures. Supreme Court held that an incompetent patient in an advanced stage of a terminal illness has right to have life-sustaining treatment withheld, a right which stems from the constitutional right of privacy and the common law right to be free of bodily invasion. Court quoted Opinion 2.18 (1986) [now Opinion 2.20] in support of the right of a terminally ill, noncomatose patient to have life-sustaining procedures withheld including the right to withhold artificial means of nutrition and hydration. *In re Grant, 109 Wash. 2d 545, 747 P.2d 445, 450, 454.*

Wis. 1992 Guardian may consent to the withholding or withdrawal of life-prolonging medical treatment on behalf of an incompetent patient and/or a patient for whom the guardian cannot reasonably make a "substituted judgment" where (1) the patient is in a persistent vegetative state with no reasonable chance of recovery, and (2) the guardian in good faith determines that it is in the patient's "best interest." The court referred to the concurring opinion in *Cruzan v. Director, Missouri Dept. of Health*, 497 U.S. 261 (1990), which quoted Opinion 2.20 (1989) in holding that medical treatment includes nutrition and hydration. Further, citing Opinion 2.18 (1986) [now Opinion 2.20], the court found the actions here consistent with current medical ethics. Thus, the state's interest in protecting the integrity of the medical profession was not implicated. *L.W. v. L.E. Phillips Career Dev. Ctr., 167 Wis. 2d 53, 71, 72, 91, 482 N.W.2d 60, 66, 74.*

Journal 2011 Analyzes the development of Italian end-of-life decision-making law. Concludes that, while Italian law more closely resembles that of the U.S. than one might predict given the countries' differing cultural backgrounds and political-legal systems, substantial differences remain. References Opinions 2.20. Cerminara, Pizzetti, & Photangtham, *Schiavo Revisited? The Struggle for Autonomy at the End of Life in Italy, 12 Marq. Elder's Advisor 295, 308 (2011).*

Journal 2010 Discusses futility disputes where a patient's surrogate wishes to prolong treatment that the physician deems medically ineffective, and the current lack of legal remedies to resolve them. Concludes that states need to establish fair, impartial, and patient-centered methods of resolving futility disputes including independent medical boards that would operate under procedural and substantive regulations. Quotes Opinions 2.02 and 2.035. References Opinions 2.17 and 2.20. Bassel, *Order at the End of Life: Establishing a Clear and Fair Mechanism for the Resolution of Futility Disputes*, 63 Vand. L. Rev. 491, 494, 523 (2010).

Journal 2010 Discusses conflicts between surrogates and health care professionals in the context of "futile" care for patients. Further, discusses how "surrogate selection" laws may be used to replace a surrogate demanding inappropriately aggressive end-of-life treatment. Concludes that while surrogate selection has resolved some futility issues, an increase in independent ethics committees would be beneficial in dispelling other major issues. Quotes and cites Opinions 2.20 and 8.081. Pope, *Surrogate Selection: An Increasingly Viable, but Limited, Solution to Intractable Futility Disputes*, 3 St. Louis U. J. Health L. & Pol'y 183, 207, 208, 211-214, 224, 228 (2010).

Journal 2010 Examines whether standards and practices regarding euthanasia, other than those which have been legally and ethically established, should be applied in extreme emergency situations. Concludes that creating an exception to the prohibition against euthanasia in such situations has no legal or ethical foundation and is not necessary as a means to cope with disasters. Argues for the development of disaster planning consistent with established legal and ethical principles. Quotes Opinion 8.08. Cites Opinions 2.20 and 2.21. Shea, *Hurricane Katrina and the Legal and Bioethical Implications of Involuntary Euthanasia as a Component of Disaster Management in Extreme Emergency Situations*, 19 Annals Health L. 133, 137-138 (2010).

Journal 2009 Argues that adults have the right to procreate using assisted reproductive technologies that create embryos, and that such embryos are morally equivalent to individuals on life support. Further argues that, just as families of an individual being removed from life support can consent to the donation of that individual's organs, parents of an embryo can consent to the donation of that embryo's cells for research. Concludes the philosophical notion that life begins at conception can be reconciled with support for embryonic stem cell research if the full humanity of the embryo is recognized throughout the process. Quotes Opinion 2.20. References Opinion 2.20. Dolin, *A Defense of Embryonic Stem Cell Research*, 84 Ind. L. J. 1203, 1223, 1227 (2009).

Journal 2009 Discusses the avoidable consequences rule in the context of awards for pain and suffering. Suggests courts should reevaluate the noneconomic nature of emotional harm to recharacterize some pain and suffering damages as medical expenses. Quotes Opinion 2.20. Noah, *Comfortably Numb: Medicalizing (and Mitigating) Pain-and-Suffering Damages*, 42 U. Mich. J. L. Reform 431, 435 (2009).

Journal 2008 Discusses medical options when the physician can do nothing further to cure the patient and examines the Texas Advance Directives Act, a medical futility statute. Concludes conflicts may be reduced if physician-patient communication is initiated when treatment begins rather than when further treatment becomes futile. Cites the Texas medical futility process as an example for providing physicians a mechanism for resolving conflicts with patients. Quotes Opinions 2.035, 2.037, and 2.20. Dahm, *Medical Futility and the Texas Medical Futility Statute: A Model to Follow or One to Avoid? 20 Health Law 25, 26 (Aug. 2008).

Journal 2008 Discusses patient autonomy, pain, and the current law governing the right to die. Argues pain management is essential to ensure patients possess the requisite autonomy to make end-of-life care decisions. Quotes Opinion 2.20. Lasken, *The Incoherent Right to Die*, 4 NAELA J. 167, 176 (2008).

Journal 2007 Compares US and international policy on end-of-life decision making. Concludes that interests of patient autonomy should be balanced with family interests and advocates a comprehensive "best interest" model. Quotes Opinion 2.037. Cites Opinions 2.035 and 2.20. Rode, *End-of-Life Decision Making for Patients in Persistent Vegetative States: A Comparative Analysis*, 30 Hastings Int'l & Comp. L. Rev. 477, 499, 500 (2007).

Journal 2007 Discusses patients' right to refuse medical treatment and the corresponding duties of health care professionals. Concludes that detailed, carefully prepared advance directives are necessary to fulfill patients' wishes. Quotes Ch. II (1940) [now Opinions 8.08 and 8.082] and Opinions 2.035, 2.037, 2.20, 2.225, 8.081, and 10.015. Cites Opinions 9.11 and 9.115. Stamatakis, *Beyond Advance Directives: Personal Autonomy and the Right to Refuse Life-Sustaining Medical Treatment*, 47 N. H. B. J. 20, 29-30 (2007).

Journal 2007 Argues that Drug Enforcement Agency (DEA) regulation of physicians has resulted in a denial of palliative care to patients. Concludes that in regulating controlled substances, federal and state government must not lose sight of patient need for palliative care. Quotes Opinion 2.20. Trehan, *Fear of Prescribing: How the DEA Is Infringing on Patients' Right to Palliative Care*, 61 U. Miami L. Rev. 961, 975 (2007).

Journal 2006 Discusses an attorney's responsibility to a client on death row who wishes to volunteer for execution. Concludes that an attorney should never assist a client in waiving an appeal. Quotes Opinions 2.20 and 2.211. Oleson, *Swilling Hemlock: The Legal Ethics of Defending a Client Who Wishes to Volunteer for Execution*, 63 Wash. & Lee L. Rev. 147, 277, 325 (2006).

Journal 2006 Examines current policy governing removal of a feeding tube from a patient in a permanent vegetative state. Proposes a policy of a rebuttable presumption that the feeding tube may be removed. References Opinion 2.20. Shepherd, *In Respect of People Living in a Permanent*

Vegetative State—And Allowing Them to Die, 16 Health Matrix 631, 671 (2006).

Journal 2006 Reviews legislation and case law governing conscience clauses for medical professionals. Concludes that conscientious objections to providing care should be permitted only when based on accepted principles of medical ethics. Quotes Opinion 2.18 (1986) [now Opinion 2.20]. References Opinion 8.032. Swartz, *"Conscience Clauses" or "Unconscionable Clauses": Personal Beliefs Versus Professional Responsibilities, 6 Yale J. Health Pol'y, L. & Ethics 269, 317, 347 (2006).*

Journal 2005 Discusses the "best interest" standard used in making end-of-life decisions. Concludes that this standard allows for humane end-of-life decisions to be made on behalf of never-competent patients. Cites Opinion 2.20. Cantor, *The Bane of Surrogate Decision-Making: Defining the Best Interests of Never-Competent Persons, 26 J. Legal Med. 155, 160 (2005).*

Journal 2005 Discusses the facts and history of the *Schiavo* case. Concludes that patient autonomy, family privacy, and patient dignity should prevail in making decisions to withhold life-sustaining treatment. References Opinion 2.20. Gostin, *Ethics, the Constitution, and the Dying Process: The Case of Theresa Marie Schiavo, 293 JAMA 2403, 2405 (2005).*

Journal 2005 Discusses the moral and ethical justifications for the Supreme Court's use of the doctrine of double effect in *Vacco v. Quill.* Concludes that the Court's use of the principle of double effect conforms with widely accepted clinical and ethical norms and is supported by American case law. Quotes Opinion 2.20. Lyons, *In Incognito—The Principle of Double Effect in American Constitutional Law, 57 Fla. L. Rev. 469, 474 (2005).*

Journal 2005 Discusses the evidentiary standards utilized to permit withdrawal of life-sustaining treatment by substitute decision-makers when patients are in a persistent vegetative state. Concludes that a futility rationale for making end-of-life decisions may represent the best approach in these situations. Quotes Opinion 2.035. Cites Opinion 2.20. Mareiniss, *A Comparison of Cruzan and Schiavo: The Burden of Proof, Due Process, and Autonomy in the Persistently Vegetative Patient, 26 J. Legal Med. 233, 248, 250 (2005).*

Journal 2004 Considers whether profoundly mentally disabled persons have the same constitutional rights as competent individuals to refuse life-sustaining medical treatment. Concludes that through the use of a surrogate, these individuals have similar but not identical rights in this context. Cites Opinion 2.20. Cantor, *The Relation Between Autonomy-Based Rights and Profoundly Mentally Disabled Persons, 13 Annals Health L. 37, 70 (2004).*

Journal 2004 Analyzes various issues relating to the role of mental health professionals in capital punishment in light of Albert Bandura's model of "mechanisms of moral disengagement." Concludes that facilitating participation of mental health professionals in executions creates conflicts with the humanistic norms of the profession. Quotes Preamble and Opinions 1.01, 1.02, 2.06, 2.067, 2.20, 2.21, 2.211, and 8.14. Judges, *The Role of Mental Health Professionals in Capital Punishment: An Exercise in Moral Disengagement, 41 Hous. L. Rev. 515, 562, 568, 569, 570, 571-72, 581, 586, 588, 598 (2004).*

Journal 2003 Discusses whether patients may assert a claim of medical malpractice for inadequate treatment of pain. Concludes courts should find that failure to adequately treat pain constitutes negligence. Quotes Opinion 2.20. Mayer, *Bergman v. Chin: Why an Elder Abuse Case Is a Stride in the Direction of Civil Culpability for Physicians Who Undertreat Patients Suffering From Terminal Pain, 37 New Eng. L. Rev. 313, 340 (2003).*

Journal 2003 Identifies legal obstacles to adequate pain care in long-term care facilities. Concludes that the government must take action to ensure effective pain management for patients in these facilities. Quotes Opinion 2.20. Seng, *Legal and Regulatory Barriers to Adequate Pain Control for Elders in Long-Term Care Facilities, 6 N. Y. City L. Rev. 95, 97 (2003).*

Journal 2002 Suggests a reconceptualization for bioethics that integrates an analysis of the history of moral change. Concludes that bioethical textbooks should include discussion about the history of bioethics and medical ethics. Quotes Opinion 2.20. References Opinions 6.02, 6.03, 6.04 [now Opinion 8.06], and 8.032. Baker, *Bioethics and History, 27 J. Med. & Phil. 447, 455, 469 (2002).*

Journal 2002 Explores the implications of withholding medical treatment when abortion results in a live birth. Concludes that, in these situations, abortive parents and physicians should not solely decide the child's best interest. Quotes Preamble, Principles I and III, and Opinions 2.035, 2.20, and 2.215. Casagrande, *Children Not Meant to Be: Protecting the Interests of the Child When Abortion Results in Live Birth, 6 Quinnipiac Health L. J. 19, 44, 45, 47-48 (2002).*

Journal 2002 Considers a judicial model to evaluate the relationship between law and bioethics. Concludes that, in this regard, ethics may justify court decisions but likely will not break new ground. Quotes Opinion 2.20. Gross, *Wagging the Watchdog: Law and the Emergence of Bioethical Norms, 21 Med. & L. 687, 702 (2002).*

Journal 2002 Considers the use of nonlegal materials in US Supreme Court decisions. Concludes that law alone cannot answer complex legal questions. Cites Opinions 2.20 and 2.211. Hasko, *Persuasion in the Court: Nonlegal Materials in U.S. Supreme Court Opinions, 94 Law Libr. J. 427, 444, 453 (2002).*

Journal 2002 Examines competing interests regarding genetic testing. Argues that testing of employees should be banned. Concludes that Congress should pass legislation prohibiting genetic testing in the workplace. Quotes Opinion 2.20. Krumm, *Genetic Discrimination: Why Congress Must Ban Genetic Testing in the Workplace, 23 J. Legal Med. 491, 506 (2002).*

Journal 2002 Evaluates pain management treatment for prisoners. Concludes that withholding treatment for, or failing to adequately treat, pain violates the Eighth Amendment. Quotes Principle V and Opinion 2.20. McGrath, *Raising the "Civilized Minimum" of Pain Amelioration for Prisoners to Avoid Cruel and Unusual Punishment, 54 Rutgers L. Rev. 649, 657, 660 (2002).*

Journal 2002 Examines key factors that led to the current palliative care crisis. Analyzes state legislative and judicial efforts to improve palliative care. Concludes with model legislation that holds physicians accountable for inadequate palliative care. Quotes Opinions 2.21 and 2.211. References Opinion 2.20. Oken, *Curing Healthcare Providers' Failure to Administer Opioids in the Treatment of Severe Pain, 23 Cardozo L. Rev. 1917, 1925-26, 1952, 1954 (2002).*

Journal 2001 Explores the similarities and differences among active voluntary euthanasia, terminal sedation, and assisted suicide. Examines the problems with making moral distinctions based on physicians' intentions. Concludes that, with proper safeguards, active voluntary euthanasia and assisted suicide are more protective of patient self-determination. Quotes Opinions 2.20 and 2.21. Gauthier, *Active Voluntary Euthanasia, Terminal Sedation, and Assisted Suicide, 12 J. Clinical Ethics 43, 43-44, 49 (2001).*

Journal 2001 Examines the role of telemedicine in end-of-life decision-making. Concludes that telemedicine should not be used as a substitute for face-to-face discussions, but as a method to supplement such discussions with input from other experienced clinicians. Cites Opinion 2.20. Pronovost & Williams, *Telemedicine and End-of-Life Care: What's Wrong With This Picture? 12 J. Clinical Ethics 64, 68 (2001).*

Journal 2001 Discusses the North Carolina case of *In Re Cartrette,* which focuses on a mother's decision to terminate life support for her incompetent daughter, who is neither terminally ill nor in a persistent vegetative state (PVS). Argues against sole reliance on a quality-of-life assessment as a predicate for surrogate decision-making for a patient who has never been competent. Urges adoption of best interests standard. Quotes Opinion 2.20. Sabo, *Limiting a Surrogate's Authority to Terminate Life-Support for an Incompetent Adult, 79 N. C. L. Rev. 1815, 1815 (2001).*

Journal 2000 Examines questions regarding the legality of such practices as voluntary stopping of eating and drinking (VSED), use of risky analgesics, and terminal sedation. Explores the distinctions between physician-assisted suicide and other palliative interventions. Concludes VSED, risky analgesics, and certain types of terminal sedation are lawful and should be made available to dying patients who make informed decisions to accept the risks involved. Quotes Opinions 2.21 and 2.211. Cites Opinions 2.18 and 2.20.

Cantor & Thomas, *The Legal Bounds of Physician Conduct Hastening Death, 48 Buff. L. Rev. 83, 110, 131, 158 (2000).*

Journal 2000 Examines various laws associated with physician-assisted suicide, including the Oregon Death with Dignity Act, the Legal Drug Abuse and Prevention Act of 1998, and the Pain Relief Promotion Act of 1999 (PRPA). Argues that the Supreme Court should declare the PRPA unconstitutional. References Opinion 2.20. Fallek, *The Pain Relief Promotion Act: Will It Spell Death to "Death With Dignity" or Is It Unconstitutional? 27 Fordham Urb. L. J. 1739, 1755 (2000).*

Journal 2000 Considers the question of whether physician-assisted suicide and euthanasia should be legalized. Concludes that, under basic moral and common law principles, the intentional taking of human life by a private person is wrong. References Opinions 2.20, 2.21, and 2.211. Gorsuch, *The Right to Assisted Suicide and Euthanasia, 23 Harv. J. L. & Pub. Pol'y 599, 653, 707 (2000).*

Journal 2000 Examines advance directive pregnancy provisions. Discusses the right to refuse medical treatment and the right to terminate pregnancy. Concludes the Minnesota advance directive pregnancy presumption balances the woman's right to terminate a pregnancy and the right to refuse medical treatment with the state interest in potential life. References Opinion 2.20. Jerdee, *Breaking Through the Silence: Minnesota's Pregnancy Presumption and the Right to Refuse Medical Treatment, 84 Minn. L. Rev. 971, 980 (2000).*

Journal 2000 Examines legal and ethical issues bearing upon pain management. Asserts that health care professionals have a legal and ethical duty to relieve pain and suffering of patients whenever possible. Suggests that this duty is legally enforceable. Quotes Principle V and Opinions 2.20 and 9.011. Rich, *A Prescription for the Pain: The Emerging Standard of Care for Pain Management, 26 Wm. Mitchell L. Rev. 1, 35-36, 85 (2000).*

Journal 2000 Examines existing law governing a parent's authority to make health care decisions for a child. Concludes that, consistent with principles of beneficence and autonomy, parents generally should retain their status as primary decision-makers for their children. Cites Opinion 2.20. Rosato, *Using Bioethics Discourse to Determine When Parents Should Make Health Care Decisions for Their Children: Is Deference Justified? 73 Temp. L. Rev. 1, 40, 44 (2000).*

Journal 1999 States that a distrust of the medical profession arose from changes in the health care system and federal law. Explains how legislation may help alleviate some of the distrust. Suggests that people need more access to information about their health plans. References Opinions 2.20 and 2.225. Cerminara, *Protecting Participants in and Beneficiaries of ERISA-Governed Managed Health Care Plans, 29 U. Mem. L. Rev. 317, 324 (1999).*

Journal 1999 Discusses use of the hierarchical decision-making model for end-of-life decisions. Proposes that a consensus-based decision-making model, which synthesizes therapeutic jurisprudence and preventive law, should replace the hierarchical decision-making model. Argues that the consensus-based model would decrease court involvement and advance the interests of those affected by the decision. Quotes Opinion 2.20. Hafemeister, *End-of-Life Decision Making, Therapeutic Jurisprudence, and Preventive Law: Hierarchical v. Consensus-Based Decision-Making Model, 41 Ariz. L. Rev. 329 (1999).*

Journal 1999 States that the Patient Self-Determination Act is the medical field's version of the Miranda warning. Suggests that, although the act is followed, many patients do not understand how to exercise their right to medical self-determination. Argues that informed consent should be required in relation to advance directives. Cites Opinion 2.20. Pope, *The Maladaptation of Miranda to Advance Directives: A Critique of the Implementation of the Patient Self-Determination Act, 9 Health Matrix 139, 178 (1999).*

Journal 1999 Examines legal and policy issues regarding physician-assisted suicide. Distinguishes between refusing treatment and assisted suicide. Concludes that there are too many dangers posed by physician-assisted suicide to warrant legalization. Quotes Opinion 2.211. Cites Opinions 2.20 and 2.21. Pratt, *Too Many Physicians: Physician-Assisted Suicide After Glucksberg/Quill, 9 Alb. L. J. Sci. & Tech. 161, 208 (1999).*

Journal 1999 Evaluates liability theories used in cases alleging failure to follow do-not-resuscitate orders and advance directives. Analyzes the impact of legal liability as a means to ensure compliance with such orders and directives. Concludes that there is an increased need for open communication among physicians, patients, and patients' family members. Quotes Opinion 2.20. Rodriguez, *Suing Health Care Providers for Saving Lives: Liability for Providing Unwanted Life-Sustaining Treatment, 20 J. Legal Med. 1, 62 (1999).*

Journal 1999 Explains the rule of double effect. Distinguishes between assisted suicide and pain control for terminally ill patients. Suggests that the rule of double effect needs to be adequately defined so physicians will understand that they can ethically give terminally ill patients drugs that will alleviate their pain, but that also may hasten their death. Cites Opinion 2.20. Sulmasy & Pellegrino, *The Rule of Double Effect: Clearing Up the Double Talk, 159 Arch. Intern. Med. 545, 550 (1999).*

Journal 1998 Explains that the US Supreme Court's decisions in *Washington* and *Vacco* left the door open for future constitutional challenges regarding the right to physician-assisted suicide. States that the Court did not explicitly deny the existence of a right to physician-assisted suicide. Quotes Opinion 2.20. Cites Opinion 2.211. Cohen, *The Open Door: Will the Right to Die Survive Washington v. Glucksberg and Vacco v. Quill? 16 In Pub. Interest 79, 94 (1998).*

Journal 1998 Describes a survey regarding physician-assisted suicide given to members of the Group for the Advancement of Psychiatry. Discusses the results of the survey, noting that most surveyed psychiatrists oppose assisting patients to die. Cites Opinions 2.06 and 2.20. Kramer, Gruenberg, & Fidler, *Psychiatrists' Attitudes Toward Physician-Assisted Suicide: A Survey, 19 Am. J. Forensic Psychiatry 81, 87, 90 (1998).*

Journal 1998 Discusses legal aspects of physician-assisted suicide. Identifies acceptable end-of-life choices and compares them to physician-assisted suicide. Points out that physician-assisted suicide has the potential for abuse and that safeguards have not been implemented to protect people from that risk. Quotes Opinion 2.211. Cites Opinions 2.20 and 8.08. Mitchell, *Physician-Assisted Suicide: A Survey of the Issues Surrounding Legalization, 74 N. D. L. Rev. 341, 349 (1998).*

Journal 1998 Points out that the court in *Vacco v. Quill* did not reject the practice of physician-assisted suicide and left the subject open for state experimentation. Discusses routes some states have taken regarding assisted suicide. Concludes that access to assisted suicide is outweighed by the risk it will be utilized by depressed and mentally ill people. Quotes Opinions 2.20 and 2.211. Moore, *Physician-Assisted Suicide: Does "The End" Justify the Means? 40 Ariz. L. Rev. 1471, 1472, 1481-82, 1491 (1998).*

Journal 1998 Discusses consequences physician-assisted suicide may have on disabled individuals. Weighs potential benefits and disadvantages stemming from physician-assisted suicide. Concludes that only a small number of people with disabilities would benefit from physician-assisted suicide and that the benefits are outweighed by the risk of abuse. Cites Opinion 2.20. National Council on Disability, *Assisted Suicide: A Disability Perspective, 14 Issues L. & Med. 273, 292 (1998).*

Journal 1998 Observes that the Patient Self-Determination Act does not obligate physicians to discuss advance directives with patients. Explains that physicians may elect not to discuss advance directives with patients because of lack of time and reimbursement for such discussions. Emphasizes that patients, physicians, and health care providers may benefit from advance directives. Quotes Opinion 2.20. Rich, *Advance Directives: The Next Generation, 19 J. Legal Med. 63, 79 (1998).*

Journal 1998 Provides a historical view on parents' rights to make medical decisions for their children. Argues that parents have the right to make medical decisions for their children when the decisions are supported by medical evidence. This right extends to decisions regarding life-sustaining medical treatment. Quotes Opinion 2.20. Walters, *Life-Sustaining Medical Decisions Involving Children: Father Knows Best, 15 T. M. Cooley L. Rev. 115, 128, 138, 151 (1998).*

Journal 1997 Reviews the criminalization of physician-assisted suicide. Discusses informed consent, the double effect, and the right to die. Explains the current state of the law and the position Illinois has taken. Advocates the adoption of a law authorizing physician-assisted suicide in Illinois. References Opinion 2.20. Comment, *An Illinois Physician-Assisted Suicide Act: A Merciful End to a Terminally Ill Criminal Tradition,* 28 Loy. U. Chi. L. J. 763, 775 (1997).

Journal 1997 Discusses Pennsylvania Supreme Court case of *In Re Fiori.* Explains that the court extended the right to refuse medical treatment to patients in permanent vegetative states. Notes that the court now allows family members to exercise this right on behalf of such patients. Quotes Opinion 2.20. Comment, *Surrogate Health Care Decision Making: The Pennsylvania Supreme Court Recognizes the Right of an Individual in a Permanent Vegetative State to Refuse Life-Sustaining Measures Through a Surrogate Decision Maker,* 35 Duq. L. Rev. 849, 859-60 (1997).

Journal 1997 Discusses goals of care included in advance directives and whether they can be used to predict specific interventions and results. Offers insights provided by survey of physicians at Massachusetts General Hospital. Cites Opinions 2.20 and 2.21. Fischer, Alpert, Stoeckle, & Emanuel, *Can Goals of Care Be Used to Predict Intervention Preferences in an Advance Directive?* 157 Arch. Intern. Med. 801, 807 (1997).

Journal 1997 Examines the evolution of the Indiana health care system. Discusses developments in Indiana jurisprudence regarding the physician-patient relationship. Explores various challenges facing the relationship and recognizes the need for legal rules to help address these challenges. Quotes Opinion 8.08. Cites Opinions 2.20, 9.06, and 9.12. Kinney & Selby, *History and Jurisprudence of the* physician-patient *Relationship in Indiana,* 30 Ind. L. Rev. 263, 269, 272, 276 (1997).

Journal 1996 Proposes a model state statute allowing and controlling physician-assisted suicide. Analyzes the constitutionality of the act and offers public policy justifications for the act's provisions. Concludes that proponents of physician-assisted suicide should provide precise, carefully tailored examples of regulations. Quotes Opinion 2.211. Cites Opinion 2.20. Baron, Bergstresser, Brock, Cole, Dorfman, Johnson, Schnipper, Vorenberg, & Wanzer, *A Model State Act to Authorize and Regulate Physician-Assisted Suicide,* 33 Harv. J. Legis. 1, 2, 7 (1996).

Journal 1996 Explores the issue of legalizing physician-assisted suicide. Opines that the current state of technology increases life expectancy but with a concomitant decrease in dignity and autonomy surrounding one's death. Notes that the elderly are committing suicide at an increasing rate. Cites Opinions 2.20, 2.21, and 2.211. Morgan & Sutherland, *Last Rights? Confronting Physician-Assisted Suicide in Law and Society: Legal Liturgies on Physician-Assisted Suicide,* 26 Stetson L. Rev. 481, 484 (1996).

Journal 1996 Considers the right to death with dignity. Suggests that the AMA's position undermines mitigation of suffering and the individuals' right to self-determination.

Concludes that restrictions on the right to death with dignity may be constitutionally impermissible. Quotes Opinion 2.211. Cites Opinion 2.20. Note, *Who Decides if There Is Triumph in the Ultimate Agony? Constitutional Theory and the Emerging Right to Die With Dignity,* 37 Wm. & Mary L. Rev. 827, 829 (1996).

Journal 1996 Discusses the physician's duty to relieve pain. Considers current attitudes toward pain management. Concludes that, consistent with principles of beneficence, physicians are obligated to provide pain relief and palliation. Quotes Opinion 2.20. Post, Blustein, Gordon, & Dubler, *Pain: Ethics, Culture, and Informed Consent to Relief,* 24 J. Law Med. & Ethics 348, 349, 356 (1996).

Journal 1996 Discusses children's rights to consent to or refuse life-sustaining medical treatment. Compares the rights of children to those of adults in a medical decision-making context. Proposes reforms to allow minors legal rights to make decisions regarding withdrawal of life-sustaining treatment. Quotes Opinion 2.20. Rosato, *The Ultimate Test of Autonomy: Should Minors Have a Right to Make Decisions Regarding Life-Sustaining Treatment?* 49 Rutgers L. Rev. 1, 80-81, 82 (1996).

Journal 1995 Explores reluctance of long-term care facilities to allow patients to forgo life-sustaining tube feeding. Concludes that policies must be adopted to ensure that patients' rights to refuse artificial nutrition and hydration are protected. Cites Opinion 2.20. Meisel, *Barriers to Forgoing Nutrition and Hydration in Nursing Homes,* XXI Am. J. Law & Med. 335, 353-54 (1995).

Journal 1995 Examines the problem of determining when a patient has lost decision-making capacity. Compares the authority of the treating physician with that of the patient's designated agent in making such a determination. Cites Opinion 2.20. Schneiderman, Teetzel, & Kalmanson, *Who Decides Who Decides? When Disagreement Occurs Between the Physician and the Patient's Appointed Proxy About the Patient's Decision-Making Capacity,* 155 Arch. Intern. Med. 793, 796 (1995).

Journal 1995 Offers relevant historical perspectives and provides comprehensive ethical and legal discussion of physician-assisted suicide and euthanasia. Highlights important legislative developments, including the Oregon Death with Dignity Act, and analyzes significant judicial opinions. Quotes Principles III, IV, and VI and Opinions 2.21 and 9.12. Cites Opinions 2.20 and 8.11. Stone & Winslade, *Physician-Assisted Suicide and Euthanasia in the United States: Legal and Ethical Observations,* 16 J. Legal Med. 481, 483, 490, 497, 498, 499 (1995).

Journal 1994 Considers how greater patient autonomy has led to situations in which medical care may be viewed as futile. Suggests that the law has intruded too far into this area of medicine. Quotes Opinion 2.035. Cites Opinions 2.03, 2.095, 2.17, 2.19, 2.20, and 2.22. Cultice, *Medical Futility: When Is Enough, Enough?* 27 J. Health & Hosp. Law 225, 230, 256 (1994).

Journal 1994 Discusses whether a patient's prior expression of treatment choices in an advance directive accurately represents future choices. Concludes that patients are capable of making stable scenario- and treatment-specific advance directives, that their choices become more stable with repeated consideration, and that illness has little effect on stability of choices. Cites Opinion 2.20. Emanuel, Emanuel, Stoeckle, Hummel, & Barry, *Advance Directives: Stability of Patients' Treatment Choices, 154 Arch. Intern. Med. 209, 217 (1994).*

Journal 1994 Analyzes physicians' attitudes about whether to initiate or withhold tube feeding when patients' preferences are unknown. Concludes that patient prognosis and quality of life are the most important influences on physician decisions about tube feeding. Cites Opinion 2.20. Hodges, Tolle, Stocking, & Cassel, *Tube Feeding: Internists' Attitudes Regarding Ethical Obligations, 154 Arch. Intern. Med. 1013, 1020 (1994).*

Journal 1994 Examines the various types of advance health care directives and reviews pertinent Arkansas law. Concludes that directives should conform to each person's values, health status, and medical prognosis. Cites Opinion 2.20. Leflar, *Advance Health Care Directives Under Arkansas Law, 1994 Ark. L. Notes 37, 42.*

Journal 1994 Examines how state laws have accommodated medical developments in the area of treatment decisions and how they serve to resolve and encourage conflict in health care decision-making. Considers the roles of physicians, hospitals, and families and how their wishes may conflict with those of the patient. Cites Opinion 2.20. Tarantino, *Withdrawal of Life Support: Conflict Among Patient Wishes, Family, Physicians, Courts and Statutes, and the Law, 42 Buff. L. Rev. 623, 638, 639, 646 (1994).*

Journal 1994 Determines that physicians are not taking the responsibility for initiating discussions about end-of-life medical treatment and that many patients falsely assume that their physicians would know what kind of treatments they would want. Concludes that physician-patient communication is improved slightly when there is an advance directive, but that there is still a lack of detailed discussion about end-of-life treatments. Cites Opinion 2.20. Virmani, Schneiderman, & Kaplan, *Relationship of Advance Directives to* physician-patient *Communication, 154 Arch. Intern. Med. 909, 913 (1994).*

Journal 1993 Analyzes the implications of giving patients and their families an absolute right to control medical treatment. Argues that courts should refrain from ordering physicians to treat patients when physicians believe that treatment would be ineffective. Quotes Fundamental Elements (5) and Opinions 2.11 (1982) [now Opinion 2.20] and 2.18 (1986) [now Opinion 2.20]. Comment, *Beyond Autonomy: Judicial Restraint and the Legal Limits Necessary to Uphold the Hippocratic Tradition and Preserve the Ethical Integrity of the Medical Profession, 9 J. Contemp. Health L. & Pol'y 451, 467, 468 (1993).*

Journal 1993 Discusses Ohio's living will statute in light of the *Cruzan* decision. Presents the medical implications of the persistent vegetative state patient. Quotes Opinion 2.18 (1986) [now Opinion 2.20]. Comment, *One Step Forward, Two Steps Back: A Constitutional and Critical Look at Ohio's New Living Will Statute, 54 Ohio St. L. J. 445, 447, 460, 470 (1993).*

Journal 1993 Discusses the problem of physicians withholding needed medical treatment from HIV-infected infants. Concludes that current law should be expanded to eliminate this discrimination. Quotes Opinions 2.09, 2.17, 2.20, 2.22, 4.04, and 8.03. Crossley, *Of Diagnoses and Discrimination: Discriminatory Nontreatment of Infants With HIV Infection, 93 Columbia L. Rev. 1581, 1620, 1621 (1993).*

Journal 1993 Discusses the relationship between a physician's professional conscience and end of life decision-making. Considers the issue of futile medical treatment. Examines case law concerning a patient's right to demand treatment and a physician's obligation to provide it. References Opinions 2.20 and 2.22. Daar, *A Clash at the Bedside: Patient Autonomy v. a Physician's Professional Conscience, 44 Hastings L. J. 1241, 1257, 1268, 1286 (1993).*

Journal 1993 Argues that society should not permit euthanasia because of lack of protection against potential abuses. Recommends that health care providers be taught to treat pain and more effectively care for dying patients, rather than to affirmatively end life. Quotes Opinions 2.17 and 2.20. Dickey, *Euthanasia: A Concept Whose Time Has Come? 8 Issues in Law & Med. 521, 523, 524 (1993).*

Journal 1993 Discusses the legal distinction between "the right to die" and physician-assisted suicide. Examines how the law is applied and whether it should be reformed in light of public opinion and changing ethical standards. References Opinion 2.20. Gostin, *Drawing a Line Between Killing and Letting Die: The Law, and Law Reform, on Medically Assisted Dying, 21 J. Law Med. & Ethics 94, 98 (1993).*

Journal 1993 Considers how life-sustaining treatments have led to prolonged life under unacceptable circumstances. Recommends quality assurance programs that promote discussion between physicians and patients regarding life-sustaining treatment problems. Cites Opinions 2.20 and 2.21. Pearlman, Cain, Patrick, Appelbaum-Maizel, Starks, Jecker, & Uhlmann, *Insights Pertaining to Patient Assessments of States Worse Than Death, 4 J. Clinical Ethics 33, 40 (1993).*

Journal 1993 Considers whether criminal penalties should be imposed on a physician who assists in the suicide of a competent, nonterminal patient who requested such assistance. Presents the arguments for and against active euthanasia, with emphasis on the "slippery slope" argument. References Opinions 2.06 and 2.20. Persels, *Forcing the Issue of Physician-Assisted Suicide: Impact of the Kevorkian Case on the Euthanasia Debate, 14 J. Legal Med. 93, 115 (1993).*

Journal 1993 Discusses legal and ethical issues raised by physician aid-in-dying. Concludes that passive euthanasia for competent, terminal adults is the accepted norm and physician aid-in-dying is the new frontier. Quotes Opinion 2.18 (1986) [now Opinion 2.20]. Risley, *Ethical and Legal Issues in the Individual's Right to Die, 20 Ohio N. U. L. Rev. 597, 605 (1993).*

Journal 1992 Considers when it is appropriate to withdraw artificial food and nutrition from an incompetent patient under the Indiana "Living Wills" statute. Concludes that, in Indiana, it is appropriate to remove artificial nutrition and hydration that only "prolongs the dying process." Quotes Opinion 2.20. Anderson, *A Medical-Legal Dilemma: When Can "Inappropriate" Nutrition and Hydration Be Removed in Indiana? 67 Ind. L. J. 479, 480 (1992).*

Journal 1992 Analyzes the arguments for and against active euthanasia, including ethical concerns, the slippery slope argument, and the proper role of the physician. Suggests that active euthanasia may be acceptable when its administration is restricted to physicians. References Opinions 2.20 and 2.21. Brock, *Voluntary Active Euthanasia, 22 Hastings Center Rep. 10 (March/April 1992).*

Journal 1992 Examines several issues regarding persistent vegetative state (PVS) patients, including whether PVS patients are really dead, whether nutrition and hydration should be withheld, whether life-sustaining treatments are futile or medically inappropriate, and whether ordinary standards for decision-making should be applied to PVS patients. Concludes that life-sustaining therapy may be withheld or continued, but that withdrawal of nutrition and hydration, as well as active euthanasia, present more difficult questions. References Opinions 2.20 and 2.22. Brody, *Special Ethical Issues in the Management of PVS Patients, 20 Law Med. & Health Care 104, 109 (1992).*

Journal 1992 Examines ethical and legal issues surrounding cardiopulmonary resuscitation and emergency cardiac care. Discusses advance directives and proxy decision-making, medical futility, resource allocation, and do-not-resuscitate orders. References Opinions 2.20 and 2.22. Comment, *Ethical Considerations in Resuscitation, 268 JAMA 2282, 2283, 2287 (1992).*

Journal 1992 Defines the right of terminally ill, competent patients to die with the assistance of a physician and argues that it is essentially the same as the right to die by refusing life-sustaining medical treatment. Concludes that courts should balance patients' rights with compelling state interests in assessing the scope of this right. Cites Opinion 2.20. Comment, *Physician Assisted Suicide and the Right to Die With Assistance, 105 Harvard L. Rev. 2021, 2027, 2035 (1992).*

Journal 1992 Discusses the Iowa living will statute, comparing it to similar laws in other states. Proposes a revised statute to address problems arising in light of recent court decisions. References Opinion 2.20. Goldman, *Revising Iowa's Life-Sustaining Procedures Act: Creating a Practical Guide to Living Wills in Iowa, 76 Iowa L. Rev. 1137, 1149 (1992).*

Journal 1992 Explores various health policy issues addressed by the Indiana state legislature. Considers Indiana lawmakers' responses to the following concerns: health care access, tort reform, the right to die, Medicaid reimbursements, and discrimination against AIDS patients. Cites Opinion 2.18 (1986) [now Opinion 2.20]. Kumar & Kinney, *Indiana Lawmakers Face National Health Policy Issues, 25 Indiana L. Rev. 1271, 1275, 1276 (1992).*

Journal 1992 Discusses the need for a policy governing life-sustaining treatment decisions for incompetent adult wards of the state. Provides a basic outline for such a policy and proposes a model policy statement. Quotes Opinion 2.20. McKnight & Bollis, *Foregoing Life-Sustaining Treatment for Adult Developmentally Disabled, Public Wards: A Proposed Statute, XVIII Am. J. Law & Med. 203, 206, 220, 227 (1992).*

Journal 1992 Observes that the fundamental question in *Cruzan* was whether there should be judicial oversight regarding decisions to forgo life-sustaining treatment. Concludes that *Cruzan* did not resolve this issue. Cites Opinion 2.18 (1986) [now Opinion 2.20]. Meisel, *A Retrospective on Cruzan, 20 Law Med. & Health Care 340, 345 (1992).*

Journal 1992 Explores evolution of the legal consensus that terminating life support is legitimate under some circumstances. Suggests that the consensus will continue to spread in the absence of opposition and may extend to mercy killing and futility cases. Quotes Opinion 2.18 (1986) [now Opinion 2.20]. Meisel, *The Legal Consensus About Forgoing Life-Sustaining Treatment: Its Status and Its Prospects, 2 Kennedy Inst. Ethics J. 309, 325 (1992).*

Journal 1992 Considers the debate surrounding medical futility. Observes that this debate is encouraging reexamination of the nature of patient entitlement to medical care as well as the "ends of medicine." References Opinions 2.20, 2.21, and 2.22. Miles, *Medical Futility, 20 Law Med. & Health Care 310, 311, 313 (1992).*

Journal 1992 Analyzes North Carolina's living will and health care power of attorney statutes in light of the *Cruzan* case. Notes recent changes to both statutes and problems that continue to exist. Quotes Opinion 2.21 (1992) [now Opinion 2.20]. Note, *Exercising the Right to Die: North Carolina's Amended Natural Death Act and the 1991 Health Care Power of Attorney Act, 70 No. Carolina L. Rev. 2108, 2116 (1992).*

Journal 1992 Explains how the "terminal condition" requirement in natural death acts may reduce the number of people who fall within the scope of coverage. Also indicates that omission of nutrition and hydration from the list of treatments that may be withdrawn limits patient choices. Quotes Opinion 2.20. References Opinion 2.22. Note, *State Natural Death Acts: Illusory Protection of Individuals'*

Life-Sustaining Treatment Decisions, 29 Harvard J. Legis. 175, 186, 194, 195, 201 (1992).

Journal 1992 Discusses the impact of physicians' values on end-of-life decision making for patients. Examines how and why physician values may become dominant. References Opinions 2.20, 2.22, and 9.121. Orentlicher, *The Illusion of Patient Choice in End-Of-Life Decisions, 267 JAMA 2101, 2102 (1992).*

Journal 1992 Contrasts physician-assisted suicide and voluntary euthanasia. Recommends legalization of physician-assisted suicide and proposes guidelines for implementation. References Opinion 2.20. Quill, Cassel, & Meier, *Care of the Hopelessly Ill: Proposed Clinical Criteria for Physician-Assisted Suicide, 327 New Eng. J. Med. 1380, 1381 (1992).*

Journal 1992 Suggests that triage and cost-benefit analysis are the most effective means to evaluate issues associated with allocating scarce medical resources to disabled infants. Concludes both that selective treatment can never be considered murder and that governmental intrusion in this area should be minimal. Quotes Opinions 2.10 (1982) [now Opinion 2.17] and 2.18 (1986) [now Opinion 2.20]. Smith, *Murder, She Wrote or Was It Merely Selective Nontreatment? 8 J. Contemp. Health L. & Pol'y 49, 53 (1992).*

Journal 1991 Discusses the manner in which competent and incompetent patients could exercise the right to refuse life-sustaining medical treatment prior to *Cruzan.* Analyzes the effect *Cruzan* had on these rights. Concludes that *Cruzan* had limited far-reaching impact and failed to answer several important questions. Cites Opinion 2.20. Albert, *Cruzan v. Director, Missouri Department of Health: Too Much Ado, 12 J. Legal Med. 331, 338, 343 (1991).*

Journal 1991 Discusses why families of persistent vegetative state patients should not make decisions regarding whether to withdraw life support. Observes that leaving decisions to families creates the possibility they will decide in opposition of the patient. References Opinion 2.20. Baron, *Why Withdrawal of Life-Support for PVS Patients Is Not a Family Decision, 19 Law Med. & Health Care 73 (1991).*

Journal 1991 Considers the issue of how courts should decide right-to-die cases in Massachusetts. Concludes that there are no clear standards for physicians to follow and recommends that physicians obtain court approval before withdrawing artificial nutrition and hydration from a patient in a persistent vegetative state. Quotes Opinion 2.20. Comment, *A Right to Die: Can a Massachusetts Physician Withdraw Artificial Nutrition and Hydration From a Persistently Vegetative Patient Following Cruzan v. Director, Missouri Department of Health? 26 New Eng. L. Rev. 199, 216, 220 (1991).*

Journal 1991 Discusses major neurologic syndromes in life-sustaining medical treatment decisions. Concludes with a survey of the major legal developments in the area since

Cruzan. References Opinion 2.20. Cranford, *Neurologic Syndromes and Prolonged Survival: When Can Artificial Nutrition and Hydration Be Foregone? 19 Law Med. & Health Care 13, 14, 16, 17 (1991).*

Journal 1991 Reports that most individuals surveyed favor use of advance directives and would not desire life-sustaining treatment if faced with a poor prognosis. Recommends that physicians routinely discuss advance directives with patients. Cites Opinion 2.20. Emanuel, Barry, Stoeckle, Ettelson, & Emanuel, *Advance Directives for Medical Care—A Case for Greater Use, 324 New Eng. J. Med. 889 (1991).*

Journal 1991 Discusses the "slippery slope" argument against expanding the right to die. Concludes that society seems to be sliding down the slippery slope toward euthanasia. Cites Opinion 2.18 (1986) [now Opinion 2.20]. Kamisar, *When Is There a Constitutional "Right to Die"? When Is There No Constitutional "Right to Live"? 25 Georgia L. Rev. 1203, 1207, 1208, 1222 (1991).*

Journal 1991 Discusses common misperceptions about legal implications of terminating life support. Emphasizes importance of educating physicians about these medical-legal considerations. References Opinion 2.20. Meisel, *Legal Myths About Terminating Life Support, 151 Arch. Intern. Med. 1497, 1499 (1991).*

Journal 1991 Discusses health care decision-making for terminally ill incompetent patients in Ohio. Argues that Ohio is one of the few remaining states that does not adequately protect the rights of incompetent terminally ill patients. Cites Opinion 2.18 (1986) [now Opinion 2.20]. Mullins, *The Need for Guidance in Decisionmaking for Terminally Ill Incompetents: Is the Ohio Legislature in a "Persistent Vegetative State"? 17 Ohio No. Univ. L. Rev. 827, 844 (1991).*

Journal 1991 Discusses the major issues contained in the *Cruzan* decision. Analyzes the legal predicates for an incompetent patient's right to refuse life-sustaining treatment. References Opinion 2.20. Note, *Cruzan v. Director, Missouri Department of Health: To Die or Not to Die: That Is the Question—But Who Decides? 51 Louisiana L. Rev. 1307, 1327, 1333 (1991).*

Journal 1991 Explores the growth of "right to die" jurisprudence with particular emphasis on post-*Cruzan* developments. Notes that the New York "Health Care Proxy Law" does not apply to situations in which a patient is incompetent, but did not appoint an agent. References Opinion 2.20. Note, *Health Care Proxies: New York's Attempt to Resolve the Right to Die Dilemma, 57 Brooklyn L. Rev. 145, 168 (1991).*

Journal 1991 Analyzes the Illinois Supreme Court case of *In re Estate of Longeway*, where the court decided that, absent an advance directive, the guardian of an incompetent patient could authorize the withdrawal of artificial nutrition and hydration. Concludes that written directives other than living wills may best secure patients' rights. Cites Opinion 2.18 (1986) [now Opinion 2.20]. Note, *Redefining the Right to Die in Illinois, 15 So. Ill. Univ. L. J. 1261, 1273 (1991).*

Journal 1991 Discusses applicable law regarding patients in a persistent vegetative state. Compares *Cruzan* with other right-to-die cases, arguing that the *Cruzan* decision makes it more difficult for individuals to secure this right. Quotes Opinion 2.20. Note, *Something Worth Writing Home About: Clear and Convincing Evidence, Living Wills, and Cruzan v. Director, Missouri Department of Health, 22 Univ. Toledo L. Rev. 871, 879 (1991).*

Journal 1991 Examines the living will and durable power of attorney as health care planning devices in South Carolina. Considers both statutory and nonstatutory forms of the living will. References Opinion 2.20. Patterson, *Planning for Health Care Using Living Wills and Durable Powers of Attorney: A Guide for the South Carolina Attorney, 42 So. Carolina L. Rev. 525, 535, 541, 547, 548 (1991).*

Journal 1991 Explains the contractual nature of the physician-patient relationship and how it has been ignored by many courts in right-to-die cases. Concludes there is a constitutional right to privacy in health care decision-making. Cites Opinion 2.18 (1986) [now Opinion 2.20]. Rich, *The Assault on Privacy on Healthcare Decisionmaking, 68 Denver L. Rev. 1, 10 (1991).*

Journal 1991 Considers the limits of patient autonomy in demanding treatment that the physician feels provides no medical benefit. Discusses these issues in light of the Helga Wanglie case. References Opinion 2.20. Rie, *The Limits of a Wish, 21 Hastings Center Rep. 24 (July/August 1991).*

Journal 1991 Analyzes three important right-to-die cases: *Cruzan, Wanglie,* and *Busalacchi.* Concludes that there should be a nationwide system to address right-to-die cases. References Opinion 2.20. Roach, *Paradox and Pandora's Box: The Tragedy of Current Right-to-Die Jurisprudence, 25 Univ. Mich. J. Law Reform 133, 137, 158 (1991).*

Journal 1990 Argues that *Roe v. Wade* not only protects a woman's right to choose, but also preserves a physician's right to treat. Observes that this protected relationship extends into the arena of right-to-die cases. Cites Opinion 2.20. Annas, Glantz, & Mariner, *The Right of Privacy Protects the Doctor-Patient Relationship, 263 JAMA 858, 861 (1990).*

Journal 1990 Discusses the connection between law and medicine in the context of health care decision-making. Presents several illustrations, noting the involvement of courts and judges. Quotes Opinion 2.18 [now Opinion 2.20]. Bellacosa, *The Fusion of Medicine and Law for In Extremis Health and Medical Decisions: Does It Produce Energy and Light or Just Cosmic Debris? 18 Bull. Am. Acad. Psychiatry Law 5, 9 (1990).*

Journal 1990 Finds that a vast majority of North Carolina nursing homes have written cardiopulmonary resuscitation policies, but that there is substantial variation among them.

Concludes that such variations risk limiting or ignoring the personal rights of residents. References Opinions 2.20 and 2.22. Brunetti, Weiss, Studenski, & Clipp, *Cardiopulmonary Resuscitation Policies and Practices: A Statewide Nursing Home Study, 150 Arch. Intern. Med. 121, 122 (1990).*

Journal 1990 Discusses the importance of living wills and society's acceptance of terminating medical care in appropriate situations. Proposes a living will that addresses the shortcomings of current living will statutes. Cites Opinion 2.18 (1986) [now Opinion 2.20]. Cantor, *My Annotated Living Will, 18 Law Med. & Health Care 114 (1990).*

Journal 1990 Discusses the "living will" and its role in American society. Concludes that legislators need to be more aware of the goals of living wills when drafting statutes. Quotes Opinion 2.20. Comment, *The Living Will: Preservation of the Right-To-Die Demands Clarity and Consistency, 95 Dickinson L. Rev. 209, 217 (1990).*

Journal 1990 Explores current law governing the right of a person to withdraw artificial hydration and nutrition, with emphasis on Oklahoma law, which omits artificial nutrition and hydration from the list of treatments that may be withdrawn. Concludes that individuals have a right to withdraw such treatment and that Oklahoma law may be unconstitutional. Quotes Opinion 2.18 (1986) [now Opinion 2.20]. Comment, *Right to Die: Oklahoma's Position on Nutrition and Hydration: Confusing or Unconstitutional? 43 Okla. L. Rev. 143, 151 (1990).*

Journal 1990 Examines the right of competent patients to refuse treatment on the basis of a common law right of bodily integrity, the right to privacy, and statutory provisions such as natural death acts. Concludes that the law is unsettled with respect to the right of incompetent, nonterminal patients to refuse medical care. Quotes Opinion 2.18 (1986) [now Opinion 2.20]. Comment, *The Right to Refuse Life Sustaining Medical Treatment and the Nonterminally Ill Patient: An Analysis of Abridgment and Anarchy, 17 Pepperdine L. Rev. 461, 462 (1990).*

Journal 1990 Discusses how the imprecise language of euthanasia muddles public discussion of the issue. Concludes that medical ethics must distinguish between acts and omissions undertaken to cause death and those considered reasonable treatment under the circumstances. Quotes Opinion 2.20 (1989). Devettere, *The Imprecise Language of Euthanasia and Causing Death, 1 J. Clinical Ethics 268, 268 (1990).*

Journal 1990 Discusses the proposition that an objective standard should govern end-of-life decision-making instead of living wills or similar instruments. Concludes that an objective standard is preferable and recommends that courts adopt such a standard. References Opinion 2.20. Dresser, *Relitigating Life and Death, 51 Ohio St. L. J. 425, 436 (1990).*

Journal 1990 Discusses the development of the law regarding the withdrawal of life-sustaining medical treatment from incompetent patients since the *Quinlan* case. Concludes that *Cruzan* did not resolve a number of important questions concerning the right to die. Quotes Opinion 2.18 (1986) [now Opinion 2.20]. McNoble, *The Cruzan Decision—A Surgeon's Perspective*, 20 Memphis State Univ. L. Rev. 569, 581, 600, 601 (1990).

Journal 1990 Considers how the case may be misperceived. Proposes that health care professionals should routinely advise patients of the necessity of making their wishes about life-sustaining treatment known. Quotes Opinion 2.18 (1986) [now Opinion 2.20]. Meisel, *Lessons From Cruzan, 1 J. Clinical Ethics 245, 248 (1990).*

Journal 1990 Discusses the right of physicians to refrain from participating in the withdrawal or removal of life-sustaining treatment. Concludes that federal and state legislation is needed to protect the right of conscience of medical personnel in this context. Quotes Opinion 2.20. Note, *I Have A Conscience, Too: The Plight of Medical Personnel Confronting the Right to Die, 65 Notre Dame L. Rev. 699, 706 (1990).*

Journal 1990 Discusses advance medical directives including living wills and durable powers of attorney. Concludes by examining the physician's role in implementing patient preferences. Cites Opinion 2.20. Orentlicher, *Advance Medical Directives, 263 JAMA 2365 (1990).*

Journal 1990 Discusses the moral dilemma in deciding whether to withdraw artificial nutrition and hydration from a patient and the appropriate role of the judiciary. Concludes that judicial decisions do not represent the moral viewpoint of society and that moral pronouncements should not be made in the courtroom. Quotes Preamble, Principles I, II, III, IV, V, VI, and VII, and Opinion 2.20. Peccarelli, *A Moral Dilemma: The Role of Judicial Intervention in Withholding or Withdrawing Nutrition and Hydration, 23 John Marshall L. Rev. 537, 539, 540, 541 (1990).*

Journal 1990 Explores how recent advances in medical science and technology have resulted in changing views concerning withdrawing and withholding of life support. Concludes that morality plays a key role in dealing with this issue and that physicians should rely upon fundamental principles of medicine for guidance. Quotes Opinion 2.20. Sprung, *Changing Attitudes and Practices in Forgoing Life-Sustaining Treatments, 263 JAMA 2211, 2213 (1990).*

Journal 1990 Looks into the appropriateness of terminating life-prolonging treatment for patients lacking decision-making abilities. Concludes that physicians do not risk serious liability for withdrawing life support. References Opinion 2.20. Weir & Gostin, *Decisions to Abate Life-Sustaining Treatment for Nonautonomous Patients: Ethical Standards and Legal Liability for Physicians After Cruzan, 264 JAMA 1846, 1849, 1850 (1990).*

Journal 1989 Challenges the notion that removal of artificial nutrition from permanently unconscious patients constitutes active euthanasia. Concludes by observing that the traditional judicial approach, which permits withdrawal of artificial nutrition, is entirely consistent with accepted medical, legal, and ethical doctrines. Cites Opinion 2.18 (1986) [now Opinion 2.20]. Cantor, *The Permanently Unconscious Patient, Non-Feeding and Euthanasia, XV Am. J. Law & Med. 381, 385 (1989).*

Journal 1989 Examines and criticizes the legal advice that was rendered by hospital counsel in the context of the Samuel Linares case, which occurred at Rush-Presbyterian-St. Luke's Medical Center in Chicago, Illinois. Focusing on such issues as whether forgoing ventilator assistance constitutes murder or child abuse and neglect, concludes that ultraconservative legal advice led to moral paralysis, thereby precipitating the tragic and unnecessary action of the child's father. References Opinion 2.20. Nelson & Cranford, *Legal Advice, Moral Paralysis and the Death of Samuel Linares, 17 Law Med. & Health Care 316, 319 (1989).*

Journal 1989 Observes that, while new policies regarding physician care of hopelessly ill patients have developed, there is a significant gap between development and implementation of those policies. Urges that this gap be closed and that an overall doctrine of flexible care be developed. References Opinion 2.20. Wanzer, Federman, Adelstein, Cassel, Cassem, Cranford, Hook, Lo, Moertel, Safar, Stone, & Van Eys, *The Physician's Responsibility Toward Hopelessly Ill Patients: A Second Look, 320 New Eng. J. Med. 844, 844 (1989).*

Journal 1988 Considers and challenges certain presumed implications of the definition of *death* as brain death. Points to the importance of the distinction between death of the person as contrasted with death of the body. References Opinion 2.18 (1986) [now Opinion 2.20]. Brody, *Ethical Questions Raised by the Persistent Vegetative Patient, 18 Hastings Center Rep. 33, 34 (Feb./March 1988).*

Journal 1988 Explores the revitalization of the hospice concept and the various structural models available for providing care to the terminally ill. Examines the cost-effectiveness of hospice care and discusses various ethical and legal problems that arise in the context of providing hospice care, including withholding or withdrawing life-prolonging medical treatment. References Opinion 2.18 (1986) [now Opinion 2.20]. Comment, *The Hospice Movement: A Renewed View of the Death Process, 4 J. Contemp. Health L. & Pol'y 295, 312 (1988).*

Journal 1988 Focuses on the issue of removal of life-sustaining medical treatment from incompetent patients whose wishes are unknown. The importance of quality-of-life considerations as an aspect of surrogate decision-making in this context is emphasized. References Opinion 2.18 (1986) [now Opinion 2.20]. Quinn, *The Best Interests of Incompetent Patients: The Capacity for Interpersonal Relationships as a Standard for Decisionmaking, 76 Cal. L. Rev. 897, 906 (1988).*

Journal 1988 Examines the meaning and scope of the phrase *artificial feeding*, the distinction between ordinary and extraordinary care, and the impact of medical condition and competency on the patient's right to refuse treatment. Concludes that the value of patient autonomy is not the controlling factor in such cases, but only one factor that must be balanced against the nature and probable results of the proposed treatment. Quotes Opinion 2.18 (1986) [now Opinion 2.20]. Snyder, *Artificial Feeding and the Right to Die: The Legal Issues, 9 J. Legal Med. 349, 351, 352, 357 (1988).*

Journal 1988 Discusses numerous judicial decisions in which the courts have focused, among other things, on the withdrawal of artificial feeding from incompetent adult patients. Practical suggestions are offered to caregivers and relevant policy implications and other unresolved issues are addressed. Quotes from Opinion 2.18 (1986) [now Opinion 2.20]. Steinbrook & Lo, *Artificial Feeding Solid Ground, Not a Slippery Slope, 318 New Eng. J. Med. 286, 288 (1988).*

Journal 1988 Discusses moral justification for limited respirator use in prolonging anencephalic infants as organ donors for neonates, problems in determining brain death, and the need for additional research relative to anencephalic newborns. Ethical justifications for withdrawal of artificial life support from adult patients who are permanently comatose are offered, by way of analogy, for the purpose of demonstrating the ethical and medical propriety of attaching volunteered, select anencephalic infants to respirators in an effort to obtain scarce organs. Cites Opinion 2.18 (1986) [now Opinion 2.20]. Walters & Ashwal, *Organ Prolongation in Anencephalic Infants: Ethical and Medical Issues, 18 Hastings Center Rep. 19, 21 (Oct./Nov. 1988).*

Journal 1987 Focuses on the issue of withholding nutrition and hydration from comatose patients with emphasis on the questions of what constitutes medical treeatment and when it may properly be withheld. Briefly discusses the often cited cases that have addressed these issues, noting the importance of the position of the AMA regarding withholding or withdrawing life-prolonging medical treatment. References Opinion 2.18 (1986) [now Opinion 2.20]. Comment, *Hold on Courts: May a Comatose Patient Be Denied Food and Water, 31 St. Louis Univ. L. J. 749, 750 (1987).*

Journal 1987 Following comprehensive analysis of existing common law, notes a trend toward granting families greater autonomy in making decisions for incompetent adult patients. Supports this trend and advocates recognition of a more prominent role for the family in these situations. References Opinion 2.18 (1986) [now Opinion 2.20]. Comment, *The Role of the Family in Medical*

Decisionmaking for Incompetent Adult Patients: A Historical Perspective and Case Analysis, 48 U. Pittsburgh L. Rev. 539, 571, 607, 610-11 (1987).

Journal 1986 Discusses the distinction between the persistent vegetative state and coma, pointing out the confusion of these concepts in various leading right-to-die cases. Addresses philosophical and ethical predicates for withholding treatment noting that, in the final analysis, a balancing of the benefits and burdens of treatment should involve the patient, the family, and the physician. Cites Opinion 2.11 (1981) [now Opinion 2.20]. Berrol, *Considerations for Management of the Persistent Vegetative State, 67 Arch. Phys. Med. Rehabil. 283, 285 (1986).*

Journal 1986 Observes that life-sustaining medical treatment includes artificial nutrition and hydration and that patients have a right to forgo such treatment under the Washington State Constitution, applicable common law, and the Washington Natural Death Act. Notes that available judicial standards for surrogate decision-making in this context are inadequate, and proposes substantive guidelines for the making of such decisions. References Opinion 2.18 (1986) [now Opinion 2.20]. Comment, *Artificial Nutrition and the Terminally Ill: How Should Washington Decide? 61 Wash. L. Rev. 419, 421, 447 (1986).*

Journal 1986 Analyzes the law's approach to death by evaluating various legal issues that arise in the context of efforts to define death. Asserts that neocortical death should be viewed as death of the person for all legal purposes. References Opinion 2.18 (1986) [now Opinion 2.20]. Smith, *Legal Recognition of Neocortical Death, 71 Cornell L. Rev. 850, 860, 876-77 (1986).*

Journal 1985 Focuses on the issue of withholding medical care and treatment from infants for whom there is little reasonable expectation of normal development. Urges that parents should assume principal decision-making responsibility and offers framework for limited state intervention. References Opinion 2.18 (1986) [now Opinion 2.20]. Haddon, *Baby Doe Cases: Compromise and Moral Dilemma, 34 Emory L. J. 545, 556 (1985).*

Journal 1984 Evaluates two divergent approaches to the legal treatment of withdrawing nourishment. Favors the patient's rights to privacy and to treatment as the primary factors in resolving the issue of withdrawing nourishment. Quotes Opinion 2.11 (1982) [now Opinion 2.20]. Horan & Grant, *The Legal Aspects of Withdrawing Nourishment, 5 J. Legal Med. 595, 626 (1984).*

5.4 Orders Not to Attempt Resuscitation (DNAR)

Kan. App. 1998 Physician was convicted of attempted murder of a terminally ill patient, and intentional and malicious second-degree murder of another terminally ill patient. The court quoted Opinion 2.22, to exemplify a physician's duty to provide cardiopulmonary resuscitation

unless the physician believes that such action would be futile. Additionally, the court referenced Opinion 2.20, in support of a physician's duty to provide a terminally ill patient adequate pain relief. The court reversed the physician's convictions, stating that the jury could not disregard the testimony of several physicians who concurred with the defendant-physician's treatment of the deceased patients. *State v. Naramore, 25 Kan. App. 2d 302, 965 P.2d 211, 214, 216.*

Journal 2006 Examines the public reaction to the Terri Schiavo case. Concludes that public fears were misplaced and that all persons benefited from the decision. Quotes Opinions 2.03, 2.035, and 2.17. Cites Opinion 2.22. Cerminara, *Musings on the Need to Convince Some People With Disabilities That End-of-Life Decision-Making Advocates Are Not Out to Get Them, 37 Loy. U. Chi. L. J. 343, 347 (2006).*

Journal 2006 Argues for an alternative framework by which health ethics, policy, and law can address equitable distribution of health care. Concludes that a new paradigm would lead to a more efficient and compassionate system. References Opinions 2.22 and 8.13. Ruger, *Health, Capability, and Justice: Toward a New Paradigm of Health Ethics, Policy and Law, 15 Cornell J. L. & Pub. Pol'y 403, 425, 465 (2006).*

Journal 2004 Examines conflicts that arise when a hospice may be obligated to resuscitate a patient who has not executed an advance directive regarding CPR. Concludes that the Patient Self-Determination Act must be amended to allow hospice providers to administer CPR in only a limited number of circumstances. References Opinions 2.035 and 2.22. Rutkow, *Dying to Live: The Effect of the Patient Self-determination Act on Hospice Care, 7 N. Y. U. J. Legis. & Pub. Pol'y 393, 413, 430 (2004).*

Journal 2001 Observes that many aspects of managed care have increased the tensions between patients and their health care providers. Notes that patient dissatisfaction is on the rise for other reasons as well. Concludes that Congress should take a comprehensive legislative approach in addressing these issues. Quotes Opinion 2.17. Cites Opinion 2.035. References Opinions 2.037 and 2.22. Sanematsu, *Taking a Broader View of Treatment Disputes Beyond Managed Care: Are Recent Legislative Efforts the Cure? 48 UCLA L. Rev. 1245, 1258, 1284 (2001).*

Journal 2000 Discusses a medical-ethical strategy for managing iatrogenic cardiac arrests in DNR patients. Suggests that many factors must be taken into account before withholding resuscitation in certain unanticipated situations, such as an iatrogenic catastrophe. References Opinion 2.22. Christensen & Orlowski, *Iatrogenic Cardiopulmonary Arrests in DNR Patients, 11 J. Clinical Ethics 14, 15, 20 (2000).*

Journal 2000 Discusses euphemisms used through medical codes in hospitals regarding end-of-life patient care. Examines how the fear of medical failure and the fear of litigation mold decision-making in critical care units. Concludes that health care providers often lack the courage to let a patient die. References Opinion 2.22. Smith, *Euphemistic Codes and Tell-Tale Hearts: Humane Assistance in End-of-Life Cases, 10 Health Matrix 175, 177 (2000).*

Journal 2000 Discusses current law governing consent to sperm retrieval and insemination after death or persistent vegetative state. Identifies gaps in the law. Concludes that sperm retrieval and insemination in these situations should be permitted, provided there is express prior consent or sufficient evidence from which consent may be implied. Cites Opinion 2.22. Strong, *Consent to Sperm Retrieval and Insemination After Death or Persistent Vegetative State, 14 J. L. & Health 243, 248 (2000).*

Journal 1998 Explains when a surrogate is required to make health care decisions. Discusses limitations of a surrogate's authority. Emphasizes that the health care provider must recognize that ultimate decision-making regarding care first belongs to the patient, and then to the surrogate. Quotes Opinion 2.035. Cites Opinion 8.11. References Opinion 2.22. O'Neill, *Surrogate Health Care Decisions for Adults in Illinois—Answers to the Legal Questions That Health Care Providers Face on a Daily Basis, 29 Loy. Univ. Chi. L. J. 411, 445, 448 (1998).*

Journal 1998 Discusses various ways theorists define medical futility. Evaluates the impact of *In re Baby K* on the correct notion of medical futility. Examines how futility affects patient autonomy. Quotes Opinion 2.22. Strasser, *The Futility of Futility? On Life, Death, and Reasoned Public Policy, 57 Md. L. Rev. 505, 523, 552, 553 (1998).*

Journal 1997 Examines case law pertaining to medical futility disputes. Reviews hospital policies regarding futility and notes a variety of definitions and guidelines. Concludes that, absent a clear consensus, physicians should not act solely to decide questions of futility. References Opinions 2.035 and 2.22. Johnson, Gibbons, Goldner, Wiener, & Eton, *Legal and Institutional Policy Responses to Medical Futility, 30 J. Health & Hosp. L. 21, 26, 31, 35, 36 (1997).*

Journal 1997 Explores the meaning of cardiopulmonary resuscitation and legal issues involving DNR orders. Considers problems created by DNR orders in operating rooms in light of patients' rights. Concludes that hospitals must adopt clear policies for their surgical teams to follow. Quotes Opinion 8.08. References Opinion 2.22. Lonchyna, *To Resuscitate or Not . . . In the Operating Room: The Need for Hospital Policies for Surgeons Regarding DNR Orders, 6 Annals Health L. 209, 215, 217 (1997).*

Journal 1997 Considers individuals' right to die and the value of a wrongful living tort. Proposes that courts should reject any cause of action for wrongful living in situations where patient advance directives are not honored by physicians. References Opinion 2.22. Milani, *Better Off Dead Than Disabled? Should Courts Recognize a Wrongful Living Cause of Action When Doctors Fail to Honor Patients' Advance Directives? 54 Wash. & Lee L. Rev. 149, 151-52 (1997).*

Journal 1994 Considers how greater patient autonomy has led to situations in which medical care may be viewed as futile. Suggests that the law has intruded too far into this area of medicine. Quotes Opinion 2.035. Cites Opinions 2.03, 2.095, 2.17, 2.19, 2.20, and 2.22. Cultice, *Medical*

Futility: When Is Enough, Enough? 27 J. Health & Hosp. Law 225, 230, 256 (1994).

Journal 1993 Discusses physician, patient, and societal concerns about futility. Concludes that futility decisions should be left to physicians. Cites Opinion 2.22. Bennett, *When Is Medical Treatment Futile? 9 Issues in Law & Med. 35, 39 (1993).*

Journal 1993 Considers how patient self-determination may be affected by cardiopulmonary resuscitation and do-not-resuscitate policies. Opposes a "futility" exception to informed consent as being violative of a physician's fiduciary duties to patients. Cites Opinion 8.07 (1986) [now Opinion 8.08]. References Opinion 2.22. Boozang, *Death Wish: Resuscitating Self-Determination for the Critically Ill, 35 Ariz. L. Rev. 23, 24, 28, 52 (1993).*

Journal 1993 Discusses the problem of physicians withholding needed medical treatment from HIV-infected infants. Concludes that current law should be expanded to eliminate this discrimination. Quotes Opinions 2.09, 2.17, 2.20, 2.22, 4.04, and 8.03. Crossley, *Of Diagnoses and Discrimination: Discriminatory Nontreatment of Infants With HIV Infection, 93 Columbia L. Rev. 1581, 1620, 1621 (1993).*

Journal 1993 Discusses the relationship between a physician's professional conscience and end-of-life decision-making. Considers the issue of futile medical treatment. Examines case law concerning a patient's right to demand treatment and a physician's obligation to provide it. References Opinions 2.20 and 2.22. Daar, *A Clash at the Bedside: Patient Autonomy v. a Physician's Professional Conscience, 44 Hastings L. J. 1241, 1257, 1268, 1286 (1993).*

Journal 1993 Discusses the American Heart Association's acknowledgment of medical futility, but questions whether its views adequately reflect current ethical perceptions. Proposes ways in which the guidelines should be reformed. References Opinion 2.22. Jecker & Schneiderman, *An Ethical Analysis of the Use of "Futility" in the 1992 American Heart Association Guidelines for Cardiopulmonary Resuscitation and Emergency Cardiac Care, 153 Arch. Intern. Med. 2195, 2197 (1993).*

Journal 1993 Examines the American Heart Association's guidelines for withholding cardiopulmonary resuscitation in emergency medical service systems and criticizes them for being too strict. Argues that a mechanism should be created to facilitate prehospital DNR orders and ensure that they are followed. References Opinion 2.22. McIntyre, *Loosening Criteria for Withholding Prehospital Cardiopulmonary Resuscitation, 153 Arch. Intern. Med. 2189, 2190 (1993).*

Journal 1992 Examines several issues regarding persistent vegetative state (PVS) patients, including whether PVS patients are really dead, whether nutrition and hydration should be withheld, whether life-sustaining treatments are futile or medically inappropriate, and whether ordinary standards for decision-making should be applied to PVS

patients. Concludes that life-sustaining therapy may be withheld or continued, but that withdrawal of nutrition and hydration, as well as active euthanasia, present more difficult questions. References Opinions 2.20 and 2.22. Brody, *Special Ethical Issues in the Management of PVS Patients, 20 Law Med. & Health Care 104, 109 (1992).*

Journal 1992 Discusses "do-not-resuscitate" (DNR) orders in light of the Patient Self-Determination Act. Proposes a policy of required reconsideration of DNR orders in hospitals when a patient enters a treatment setting in which discreet, time-limited therapies are offered that may precipitate cardiac arrest. References Opinion 2.22. Cohen & Cohen, *Required Reconsideration of "Do-Not-Resuscitate" Orders in the Operating Room and Certain Other Treatment Settings, 20 Law Med. & Health Care 354, 356 (1992).*

Journal 1992 Examines ethical and legal issues surrounding cardiopulmonary resuscitation and emergency cardiac care. Discusses advance directives and proxy decision-making, medical futility, resource allocation, and do-not-resuscitate orders. References Opinions 2.20 and 2.22. Comment, *Ethical Considerations in Resuscitation, 268 JAMA 2282, 2283, 2287 (1992).*

Journal 1992 Considers the debate surrounding medical futility. Observes that this debate is encouraging reexamination of the nature of patient entitlement to medical care as well as the "ends of medicine." References Opinions 2.20, 2.21, and 2.22. Miles, *Medical Futility, 20 Law Med. & Health Care 310, 311, 313 (1992).*

Journal 1992 Explains how the "terminal condition" requirement in natural death acts may reduce the number of people who fall within the scope of coverage. Also indicates that omission of nutrition and hydration from the list of treatments that may be withdrawn limits patient choices. Quotes Opinion 2.20. References Opinion 2.22. Note, *State Natural Death Acts: Illusory Protection of Individuals' Life-Sustaining Treatment Decisions, 29 Harvard J. Legis. 175, 186, 194, 195, 201 (1992).*

Journal 1992 Discusses the impact of physicians' values on end-of-life decision making for patients. Examines how and why physician values may become dominant. References Opinions 2.20, 2.22, and 9.121. Orentlicher, *The Illusion of Patient Choice in End-of-Life Decisions, 267 JAMA 2101, 2102 (1992).*

Journal 1992 Discusses results of a study that evaluated the impact of ethics education on do-not-resuscitate (DNR) practices by house officers. Concludes that educational programs improve care for DNR patients. References Opinion 2.22. Sulmasy, Geller, Faden, & Levine, *The Quality of Mercy: Caring for Patients With "Do-Not-Resuscitate" Orders, 267 JAMA 682 (1992).*

Journal 1991 Examines the involvement of the legal system in end-of-life medical decision-making. Questions whether the law should intrude into the domain. Concludes that judges should become involved primarily to address the "terms of reconciliation" between physicians and patients. References Opinion 2.22. Flick, *The Due Process of Dying, 79 Cal. L. Rev. 1121, 1152 (1991)*.

Journal 1990 Finds that a vast majority of North Carolina nursing homes have written cardiopulmonary resuscitation policies, but that there is substantial variation among them. Concludes that such variations risk limiting or ignoring the personal rights of residents. References Opinions 2.20 and 2.22. Brunetti, Weiss, Studenski, & Clipp, *Cardiopulmonary Resuscitation Policies and Practices: A Statewide Nursing Home Study, 150 Arch. Intern. Med. 121, 122 (1990)*.

5.5 Medically Ineffective Interventions

Journal 2010 Discusses futility disputes where a patient's surrogate wishes to prolong treatment that the physician deems medically ineffective, and the current lack of legal remedies to resolve them. Concludes that states need to establish fair, impartial, and patient-centered methods of resolving futility disputes including independent medical boards that would operate under procedural and substantive regulations. Quotes Opinions 2.02 and 2.035. References Opinions 2.17 and 2.20. *Bassel, Order at the End of Life: Establishing a Clear and Fair Mechanism for the Resolution of Futility Disputes, 63 Vand. L. Rev. 491, 494, 523 (2010)*.

Journal 2009 Examines criteria defining when renal dialysis becomes futile. Concludes that uniform guidelines should be adopted defining when medical care is futile and should be withheld. Cites Opinion 2.035. Fink, *Time to Stop Dialyzing the Dead (and Treating Other Patients Too Aggressively, Too), 38 Dialysis & Transplantation 184, 185 (May 2009, 1, 1)*.

Journal 2009 Explores the nature of the physician-patient relationship and the impact of increased availability of medical information on patient autonomy and physician responsibility to exercise independent judgment. Concludes physicians must treat patients in accordance with their fiduciary obligation to use their own judgment when confronted with a patient demanding unnecessary medical services. Quotes Preamble, Principles I and VIII, and Opinions 2.035, 8.03, and 10.015. Hafemeister, *The Fiduciary Obligation of Physicians to "Just Say No" if an "Informed" Patient Demands Services That Are Not Medically Indicated, 39 Seton Hall L. Rev. 335, 372, 373, 374 (2009)*.

Journal 2008 Discusses medical options when the physician can do nothing further to cure the patient and examines the Texas Advance Directives Act, a medical futility statute. Concludes conflicts may be reduced if physician-patient communication is initiated when treatment begins rather than when further treatment becomes futile. Cites the Texas medical futility process as an example for providing physicians a mechanism for resolving conflicts with patients. Quotes Opinions 2.035, 2.037, and 2.20. Dahm, *Medical Futility and the Texas Medical Futility Statute: A Model to Follow or One to Avoid? 20 Health Law 25, 26 (Aug. 2008)*.

Journal 2007 Argues that it is unethical for a physician to withhold CPR without seeking consent of the patient. Concludes that standards for withholding care should be agreed upon by society and passed into law. Cites Opinion 2.035. Manthous, *Counterpoint: Is It Ethical to Order "Do Not Resuscitate" Without Patient Consent? 132 Chest 751, 753 (2007)*.

Journal 2007 Compares US and international policy on end-of-life decision making. Concludes that interests of patient autonomy should be balanced with family interests and advocates a comprehensive "best interest" model. Quotes Opinion 2.037. Cites Opinions 2.035 and 2.20. Rode, *End-of-Life Decision Making for Patients in Persistent Vegetative States: A Comparative Analysis, 30 Hastings Int'l & Comp. L. Rev. 477, 499, 500 (2007)*.

Journal 2007 Discusses patients' right to refuse medical treatment and the corresponding duties of health care professionals. Concludes that detailed, carefully prepared advance directives are necessary to fulfill patients' wishes. Quotes Ch. II (1940) [now Opinions 8.08 and 8.082] and Opinions 2.035, 2.037, 2.20, 2.225, 8.081, and 10.015. Cites Opinions 9.11 and 9.115. Stamatakis, *Beyond Advance Directives: Personal Autonomy and the Right to Refuse Life-Sustaining Medical Treatment, 47 N. H. B. J. 20, 29-30 (2007)*.

Journal 2006 Examines ethical dilemmas physicians may face as providers of pay-for-performance medical care. Concludes that this strategy offers a benefit to patients as long as physicians uphold stringent ethical standards and work together to ensure optimum patient care. Cites Principles I, V, VIII, and IX and Opinions 2.035, 2.095, 6.01, 8.021, 8.03, 8.0501, 8.053, 8.054, and 8.121. Bostick, Sade, & McMahon, *Report of the Council on Ethical and Judicial Affairs: Physician Pay-For-Performance Programs, 3 Ind. Health L. Rev. 429, 430, 431, 432-33, 434, 435, 436 (2006)*.

Journal 2006 Examines the public reaction to the Terri Schiavo case. Concludes that public fears were misplaced and that all persons benefited from the decision. Quotes Opinions 2.03, 2.035, and 2.17. Cites Opinion 2.22. Cerminara, *Musings on the Need to Convince Some People With Disabilities That End-of-Life Decision-Making Advocates Are Not Out to Get Them, 37 Loy. U. Chi. L. J. 343, 347 (2006)*.

Journal 2006 Reviews policy surrounding medical futility in the US and UK. Concludes that communication and collaboration with patients and their families is the best solution for addressing decisions about futile care. Quotes Opinion 2.035. Cites Opinion 2.03. Rowland, *Communicating Past the Conflict: Solving the Medical Futility Controversy With*

Process-Based Approaches, 14 U. Miami Int'l & Comp. L. Rev. 271, 278-79 (2006).

Journal 2006 Discusses the ethical controversy surrounding physician-assisted suicide. Concludes that natural law and individual autonomy are important considerations in the ethical debate. Quotes Opinion 2.211. Cites Opinion 2.035. Wong, *Whose Life Is It Anyway? 5 Cardozo Pub. L. Pol'y & Ethics J. 233, 271-72 (2006).*

Journal 2005 Examines ethical rules governing various forms of alternative dispute resolution. Concludes that a unique set of guidelines is needed for negotiation which encourages greater disclosure, communication, and trust between parties. References Opinion 2.035. Bordone, *Fitting the Ethics to the Forum: A Proposal for Process-Enabling Ethical Codes, 21 Ohio St. J. on Disp. Resol. 1, 35 (2005).*

Journal 2005 Discusses the evidentiary standards utilized to permit withdrawal of life-sustaining treatment by substitute decision-makers when patients are in a persistent vegetative state. Concludes that a futility rationale for making end-of-life decisions may represent the best approach in these situations. Quotes Opinion 2.035. Cites Opinion 2.20. Mareiniss, *A Comparison of Cruzan and Schiavo: The Burden of Proof, Due Process, and Autonomy in the Persistently Vegetative Patient, 26 J. Legal Med. 233, 248, 250 (2005).*

Journal 2004 Discusses a physician's conflict of interest in making end-of-life decisions when there is pressure to maximize ICU profits. Concludes that formal guidelines are needed to ensure that proper life-ending decisions are made in the ICU. Quotes Opinion 2.035. Fleming, *Healthcare Access: Conflicts of Interest Presented by Managed Care ICU Bedside Rationing and Their Impact on Minorities and Women, 5 Geo. J. Gender & L. 663, 667 (2004).*

Journal 2004 Examines conflicts that arise when a hospice may be obligated to resuscitate a patient who has not executed an advance directive regarding CPR. Concludes that the Patient Self-Determination Act must be amended to allow hospice providers to administer CPR in only a limited number of circumstances. References Opinions 2.035 and 2.22. Rutkow, *Dying to Live: The Effect of the Patient Self-Determination Act on Hospice Care, 7 N. Y. U. J. Legis. & Pub. Pol'y 393, 413, 430 (2004).*

Journal 2004 Discusses the law in Tennessee regarding surrogate decision-making. Concludes that recent legislation passed in Tennessee will assist those who care for incapacitated patients. Cites Opinions 2.035, 8.081, and 8.115. Wampler, *To Be or Not to Be in Tennessee: Deciding Surrogate Issues, 34 U. Mem. L. Rev. 333, 365 (2004).*

Journal 2002 Explores the implications of withholding medical treatment when abortion results in a live birth. Concludes that, in these situations, abortive parents and physicians should not solely decide the child's best interest. Quotes Preamble, Principles I and III, and Opinions 2.035, 2.20, and 2.215. Casagrande, *Children Not Meant*

to Be: Protecting the Interests of the Child When Abortion Results in Live Birth, 6 Quinnipiac Health L. J. 19, 44, 45, 47-48 (2002).

Journal 2002 Discusses the precautions lawyers must take when advising clients about living wills. Concludes clients must be reminded that medical advances or changes in circumstances may affect their living wills. Quotes Opinion 2.035. Kruse, *A Call for New Perspectives for Living Wills (You Might Like It Here), 37 Real Prop., Prob. & Tr. J. 545, 550 (2002).*

Journal 2001 Observes that many aspects of managed care have increased the tensions between patients and their health care providers. Notes that patient dissatisfaction is on the rise for other reasons as well. Concludes that Congress should take a comprehensive legislative approach in addressing these issues. Quotes Opinion 2.17. Cites Opinion 2.035. References Opinions 2.037 and 2.22. Sanematsu, *Taking a Broader View of Treatment Disputes Beyond Managed Care: Are Recent Legislative Efforts the Cure? 48 UCLA L. Rev. 1245, 1258, 1284 (2001).*

Journal 2000 Considers whether age is a sufficient justification to limit or deny access to health care. Concludes that the use of advance care directives, further research, and educational programs can help physicians address this ethical challenge. Quotes Opinion 2.035. Tadd & Bayer, *Commentary: Medical Decision Making Based on Chronological Age—Cause for Concern, 11 J. Clinical Ethics 328, 330 (2000).*

Journal 1998 Explains when a surrogate is required to make health care decisions. Discusses limitations of a surrogate's authority. Emphasizes that the health care provider must recognize that ultimate decision-making regarding care first belongs to the patient, and then to the surrogate. Quotes Opinion 2.035. Cites Opinion 8.11. References Opinion 2.22. O'Neill, *Surrogate Health Care Decisions for Adults in Illinois—Answers to the Legal Questions That Health Care Providers Face on a Daily Basis, 29 Loy. Univ. Chi. L. J. 411, 445, 448 (1998).*

Journal 1997 Examines case law pertaining to medical futility disputes. Reviews hospital policies regarding futility and notes a variety of definitions and guidelines. Concludes that, absent a clear consensus, physicians should not act solely to decide questions of futility. References Opinions 2.035 and 2.22. Johnson, Gibbons, Goldner, Wiener, & Eton, *Legal and Institutional Policy Responses to Medical Futility, 30 J. Health & Hosp. L. 21, 26, 31, 35, 36 (1997).*

Journal 1995 Considers how the judiciary, legislatures, and provider institutions balance the values of patients and their physicians. Recommends that physicians and hospitals promulgate written policies outlining their preferred treatment parameters in any given circumstance. Quotes Opinion 2.035. Daar, *Medical Futility and Implications for Physician Autonomy, XXI Am. J. Law & Med. 221, 234 (1995).*

Journal 1995 Examines the rights of health care professionals to refuse to participate in patient care on the basis of conscientious objection. Suggests steps that health care facilities may take when dealing with health care professionals who object to participating in patient care. Quotes Principles I and VI and Opinions 1.02, 2.035, and 9.055. Dellinger & Vickery, *When Staff Object to Participating in Care, 28 J. Health & Hospital Law 269, 272, 276 (1995).*

Journal 1994 Considers how greater patient autonomy has led to situations in which medical care may be viewed as futile. Suggests that the law has intruded too far into this area of medicine. Quotes Opinion 2.035. Cites Opinions 2.03, 2.095, 2.17, 2.19, 2.20, and 2.22. Cultice, *Medical Futility: When Is Enough, Enough? 27 J. Health & Hosp. Law 225, 230, 256 (1994).*

Journal 2006 Examines US and UK terminal illness jurisprudence. Proposes new legislation should be drafted to allow for palliative care when curative treatments are no longer appropriate. Cites Opinions 2.037 and 9.115. Feldhammer, *Medical Torture: End of Life Decision-Making in the United Kingdom and United States, 14 Cardozo J. Int'l & Comp. L. 511, 514-15, 532 (2006).*

Journal 2006 Reviews Texas statutory policies related to the handling of cases of medical futility. Concludes that effective communication is the best means of resolving a conflict over treatment and that statutory guidelines are best used as a last resort. Cites Opinion 2.037. Halevy & McGuire, *The History, Successes and Controversies of the Texas "Futility" Policy, 43 Houston Lawyer 38, 39 (2006).*

Journal 2006 Discusses decision-making authority in cases of medical futility. Concludes that unilateral decision-making by the health care provider poses numerous ethical and legal problems. Quotes Opinion 2.037. Kwiecinski, *To Be or Not to Be, Should Doctors Decide? Ethical and Legal Aspects of Medical Futility Policies, 7 Marq. Elder's Advisor 313, 323-24 (2006).*

Journal 2002 Critiques Daniel Callahan's theory of rationing health resources according to age. Concludes age

should not be a controlling factor in end-of-life decision-making. References Opinion 2.037. Cohen-Almagor, *A Critique of Callahan's Utilitarian Approach to Resource Allocation in Health Care, 17 Issues L. & Med. 247, 261 (2002).*

Journal 2002 Analyzes ethical positions on futility in light of the California Uniform Health Care Decisions Act. Concludes the Act provides only a preliminary framework and considers AMA guidelines on medical futility in offering suggestions for change. Quotes Opinion 2.037. Ferguson, *Ethical Postures of Futility and California's Uniform Health Care Decisions Act, 75 S. Cal. L. Rev. 1217, 1252-53 (2002).*

Journal 2000 Discusses the rise and fall of the futility movement. Focuses on attempts to define and develop a process for resolving futility disputes. Concludes that the decision-making dilemma surrounding treatments of minimal benefit still exists and that talking to patients and families should be viewed as the primary method by which physicians may address this problem. References Opinion 2.037. Helft, Siegler, & Lantos, *The Rise and Fall of the Futility Movement, 343 New Eng. J. Med. 293, 294 (2000).*

Journal 2000 Evaluates documentation of decision-making in the treatment of hospitalized elderly trauma patients who died. Considers the frequency of withdrawal of therapy and who made the decisions. Concludes that further research is needed regarding methods to resolve disputes involving futility and withdrawal of therapy. References Opinion 2.037. Trunkey, Cahn, Lenfesty, & Mullins, *Management of the Geriatric Trauma Patient at Risk of Death: Therapy Withdrawal Decision Making, 135 Arch. Surg. 34, 35 (2000).*

Journal 2000 Discusses medical futility and offers a case-based assessment of circumstances under which continued use of treatment may exceed the boundaries of reasonableness. Suggests a procedural approach for making decisions on a case-by-case basis. References Opinion 2.037. Truog, *Futility in Pediatrics: From Case to Policy, 11 J. Clinical Ethics 136, 139, 141 (2000).*

5.7 Physician-Assisted Suicide

U.S. 2006 State of Oregon brought suit seeking declaratory and injunctive relief from enforcement of an interpretive rule of a US Attorney General's opinion, which stated that physicians who assist patients in suicide under the authority of the Oregon Death with Dignity Act (ODWDA) violate the federal Controlled Substances Act (CSA). The Ninth Circuit Court of Appeals found the rule invalid. Appeal to the Supreme Court followed. In affirming, the majority held that the interpretive rule is not entitled to deference and that the CSA does not allow the attorney general to prohibit physicians from prescribing drugs for use in assisted suicide pursuant to state law. Quoting Opinion 2.211, the dissent stated that assisted suicide is incompatible with a physician's

role as a healer and does not serve a legitimate medical purpose. *Gonzales v. Oregon, 126 S. Ct. 904, 932.*

U.S. 1997 Several physicians and terminally ill patients sued the state seeking a declaration that its prohibition against physician-assisted suicide violates the Fourteenth Amendment's Equal Protection Clause. The trial court disagreed, but the Second Circuit reversed, holding that the state accords different treatment to those terminally ill patients who wish to hasten their death by self-administering prescribed drugs and to those patients who wish to do so by directing the removal of life support systems. The Supreme Court reversed holding that the prohibition against assisting suicide does not violate the Equal Protection Clause. The Court concluded that there is a distinction between assisting suicide and withdrawing treatment, quoting reports of the AMA Council on Ethical and Judicial Affairs [now Opinions 2.20 and 2.211]. *Vacco v. Quill, 117 S. Ct. 2293, 2298, 138 L. Ed. 2d 834.*

U.S. 1997 Several Washington physicians, terminally ill patients, and a not-for-profit organization that counsels people considering physician-assisted suicide sued the state seeking to have statutory ban on physician-assisted suicide declared unconstitutional. The trial court agreed and the Ninth Circuit affirmed. The Supreme Court, in reversing the decision, held that prohibition against causing or aiding a suicide does not violate the Due Process Clause. The Court also noted that the prohibition was rationally related to legitimate state interests in protecting the integrity and ethics of the medical profession, quoting from Opinion 2.211. *Washington v. Glucksberg, 117 S. Ct. 2258, 2273, 138 L. Ed. 2d 772.*

9th Cir. 1996 Suit was brought by several physicians and a not-for-profit corporation which provides information, assistance, and counseling to competent terminally ill adult patients contemplating suicide, asserting that a state statute making it a crime to aid anyone in attempting to commit suicide unconstitutionally prevents terminally ill patients from exercising their protected liberty interests. Appeals court, en banc, held that the choice of how and when to die is a liberty interest and that the statute violates the due process rights of competent, terminally ill adults who wish to hasten their deaths by obtaining medication prescribed by their physicians. Stating that physician-assisted suicide runs counter to medical ethics, the dissent cited Opinions 2.20, 2.21, and 2.211 and quoted Opinion 2.211. *Compassion in Dying v. Washington, 79 F.3d 790, 840, 855 replacing, 49 F.3d 586 (9th Cir. 1995).*

9th Cir. 1995 A not-for-profit corporation organized to assist terminally ill persons in committing suicide and several physicians alleged that a state statute making aiding a suicide attempt a crime violated 42 USC § 1983 and the Constitution. In upholding the statute, the court quoted Opinion 2.211 as articulating the ethical position of the medical profession against assisted suicide. In turn, the court found upholding the ethical integrity of the medical profession to be one of the many state interests outweighing the alleged liberty interest in medically assisted suicide. *Compassion in Dying v. Washington, 49 F.3d 586, 592, replaced, 79 F.3d 790 (9th Cir. 1996).*

Alaska 2001 Two mentally competent, terminally ill adults filed suit, asking the superior court to declare Alaska's manslaughter statute invalid so that their physicians could assist them in committing suicide. The superior court entered summary judgment against the patients and the Alaska Supreme Court affirmed. In concluding that Alaska's constitutional rights of privacy and liberty do not afford terminally ill patients the right to a physician's assistance in committing suicide, the court quoted Opinion 2.211 in support of the

state's interest in protecting the integrity of the medical profession. *Sampson v. State, 31 P.3d 88, 96, 97.*

Fla. 1997 A patient, suffering from acquired immune deficiency syndrome (AIDS), and his physician filed suit for a declaratory judgment that state law prohibiting assisted suicide violated the privacy clause of the state constitution, as well as the due process and equal protection clauses of the Fourteenth Amendment to the US Constitution. The trial court concluded that the law was unconstitutional. On appeal the state Supreme Court, relying on the US Supreme Court's rulings in *Washington v. Glucksberg*, 117 S.Ct. 2258 (1997) and *Vacco v. Quill*, 117 S.Ct. 2293 (1997), held that the state's ban was not unconstitutional. In determining that the right to assisted suicide is not included in the state's guarantee of privacy, the court quoted from Opinion 2.211. *Krischer v. McIver, 697 So. 2d 97, 103.*

Mich. App. 2001 State brought criminal action against physician for the murder of a patient by lethal injection. The trial court convicted the physician of second-degree murder and delivering a controlled substance. On appeal, the trial court decision was affirmed. The physician asked the appellate court to conclude that euthanasia is legal and to reverse his conviction on constitutional grounds. The appellate court relied on *Washington v. Glucksberg*, 521 U.S. 702 (1997) in determining there is no constitutional right to commit euthanasia, so that an individual can be free from intolerable and irremediable suffering. In discussing *Glucksberg*, the court observed that a state has a legitimate interest in protecting the integrity and ethics of the medical profession. The court noted *Glucksberg's* reference to Opinions 2.20, 2.21, and 2.211 in this regard. *People v. Kevorkian, 248 Mich. App. 373, 639 N.W.2d 291, 305 n. 42.*

Journal 2011 Discusses physician-assisted suicide as permitted in Oregon and Washington and examines 2009 legislative proposal allowing physician-assisted suicide in Vermont. Concludes that legalizing physician-assisted suicides would promote elder abuse and would also devalue the lives of the disabled. Quotes Opinion 2.211. Dore, *Physician-Assisted Suicide: A Recipe for Elder Abuse and the Illusion of Personal Choice, 36 Vt. B. J. 53, 53 (Winter 2011).*

Journal 2011 Argues physicians should have the choice to participate in lethal injection executions. Concludes that although executions may proceed without physician involvement and the integrity and ethics of the medical profession must be protected, because executions performed without a physician have been mishandled, physician involvement is needed. Quotes Opinion 2.211. References Opinion 2.06. Nelson & Ashby, *Rethinking the Ethics of Physician Participation in Lethal Injection Execution, 41 Hastings Center Rep., 28, 29, 35 (May-June 2011).*

Journal 2011 Analyzes and criticizes changes in Britain's assisted suicide law and policy. Argues that recent changes mistakenly view the value of human life from a human-centered, morally relative legal positivist perspective. Cites

Opinion 2.211. Wagner, Kane, & Kallman, *Suicide Killing of Human Life as a Human Right*, 6 Liberty U. L. Rev. 27, 38 (2011).

Journal 2010 Examines aid in dying or physician-assisted suicide in Idaho. Concludes physician-assisted suicide is not legal in Idaho and any physician engaging in this practice may face criminal and civil liability. Quotes Opinion 2.211. Dore, *Aid in Dying: Not Legal in Idaho; Not About Choice*, 53 The Advocate 18 (Sept. 2010).

Journal 2010 Discusses the need for statutory regulation in the context of physician-assisted death. Concludes that states should proactively regulate this practice to prevent abuse and misuse and proposes a statutory framework. Quotes Opinion 2.211. Mason, *Ignoring It Will Not Make It Go Away: Guidelines for Statutory Regulation of Physician-Assisted Death*, 45 New Eng. L. Rev. 139, 142 (2010).

Journal 2009 Argues there is no basis for distinguishing the right to refuse life-sustaining treatment and the right to physician-assisted suicide. Concludes physician-assisted suicide should be permitted as a constitutionally protected right for mentally competent, terminally ill patients, in accordance with the American values of individualism and self-determination. Quotes Opinion 2.211. Chamberlain, *Looking for a "Good Death": The Elderly Terminally Ill's Right to Die by Physician-Assisted Suicide*, 17 Elder L. J. 61, 81 (2009).

Journal 2008 Explores the question of whether physician-assisted dying is ethically and legally appropriate by using empirical research to address concerns and objections. Concludes more research is needed to better understand the pressures experienced by patients facing end-of-life decisions. Quotes Opinions 2.21 and 2.211. Battin, *Physician-Assisted Dying and the Slippery Slope: The Challenge of Empirical Evidence*, 45 Willamette L. Rev. 91, 98-99 (2008).

Journal 2008 Examines patient-familial concerns in physician-assisted suicide (PAS) and existing case law. Concludes legislators must focus on families of terminally ill patients when proposing PAS legislation. Quotes Opinion 2.211. Economou, *What About Families? A Different Perspective on Physician Assisted Suicide in California*, 7 Whittier J. Child & Fam. Advoc. 253, 259 (2008).

Journal 2007 Examines the role of the medical profession in participating in state-sanctioned lethal injection. Concludes that any participation is unethical because it causes harm and undermines trust. Cites Opinion 2.06. References Opinions 2.211 and 9.02. Black & Sade, *Lethal Injection and Physicians: State Law vs Medical Ethics*, 298 JAMA 2779, 2780, 2781 (2007).

Journal 2007 Discusses the impact of *Gonzales v. Oregon* on palliative care policies. Concludes Gonzales paves the way for ethical provision of palliative care. Quotes Opinion 2.211. Hilliard, *The Politics of Palliative Care and the*

Ethical Boundaries of Medicine: Gonzales v. Oregon as a Cautionary Tale, 35 J. L. Med. & Ethics 158, 170 (2007).

Journal 2007 Reviews recent US Supreme Court decisions on physician-assisted suicide. Concludes that the most important public policy question to be considered is the motivation of patients in electing to end their lives. Quotes Opinion 2.211. Levy, *Gonzales v. Oregon and Physician-Assisted Suicide: Ethical and Policy Issues*, 42 Tulsa L. Rev. 699, 699 (2007).

Journal 2007 Examines the existence of a right to physician-assisted suicide. Concludes that terminally ill patients deserve the availability of a means to alleviate their suffering and preserve their dignity. Quotes Opinion 2.211. Urofsky, *Do Go Gentle Into That Good Night: Thoughts on Death, Suicide, Morality and the Law*, 59 Ark. L. Rev. 819, 832 (2007).

Journal 2006 Discusses legal and political issues surrounding physician-assisted suicide. Concludes that palliative care is sufficient to allow for a death with dignity. Quotes Opinion 2.211. Aden, *End of Life Decision Making: The Right to Die? You Can Go Your Own Way: Exploring the Relationship Between Personal and Political Autonomy in Gonzales v. Oregon*, 15 Temp. Pol. & Civ. Rts. L. Rev. 323, 329 (2006).

Journal 2006 Analyzes the proceedings and decision in *Gonzales v. Oregon*. Concludes the Court's holding is correct and that other states should adopt statutes similar to the Oregon Death with Dignity Act. Quotes Opinion 2.211. Chand, *Deconstructing Gonzales v. Oregon: When Political Agendas Yield to Rudimentary Notions of Federalism and Statutory Interpretation*, 50 How. L. J. 229, 239-40 (2006).

Journal 2006 Reviews government responses to euthanasia after passage of Oregon's Death with Dignity Act. Concludes that palliative care should be embraced by lawmakers as an alternative to euthanasia. References Opinion 2.211. Clark, *Oregon's Death with Dignity Act and Alleged Patient Euthanasia After Hurricane Katrina—The Government's Role*, 18 Health Lawyer 1, 8 (2006).

Journal 2006 Reviews physician-assisted suicide jurisprudence. Predicted that the Supreme Court would likely strike down Oregon's Death with Dignity Act in 2006. Quotes Opinion 2.211. Danino, *Dodging the Issue of Physician Assisted Suicide: The Supreme Court's Likely Response in Gonzales v. Oregon*, 10 Mich. St. U. J. Med. & L. 299, 305 (2006).

Journal 2006 Reviews *Gonzales v. Oregon* and discusses its impact on the field of medicine. Concludes that palliative care is an important consideration in end-of-life care. Quotes Opinion 2.211 (1993). Gostin, *Physician-Assisted Suicide: A Legitimate Medical Practice?* 295 JAMA 1941, 1942 (2006).

Journal 2006 Reviews the role of the judiciary and the medical profession in deciding what purposes medicine should serve. Concludes the medical profession's ability to address patient need rests on its authority to act as a self-governing profession. References Opinion 2.211. Gregg, *The Supreme Court and the Purposes of Medicine, 354 New Eng. J. Med. 993, 994 (2006).*

Journal 2006 Discusses whether, under the Oregon Death with Dignity Act, physician-assisted suicide serves a "legitimate medical purpose" within the meaning of the Controlled Substances Act. Concludes that it does. Quotes Opinion 2.211. Hughes, *The Oregon Death with Dignity Act: Relief of Suffering at the End of Medicine's Ability to Heal, 95 Geo. L. J. 207, 219 (2006).*

Journal 2006 Discusses surrogate decision making and an individual's right to refuse medical treatment. Concludes that the *Cruzan* clear and convincing evidence standard should serve as the constitutional minimum test for withdrawing life support. References Opinion 2.211. Lapertosa, *End of Life Decision Making: The Right to Die? Preventing the "Right to Refuse" From Becoming a License to Kill: Adopting a Constitutional Minimum Standard for Approving Withdrawal of Life Support for Legally Incompetent Patients, 15 Temp. Pol. & Civ. Rts. L. Rev. 483, 488 (2006).*

Journal 2006 Considers current laws governing physician-assisted suicide. Concludes that Hawaii should adopt a law analogous to Oregon's Death with Dignity Act. Quotes Opinion 2.211. McAneeley, *Physician-Assisted Suicide: Expanding the Laboratory to the State of Hawai'i, 29 Hawaii L. Rev. 269, 294 (2006).*

Journal 2006 Discusses political philosophies which support an individual's constitutional right to die. Concludes that individuals past the age of retirement should be able to choose physician-assisted suicide. References Opinion 2.211. Mitchell, *My Father, John Locke, and Assisted Suicide: The Real Constitutional Right, 3 Ind. Health L. Rev. 45, 60 (2006).*

Journal 2006 Discusses an attorney's responsibility to a client on death row who wishes to volunteer for execution. Concludes that an attorney should never assist a client in waiving an appeal. Quotes Opinions 2.20 and 2.211. Oleson, *Swilling Hemlock: The Legal Ethics of Defending a Client Who Wishes to Volunteer for Execution, 63 Wash. & Lee L. Rev. 147, 277, 325 (2006).*

Journal 2006 Discusses the ethical controversy surrounding physician-assisted suicide. Concludes that natural law and individual autonomy are important considerations in the ethical debate. Quotes Opinion 2.211. Cites Opinion 2.035. Wong, *Whose Life Is It Anyway? 5 Cardozo Pub. L. Pol'y & Ethics J. 233, 271-72 (2006).*

Journal 2005 Provides the moral rationale for the Partial-Birth Abortion Ban Act of 2003. Concludes that the Supreme Court's decision in *Lawrence v. Texas* does not prohibit morals legislation where the proscribed conduct may broadly affect societal morals. Quotes 2.211. Johnson, *Habit and Discernment in Abortion Practice: The Partial-Birth Abortion Ban Act of 2003 as Morals Legislation, 36 Rutgers L. J. 549, 582 (2005).*

Journal 2004 Analyzes various issues relating to the role of mental health professionals in capital punishment in light of Albert Bandura's model of "mechanisms of moral disengagement." Concludes that facilitating participation of mental health professionals in executions creates conflicts with the humanistic norms of the profession. Quotes Preamble and Opinions 1.01, 1.02, 2.06, 2.067, 2.20, 2.21, 2.211, and 8.14. Judges, *The Role of Mental Health Professionals in Capital Punishment: An Exercise in Moral Disengagement, 41 Hous. L. Rev. 515, 562, 568, 569, 570, 571-72, 581, 586, 588, 598 (2004).*

Journal 2003 Analyzes the objective and subjective tests used to determine which individuals qualify for PAS and euthanasia in the US and the Netherlands. Concludes that both tests provide sufficient safeguards to protect vulnerable groups. Quotes Opinions 2.21 and 2.211. Green, *Physician-Assisted Suicide and Euthanasia: Safeguarding Against the "Slippery Slope"—The Netherlands Versus the United States, 13 Ind. Int'l & Comp. L. Rev. 639, 662 (2003).*

Journal 2003 Discusses the inconsistent governmental regulation of drugs used in physician-assisted suicide (PAS) and lethal injections. Concludes that the FDA should regulate drugs used in lethal injections in the same manner it has attempted to regulate drugs used in PAS. Quotes Opinions 2.06 and 2.211. Miller, *A Death by Any Other Name: The Federal Government's Inconsistent Treatment of Drugs Used in Lethal Injections and Physician-Assisted Suicide, 17 J. L. & Health 217, 234-35 (2003).*

Journal 2003 Considers societal harm as a justification for statutes prohibiting otherwise harmless conduct. Concludes that moral reaction patterns, which typically prevent humans from injuring one another, are important fibers in the fabric of society. Quotes Opinion 2.211. Johnson, *Harm to the "Fabric of Society" as a Basis for Regulating Otherwise Harmless Conduct: Notes on a Theme From Ravin v. State, 27 Seattle U. L. Rev. 41, 55 (2003).*

Journal 2003 Examines the individual rights arguments in the physician-assisted suicide and euthanasia debate. Concludes that collective rather than individual rationality should determine the path that society takes on these issues. Quotes Opinion 2.211. Wong, *A Matter of Life and Death: A Very Personal Discourse, 1 Geo. J. L. & Pub. Pol'y 339, 350 (2003).*

Journal 2002 Considers the use of nonlegal materials in US Supreme Court decisions. Concludes that law alone cannot answer complex legal questions. Cites Opinions 2.20 and 2.211. Hasko, *Persuasion in the Court: Nonlegal Materials in U.S. Supreme Court Opinions, 94 Law Libr. J. 427, 444, 453 (2002).*

Journal 2002 Examines key factors that led to the current palliative care crisis. Analyzes state legislative and judicial efforts to improve palliative care. Concludes with model legislation that holds physicians accountable for inadequate palliative care. Quotes Opinions 2.21 and 2.211. References Opinion 2.20. Oken, *Curing Healthcare Providers' Failure* *to Administer Opioids in the Treatment of Severe Pain, 23 Cardozo L. Rev. 1917, 1925-26, 1952, 1954 (2002).*

Journal 2002 Proposes an ethical argument for suppressing agonal respiration in dying patients under rare circumstances. Concludes that using neuromuscular block agents in terminally ill, well-sedated, gasping patients can allow for a good death. References Opinion 2.211. Perkin & Resnik, *The Agony of Agonal Respiration: Is the Last Gasp Necessary? 28 J. Med. Ethics 164, 169 (2002).*

Journal 2002 Reviews the ethical and legal issues arising in connection with the development of standards for pain management. Concludes that appropriate guidelines for pain management should be established by the medical profession. Cites Opinions 2.21 and 2.211. Stark, *Bio-Ethics and Physician Liability: The Liability Effects of Developing Pain Management Standards, 14 St. Thomas L. Rev. 601, 631 (2002).*

Journal 2000 Examines questions regarding the legality of such practices as voluntary stopping of eating and drinking (VSED), use of risky analgesics, and terminal sedation. Explores the distinctions between physician-assisted suicide and other palliative interventions. Concludes VSED, risky analgesics, and certain types of terminal sedation are lawful and should be made available to dying patients who make informed decisions to accept the risks involved. Quotes Opinions 2.21 and 2.211. Cites Opinions 2.18 and 2.20. Cantor & Thomas, *The Legal Bounds of Physician Conduct Hastening Death, 48 Buff. L. Rev. 83, 110, 131, 158 (2000).*

Journal 2000 Considers the question of whether physician-assisted suicide and euthanasia should be legalized. Concludes that, under basic moral and common law principles, the intentional taking of human life by a private person is wrong. References Opinions 2.20, 2.21, and 2.211. Gorsuch, *The Right to Assisted Suicide and Euthanasia, 23 Harv. J. L. & Pub. Pol'y 599, 653, 707 (2000).*

Journal 2000 Examines British pharmacists' views on physician-assisted suicide (PAS), including such topics as professional responsibility, personal beliefs, and relevant legal and ethical guidelines. Concludes that most pharmacists view their professional responsibilities regarding PAS differently from physicians. Cites Opinion 2.211. Hanlon, Weiss, & Rees, *British Community Pharmacists' Views of Physician-Assisted Suicide (PAS), 26 J. Med. Ethics 363, 367, 369 (2000).*

Journal 2000 Discusses ways in which courts and society can take steps to ensure ethical integrity in the medical profession (EIMP). Reviews the case of *Washington v. Glucksberg*, discussing its role in advocating EIMP as a state interest in assisted suicide law. Quotes Opinion 2.211. Kalt, *Death, Ethics, and the State, 23 Harv. J. L. & Pub. Pol'y 487, 537, 539 (2000).*

Journal 2000 Discusses the debate regarding whether physicians should legally participate in hastening or causing death. Explores laws against assisted suicide. Evaluates ethical and social concerns associated with assisted suicide.

Quotes Opinion 2.211. Larson, *Tales of Death: Storytelling in the Physician-Assisted Suicide Litigation, 39 Washburn L. J. 159, 177 (2000).*

Journal 2000 Explores the ongoing debate surrounding the legalization of assisted suicide. Defines and distinguishes assisted suicide and euthanasia from other ethical acts. Concludes most of the critical research questions that bear on current policy debates regarding legalization of assisted suicide remain unanswered. References Opinions 2.21 and 2.211. Rosenfeld, *Assisted Suicide, Depression, and the Right to Die, 6 Psychol. Pub. Pol'y & L. 467, 469 (2000).*

Journal 2000 Examines the background of assisted suicide and Michigan's attempt to ban it. Discusses *Cooley v. Granholm*, which is Michigan's most recent constitutional challenge. Concludes that the issue of physician-assisted suicide likely would not arise if society did a better job of providing end-of-life care. Quotes Opinion 2.211. Santayana, *The Michigan Legislature Persists in Prohibiting Assisted Suicide, 77 U. Det. Mercy L. Rev. 875, 886 (2000).*

Journal 2000 Explores the debate regarding physician-assisted suicide. Concludes that autonomy should be respected and that an individual's wishes for assisted suicide should be honored, unless the individual is misinformed or legally incompetent. Quotes Opinion 2.211. References Opinion 2.06. Urofsky, *Justifying Assisted Suicide: Comments on the Ongoing Debate, 14 Notre Dame J. L. Ethics & Pub. Pol'y 893, 918, 923 (2000).*

Journal 1999 Points out that a majority of people favor legalizing physician-assisted suicide. Discusses the right to die under the Ninth Amendment. Explains that a Ninth Amendment claim to the right to die has not been addressed by the US Supreme Court. Quotes Opinion 2.211. Hardaway, Peterson, & Mann, *The Right to Die and the Ninth Amendment: Compassion and Dying After Glucksberg and Vacco, 7 Geo. Mason L. Rev. 313, 342 (1999).*

Journal 1999 Examines legal and policy issues regarding physician-assisted suicide. Distinguishes between refusing treatment and assisted suicide. Concludes that there are too many dangers posed by physician-assisted suicide to warrant legalization. Quotes Opinion 2.211. Cites Opinions 2.20 and 2.21. Pratt, *Too Many Physicians: Physician-Assisted Suicide After Glucksberg/Quill, 9 Alb. L. J. Sci. & Tech. 161, 208 (1999).*

Journal 1998 Evaluates recent Supreme Court decisions denying a constitutional right to physician-assisted suicide. Explains that, if society adopts Oregon's view on physician-assisted suicide, then the focus will shift to when it is acceptable to end someone's life. Suggests that the debate over physician-assisted suicide does not concern death, but rather how society will care for people at the end of their lives. Quotes Opinion 2.211. Chopko, *Responsible Public Policy at the End of Life, 75 U. Det. Mercy L. Rev. 557, 573 (1998).*

Journal 1998 Explains that the US Supreme Court's decisions in *Washington* and *Vacco* left the door open for future constitutional challenges regarding the right to physician-assisted suicide. States that the Court did not explicitly deny the existence of a right to physician-assisted suicide. Quotes Opinion 2.20. Cites Opinion 2.211. Cohen, *The Open Door: Will the Right to Die Survive Washington v. Glucksberg and Vacco v. Quill?* 16 In Pub. Interest 79, 94 (1998).

Journal 1998 Examines ethical issues surrounding physician-assisted suicide. Explores physician-assisted suicide in the context of the influence of psychodynamic psychiatry on the physician-patient relationship. Concludes that if physicians approved of physician-assisted suicide, then it would undermine the physician-patient relationship. Quotes Opinion 2.211. Hamilton, Edwards, Boehnlein, & Hamilton, *The Doctor-Patient Relationship and Assisted Suicide: A Contribution From Dynamic Psychiatry,* 19 Am. J. Forensic Psychiatry 59, 60 (1998).

Journal 1998 Analyzes recent US Supreme Court decisions on physician-assisted suicide. Discusses amicus briefs that may have affected the Supreme Court's decisions. Theorizes that the Supreme Court will confront the subject of physician-assisted suicide in the future. References Opinion 2.211. Kamisar, *On the Meaning and Impact of the Physician-Assisted Suicide Cases,* 82 Minn. L. Rev. 895, 909, 918 (1998).

Journal 1998 Explains that a determination of mental capacity to consent must be made when a person requests physician-assisted suicide in a jurisdiction where such practice is legal. Explores the potential for liability in the context of making such a determination. Argues that standards regarding determination of mental capacity must be established by case law or legislation. Cites Opinion 2.211. References Opinion 2.06. Lipschitz, *Psychiatry and Consent for Physician-Assisted Suicide,* 19 Am. J. Forensic Psychiatry 91, 103, 104 (1998).

Journal 1998 Discusses legal aspects of physician-assisted suicide. Identifies acceptable end-of-life choices and compares them to physician-assisted suicide. Points out that physician-assisted suicide has the potential for abuse and that safeguards have not been implemented to protect people from that risk. Quotes Opinion 2.211. Cites Opinions 2.20 and 8.08. Mitchell, *Physician-Assisted Suicide: A Survey of the Issues Surrounding Legalization,* 74 N. D. L. Rev. 341, 349 (1998).

Journal 1998 Points out that the court in *Vacco v. Quill* did not reject the practice of physician-assisted suicide and left the subject open for state experimentation. Discusses routes some states have taken regarding assisted suicide. Concludes that access to assisted suicide is outweighed by the risk it will be utilized by depressed and mentally ill people. Quotes Opinions 2.20 and 2.211. Moore, *Physician-Assisted Suicide: Does "The End" Justify the Means?* 40 Ariz. L. Rev. 1471, 1472, 1481-82, 1491 (1998).

Journal 1998 Points out that psychiatrists have a limited ability to make assessments regarding the requests of terminally ill patients for physician-assisted suicide. Argues

that psychiatrists must oppose physician-assisted suicide because its practice would be detrimental to the profession of medicine and would adversely affect the practice of psychiatry. Quotes Opinion 2.211. Orr & Bishop, *Why Psychiatrists Should Not Participate in Euthanasia and Physician-Assisted Suicide,* 19 Am. J. Forensic Psychiatry 35, 36 (1998).

Journal 1998 Analyzes arguments for and against physician-assisted suicide. Distinguishes between killing and allowing a person to die. Concludes that the issue of assisted suicide should be addressed in the political arena rather than in the federal court system. Cites Opinion 2.211. Park, *Physician-Assisted Suicide: State Legislation Teetering at the Pinnacle of a Slippery Slope,* 7 Wm. & Mary Bill Rts. J. 277, 292, 293 (1998).

Journal 1998 Argues that physician-assisted suicide should be available for terminally ill patients whose pain is not alleviated through medications. Analyzes the effects of state regulation of physician-assisted suicide. Explores the possibility of using Thirteenth Amendment claims to abolish possible racially discriminatory use of physician-assisted suicide. Quotes Opinion 2.211. Pittman, *Physician-Assisted Suicide in the Dark Ward: The Intersection of the Thirteenth Amendment and Health Care Treatments Having Disproportionate Impacts on Disfavored Groups,* 28 Seton Hall L. Rev. 774, 784 (1998).

Journal 1998 Explains that physician-assisted suicide diametrically opposes the ideals of the medical profession. States that referendums are not good ways to make public policy. Suggests that patients should discuss their wishes regarding withholding or withdrawing life-sustaining medical treatment with their physicians and families. References Opinion 2.211. Reardon, *American Medical Association Perspective on Physician Assisted Suicide,* 75 U. Det. Mercy L. Rev. 515 (1998).

Journal 1998 Analyzes the Supreme Court's decision in *Washington v. Glucksberg.* Explains how the state's interest in preserving life can be viewed as an interest in preserving the sanctity of personal autonomy. Argues that physician-assisted suicide would preserve individual freedom and the sanctity of life. Quotes Opinion 2.211. Staihar, *The State's Unqualified Interest in Preserving Life: A Critique of the Formulations of Life's Sanctity in Washington v. Glucksberg,* 34 Idaho L. Rev. 401, 415 (1998).

Journal 1998 Discusses the US Supreme Court's decision in *Washington v. Glucksberg.* Points out that the Supreme Court left many unresolved issues concerning physician-assisted suicide. Provides criteria that could be used by state legislatures in drafting pertinent statutes. Cites Opinion 2.211. Testa, *Sentenced to Life? An Analysis of the United States Supreme Court's Decision in Washington v. Glucksberg,* 22 Nova L. Rev. 821, 839 (1998).

Journal 1998 Examines society's increasing acceptance of the belief in an individual's right to die. Discusses issues surrounding physician-assisted suicide. Evaluates the impact of

US Supreme Court decisions on physician-assisted suicide. Quotes Opinion 2.211. Urofsky, *Leaving the Door Ajar: The Supreme Court and Assisted Suicide, 32 U. Rich. L. Rev. 313, 336 (1998).*

Journal 1997 Reviews the arguments made in *amicus curiae* briefs submitted to the Supreme Court on the topic of assisted suicide. Focuses on key insights into the debate offered by the various *amici curiae*. Quotes Opinion 2.211. Coleson, *The Glucksberg & Quill Amicus Curiae Briefs: Verbatim Arguments Opposing Assisted Suicide, 13 Issues in Law & Med. 3, 67 (1997).*

Journal 1997 Considers the legal and ethical issues involved with physician-assisted suicide and euthanasia. Explores recent legal developments in the courts. Opines that Texas should allow physician-assisted suicide, at least for the terminally ill. Asserts that banning such a practice is unconstitutional. Quotes Opinion 2.211. References Opinion 2.21. Comment, *Physician-Assisted Suicide: Should Texas Be Different? 33 Hous. L. Rev. 1475, 1480, 1488 (1997).*

Journal 1997 Discusses the consequences of physician-assisted suicide. Argues that assisted suicide would divide the medical community. Concludes that physician-assisted suicide does not enhance freedom. Quotes Opinion 2.211. FitzGibbon, *The Failure of the Freedom-Based and Utilitarian Arguments for Assisted Suicide, 42 Am. J. Juris. 211, 252 (1997).*

Journal 1997 Explores a model physician-assisted suicide statute. Explains its history, provisions, and effects. Posits that the Act reaches further than one may suspect. Notes the AMA's position on assisted death and concludes that the Act fails to account for moral tradition. Quotes Opinion 2.211. FitzGibbon & Lai, *The Model Physician-Assisted Suicide Act and the Jurisprudence of Death, 13 Issues in Law & Med. 173, 203-04 (1997).*

Journal 1997 Considers US Supreme Court decisions regarding physician-assisted suicide. Argues that state legislatures should enact statutes to legalize physician-assisted suicide. Proposes a model act on physician-assisted suicide. Cites Opinion 2.211. Glynn, *Turning to State Legislatures to Legalize Physician-Assisted Suicide for Seriously Ill, Non-Terminal Patients After Vacco v. Quill and Washington v. Glucksberg, 6 J. L. & Pol'y. 329, 345 (1997).*

Journal 1997 Considers the right to die. Discusses the extension of the right to refuse treatment to decisions affecting life and death. Explains that courts distinguish between withdrawing life-sustaining treatment and euthanasia or assisted suicide. Emphasizes the importance of quality end-of-life care. Cites Opinion 2.211. Gostin, *Deciding Life and Death in the Courtroom: From Quinlan to Cruzan, Glucksberg, and Vacco—A Brief History and Analysis of Constitutional Protection of the Right to Die, 278 JAMA 1523, 1525, 1528 (1997).*

Journal 1997 States that the US Supreme Court has ended the *Roe v. Wade* era in which the Court made decisions on

social policy based on normative judgments. Discusses the dangers posed by physician-assisted suicide. Argues that the decision in *Washington v. Glucksberg* averted the danger of abuse posed by physician-assisted suicide. Quotes Opinion 2.211. McConnell, *The Right to Die and the Jurisprudence of Tradition, 1997 Utah L. Rev. 665, 703-04 (1997).*

Journal 1997 Examines possible legalization of euthanasia, observing that any form of euthanasia will be a step toward horrible death. Posits that legalizing euthanasia will create unsolvable mortal dangers that conflict with universal values of life. Concludes that physician-assisted suicide would create many victims. Cites Opinion 2.211. McGonnigal, *This Is Who Will Die When Doctors Are Allowed to Kill Their Patients, 31 J. Marshall L. Rev. 95, 103 (1997).*

Journal 1997 Explores the ethical and legal debate over assisted suicide. Examines cases dealing with prohibitions against physician-assisted suicide. Considers the Oregon Death with Dignity Act in light of the ruling in *Lee v. Oregon.* Quotes Opinion 2.211. Note, *Constitutional Aspects of Physician-Assisted Suicide After Lee v. Oregon, XXIII Am. J. Law & Med. 69 (1997).*

Journal 1997 Discusses the difference between physician-assisted suicide and the withdrawal of life-sustaining medical treatment. Posits that traditional moral arguments cannot justify the distinction. Examines how a right to assisted suicide for terminal patients brings right-to-die laws into alignment with underlying ethical precepts. References Opinion 2.211. Orentlicher, *The Legalization of Physician Assisted Suicide: A Very Modest Revolution, 38 B. C. L. Rev. 443, 459-60 (1997).*

Journal 1997 Considers the perspectives of medical residents about end-of-life issues. Investigates the differences of opinion held by residents in psychiatry, internal medicine, and emergency medicine. References Opinion 2.211. Roberts, Roberts, Warner, Solomon, Hardee, & McCarty, *Internal Medicine, Psychiatry, and Emergency Medicine Residents' Views of Assisted Death Practices, 157 Arch. Intern. Med. 1603, 1609 (1997).*

Journal 1996 Proposes a model state statute allowing and controlling physician-assisted suicide. Analyzes the constitutionality of the act and offers public policy justifications for the act's provisions. Concludes that proponents of physician-assisted suicide should provide precise, carefully tailored examples of regulations. Quotes Opinion 2.211. Cites Opinion 2.20. Baron, Bergstresser, Brock, Cole, Dorfman, Johnson, Schnipper, Vorenberg, & Wanzer, *A Model State Act to Authorize and Regulate Physician-Assisted Suicide, 33 Harv. J. Legis. 1, 2, 7 (1996).*

Journal 1996 Examines the issue of physician-assisted suicide. Observes that it is important to consider not only whether some form of physician-assisted suicide should enjoy legal and ethical support in our society, but also whether physicians should be involved. Concludes that physicians, as a profession, probably are not the proper individuals to perform this function. Cites Opinions 2.21

and 2.211. Clark, *Autonomy and Death, 71 Tul. L. Rev. 45, 89 (1996).*

Journal 1996 Criticizes the circuit court's opinion in *Compassion in Dying.* Suggests that the opinion fails to fully consider the ethical prohibitions against physician-assisted suicide. Concludes that the court's opinion is not based on a complete and accurate presentation of historical views and attitudes about suicide. Quotes Opinion 2.211. Duncan & Lubin, *The Use and Abuse of History in Compassion in Dying, 20 Harv. J. L. & Pub. Pol'y 175, 183 (1996).*

Journal 1996 Examines ethical and legal issues involved in physician-assisted suicide. Asserts that the judiciary is not the proper forum for establishing guidelines regarding these issues. Concludes that individual state legislative enactments are the proper vehicles for delineating appropriate guidelines. Quotes Opinion 2.211. Kass & Lund, *Physician-Assisted Suicide, Medical Ethics and the Future of the Medical Profession, 35 Duq. L. Rev. 395, 404 (1996).*

Journal 1996 Discusses the historical development of the right to die. Considers patient autonomy and paternalism and the role physicians play in end-of-life decisions. Explains the issue in the context of federal cases. Examines the true extent of a protected right to die. Cites Opinion 2.211. Kelly, *The "Right to Die" in America: The Ninth Circuit's Decision in Compassion in Dying v. the State of Washington, 29 J. Health & Hosp. L. 246, 255 (1996).*

Journal 1996 Explores the issue of legalizing physician-assisted suicide. Opines that the current state of technology increases life expectancy but with a concomitant decrease in dignity and autonomy surrounding one's death. Notes that the elderly are committing suicide at an increasing rate. Cites Opinions 2.20, 2.21, and 2.211. Morgan & Sutherland, *Last Rights? Confronting Physician-Assisted Suicide in Law and Society: Legal Liturgies on Physician-Assisted Suicide, 26 Stetson L. Rev. 481, 484 (1996).*

Journal 1996 Considers the right to death with dignity. Suggests that the AMA's position undermines mitigation of suffering and the individuals' right to self-determination. Concludes that restrictions on the right to death with dignity may be constitutionally impermissible. Quotes Opinion 2.211. Cites Opinion 2.20. Note, *Who Decides if There Is Triumph in the Ultimate Agony? Constitutional Theory and the Emerging Right to Die With Dignity, 37 Wm. & Mary L. Rev. 827, 829 (1996).*

Journal 1996 Explores ethical problems accompanying the power to prolong and preserve life past points previously achievable. Questions whether physician-assisted suicide is a proper and ethically desirable course of treatment. Discusses recent developments and arguments surrounding physician-assisted suicide. References Opinion 2.211. Thomasma, *When Physicians Choose to Participate in the Death of Their Patients: Ethics and Physician-Assisted Suicide, 24 J. Law Med. & Ethics 183, 184, 195 (1996).*

Journal 1995 Suggests that people seeking suicide need life-affirming treatment, not aid in dying. Concludes that the US Constitution does not require society to stand by while a person seeks suicide. Cites Opinion 2.211. Bopp & Coleson, *The Constitutional Case Against Permitting Physician-Assisted Suicide for Competent Adults With Terminal Conditions, 11 Issues in Law & Med. 239, 250 (1995).*

Journal 1995 Examines four essential principles of bioethics—patient autonomy, nonmaleficence, beneficence. and justice—and describes the application of these in clinical settings according to bioethical norms and AMA opinions. Concludes that such an approach promotes compassionate medical caregiving and that laws should reflect these values. Quotes Opinions 2.01 and 8.18. References Opinion 2.211. Cohen, *Toward a Bioethics of Compassion, 28 Ind. L. Rev. 667, 673, 681-82, 683 (1995).*

Journal 1995 Analyzes the case of *Compassion in Dying v. Washington,* in which a federal district court judge held that certain people have a constitutional right to physician-assisted suicide. Criticizes the decision for being too broad in that it would protect active euthanasia by physicians on patients who are physically unable to perform the act themselves. Quotes Opinion 2.21. References Opinion 2.211. Larson, *Prescription for Death: A Second Opinion, 44 DePaul L. Rev. 461, 472 (1995).*

Journal 1994 Argues that assisted suicide is not an implicit right under the Fourteenth Amendment's liberty guarantee. Suggests that giving physicians the authority to determine the appropriateness of assisted suicide furthers no legitimate state interest. Cites Opinion 2.06. References Opinion 2.211. Marzen, *Out, Out Brief Candle: Constitutionally Prescribed Suicide for the Terminally Ill, 21 Hastings Const. L. Q. 799, 821 (1994).*

Journal 1992 Examines the history of the right an individual has over his or her own body, and how the right to commit suicide has evolved from that concept. Concludes that the right of an incurably ill person to commit suicide is a personal issue to be decided outside of the judicial system. References Opinions 2.21 and 2.211. Morgan, Marks, & Harty-Golder, *The Issue of Personal Choice: The Competent Incurable Patient and the Right to Commit Suicide? 57 Mo. L. Rev. 1, 44, 45 (1992).*

Journal 1992 Discusses the historical, legal, and social arguments both for and against assisted suicide and voluntary active euthanasia. Concludes that only physician-assisted suicide should be legalized. References Opinion 2.211. Note, *Aid-in-Dying: Should We Decriminalize Physician-Assisted Suicide and Physician-Committed Euthanasia? XVIII Am. J. Law & Med. 369, 370 (1992).*

5.8 Euthanasia

9th Cir. 1996 Suit was brought by several physicians and a not-for-profit corporation which provides information, assistance, and counseling to competent terminally ill adult patients contemplating suicide, asserting that a state statute making it a crime to aid anyone in attempting to commit suicide unconstitutionally prevents terminally ill patients from exercising their protected liberty interests. Appeals court, en banc, held that the choice of how and when to die is a liberty interest and that the statute violates the due process rights of competent, terminally ill adults who wish to hasten their deaths by obtaining medication prescribed by their physicians. Stating that physician-assisted suicide runs counter to medical ethics, the dissent cited Opinions 2.20, 2.21, and 2.211 and quoted Opinion 2.211. *Compassion in Dying v. Washington, 79 F.3d 790, 840, 855 replacing, 49 F.3d 586 (9th Cir. 1995).*

Mich. App. 2001 State brought criminal action against physician for the murder of a patient by lethal injection. The trial court convicted the physician of second-degree murder and delivering a controlled substance. On appeal, the trial court decision was affirmed. The physician asked the appellate court to conclude that euthanasia is legal and to reverse his conviction on constitutional grounds. The appellate court relied on *Washington v. Glucksberg*, 521 U.S. 702 (1997) in determining there is no constitutional right to commit euthanasia, so that an individual can be free from intolerable and irremediable suffering. In discussing *Glucksberg*, the court observed that a state has a legitimate interest in protecting the integrity and ethics of the medical profession. The court noted *Glucksberg's* reference to Opinions 2.20, 2.21, and 2.211 in this regard. *People v. Kevorkian, 248 Mich. App. 373, 639 N.W.2d 291, 305 n. 42.*

Journal 2010 Examines whether standards and practices regarding euthanasia, other than those which have been legally and ethically established, should be applied in extreme emergency situations. Concludes that creating an exception to the prohibition against euthanasia in such situations has no legal or ethical foundation and is not necessary as a means to cope with disasters. Argues for the development of disaster planning consistent with established legal and ethical principles. Quotes Opinion 8.08. Cites Opinions 2.20 and 2.21. Shea, *Hurricane Katrina and the Legal and Bioethical Implications of Involuntary Euthanasia as a Component of Disaster Management in Extreme Emergency Situations, 19 Annals Health L. 133, 137-138 (2010).*

Journal 2008 Explores the question of whether physician-assisted dying is ethically and legally appropriate by using empirical research to address concerns and objections. Concludes more research is needed to better understand the pressures experienced by patients facing end-of-life decisions. Quotes Opinions 2.21 and 2.211. Battin, *Physician-Assisted Dying and the Slippery Slope: The Challenge of Empirical Evidence, 45 Willamette L. Rev. 91, 98-99 (2008).*

Journal 2006 Argues that current law and ethics governing physician-assisted suicide are too simplistic. Concludes there are a number of legal ways for terminally ill patients to hasten death. Quotes Opinion 2.21. Cantor, *On Hastening Death Without Violating Legal and Moral Prohibitions, 37 Loy. U. Chi. L. J. 407, 427 (2006).*

Journal 2005 Examines the legal and ethical aspects of physician participation in capital punishment. Concludes that federal and state laws addressing this practice must be amended to harmonize the law with applicable principles of medical ethics. Quotes Opinion 2.06. Cites Opinion 2.21. References Opinion 2.01. Levy, *Conflict of Duty: Capital Punishment Regulations and AMA Medical Ethics, 26 J. Legal Med. 261, 268, 269, 270, 273 (2005).*

Journal 2004 Reviews empirical data and the arguments on both sides of the physician-assisted suicide debate. Concludes that weighing the costs and benefits associated with legalizing assisted suicide likely will not resolve the debate. References Opinion 2.211. Gorsuch, *The Legalization of Assisted Suicide and the Law of Unintended Consequences: A Review of the Dutch and Oregon Experiments and Leading Utilitarian Arguments for Legal Change, 2004 Wis. L. Rev. 1347, 1379 (2004).*

Journal 2004 Analyzes various issues relating to the role of mental health professionals in capital punishment in light of Albert Bandura's model of "mechanisms of moral disengagement." Concludes that facilitating participation of mental health professionals in executions creates conflicts with the humanistic norms of the profession. Quotes Preamble and Opinions 1.01, 1.02, 2.06, 2.067, 2.20, 2.21, 2.211, and 8.14. Judges, *The Role of Mental Health Professionals in Capital Punishment: An Exercise in Moral Disengagement, 41 Hous. L. Rev. 515, 562, 568, 569, 570, 571-72, 581, 586, 588, 598 (2004).*

Journal 2003 Analyzes the objective and subjective tests used to determine which individuals qualify for physician-assisted suicide (PAS) and euthanasia in the US and the Netherlands. Concludes that both tests provide sufficient safeguards to protect vulnerable groups. Quotes Opinions 2.21 and 2.211. Green, *Physician-Assisted Suicide and Euthanasia: Safeguarding Against the "Slippery Slope"— The Netherlands Versus the United States, 13 Ind. Int'l & Comp. L. Rev. 639, 662 (2003).*

Journal 2002 Examines key factors that led to the current palliative care crisis. Analyzes state legislative and judicial efforts to improve palliative care. Concludes with model legislation that holds physicians accountable for inadequate palliative care. Quotes Opinions 2.21 and 2.211. References Opinion 2.20. Oken, *Curing Healthcare Providers' Failure to Administer Opioids in the Treatment of Severe Pain, 23 Cardozo L. Rev. 1917, 1925-26, 1952, 1954 (2002).*

Journal 2002 Reviews the ethical and legal issues arising in connection with the development of standards for pain management. Concludes that appropriate guidelines for pain management should be established by the medical profession. Cites Opinions 2.21 and 2.211. Stark, *Bio-Ethics and Physician Liability: The Liability Effects of Developing Pain Management Standards, 14 St. Thomas L. Rev. 601, 631 (2002).*

Journal 2001 Explores the similarities and differences among active voluntary euthanasia, terminal sedation, and assisted suicide. Examines the problems with making moral distinctions based on physicians' intentions. Concludes that, with proper safeguards, active voluntary euthanasia and assisted suicide are more protective of patient self-determination. Quotes Opinions 2.20 and 2.21. Gauthier, *Active Voluntary Euthanasia, Terminal Sedation, and Assisted Suicide, 12 J. Clinical Ethics 43, 43-44, 49 (2001).*

Journal 2000 Examines questions regarding the legality of such practices as voluntary stopping of eating and drinking (VSED), use of risky analgesics, and terminal sedation. Explores the distinctions between physician-assisted suicide and other palliative interventions. Concludes VSED, risky analgesics, and certain types of terminal sedation are lawful and should be made available to dying patients who make informed decisions to accept the risks involved. Quotes Opinions 2.21 and 2.211. Cites Opinions 2.18 and 2.20. Cantor & Thomas, *The Legal Bounds of Physician Conduct Hastening Death, 48 Buff. L. Rev. 83, 110, 131, 158 (2000).*

Journal 2000 Considers the question of whether physician-assisted suicide and euthanasia should be legalized. Concludes that, under basic moral and common law principles, the intentional taking of human life by a private person is wrong. References Opinions 2.20, 2.21, and 2.211. Gorsuch, *The Right to Assisted Suicide and Euthanasia, 23 Harv. J. L. & Pub. Pol'y 599, 653, 707 (2000).*

Journal 2000 Explores the ongoing debate surrounding the legalization of assisted suicide. Defines and distinguishes assisted suicide and euthanasia from other ethical acts. Concludes most of the critical research questions that bear on current policy debates regarding legalization of assisted suicide remain unanswered. References Opinions 2.21 and 2.211. Rosenfeld, *Assisted Suicide, Depression, and the Right to Die, 6 Psychol. Pub. Pol'y & L. 467, 469 (2000).*

Journal 1999 Examines legal and policy issues regarding physician-assisted suicide. Distinguishes between refusing treatment and assisted suicide. Concludes that there are too many dangers posed by physician-assisted suicide to warrant legalization. Quotes Opinion 2.211. Cites Opinions 2.20 and 2.21. Pratt, *Too Many Physicians: Physician-Assisted Suicide After Glucksberg/Quill, 9 Alb. L. J. Sci. & Tech. 161, 208 (1999).*

Journal 1997 Considers the legal and ethical issues involved with physician-assisted suicide and euthanasia. Explores recent legal developments in the courts. Opines that Texas should allow physician-assisted suicide, at least for the terminally ill. Asserts that banning such a practice is unconstitutional. Quotes Opinion 2.211. References Opinion 2.21.

Comment, *Physician-Assisted Suicide: Should Texas Be Different? 33 Hous. L. Rev. 1475, 1480, 1488 (1997).*

Journal 1997 Discusses goals of care included in advance directives and whether they can be used to predict specific interventions and results. Offers insights provided by survey of physicians at Massachusetts General Hospital. Cites Opinions 2.20 and 2.21. Fischer, Alpert, Stoeckle, & Emanuel, *Can Goals of Care Be Used to Predict Intervention Preferences in an Advance Directive? 157 Arch. Intern. Med. 801, 807 (1997).*

Journal 1996 Examines the issue of physician-assisted suicide. Observes that it is important to consider not only whether some form of physician-assisted suicide should enjoy legal and ethical support in our society, but also whether physicians should be involved. Concludes that physicians, as a profession, probably are not the proper individuals to perform this function. Cites Opinions 2.21 and 2.211. Clark, *Autonomy and Death, 71 Tul. L. Rev. 45, 89 (1996).*

Journal 1996 Explores the issue of legalizing physician-assisted suicide. Opines that the current state of technology increases life expectancy but with a concomitant decrease in dignity and autonomy surrounding one's death. Notes that the elderly are committing suicide at an increasing rate. Cites Opinions 2.20, 2.21, and 2.211. Morgan & Sutherland, *Last Rights? Confronting Physician-Assisted Suicide in Law and Society: Legal Liturgies on Physician-Assisted Suicide, 26 Stetson L. Rev. 481, 484 (1996).*

Journal 1995 Analyzes the case of *Compassion in Dying v. Washington,* in which a federal district court judge held that certain people have a constitutional right to physician-assisted suicide. Criticizes the decision for being too broad in that it would protect active euthanasia by physicians on patients who are physically unable to perform the act themselves. Quotes Opinion 2.21. References Opinion 2.211. Larson, *Prescription for Death: A Second Opinion, 44 DePaul L. Rev. 461, 472 (1995).*

Journal 1995 Offers relevant historical perspectives and provides comprehensive ethical and legal discussion of physician-assisted suicide and euthanasia. Highlights important legislative developments, including the Oregon Death with Dignity Act, and analyzes significant judicial opinions. Quotes Principles III, IV, and VI and Opinions 2.21 and 9.12. Cites Opinions 2.20 and 8.11. Stone & Winslade, *Physician-Assisted Suicide and Euthanasia in the United States: Legal and Ethical Observations, 16 J. Legal Med. 481, 483, 490, 497, 498, 499 (1995).*

Journal 1993 Considers how life-sustaining treatments have led to prolonged life under unacceptable circumstances. Recommends quality assurance programs that promote discussion between physicians and patients regarding life-sustaining treatment problems. Cites Opinions 2.20 and 2.21. Pearlman, Cain, Patrick, Appelbaum-Maizel, Starks, Jecker, & Uhlmann, *Insights Pertaining to Patient Assessments of States Worse Than Death, 4 J. Clinical Ethics 33, 40 (1993).*

Journal 1992 Analyzes the arguments for and against active euthanasia, including ethical concerns, the slippery slope argument, and the proper role of the physician. Suggests that active euthanasia may be acceptable when its administration is restricted to physicians. References Opinions 2.20 and 2.21. Brock, *Voluntary Active Euthanasia, 22 Hastings Center Rep. 10 (March/April 1992).*

Journal 1992 Considers the debate surrounding medical futility. Observes that this debate is encouraging reexamination of the nature of patient entitlement to medical care as well as the "ends of medicine." References Opinions 2.20,

2.21, and 2.22. Miles, *Medical Futility, 20 Law Med. & Health Care 310, 311, 313 (1992).*

Journal 1992 Examines the history of the right an individual has over his or her own body, and how the right to commit suicide has evolved from that concept. Concludes that the right of an incurably ill person to commit suicide is a personal issue to be decided outside of the judicial system. References Opinions 2.21 and 2.211. Morgan, Marks, & Harty-Golder, *The Issue of Personal Choice: The Competent Incurable Patient and the Right to Commit Suicide? 57 Mo. L. Rev. 1, 44, 45 (1992).*

6 Organ Procurement and Transplantation

6.1.1 Transplantation of Organs from Living Donors

Journal 2005 Discusses policy issues and moral and ethical dilemmas associated with facial transplant surgery. Concludes that while the government should not stall the progress of biomedical science, facial transplantation practices must be regulated to ensure that progress is consistent with social norms. References Opinion 2.15. Hartman, *Face Value: Challenges of Transplant Technology, 31 Am. J. L. & Med. 7, 25, 31 (2005).*

Journal 2004 Explores the moral and political rationales for current organ acquisition policies. Concludes that, in a secular society, no plausible moral reason exists to ban the sale of organs. Quotes Opinions 2.15 and 2.151. Engelhardt, Jr, *Giving, Selling, and Having Taken: Conflicting Views of Organ Transfer, 1 Ind. Health L. Rev. 29, 33-34 (2004).*

Journal 2004 Examines state laws dealing with a minor's right to consent to medical treatment. Concludes that physicians must be aware of these laws for purposes of compliance, protection against liability, and providing minors the highest level of care. Quotes Opinion 2.015. Vukadinovich, *Minors' Rights to Consent to Treatment: Navigating the Complexity of State Laws, 37 J. Health L. 667, 689-90 (2004).*

Journal 2003 Proposes a moral, communitarian approach to address organ shortages. Concludes the next step should involve a demonstration that the communitarian approach can succeed. Quotes Opinion 2.155. Cites Opinion 2.15.

Etzioni, *Organ Donation: A Communitarian Approach, 13 Kennedy Inst. Ethics J. 1, 3, 4, 16 (March 2003).*

Journal 2003 Examines the benefits of paired organ exchanges and proposes a statutory framework for implementation. Concludes this approach supplements the current US organ procurement system without resorting to use of financial incentives. Quotes Opinion 2.15. Morley, *Increasing the Supply of Organs for Transplantation Through Paired Organ Exchanges, 21 Yale L. & Pol'y Rev. 221, 255 (2003).*

Journal 2003 Suggests that financial incentives for organ procurement should be reconsidered. Concludes that the ban on marketing organs should be lifted. References Opinion 2.15. Veatch, *Why Liberals Should Accept Financial Incentives for Organ Procurement, 13 Kennedy Inst. Ethics J. 19, 34 (March 2003).*

Journal 1995 Examines legal and ethical issues surrounding organ transplant procurement practices, with emphasis on a possible commercial system. Concludes that adequate market safeguards need to be developed to protect vulnerable donors and citizens. References Opinions 2.15 and 2.167. Banks, *Legal and Ethical Safeguards: Protection of Society's Most Vulnerable Participants in a Commercialized Organ Transplantation System, XXI Am. J. Law & Med. 45, 77, 79, 95-96, 103-04 (1995).*

6.1.2 Organ Donation after Cardiac Death

Journal 2010 Argues that a precise definition of death is needed to counteract the focus on reducing medical costs and increasing organ supplies for transplantations. Concludes that allowing dying patients more autonomy

to determine conditions for organ donation will foster an atmosphere of trust in which more people will be willing to donate earlier in the dying process. Quotes Opinion 2.157. Cites Opinion 10.01. Fry-Revere, Ray, & Reher, *Death: A*

New Legal Perspective, 27 J. Contemp. Health L. & Pol'y 1, 11, 50, 53 (2010).

Journal 2008 Argues preservation of individuals who die of uncontrolled cardiac death is authorized by the Uniform Anatomical Gift Act and does not violate the rights of family members. Concludes that organ donor population should

be expanded to include individuals who die uncontrolled cardiac deaths to increase the number of organs available for transplant. Cites Opinions 2.157 and 8.181. Bonnie, Wright, & Dineen, *Legal Authority to Preserve Organs in Cases of Uncontrolled Cardiac Death: Preserving Family Choice, 36 J. L. Med. & Ethics 741, 743 (2008).*

6.1.3 Studying Financial Incentives for Cadaveric Organ Donation

Journal 2007 Reviews major medical and legal developments in the field of organ transplantation. Concludes that introducing a policy of donor payments would be another major success. References Opinion 2.151. Kaserman, *Fifty Years of Organ Transplants: The Successes and the Failures, 23 Issues L. & Med. 45, 60 (2007).*

Journal 2007 Considers the benefits and risks associated with commodification of organs. Concludes that risks can likely be minimized and that the legal and medical communities should undertake extensive research into the benefits of commodification. References Opinion 2.151. Woan, *Buy Me a Pound of Flesh: China's Sale of Death Row Organs on the Black Market and What Americans Can Learn From It, 47 Santa Clara L. Rev. 413, 439 (2007).*

Journal 2006 Examines federal law governing organ procurement. Suggests that Congress should reconsider its policy banning financial incentives for cadaveric organ donation. References Opinion 2.151. Carlson, *Organ Donation Recovery and Improvement Act: How Congress Missed an Opportunity to Say "Yes" to Financial Incentives for Organ Donation, 23 J. Contemp. Health L. & Pol'y 136, 145 (2006).*

Journal 2006 Examines the problem of organ donor shortage in New York. Concludes that the legislature should establish a financial incentive program of "modest value" to increase the rate of donations. References Opinions 2.151 and 2.16. Flamholz, *A Penny for Your Organs: Revising New York's Policy on Offering Financial Incentives for Organ Donation, 14 J. L. & Pol'y 329, 330, 374 (2006).*

Journal 2004 Explores the moral and political rationales for current organ acquisition policies. Concludes that, in a secular society, no plausible moral reason exists to ban the sale of organs. Quotes Opinions 2.15 and 2.151. Engelhardt, Jr, *Giving, Selling, and Having Taken: Conflicting Views of Organ Transfer, 1 Ind. Health L. Rev. 29, 33-34 (2004).*

Journal 2004 Discusses regulations prohibiting financial incentives for organ donation. Concludes that repealing regulations prohibiting financial incentives for organ donation will lead to the exploitation of the poor. References Opinion 2.151. Hurley, *Cashing in on the Transplant List: An Argument Against Offering Valuable Compensation for the Donation of Organs, 4 J. High Tech. L. 117, 130 (2004).*

6.1.4 Presumed Consent and Mandated Choice for Organs from Deceased Donors

Journal 2011 Analyzes mandated choice as a method of alleviating the shortage of organs for transplant in the US. Concludes that mandated choice, with appropriate safeguards, is the best option for increasing organ donation in the US. Cites Opinion 2.155. Cotter, *Increasing Consent for Organ Donation: Mandated Choice, Individual Autonomy, and Informed Consent, 21 Health Matrix 599, 606, 607 (2011).*

Journal 2007 Argues for a policy allowing tax deductions for expenses associated with organ donation by living donors. Concludes that such a policy would properly compensate donors and reward them for reducing the cost of medical care. References Opinion 2.155. Molen, *Recognizing the Larger Sacrifice: Easing the Burdens Borne by Living Organ Donors Through Federal Tax Deductions, 21 BYU J. Pub. L. 459, 463 (2007).*

Journal 2006 Discusses federal organ procurement policies. Proposes a plan under which the federal government

guarantees equal distribution of organs, requires that all citizens act as default donors unless they opt out, and assumes all costs associated with transplantation. Quotes Opinion 2.155. Siegal & Bonnie, *Closing the Organ Gap: A Reciprocity-Based Social Contract Approach, 34 J. L. Med. & Ethics 415, 415 (2006).*

Journal 2006 Examines the organ donation system in the US. Concludes that a mandated choice system should be adopted along with an optimized allocation system. References Opinion 2.155. Spellman, *Encouragement Is Not Enough: The Benefits of Instituting a Mandated Choice Organ Procurement System, 56 Syracuse L. Rev. 353, 371 (2006).*

Journal 2003 Explores the ethical, legal, and clinical implications of non–heart-beating organ donation. Concludes that, if ambiguities are clarified, non–heart-beating organ donation can achieve an ethical good. References Opinions 2.155 and 2.162. Bell, *Non–Heart Beating Organ Donation:*

Old Procurement Strategy—New Ethical Problems, 29 J. Med. Ethics 176, 181 (2003).

Journal 2003 Recommends a modified version of mandated choice for organ procurement. Concludes that the modified version recognizes arguments favoring mandated donation while still relying on the importance of individual consent. References Opinion 2.155. Chouhan & Draper, *Modified Mandated Choice for Organ Procurement, 29 J. Med. Ethics 157, 162 (2003).*

Journal 2003 Proposes a moral, communitarian approach to address organ shortages. Concludes the next step should involve a demonstration that the communitarian approach can succeed. Quotes Opinion 2.155. Cites Opinion 2.15. Etzioni, *Organ Donation: A Communitarian Approach, 13 Kennedy Inst. Ethics J. 1, 3, 4, 16 (March 2003).*

Journal 2002 Considers ethical incentives to increase organ donation. Concludes that market-based incentives are unethical. References Opinion 2.155. Delmonico, Arnold,

Scheper-Hughes, Siminoff, Kahn, & Youngner, *Ethical Incentives—Not Payment—for Organ Donation, 346 New Eng. J. Med. 2002, 2005 (2002).*

Journal 2001 Explores ways to overcome barriers to organ donation. Clarifies ethical constraints affecting societal efforts to increase the supply of organs. Supports the rights of individuals to make organ donation decisions, but emphasizes the importance of doing so as members of communities—particularly small communities of families. Quotes Opinion 2.155. Childress, *The Failure to Give: Reducing Barriers to Organ Donation, 11 Kennedy Inst. Ethics J. 1, 13, 14 (2001).*

Journal 1997 Explores the current policies on cadaveric organ procurement in the US. Offers improvements to help save lives and end the waste of suitable organs. Discusses pertinent ethical and legal issues. References Opinion 2.155. MacDonald, *Organ Donation: The Time Has Come to Refocus the Ethical Spotlight, 8 Stan. L. & Pol'y Rev. 177, 179, 185 (1997).*

6.1.5 Umbilical Cord Blood Banking

Journal 2011 Discusses the physician's role in educating and counseling patients on the donation and storage of umbilical cord blood. Concludes physicians should encourage patients to donate their newborn's umbilical cord blood to public banks or use the Related Donor Cord Blood Program to bank blood for the newborn's sibling, but cord blood should not be banked for an unidentified possible future use. Cites Opinion 2.165. Martin, Kurtzberg, & Hesse, *Umbilical Cord Blood: A Guide for Primary Care Physicians, 84 Am. Fam. Physician 661, 661 (2011).*

6.1.6 Anencephalic Newborns as Organ Donors

Journal 2009 Explores ethical concerns surrounding organ donation from anencephalic infants. Concludes that, by viewing anencephalic infants as having been born into a state of death, an infant's organs may be donated without violating the dead donor rule. Cites Opinion 2.147. References Opinion 2.162. Khan & Lea, *Paging King Solomon: Towards Allowing Organ Donation From Anencephalic Infants, 6 Ind. Health L. Rev. 17, 38 (2009).*

Journal 2007 Explores the idea of "legal personhood" in the context of scientific advancement. Concludes that this concept is still developing and suggests that a creative approach to this area of jurisprudence is required. Cites Opinion 2.162 and Opinion 2.162 (1994). Berg, *Of Elephants and Embryos: A Proposed Framework for Legal Personhood, 59 Hastings L. J. 369, 377-78 (2007).*

Journal 2007 Argues that death for potential organ donors should not be defined as brain death. Concludes that the current definition is likely to remain the same until new technology makes transplants from animals possible. References Opinion 2.162. Truog, *Brain Death—Too Flawed to Endure, Too Ingrained to Abandon, 35 J. L. Med. & Ethics 273, 280 (2007).*

Journal 2003 Explores the ethical, legal, and clinical implications of non–heart-beating organ donation. Concludes that, if ambiguities are clarified, non–heart-beating organ donation can achieve an ethical good. References Opinions 2.155 and 2.162. Bell, *Non–Heart Beating Organ Donation: Old Procurement Strategy—New Ethical Problems, 29 J. Med. Ethics 176, 181 (2003).*

Journal 2003 Discusses how legal norms can be challenged by advances in medical knowledge. Concludes that sources beyond the law should be considered to prevent untoward legal outcomes. References Opinion 2.162. Mayo, *Sex, Marriage, Medicine, and Law: "What Hope of Harmony?" 42 Washburn L. J. 269, 271 (2003).*

Journal 1999 Discusses legal, medical, social, and ethical issues regarding organ donation by anencephalic infants. Points out the dangers surrounding anencephalic organ donation versus parents' needs for good to come out of the lives of their anencephalic children. References Opinion 2.162. Bard, *The Diagnosis Is Anencephaly and the Parents Ask About Organ Donation: Now What? A Guide for Hospital Counsel and Ethics Committees, 21 W. New Eng. L. Rev. 49, 62 (1999).*

Journal 1999 Discusses the Uniform Declaration of Death Act and the dead-donor rule. Provides ethical justifications for sustaining current policies on non–heart-beating organ donation. Cites Opinions 2.06 and 2.162. DuBois, *Non–Heart-Beating Organ Donation: A Defense of the Required Determination of Death*, 27 J. Law Med. & Ethics 126, 128 (1999).

Journal 1999 Explains that shortages in available organs have prompted a movement that favors modifying the dead-donor rule. Discusses different proposals to amend the dead-donor rule. Suggests that even the slightest modification of the rule will prompt strong opposition. References Opinion 2.162. Robertson, *The Dead Donor Rule*, 29 Hastings Center Rep. 6, 13 (Nov./Dec. 1999).

Journal 1999 Discusses national and international legislative proposals addressing human cloning. Considers human cloning for reproductive and nonreproductive reasons. Undertakes legal analysis and concludes that human cloning should not be banned completely. Cites Opinion 2.162. Smith, *Ignorance Is Not Bliss: Why a Ban on Human Cloning Is Unacceptable*, 9 Health Matrix. 311, 330, 331 (1999).

Journal 1998 Examines American and British views on the brain death test and advance directives. Points out that the brain death test has been criticized in cases where patients woke up after being in a coma for long periods of time. Argues that better utilization of advance directives may dissipate arguments for euthanasia. References Opinion 2.162. Trew, *Regulating Life and Death: The Modification and Commodification of Nature*, 29 U. Tol. L. Rev. 271, 292 (1998).

Journal 1996 Explores courses of treatment for infants born with hypoplastic left heart syndrome. Discusses the various treatment options available to infants and their frequency. Notes the controversy surrounding the AMA's opinion on anencephalic infants as organ donors. References Opinion 2.162 [subsequently amended]. Caplan, Cooper, Garcia-Prats, & Brody, *Diffusion of Innovative Approaches to Managing Hypoplastic Left Heart Syndrome*, 150 Arch. Pediatr. Adolesc. Med. 487, 490 (1996).

Journal 1996 Describes the impact of federal laws on medical decisions for anencephalic infants. Discusses selective nontreatment of such infants and the debate regarding availability of their organs for transplantation. Quotes Opinions 2.162 (1994) [subsequently amended] and 2.17. Crossley, *Infants With Anencephaly, the ADA, and the Child Abuse Amendments*, 11 Issues in Law & Med. 379, 385, 409 (1996).

Journal 1996 Proposes an alternative method of capital punishment to allow for organ donation by executed prisoners. Provides justifications for this proposal. Concludes that physicians should be able to ethically participate in this process. Quotes Principle VII. Cites Opinion 2.06. References Opinion 2.162 (1994) [subsequently amended]. Patton, *A Call for Common Sense: Organ Donation and the Executed Prisoner*, 3 Va. J. Soc. Pol'y & L. 387, 404, 405, 407-10 (1996).

Journal 1996 Examines the recent trend in health care laws and ethics to focus on the alleviation of suffering. Expresses concern that such a focus may result in the valuation of one life over another. Emphasizes the need to evaluate multiple, diverse responses to suffering. Quotes Principle VI. References Opinion 2.162. Shepherd, *Sophie's Choices: Medical and Legal Responses to Suffering*, 72 Notre Dame L. Rev. 103, 106, 133 (1996).

Journal 1994 Criticizes both the White House's proposed National Bioethics Advisory Commission and certain purely private ethical advisory bodies. Proposes that an appropriately organized new federal advisory body could provide essential guidance in developing public bioethical policies, particularly if the meaningful input of ethics scholars at universities, ethics centers, and other private organizations and public commissions were sought. Cites Opinion 2.162. Capron, *Ethics: Public and Private*, 24 Hastings Center Rep. 26, 27 (Nov./Dec. 1994).

6.2.1 Guidance for Organ Transplantation from Deceased Donors

Journal 2006 Examines the problem of organ donor shortage in New York. Concludes that the legislature should establish a financial incentive program of "modest value" to increase the rate of donations. References Opinions 2.151 and 2.16. Flamholz, *A Penny for Your Organs: Revising New York's Policy on Offering Financial Incentives for Organ Donation*, 14 J. L. & Pol'y 329, 330, 374 (2006).

Journal 2003 Considers the cause of persistent shortages of vaccines and other critical drugs. Concludes that government should take specific steps to encourage pharmaceutical manufacturers to supply these essential products. References Opinion 2.16. Noah, *Triage in the Nation's Medicine Cabinet: The Puzzling Scarcity of Vaccines and Other Drugs*, 54 S. C. L. Rev. 741, 755 (2003).

Journal 2003 Provides a moral and legal framework for considering the possibility of progress in managing technology applicable to organ transplantation. Concludes that progress in increasing the supply of organs will require an evolution in moral thinking. Quotes Opinion 2.16. Shapiro, *On the Possibility of "Progress" in Managing Biomedical Technologies: Markets, Lotteries, and Rational Moral Standards in Organ Transplantation*, 31 Cap. U. L. Rev. 13, 29 (2003).

Journal 2002 Provides ethical arguments in favor of transplantation in HIV-infected patients. Concludes that preventing such transplants is unethical and discriminatory. References Opinions 2.16 and 9.131. Halpern, Ubel, & Caplan, *Solid-Organ Transplantation in HIV-Infected Patients, 347 New Eng. J. Med. 284, 287 (2002).*

Journal 2000 Examines the criteria for organ transplantation. Explores the use of cognitive ability as an exclusion criterion for organ transplantation in children. Concludes that other useful neurologic criteria can be established to inform equitable allocation decisions. References Opinion 2.16. Orr, Johnston, Ashwal, & Bailey, *Should Children With Severe Cognitive Impairment Receive Solid Organ Transplants? 11 J. Clinical Ethics 219, 222-23, 228 (2000).*

Journal 1999 Examines the new federal rule mandating broader organ allocation. Raises various constitutional questions, particularly with respect to state laws regulating allocation of organs. Suggests that Congress needs to develop clearer guidelines in this area. Quotes Opinion 2.16. Chen, *Organ Allocation and the States: Can the States Restrict Broader Organ Sharing? 49 Duke L. J. 261, 273 (1999).*

Journal 1999 Attributes distrust and dissatisfaction with managed care organizations to individualism and cynicism in society. Argues that proposed reforms will not solve society's problems with managed care organizations. Recommends an alternative health care system that would strike a balance between considerations of patient autonomy and cost containment. References Opinion 2.16. Harris, *The Regulation of Managed Care: Conquering Individualism and Cynicism in America, 6 Va. J. Soc. Pol'y. & L. 315, 329 (1999).*

Journal 1999 Discusses the need for physicians to advocate on behalf of patients' rights in the context of health care delivery. Evaluates the nature and scope of the physician's role as advocate, noting that physicians cannot be expected to engage in attorney-like advocacy. Quotes Principles IV and VI, Fundamental Elements (2), (4), and (6) [now Opinion 10.01], Patient Responsibilities 5 [now Opinion 10.02], and Opinions 2.03, 2.07, 2.09, 2.16, 2.19, 3.06, 4.01, 4.04, 6.01, 7.02, 8.02, 8.03, 8.13, 8.132, 9.06, 9.07, and 9.131. Cites Opinions 5.05, 5.09, 7.01, 8.135, and 9.02. Sage, *Physicians as Advocates, 35 Hous. L. Rev. 1529, 1537, 1541, 1542, 1552-53, 1554, 1556, 1557, 1559, 1561-62, 1564, 1571, 1574, 1576, 1580 (1999).*

Journal 1987 Discusses the issue of the right of the individual to consent to organ removal and then examines the doctrine of informed consent as it is applied in the context of live organ donation. Evaluates the extent to which removal of nonregenerative organs disrupts the basis for application of the traditional informed consent model with special attention to children and incompetent patients. Quotes Opinion 2.15 (1986) [now Opinion 2.16]. Adams, *Live Organ Donors and Informed Consent: A Difficult Minuet, 8 J. Legal Med. 555, 560-61 (1987).*

7 Research and Innovation

7.1.1 Physician Involvement in Research

N.J. 1980 Physician employed to do research sued pharmaceutical company for wrongful discharge claiming that as an employee at will she had a cause of action for termination following her refusal to continue research she viewed as medically unethical. The court held that an employee has a cause of action when discharged contrary to a clearly mandated public policy. However, the court affirmed summary judgment because human testing was not imminent and because plaintiff failed to demonstrate the existence of a clear public policy based upon any statements of medical ethics to support her refusal to continue work on controversial drug. The dissent argued that the Opinions and Reports of the Judicial Council 5.03 and 5.18 (1979) [now Opinion 2.07] and other medical ethical statements did provide a clear expression of public policy and that plaintiff's failure to specifically cite them was merely a technical defect, and not fatal. *Pierce v. Ortho Pharmaceutical Corp., 84 N. J. 58, 417 A.2d 505, 516, 518.*

Wyo. 2000 Physician sought judicial review of board of medicine's disciplinary order. Among its holdings, the board found the physician's participation in a patient case study using testing and treatment procedures of no proven medical efficacy was unprofessional conduct contrary to recognized standards of medical ethics. The board quoted and relied on Opinion 2.07. The Supreme Court reversed the board's decision for failure to provide expert testimony regarding whether the physician's conduct was contrary to the standards set out in Opinion 2.07. *Painter v. Abels, 998 P.2d 931, 935, 939.*

Journal 2010 Discusses the shortfalls and inadequacies of current informed consent protocols in the context of sham surgery–controlled trials. Concludes that investigating institutions should strengthen their informed consent protocols in this area. Cites Opinions 2.07 and 2.076. Bertram, *How Current Informed Consent Protocols Flunk the Sham Surgery Test: A New Frontier in Medicine and Ethics, 14 Quinnipiac Health L. J. 131, 133, 161-162 (2010).*

Journal 2007 Reviews recent essays on the regulation of biomedical research and laws governing conflicts of interest. Concludes that all aspects of research are financially driven and that civil liability is a strong deterrent to unethical practice. Quotes Opinion 2.07. Bergin, *Book Review: Law and Ethics in Biomedical Research: Regulation, Conflict of Interest, and Liability,* 23 Windsor Rev. Legal & Soc. Issues 117, 122 (2007).

Journal 2005 Proposes a therapeutic approach to be used by insurers in making decisions and communicating with patients about coverage for last-chance therapies. Concludes that an approach based upon conflict management rather than dispute resolution is better equipped to treat insureds as individuals. Cites Opinion 2.07. Cerminara, *Dealing With Dying: How Insurers Can Help Patients Seeking Last-Chance Therapies (Even When the Answer is "NO"),* 15 Health Matrix 285, 293-94 (2005).

Journal 2005 Examines potential legal issues that physician investigators face in conducting placebo-controlled trials. Concludes that physician investigators who harm patients by giving them a placebo may be subject to liability. Quotes Opinion 2.07. Glass & Waring, *The Physician/ Investigator's Obligation to Patients Participating in Research: The Case of Placebo Controlled Trials,* 33 J. L. Med. & Ethics, 575, 576 (2005).

Journal 2002 Challenges the general use of special informed consent disclosure rules in experimental therapy. Discusses the lack of a bright-line distinction between standard and experimental interventions. Concludes that focus should be placed on the distinctiveness of experimentation. Quotes Opinion 2.07. References Opinion 9.032. Noah, *Informed Consent and the Elusive Dichotomy Between Standard and Experimental Therapy,* 28 Am. J. L. & Med. 361, 394, 395 (2002).

Journal 2001 Considers conflicts of interest in clinical research and other types of medical practice. Compares the way in which doctors and lawyers address conflicts of interest in professional practice. Concludes that physicians are unaware of the need to create a meaningful conflict-of-interest doctrine for medical practice. Quotes Preamble, Principle IV, and Opinions 2.07, 8.03, 8.031, and 10.01. Moore, *What Doctors Can Learn From Lawyers About Conflicts of Interest,* 81 B. U. L. Rev. 445, 447, 449-50 (2001).

Journal 1999 Explores the duty to disclose genetic test results in research and clinical settings. Characterizes the legal duty to disclose. Concludes with guidelines regarding ways that medical researchers can reduce the potential for liability in this context. Quotes Opinion 2.07. Furman, *Genetic Test Results and the Duty to Disclose: Can Medical Researchers Control Liability?* 23 Seattle Univ. L. R. 391, 408-09 (1999).

Journal 1999 Discusses the need for physicians to advocate on behalf of patients' rights in the context of health care delivery. Evaluates the nature and scope of the physician's

role as advocate, noting that physicians cannot be expected to engage in attorney-like advocacy. Quotes Principles IV and VI, Fundamental Elements (2), (4), and (6) [now Opinion 10.01], Patient Responsibilities 5 [now Opinion 10.02], and Opinions 2.03, 2.07, 2.09, 2.16, 2.19, 3.06, 4.01, 4.04, 6.01, 7.02, 8.02, 8.03, 8.13, 8.132, 9.06, 9.07, and 9.131. Cites Opinions 5.05, 5.09, 7.01, 8.135, and 9.02. Sage, *Physicians as Advocates,* 35 Hous. L. Rev. 1529, 1537, 1541, 1542, 1552-53, 1554, 1556, 1557, 1559, 1561-62, 1564, 1571, 1574, 1576, 1580 (1999).

Journal 1998 Discusses conflicts of interest in the physician-patient relationship arising out of use of financial incentives by managed care organizations. Considers how such conflicts are dealt with in the attorney-client relationship. Suggests that a financial incentive should be legally denounced if it unreasonably interferes with a physician's duty to properly care for and treat patients. Quotes Preamble, Fundamental Elements (1) [now Opinion 10.01], and Opinions 4.04, 5.01, 8.03, 8.13, and 9.06. Cites Fundamental Elements (4) [now Opinion 10.01] and Opinions 2.07, 2.08, and 2.132. Hall, *Third-Party Payor Conflicts of Interest in Managed Care: A Proposal for Regulation Based on the Model Rules of Professional Conduct,* 29 Seton Hall L. Rev. 95, 96, 107, 108, 109, 110, 111, 112, 134, 135, 136 (1998).

Journal 1998 Discusses the use of mentally impaired individuals as research subjects. Argues that a common set of rules needs to be promulgated to protect the decisionally impaired from certain risks of human research. Quotes Opinion 2.07. Sundram, *In Harm's Way: Research Subjects Who Are Decisionally Impaired,* 1 J. Health Care L. & Pol'y 36, 43-44 (1998).

Journal 1997 Considers emergency room research informed consent standards. Reviews new federal regulations and related moral and ethical concerns. Concludes that regulations will require a case-by-case approach to balancing competing interests between research and ethics. References Opinion 2.07. Brody, *New Perspectives on Emergency Room Research,* 27 Hastings Center Rep. 7, 9 (Jan./Feb. 1997).

Journal 1997 Considers informed consent and the principle of self-determination. Analyzes the tradition of informed consent in medical research, with emphasis on international considerations. Concludes that research subjects need better protection. Cites Opinion 2.07. Note, *The Informed-Consent Policy of the International Conference on Harmonization of Technical Requirements for Registrations of Pharmaceuticals for Human Use: Knowledge Is the Best Medicine,* 30 Cornell Int'l L. J. 203, 209 (1997).

Journal 1993 Considers the legitimacy of neonatal HIV screening studies conducted without parental notice or consent. Asserts that such testing is morally and legally questionable. Quotes Opinion 2.07. Isaacman & Miller, *Neonatal HIV Seroprevalence Studies,* 14 J. Legal Med. 413, 428 (1993).

Journal 1989 Discusses various social control mechanisms that have an impact upon biomedical research. Emphasis is placed upon a comparison of the effectiveness of intra- and extraprofessional methods of control. References Opinion 2.07. Benson, *The Social Control of Human Biomedical Research: An Overview and Review of the Literature, 29 Soc. Sci. Med. 1, 3 (1989).*

Journal 2004 Evaluates weaknesses in institutional review board (IRB) protection of human subjects. Concludes that one vehicle for enhancing human subjects protection is to hold IRBs legally accountable for negligent conduct. Cites Opinions 2.071, 2.075, and 8.0315. Noah, *Bioethical Malpractice: Risk and Responsibility in Human Research, 7 J. Health Care L. & Pol'y 175, 183, 235 (2004).*

Journal 2003 Provides an update on the Declaration of Helsinki and the FDA's position on placebo-controlled medical research. Concludes that the FDA should reconsider its position in light of the principles articulated in the Declaration. Quotes Opinion 2.075. Michels & Rothman, *Update on Unethical Use of Placebos in Randomised Trials, 17 Bioethics 188, 200 (2003).*

Journal 2001 Reviews federal regulations and discusses challenges associated with developing guidelines relating to the use of placebos. Concludes that the use of placebo controls in human subjects research must be carefully regulated. Quotes Opinion 2.075. Hoffman, *The Use of Placebos in Clinical Trials: Responsible Research or Unethical Practice? 33 Conn. L. Rev. 449, 454-55, 496 (2001).*

Journal 2011 Reviews the responsible conduct of research (RCR) domains of publication practices and authorship, conflicts of interest, and research misconduct. Concludes that because the accuracy, completeness, and value of the scientific record impacts the health of society, scientists are obligated to use the highest possible standards of research conduct. Quotes Principle VIII and Opinion 8.031. Horner & Minifie, *Research Ethics III: Publication Practices and Authorship, Conflicts of Interest, and Research Misconduct, 54 J. Speech, Language, & Hearing Res. S346, S351, S352 (2011).*

Journal 2008 Examines the ethical issues surrounding stem cell research. Concludes science, religion, and politics are all important in appropriately addressing the ethics of scientific innovation. Cites Opinion 8.031. Packer, *Embryonic Stem Cells, Intellectual Property, and Patents: Ethical Concerns, 37 Hofstra L. Rev. 487, 495 (2008).*

Journal 2007 Analyzes scientific, ethical, and legal issues raised in the exhumation and genetic analysis of historical figures. Concludes that biohistorical review boards should be created to generate guidelines for such research. Quotes Preamble and Opinion 2.08. Cites Opinions 2.079, 2.105, 5.05, 5.051, 5.075, 8.03, 8.031, 9.095, and 9.10. Paradise & Andrews, *Tales From the Crypt: Scientific, Ethical, and Legal Considerations for Biohistorical Analysis of Deceased Historical Figures, 26 Temp. J. Sci. Tech. & Envtl. L. 223, 287-88 (2007).*

Journal 2005 Discusses ethical, legal, and policy issues associated with treatment and research involving patients who are in a persistent vegetative or minimally conscious state. Concludes that patients in these states are at risk for therapeutic failures until physicians can more accurately determine which patients will benefit from treatment and accurately convey such information to families or surrogates. Quotes Principles VII and IX and Opinions 8.031, 8.0315, 9.065, 10.01, and 10.015. Tovino & Winslade, *A Primer on the Law and Ethics of Treatment, Research, and Public Policy in the Context of Severe Traumatic Brain Injury, 14 Ann. Health L. 1, 18, 38, 39, 40, 41 (2005).*

Journal 2004 Examines the requirements of the Privacy Rule regarding use and disclosure of a patient's identifiable health information in the context of research. Concludes that the Rule's burdensome administrative requirements may discourage research and thus outweigh any benefits for research subject autonomy. Quotes Principle VIII and Opinions 5.051, 8.031, and 10.015. Tovino, *The Use and Disclosure of Protected Health Information for Research Under the HIPAA Privacy Rule: Unrealized Patient Autonomy and Burdensome Government Regulation, 49 S. D. L. Rev. 447, 496, 502 (2004).*

Journal 2003 Discusses financial incentive programs for physicians who enroll patients in clinical trials. Concludes that more regulatory oversight is needed to protect research subjects and the integrity of the medical research process. Quotes Opinion 6.03 and 8.031. Lemmens & Miller, *The Human Subjects Trade: Ethical and Legal Issues Surrounding Recruitment Incentives, 31 J. L. Med. & Ethics 398, 407 (2003).*

Journal 2002 Considers the implications of using pharmacogenomics in drug development and health care delivery. Emphasizes various legal, economic, and social issues. Concludes that these issues must be meaningfully addressed given the benefits of pharmacogenomics. Cites Opinion 8.031. Malinowski, *Law, Policy, and Market Implications of Genetic Profiling in Drug Development, 2 Hous. J. Health L. & Pol'y 31, 51 (2002).*

Journal 2002 Discusses ethical and legal issues involving acquisition of biological specimens by commercial biobanks. Sets forth areas of inquiry for institutional review boards in evaluating the propriety of research collaborations with commercial biobanks. Cites Opinion 8.031. Rothstein, *The Role of IRBs in Research Involving Commercial Biobanks, 30 J. Law Med. & Ethics 105, 106, 108 (2002).*

Journal 2001 Explores institutional conflicts of interest arising from the impact of biotechnology and the genetics revolution on clinical research. Concludes that federal oversight changes should be implemented in order to maintain the public's trust in health science. Quotes Opinion 8.031. Malinowski, *Conflicts of Interest in Clinical Research: Legal and Ethical Issues: Institutional Conflicts and Responsibilities in an Age of Academic-Industry Alliances, 8 Wid. L. Symp. J. 47, 70 (2001).*

Journal 2001 Examines financial conflict of interest issues that arise in the context of clinical research. Concludes that open communication among stakeholders is necessary to resolve these issues. Quotes Opinions 8.03 and 8.031. Rose, *Financial Conflicts of Interest: How Are We Managing? 8 Wid. L. Symp. J. 1, 24 (2001).*

Journal 1996 Explores biotechnology advances made possible through cooperation between universities and industries. Observes that clinical investigators involved in company research are ethically prohibited from buying or selling company stock, until results are published. Concludes that cooperation in the biotechnology field will benefit society. Cites Opinion 8.031. Comment, *Alliances for the Future: Cultivating a Cooperative Environment for Biotech Success, 11 Berkeley Tech. L. J. 311, 344 (1996).*

Journal 1991 Considers whether patients should be permitted or required to pay for research in which they participate. Concludes that patient-funded research may be useful, so long as the potential for individual harm and abuse can be minimized. References Opinion 8.031. Morreim, *Patient-Funded Research: Paying the Piper or Protecting the Patient? 13 IRB 1, 2 (May/June 1991).*

Journal 1991 Discusses the ethical issues involved when physicians and scientists enroll patients in drug company–sponsored clinical trials in exchange for reimbursement. Concludes that financial arrangements between drug companies and scientists give the appearance and the opportunity for conflict of interest; thus physicians should be required to disclose funding sources to patients. References Opinion 8.031. Shimm & Spece, *Conflict of Interest and Informed Consent in Industry-Sponsored Clinical Trials, 12 J. Legal Med. 477, 481, 507, 510 (1991).*

Journal 2004 Discusses the effect of state regulatory requirements on drug companies conducting clinical research. Concludes that, although FDA requirements are compelling, drug companies also must carefully consider applicable state regulations. Quotes Opinion 8.0315. Gibbs, *State Regulation of Pharmaceutical Clinical Trials, 59 Food & Drug L. J. 265, 279 (2004).*

7.1.2 Informed Consent in Research

N.J. 1980 Physician employed to do research sued pharmaceutical company for wrongful discharge claiming that as an employee at will she had a cause of action for termination following her refusal to continue research she viewed as medically unethical. The court held that an employee has a cause of action when discharged contrary to a clearly mandated public policy. However, the court affirmed summary judgment because human testing was not imminent and because plaintiff failed to demonstrate the existence of a clear public policy based upon any statements of medical ethics to support her refusal to continue work on controversial drug. The dissent argued that the Opinions and Reports of the Judicial Council 5.03 and 5.18 (1979) [now Opinion 2.07] and other medical ethical statements did provide a clear expression of public policy and that plaintiff's failure to specifically cite them was merely a technical defect, and not fatal. *Pierce v. Ortho Pharmaceutical Corp., 84 N. J. 58, 417 A.2d 505, 516, 518.*

Wyo. 2000 Physician sought judicial review of board of medicine's disciplinary order. Among its holdings, the board found the physician's participation in a patient case study using testing and treatment procedures of no proven medical efficacy was unprofessional conduct contrary to recognized standards of medical ethics. The board quoted and relied on Opinion 2.07. The Supreme Court reversed the board's decision for failure to provide expert testimony regarding whether the physician's conduct was contrary to the standards set out in Opinion 2.07. *Painter v. Abels, 998 P.2d 931, 935, 939.*

Journal 2010 Discusses the shortfalls and inadequacies of current informed consent protocols in the context of sham surgery–controlled trials. Concludes that investigating institutions should strengthen their informed consent protocols in this area. Cites Opinions 2.07 and 2.076. Bertram, *How Current Informed Consent Protocols Flunk the Sham Surgery Test: A New Frontier in Medicine and Ethics, 14 Quinnipiac Health L. J. 131, 133, 161-162 (2010).*

Journal 2007 Reviews recent essays on the regulation of biomedical research and laws governing conflicts of interest. Concludes that all aspects of research are financially driven and that civil liability is a strong deterrent to unethical practice. Quotes Opinion 2.07. Bergin, *Book Review: Law and Ethics in Biomedical Research: Regulation, Conflict of Interest, and Liability, 23 Windsor Rev. Legal & Soc. Issues 117, 122 (2007).*

Journal 2005 Proposes a therapeutic approach to be used by insurers in making decisions and communicating with patients about coverage for last-chance therapies. Concludes that an approach based upon conflict management rather than dispute resolution is better equipped to treat insureds as individuals. Cites Opinion 2.07. Cerminara, *Dealing With Dying: How Insurers Can Help Patients Seeking Last-Chance Therapies (Even When the Answer is "NO"), 15 Health Matrix 285, 293-94 (2005).*

Journal 2005 Examines potential legal issues that physician investigators face in conducting placebo-controlled trials. Concludes that physician investigators who harm patients by giving them a placebo may be subject to liability. Quotes Opinion 2.07. Glass & Waring, *The Physician/ Investigator's Obligation to Patients Participating in Research: The Case* *of Placebo Controlled Trials, 33 J. L. Med. & Ethics, 575, 576 (2005).*

Journal 2002 Challenges the general use of special informed consent disclosure rules in experimental therapy. Discusses the lack of a bright-line distinction between standard and experimental interventions. Concludes that focus should be placed on the distinctiveness of experimentation. Quotes Opinion 2.07. References Opinion 9.032. Noah, *Informed Consent and the Elusive Dichotomy Between Standard and Experimental Therapy, 28 Am. J. L. & Med. 361, 394, 395 (2002).*

Journal 2001 Considers conflicts of interest in clinical research and other types of medical practice. Compares the way in which doctors and lawyers address conflicts of interest in professional practice. Concludes that physicians are unaware of the need to create a meaningful conflict-of-interest doctrine for medical practice. Quotes Preamble, Principle IV, and Opinions 2.07, 8.03, 8.031, and 10.01. Moore, *What Doctors Can Learn From Lawyers About Conflicts of Interest, 81 B. U. L. Rev. 445, 447, 449-50 (2001).*

Journal 1999 Explores the duty to disclose genetic test results in research and clinical settings. Characterizes the legal duty to disclose. Concludes with guidelines regarding ways that medical researchers can reduce the potential for liability in this context. Quotes Opinion 2.07. Furman, *Genetic Test Results and the Duty to Disclose: Can Medical Researchers Control Liability? 23 Seattle Univ. L. R. 391, 408-09 (1999).*

Journal 1999 Discusses the need for physicians to advocate on behalf of patients' rights in the context of health care delivery. Evaluates the nature and scope of the physician's role as advocate, noting that physicians cannot be expected to engage in attorney-like advocacy. Quotes Principles IV and VI, Fundamental Elements (2), (4), and (6) [now Opinion 10.01], Patient Responsibilities 5 [now Opinion 10.02], and Opinions 2.03, 2.07, 2.09, 2.16, 2.19, 3.06, 4.01, 4.04, 6.01, 7.02, 8.02, 8.03, 8.13, 8.132, 9.06, 9.07, and 9.131. Cites Opinions 5.05, 5.09, 7.01, 8.135, and 9.02. Sage, *Physicians as Advocates, 35 Hous. L. Rev. 1529, 1537, 1541, 1542, 1552-53, 1554, 1556, 1557, 1559, 1561-62, 1564, 1571, 1574, 1576, 1580 (1999).*

Journal 1998 Discusses conflicts of interest in the physician-patient relationship arising out of use of financial incentives by managed care organizations. Considers how such conflicts are dealt with in the attorney-client relationship. Suggests that a financial incentive should be legally denounced if it unreasonably interferes with a physician's duty to properly care for and treat patients. Quotes Preamble, Fundamental Elements (1) [now Opinion 10.01], and Opinions 4.04, 5.01, 8.03, 8.13, and 9.06. Cites Fundamental Elements (4) [now Opinion 10.01] and Opinions 2.07, 2.08, and 2.132. Hall, *Third-Party Payor Conflicts of Interest in Managed Care: A Proposal for Regulation Based on the*

Model Rules of Professional Conduct, 29 Seton Hall L. Rev. 95, 96, 107, 108, 109, 110, 111, 112, 134, 135, 136 (1998).

Journal 1998 Discusses the use of mentally impaired individuals as research subjects. Argues that a common set of rules needs to be promulgated to protect the decisionally impaired from certain risks of human research. Quotes Opinion 2.07. Sundram, *In Harm's Way: Research Subjects Who Are Decisionally Impaired, 1 J. Health Care L. & Pol'y 36, 43-44 (1998).*

Journal 1997 Considers emergency room research informed consent standards. Reviews new federal regulations and related moral and ethical concerns. Concludes that regulations will require a case-by-case approach to balancing competing interests between research and ethics. References Opinion 2.07. Brody, *New Perspectives on Emergency Room Research, 27 Hastings Center Rep. 7, 9 (Jan./Feb. 1997).*

Journal 1997 Considers informed consent and the principle of self-determination. Analyzes the tradition of informed consent in medical research, with emphasis on international considerations. Concludes that research subjects need better protection. Cites Opinion 2.07. Note, *The Informed-Consent Policy of the International Conference on Harmonization of Technical Requirements for Registrations of Pharmaceuticals for Human Use: Knowledge Is the Best Medicine, 30 Cornell Int'l L. J. 203, 209 (1997).*

Journal 1993 Considers the legitimacy of neonatal HIV screening studies conducted without parental notice or consent. Asserts that such testing is morally and legally questionable. Quotes Opinion 2.07. Isaacman & Miller, *Neonatal HIV Seroprevalence Studies, 14 J. Legal Med. 413, 428 (1993).*

Journal 1989 Discusses various social control mechanisms that have an impact upon biomedical research. Emphasis is placed upon a comparison of the effectiveness of intra- and extraprofessional methods of control. References Opinion 2.07. Benson, *The Social Control of Human Biomedical Research: An Overview and Review of the Literature, 29 Soc. Sci. Med. 1, 3 (1989).*

Journal 2005 Discusses ethical, legal, and policy issues associated with treatment and research involving patients who are in a persistent vegetative or minimally conscious state. Concludes that patients in these states are at risk for therapeutic failures until physicians can more accurately determine which patients will benefit from treatment and accurately convey such information to families or surrogates. Quotes Principles VII and IX and Opinions 8.031, 8.0315, 9.065, 10.01, and 10.015. Tovino & Winslade, *A Primer on the Law and Ethics of Treatment, Research, and Public Policy in the Context of Severe Traumatic Brain Injury, 14 Ann. Health L. 1, 18, 38, 39, 40, 41 (2005).*

Journal 2004 Discusses the effect of state regulatory requirements on drug companies conducting clinical research. Concludes that, although FDA requirements are compelling, drug companies also must carefully consider applicable state regulations. Quotes Opinion 8.0315. Gibbs, *State Regulation of Pharmaceutical Clinical Trials, 59 Food & Drug L. J. 265, 279 (2004).*

Journal 2004 Evaluates weaknesses in institutional review board (IRB) protection of human subjects. Concludes that one vehicle for enhancing human subjects protection is to hold IRBs legally accountable for negligent conduct. Cites Opinions 2.071, 2.075, and 8.0315. Noah, *Bioethical*

Malpractice: Risk and Responsibility in Human Research, 7 J. Health Care L. & Pol'y 175, 183, 235 (2004).

Journal 2006 Discusses the evolution of health law in Virginia. Concludes that the area of health law continues to expand, develop, and be refined. Cites Opinions 3.03, 3.08, 5.01, 5.015, 5.02, 5.04, 5.055, 6.02, 6.021, 6.03, 6.04, 7.03, 7.04, 7.05, 8.054, 8.08, 8.081, 8.085, 8.115, 8.12, 8.14, 8.145, 8.19, and 9.045. Guanzon, *Health Care Law, 41 U. Rich. L. Rev. 179, 199 (2006).*

7.1.3 Study Design and Sampling

N.J. 1980 Physician employed to do research sued pharmaceutical company for wrongful discharge claiming that as an employee at will she had a cause of action for termination following her refusal to continue research she viewed as medically unethical. The court held that an employee has a cause of action when discharged contrary to a clearly mandated public policy. However, the court affirmed summary judgment because human testing was not imminent and because plaintiff failed to demonstrate the existence of a clear public policy based upon any statements of medical ethics to support her refusal to continue work on controversial drug. The dissent argued that the Opinions and Reports of the Judicial Council 5.03 and 5.18 (1979) [now Opinion 2.07] and other medical ethical statements did provide a clear expression of public policy and that plaintiff's failure to specifically cite them was merely a technical defect, and not fatal. *Pierce v. Ortho Pharmaceutical Corp., 84 N. J. 58, 417 A.2d 505, 516, 518.*

Wyo. 2000 Physician sought judicial review of board of medicine's disciplinary order. Among its holdings, the board found the physician's participation in a patient case study using testing and treatment procedures of no proven medical efficacy was unprofessional conduct contrary to recognized standards of medical ethics. The board quoted and relied on Opinion 2.07. The Supreme Court reversed the board's decision for failure to provide expert testimony regarding whether the physician's conduct was contrary to the standards set out in Opinion 2.07. *Painter v. Abels, 998 P.2d 931, 935, 939.*

Journal 2010 Discusses the shortfalls and inadequacies of current informed consent protocols in the context of sham surgery–controlled trials. Concludes that investigating institutions should strengthen their informed consent protocols in this area. Cites Opinions 2.07 and 2.076. Bertram, *How Current Informed Consent Protocols Flunk the Sham Surgery Test: A New Frontier in Medicine and Ethics, 14 Quinnipiac Health L. J. 131, 133, 161-162 (2010).*

Journal 2007 Reviews recent essays on the regulation of biomedical research and laws governing conflicts of interest. Concludes that all aspects of research are financially driven and that civil liability is a strong deterrent to unethical practice. Quotes Opinion 2.07. Bergin, *Book Review: Law*

and Ethics in Biomedical Research: Regulation, Conflict of Interest, and Liability, 23 Windsor Rev. Legal & Soc. Issues 117, 122 (2007).

Journal 2005 Proposes a therapeutic approach to be used by insurers in making decisions and communicating with patients about coverage for last-chance therapies. Concludes that an approach based upon conflict management rather than dispute resolution is better equipped to treat insureds as individuals. Cites Opinion 2.07. Cerminara, *Dealing With Dying: How Insurers Can Help Patients Seeking Last-Chance Therapies (Even When the Answer is "NO"), 15 Health Matrix 285, 293-94 (2005).*

Journal 2005 Examines potential legal issues that physician investigators face in conducting placebo-controlled trials. Concludes that physician investigators who harm patients by giving them a placebo may be subject to liability. Quotes Opinion 2.07. Glass & Waring, *The Physician/ Investigator's Obligation to Patients Participating in Research: The Case of Placebo Controlled Trials, 33 J. L. Med. & Ethics, 575, 576 (2005).*

Journal 2002 Challenges the general use of special informed consent disclosure rules in experimental therapy. Discusses the lack of a bright-line distinction between standard and experimental interventions. Concludes that focus should be placed on the distinctiveness of experimentation. Quotes Opinion 2.07. References Opinion 9.032. Noah, *Informed Consent and the Elusive Dichotomy Between Standard and Experimental Therapy, 28 Am. J. L. & Med. 361, 394, 395 (2002).*

Journal 2001 Considers conflicts of interest in clinical research and other types of medical practice. Compares the way in which doctors and lawyers address conflicts of interest in professional practice. Concludes that physicians are unaware of the need to create a meaningful conflict-of-interest doctrine for medical practice. Quotes Preamble, Principle IV, and Opinions 2.07, 8.03, 8.031, and 10.01. Moore, *What Doctors Can Learn From Lawyers About Conflicts of Interest, 81 B. U. L. Rev. 445, 447, 449-50 (2001).*

Journal 1999 Explores the duty to disclose genetic test results in research and clinical settings. Characterizes the legal duty to disclose. Concludes with guidelines regarding ways that medical researchers can reduce the potential for liability in this context. Quotes Opinion 2.07. Furman, *Genetic Test Results and the Duty to Disclose: Can Medical Researchers Control Liability? 23 Seattle Univ. L. R. 391, 408-09 (1999)*.

Journal 1999 Discusses the need for physicians to advocate on behalf of patients' rights in the context of health care delivery. Evaluates the nature and scope of the physician's role as advocate, noting that physicians cannot be expected to engage in attorney-like advocacy. Quotes Principles IV and VI, Fundamental Elements (2), (4), and (6) [now Opinion 10.01], Patient Responsibilities 5 [now Opinion 10.02], and Opinions 2.03, 2.07, 2.09, 2.16, 2.19, 3.06, 4.01, 4.04, 6.01, 7.02, 8.02, 8.03, 8.13, 8.132, 9.06, 9.07, and 9.131. Cites Opinions 5.05, 5.09, 7.01, 8.135, and 9.02. Sage, *Physicians as Advocates, 35 Hous. L. Rev. 1529, 1537, 1541, 1542, 1552-53, 1554, 1556, 1557, 1559, 1561-62, 1564, 1571, 1574, 1576, 1580 (1999)*.

Journal 1998 Discusses conflicts of interest in the physician-patient relationship arising out of use of financial incentives by managed care organizations. Considers how such conflicts are dealt with in the attorney-client relationship. Suggests that a financial incentive should be legally denounced if it unreasonably interferes with a physician's duty to properly care for and treat patients. Quotes Preamble, Fundamental Elements (1) [now Opinion 10.01], and Opinions 4.04, 5.01, 8.03, 8.13, and 9.06. Cites Fundamental Elements (4) [now Opinion 10.01] and Opinions 2.07, 2.08, and 2.132. Hall, *Third-Party Payor Conflicts of Interest in Managed Care: A Proposal for Regulation Based on the Model Rules of Professional Conduct, 29 Seton Hall L. Rev. 95, 96, 107, 108, 109, 110, 111, 112, 134, 135, 136 (1998)*.

Journal 1998 Discusses the use of mentally impaired individuals as research subjects. Argues that a common set of rules needs to be promulgated to protect the decisionally impaired from certain risks of human research. Quotes Opinion 2.07. Sundram, *In Harm's Way: Research Subjects Who Are Decisionally Impaired, 1 J. Health Care L. & Pol'y 36, 43-44 (1998)*.

Journal 1997 Considers emergency room research informed consent standards. Reviews new federal regulations and related moral and ethical concerns. Concludes that regulations will require a case-by-case approach to balancing competing interests between research and ethics. References Opinion 2.07. Brody, *New Perspectives on Emergency Room Research, 27 Hastings Center Rep. 7, 9 (Jan./Feb. 1997)*.

Journal 1997 Considers informed consent and the principle of self-determination. Analyzes the tradition of informed consent in medical research, with emphasis on international considerations. Concludes that research subjects need better protection. Cites Opinion 2.07. Note, *The Informed-Consent Policy of the International Conference on Harmonization of Technical Requirements for Registrations of Pharmaceuticals for Human Use: Knowledge Is the Best Medicine, 30 Cornell Int'l L. J. 203, 209 (1997)*.

Journal 1993 Considers the legitimacy of neonatal HIV screening studies conducted without parental notice or consent. Asserts that such testing is morally and legally questionable. Quotes Opinion 2.07. Isaacman & Miller, *Neonatal HIV Seroprevalence Studies, 14 J. Legal Med. 413, 428 (1993)*.

Journal 1989 Discusses various social control mechanisms that have an impact upon biomedical research. Emphasis is placed upon a comparison of the effectiveness of intra- and extraprofessional methods of control. References Opinion 2.07. Benson, *The Social Control of Human Biomedical Research: An Overview and Review of the Literature, 29 Soc. Sci. Med. 1, 3 (1989)*.

Journal 2004 Evaluates weaknesses in institutional review board (IRB) protection of human subjects. Concludes that one vehicle for enhancing human subjects protection is to hold IRBs legally accountable for negligent conduct. Cites Opinions 2.071, 2.075, and 8.0315. Noah, *Bioethical Malpractice: Risk and Responsibility in Human Research, 7 J. Health Care L. & Pol'y 175, 183, 235 (2004)*.

7.1.4 Conflicts of Interest in Research

Journal 2011 Reviews the responsible conduct of research (RCR) domains of publication practices and authorship, conflicts of interest, and research misconduct. Concludes that because the accuracy, completeness, and value of the scientific record impacts the health of society, scientists are obligated to use the highest possible standards of research conduct. Quotes Principle VIII and Opinion 8.031. Horner & Minifie, *Research Ethics III: Publication Practices and Authorship, Conflicts of Interest, and Research Misconduct, 54 J. Speech, Language, & Hearing Res. S346, S351, S352 (2011)*.

Journal 2008 Examines the ethical issues surrounding stem cell research. Concludes science, religion, and politics are all important in appropriately addressing the ethics of scientific innovation. Cites Opinion 8.031. Packer, *Embryonic Stem Cells, Intellectual Property, and Patents: Ethical Concerns, 37 Hofstra L. Rev. 487, 495 (2008)*.

Journal 2007 Analyzes scientific, ethical, and legal issues raised in the exhumation and genetic analysis of historical figures. Concludes that biohistorical review boards should be created to generate guidelines for such research. Quotes Preamble and Opinion 2.08. Cites Opinions 2.079, 2.105, 5.05, 5.051, 5.075, 8.03, 8.031, 9.095, and 9.10. Paradise

& Andrews, *Tales From the Crypt: Scientific, Ethical, and Legal Considerations for Biohistorical Analysis of Deceased Historical Figures*, 26 Temp. J. Sci. Tech. & Envtl. L. 223, 287-88 (2007).

Journal 2005 Discusses ethical, legal, and policy issues associated with treatment and research involving patients who are in a persistent vegetative or minimally conscious state. Concludes that patients in these states are at risk for therapeutic failures until physicians can more accurately determine which patients will benefit from treatment and accurately convey such information to families or surrogates. Quotes Principles VII and IX and Opinions 8.031, 8.0315, 9.065, 10.01, and 10.015. Tovino & Winslade, *A Primer on the Law and Ethics of Treatment, Research, and Public Policy in the Context of Severe Traumatic Brain Injury*, 14 Ann. Health L. 1, 18, 38, 39, 40, 41 (2005).

Journal 2004 Examines the requirements of the Privacy Rule regarding use and disclosure of a patient's identifiable health information in the context of research. Concludes that the Rule's burdensome administrative requirements may discourage research and thus outweigh any benefits for research subject autonomy. Quotes Principle VIII and Opinions 5.051, 8.031, and 10.015. Tovino, *The Use and Disclosure of Protected Health Information for Research Under the HIPAA Privacy Rule: Unrealized Patient Autonomy and Burdensome Government Regulation*, 49 S. D. L. Rev. 447, 496, 502 (2004).

Journal 2003 Discusses financial incentive programs for physicians who enroll patients in clinical trials. Concludes that more regulatory oversight is needed to protect research subjects and the integrity of the medical research process. Quotes Opinion 6.03 and 8.031. Lemmens & Miller, *The Human Subjects Trade: Ethical and Legal Issues Surrounding Recruitment Incentives*, 31 J. L. Med. & Ethics 398, 407 (2003).

Journal 2002 Considers the implications of using pharmacogenomics in drug development and health care delivery. Emphasizes various legal, economic, and social issues. Concludes that these issues must be meaningfully addressed given the benefits of pharmacogenomics. Cites Opinion 8.031. Malinowski, *Law, Policy, and Market Implications of Genetic Profiling in Drug Development*, 2 Hous. J. Health L. & Pol'y 31, 51 (2002).

Journal 2002 Discusses ethical and legal issues involving acquisition of biological specimens by commercial biobanks. Sets forth areas of inquiry for institutional review boards in evaluating the propriety of research collaborations with commercial biobanks. Cites Opinion 8.031. Rothstein, *The Role of IRBs in Research Involving Commercial Biobanks*, 30 J. Law Med. & Ethics 105, 106, 108 (2002).

Journal 2001 Explores institutional conflicts of interest arising from the impact of biotechnology and the genetics revolution on clinical research. Concludes that federal oversight changes should be implemented in order to maintain the public's trust in health science. Quotes Opinion 8.031.

Malinowski, *Conflicts of Interest in Clinical Research: Legal and Ethical Issues: Institutional Conflicts and Responsibilities in an Age of Academic-Industry Alliances*, 8 Wid. L. Symp. J. 47, 70 (2001).

Journal 2001 Considers conflicts of interest in clinical research and other types of medical practice. Compares the way in which doctors and lawyers address conflicts of interest in professional practice. Concludes that physicians are unaware of the need to create a meaningful conflict-of-interest doctrine for medical practice. Quotes Preamble, Principle IV, and Opinions 2.07, 8.03, 8.031, and 10.01. Moore, *What Doctors Can Learn From Lawyers About Conflicts of Interest*, 81 B. U. L. Rev. 445, 447, 449-50 (2001).

Journal 2001 Examines financial conflict of interest issues that arise in the context of clinical research. Concludes that open communication among stakeholders is necessary to resolve these issues. Quotes Opinions 8.03 and 8.031. Rose, *Financial Conflicts of Interest: How Are We Managing?* 8 Wid. L. Symp. J. 1, 24 (2001).

Journal 1996 Explores biotechnology advances made possible through cooperation between universities and industries. Observes that clinical investigators involved in company research are ethically prohibited from buying or selling company stock, until results are published. Concludes that cooperation in the biotechnology field will benefit society. Cites Opinion 8.031. Comment, *Alliances for the Future: Cultivating a Cooperative Environment for Biotech Success*, 11 Berkeley Tech. L. J. 311, 344 (1996).

Journal 1991 Considers whether patients should be permitted or required to pay for research in which they participate. Concludes that patient-funded research may be useful, so long as the potential for individual harm and abuse can be minimized. References Opinion 8.031. Morreim, *Patient-Funded Research: Paying the Piper or Protecting the Patient?* 13 IRB 1, 2 (May/June 1991).

Journal 1991 Discusses the ethical issues involved when physicians and scientists enroll patients in drug company–sponsored clinical trials in exchange for reimbursement. Concludes that financial arrangements between drug companies and scientists give the appearance and the opportunity for conflict of interest; thus physicians should be required to disclose funding sources to patients. References Opinion 8.031. Shimm & Spece, *Conflict of Interest and Informed Consent in Industry-Sponsored Clinical Trials*, 12 J. Legal Med. 477, 481, 507, 510 (1991).

Journal 2004 Discusses the effect of state regulatory requirements on drug companies conducting clinical research. Concludes that, although FDA requirements are compelling, drug companies also must carefully consider applicable state regulations. Quotes Opinion 8.0315. Gibbs, *State Regulation of Pharmaceutical Clinical Trials*, 59 Food & Drug L. J. 265, 279 (2004).

Journal 2004 Evaluates weaknesses in institutional review board (IRB) protection of human subjects. Concludes that one vehicle for enhancing human subjects protection is to hold IRBs legally accountable for negligent conduct.

Cites Opinions 2.071, 2.075, and 8.0315. Noah, *Bioethical Malpractice: Risk and Responsibility in Human Research, 7 J. Health Care L. & Pol'y 175, 183, 235 (2004).*

7.1.5 Misconduct in Research

NJ 1980 Physician employed to do research sued pharmaceutical company for wrongful discharge claiming that as an employee at will she had a cause of action for termination following her refusal to continue research she viewed as medically unethical. The court held that an employee has a cause of action when discharged contrary to a clearly mandated public policy. However, the court affirmed summary judgment because human testing was not imminent and because plaintiff failed to demonstrate the existence of a clear public policy based upon any statements of medical ethics to support her refusal to continue work on controversial drug. The dissent argued that the Opinions and Reports of the Judicial Council 5.03 and 5.18 (1979) [now Opinion 2.07] and other medical ethical statements did provide a clear expression of public policy and that plaintiff's failure to specifically cite them was merely a technical defect, and not fatal. *Pierce v. Ortho Pharmaceutical Corp., 84 N. J. 58, 417 A.2d 505, 516, 518.*

Wyo. 2000 Physician sought judicial review of board of medicine's disciplinary order. Among its holdings, the board found the physician's participation in a patient case study using testing and treatment procedures of no proven medical efficacy was unprofessional conduct contrary to recognized standards of medical ethics. The board quoted and relied on Opinion 2.07. The Supreme Court reversed the board's decision for failure to provide expert testimony regarding whether the physician's conduct was contrary to the standards set out in Opinion 2.07. *Painter v. Abels, 998 P.2d 931, 935, 939.*

Journal 2010 Discusses the shortfalls and inadequacies of current informed consent protocols in the context of sham surgery–controlled trials. Concludes that investigating institutions should strengthen their informed consent protocols in this area. Cites Opinions 2.07 and 2.076. Bertram, *How Current Informed Consent Protocols Flunk the Sham Surgery Test: A New Frontier in Medicine and Ethics, 14 Quinnipiac Health L. J. 131, 133, 161-162 (2010).*

Journal 2007 Reviews recent essays on the regulation of biomedical research and laws governing conflicts of interest. Concludes that all aspects of research are financially driven and that civil liability is a strong deterrent to unethical practice. Quotes Opinion 2.07. Bergin, *Book Review: Law and Ethics in Biomedical Research: Regulation, Conflict of Interest, and Liability, 23 Windsor Rev. Legal & Soc. Issues 117, 122 (2007).*

Journal 2005 Proposes a therapeutic approach to be used by insurers in making decisions and communicating with patients about coverage for last-chance therapies. Concludes that an approach based upon conflict management rather than dispute resolution is better equipped to treat insureds as individuals. Cites Opinion 2.07. Cerminara, *Dealing With Dying: How Insurers Can Help Patients Seeking Last-Chance Therapies (Even When the Answer is "NO"), 15 Health Matrix 285, 293-94 (2005).*

Journal 2005 Examines potential legal issues that physician investigators face in conducting placebo-controlled trials. Concludes that physician investigators who harm patients by giving them a placebo may be subject to liability. Quotes Opinion 2.07. Glass & Waring, *The Physician/ Investigator's Obligation to Patients Participating in Research: The Case of Placebo Controlled Trials, 33 J. L. Med. & Ethics, 575, 576 (2005).*

Journal 2002 Challenges the general use of special informed consent disclosure rules in experimental therapy. Discusses the lack of a bright-line distinction between standard and experimental interventions. Concludes that focus should be placed on the distinctiveness of experimentation. Quotes Opinion 2.07. References Opinion 9.032. Noah, *Informed Consent and the Elusive Dichotomy Between Standard and Experimental Therapy, 28 Am. J. L. & Med. 361, 394, 395 (2002).*

Journal 2001 Considers conflicts of interest in clinical research and other types of medical practice. Compares the way in which doctors and lawyers address conflicts of interest in professional practice. Concludes that physicians are unaware of the need to create a meaningful conflict-of-interest doctrine for medical practice. Quotes Preamble, Principle IV, and Opinions 2.07, 8.03, 8.031, and 10.01. Moore, *What Doctors Can Learn From Lawyers About Conflicts of Interest, 81 B. U. L. Rev. 445, 447, 449-50 (2001).*

Journal 1999 Explores the duty to disclose genetic test results in research and clinical settings. Characterizes the legal duty to disclose. Concludes with guidelines regarding ways that medical researchers can reduce the potential for liability in this context. Quotes Opinion 2.07. Furman, *Genetic Test Results and the Duty to Disclose: Can Medical Researchers Control Liability? 23 Seattle Univ. L. R. 391, 408-09 (1999).*

Journal 1999 Discusses the need for physicians to advocate on behalf of patients' rights in the context of health care delivery. Evaluates the nature and scope of the physician's role as advocate, noting that physicians cannot be expected to engage in attorney-like advocacy. Quotes Principles IV and VI, Fundamental Elements (2), (4), and (6) [now Opinion 10.01], Patient Responsibilities 5 [now Opinion 10.02], and Opinions 2.03, 2.07, 2.09, 2.16, 2.19, 3.06, 4.01, 4.04, 6.01, 7.02, 8.02, 8.03, 8.13, 8.132, 9.06, 9.07, and 9.131. Cites Opinions 5.05, 5.09, 7.01, 8.135, and 9.02. Sage, *Physicians as Advocates, 35 Hous. L. Rev. 1529, 1537, 1541, 1542, 1552-53, 1554, 1556, 1557, 1559, 1561-62, 1564, 1571, 1574, 1576, 1580 (1999).*

Journal 1998 Discusses conflicts of interest in the physician-patient relationship arising out of use of financial incentives by managed care organizations. Considers how such conflicts are dealt with in the attorney-client relationship. Suggests that a financial incentive should be legally denounced if it unreasonably interferes with a physician's duty to properly care for and treat patients. Quotes Preamble, Fundamental Elements (1) [now Opinion 10.01], and Opinions 4.04, 5.01, 8.03, 8.13, and 9.06. Cites Fundamental Elements (4) [now Opinion 10.01] and Opinions 2.07, 2.08, and 2.132. Hall, *Third-Party Payor Conflicts of Interest in Managed Care: A Proposal for Regulation Based on the Model Rules of Professional Conduct, 29 Seton Hall L. Rev. 95, 96, 107, 108, 109, 110, 111, 112, 134, 135, 136 (1998).*

Journal 1998 Discusses the use of mentally impaired individuals as research subjects. Argues that a common set of rules needs to be promulgated to protect the decisionally impaired from certain risks of human research. Quotes Opinion 2.07. Sundram, *In Harm's Way: Research Subjects Who Are Decisionally Impaired, 1 J. Health Care L. & Pol'y 36, 43-44 (1998).*

Journal 1997 Considers emergency room research informed consent standards. Reviews new federal regulations and related moral and ethical concerns. Concludes that regulations will require a case-by-case approach to balancing competing interests between research and ethics. References Opinion 2.07. Brody, *New Perspectives on Emergency Room Research, 27 Hastings Center Rep. 7, 9 (Jan./Feb. 1997).*

Journal 1997 Considers informed consent and the principle of self-determination. Analyzes the tradition of informed consent in medical research, with emphasis on international considerations. Concludes that research subjects need better protection. Cites Opinion 2.07. Note, *The Informed-Consent Policy of the International Conference on Harmonization of Technical Requirements for Registrations of Pharmaceuticals for Human Use: Knowledge Is the Best Medicine, 30 Cornell Int'l L. J. 203, 209 (1997).*

Journal 1993 Considers the legitimacy of neonatal HIV screening studies conducted without parental notice or consent. Asserts that such testing is morally and legally questionable. Quotes Opinion 2.07. Isaacman & Miller, *Neonatal HIV Seroprevalence Studies, 14 J. Legal Med. 413, 428 (1993).*

Journal 1989 Discusses various social control mechanisms that have an impact upon biomedical research. Emphasis is placed upon a comparison of the effectiveness of intra- and extraprofessional methods of control. References Opinion 2.07. Benson, *The Social Control of Human Biomedical Research: An Overview and Review of the Literature, 29 Soc. Sci. Med. 1, 3 (1989).*

7.2.1 Principles for Disseminating Research Results

N.J. 1980 Physician employed to do research sued pharmaceutical company for wrongful discharge claiming that as an employee at will she had a cause of action for termination following her refusal to continue research she viewed as medically unethical. The court held that an employee has a cause of action when discharged contrary to a clearly mandated public policy. However, the court affirmed summary judgment because human testing was not imminent and because plaintiff failed to demonstrate the existence of a clear public policy based upon any statements of medical ethics to support her refusal to continue work on controversial drug. The dissent argued that the Opinions and Reports of the Judicial Council 5.03 and 5.18 (1979) [now Opinion 2.07] and other medical ethical statements did provide a clear expression of public policy and that plaintiff's failure to specifically cite them was merely a technical defect, and not fatal. *Pierce v. Ortho Pharmaceutical Corp., 84 N. J. 58, 417 A.2d 505, 516, 518.*

Wyo. 2000 Physician sought judicial review of board of medicine's disciplinary order. Among its holdings, the board found the physician's participation in a patient case

study using testing and treatment procedures of no proven medical efficacy was unprofessional conduct contrary to recognized standards of medical ethics. The board quoted and relied on Opinion 2.07. The Supreme Court reversed the board's decision for failure to provide expert testimony regarding whether the physician's conduct was contrary to the standards set out in Opinion 2.07. *Painter v. Abels, 998 P.2d 931, 935, 939.*

Journal 2010 Discusses the shortfalls and inadequacies of current informed consent protocols in the context of sham surgery–controlled trials. Concludes that investigating institutions should strengthen their informed consent protocols in this area. Cites Opinions 2.07 and 2.076. Bertram, *How Current Informed Consent Protocols Flunk the Sham Surgery Test: A New Frontier in Medicine and Ethics, 14 Quinnipiac Health L. J. 131, 133, 161-162 (2010).*

Journal 2007 Reviews recent essays on the regulation of biomedical research and laws governing conflicts of interest. Concludes that all aspects of research are financially driven and that civil liability is a strong deterrent to unethical practice. Quotes Opinion 2.07. Bergin, *Book Review: Law* *and Ethics in Biomedical Research: Regulation, Conflict of Interest, and Liability,* 23 Windsor Rev. Legal & Soc. Issues 117, 122 (2007).

Journal 2005 Proposes a therapeutic approach to be used by insurers in making decisions and communicating with patients about coverage for last-chance therapies. Concludes that an approach based upon conflict management rather than dispute resolution is better equipped to treat insureds as individuals. Cites Opinion 2.07. Cerminara, *Dealing With Dying: How Insurers Can Help Patients Seeking Last-Chance Therapies (Even When the Answer is "NO"),* 15 Health Matrix 285, 293-94 (2005).

Journal 2005 Examines potential legal issues that physician investigators face in conducting placebo-controlled trials. Concludes that physician investigators who harm patients by giving them a placebo may be subject to liability. Quotes Opinion 2.07. Glass & Waring, *The Physician/ Investigator's Obligation to Patients Participating in Research: The Case of Placebo Controlled Trials,* 33 J. L. Med. & Ethics, 575, 576 (2005).

Journal 2002 Challenges the general use of special informed consent disclosure rules in experimental therapy. Discusses the lack of a bright-line distinction between standard and experimental interventions. Concludes that focus should be placed on the distinctiveness of experimentation. Quotes Opinion 2.07. References Opinion 9.032. Noah, *Informed Consent and the Elusive Dichotomy Between Standard and Experimental Therapy,* 28 Am. J. L. & Med. 361, 394, 395 (2002).

Journal 2001 Considers conflicts of interest in clinical research and other types of medical practice. Compares the way in which doctors and lawyers address conflicts of interest in professional practice. Concludes that physicians are unaware of the need to create a meaningful conflict-of-interest doctrine for medical practice. Quotes Preamble, Principle IV, and Opinions 2.07, 8.03, 8.031, and 10.01. Moore, *What Doctors Can Learn From Lawyers About Conflicts of Interest,* 81 B. U. L. Rev. 445, 447, 449-50 (2001).

Journal 1999 Explores the duty to disclose genetic test results in research and clinical settings. Characterizes the legal duty to disclose. Concludes with guidelines regarding ways that medical researchers can reduce the potential for liability in this context. Quotes Opinion 2.07. Furman, *Genetic Test Results and the Duty to Disclose: Can Medical Researchers Control Liability?* 23 Seattle Univ. L. R. 391, 408-09 (1999).

Journal 1999 Discusses the need for physicians to advocate on behalf of patients' rights in the context of health care delivery. Evaluates the nature and scope of the physician's role as advocate, noting that physicians cannot be expected to engage in attorney-like advocacy. Quotes Principles IV and VI, Fundamental Elements (2), (4), and (6) [now Opinion 10.01], Patient Responsibilities 5 [now Opinion 10.02], and Opinions 2.03, 2.07, 2.09, 2.16, 2.19, 3.06, 4.01, 4.04, 6.01, 7.02, 8.02, 8.03, 8.13, 8.132, 9.06, 9.07, and 9.131. Cites

Opinions 5.05, 5.09, 7.01, 8.135, and 9.02. Sage, *Physicians as Advocates,* 35 Hous. L. Rev. 1529, 1537, 1541, 1542, 1552-53, 1554, 1556, 1557, 1559, 1561-62, 1564, 1571, 1574, 1576, 1580 (1999).

Journal 1998 Discusses conflicts of interest in the physician-patient relationship arising out of use of financial incentives by managed care organizations. Considers how such conflicts are dealt with in the attorney-client relationship. Suggests that a financial incentive should be legally denounced if it unreasonably interferes with a physician's duty to properly care for and treat patients. Quotes Preamble, Fundamental Elements (1) [now Opinion 10.01], and Opinions 4.04, 5.01, 8.03, 8.13, and 9.06. Cites Fundamental Elements (4) [now Opinion 10.01] and Opinions 2.07, 2.08, and 2.132. Hall, *Third-Party Payor Conflicts of Interest in Managed Care: A Proposal for Regulation Based on the Model Rules of Professional Conduct,* 29 Seton Hall L. Rev. 95, 96, 107, 108, 109, 110, 111, 112, 134, 135, 136 (1998).

Journal 1998 Discusses the use of mentally impaired individuals as research subjects. Argues that a common set of rules needs to be promulgated to protect the decisionally impaired from certain risks of human research. Quotes Opinion 2.07. Sundram, *In Harm's Way: Research Subjects Who Are Decisionally Impaired,* 1 J. Health Care L. & Pol'y 36, 43-44 (1998).

Journal 1997 Considers emergency room research informed consent standards. Reviews new federal regulations and related moral and ethical concerns. Concludes that regulations will require a case-by-case approach to balancing competing interests between research and ethics. References Opinion 2.07. Brody, *New Perspectives on Emergency Room Research,* 27 Hastings Center Rep. 7, 9 (Jan./Feb. 1997).

Journal 1997 Considers informed consent and the principle of self-determination. Analyzes the tradition of informed consent in medical research, with emphasis on international considerations. Concludes that research subjects need better protection. Cites Opinion 2.07. Note, *The Informed-Consent Policy of the International Conference on Harmonization of Technical Requirements for Registrations of Pharmaceuticals for Human Use: Knowledge Is the Best Medicine,* 30 Cornell Int'l L. J. 203, 209 (1997).

Journal 1993 Considers the legitimacy of neonatal HIV screening studies conducted without parental notice or consent. Asserts that such testing is morally and legally questionable. Quotes Opinion 2.07. Isaacman & Miller, *Neonatal HIV Seroprevalence Studies,* 14 J. Legal Med. 413, 428 (1993).

Journal 1989 Discusses various social control mechanisms that have an impact upon biomedical research. Emphasis is placed upon a comparison of the effectiveness of intra- and extraprofessional methods of control. References Opinion 2.07. Benson, *The Social Control of Human Biomedical Research: An Overview and Review of the Literature,* 29 Soc. Sci. Med. 1, 3 (1989).

Journal 2011 Examines patentable subject matter exclusion standards in light of the Supreme Court's decision in Bilski v. Kappos, as well as recent lower court eligibility decisions involving medical and biotechnological inventions. Argues for a greater degree of understanding and consensus regarding the degree of creativity in the applications of newly identified, fundamental knowledge to support patent rights for such inventions. Quotes Opinion 9.08. Sarnoff, *Patent Eligible Medical and Biotechnology Inventions After Bilski, Prometheus, and Myriad, 19 Tex. Intell. Prop. L. J. 393, 407 (2011).*

Journal 2010 Analyzes the federal courts' treatment of process patents and the mental steps associated with them. Concludes that medical diagnostic techniques have properly emerged from recent subject matter challenges as a viable candidate for patentability, despite the historical resistance to give protection to process patent claims incorporating mental steps. Quotes Opinion 9.08. Pessagno, *Prometheus and Bilski: Pushing the Bounds of Patentable Subject Matter in Medical Diagnostic Techniques With the Machine-or-Transformation Test, 36 Am. J. L. & Med. 619, 620 (2010).*

Journal 2010 Explores how participation in online social networks may blur boundaries between personal and professional relationships for health care professionals and how such risks may be mitigated by use of network privacy and security settings. Suggests that health care institutions are likely to institute online social-networking policies for employees. Quotes Opinions 5.026, 5.027, 5.045, 5.046, 5.05, 5.059, 5.0591, 8.14, 9.08, and 9.123. Cites Opinions 5.026, 9.031, and 9.12. Terry, *Physicians and Patients Who "Friend" or "Tweet": Constructing a Legal Framework for Social Networking in a Highly Regulated Domain, 43 Ind. L. Rev. 285, 314-16, 319, 334-36, 338 (2010).*

Journal 2009 Argues against the federal Physician Immunity Statute protecting physicians from infringement liability in certain situations involving patented medical procedures. Concludes the fundamental principles of the patent system can accommodate advances in biotechnology. Quotes Opinion 9.09. References Opinion 9.08. Rundle, *The Physician's Immunity Statute: A Botched Operation or a Model Procedure? 34 J. Corp. L. 943, 947 (2009).*

Journal 2008 Examines natural principles and relationships and the patentability of medical and diagnostic processes. Concludes patent laws should be strictly upheld to incentivize disclosure of medical innovations. Quotes Opinion 9.08. Anderson, *Distinguishing Patentable Process Claims From Unpatentable Laws of Nature in the Medical Technology Field, 59 Ala. L. Rev. 1203, 1216 (2008).*

Journal 2008 Discusses whether the current patent system fulfills the interests of incentivizing innovation in the medical device industry while making the devices available at a reasonable cost. Concludes a reform of the system to include an alternative compensation regimen is necessary to balance ethical and economic interests. Quotes Opinion

9.08. Nugent, *Patenting Medical Devices: The Economic Implications of Ethically Motivated Reform, 17 Ann. Health L. 135, 160 (2008).*

Journal 2002 Evaluates the application of biomedical knowledge in clinical practice. Concludes that serious inadequacies exist in the current practice of evidence-based medicine. Quotes Principle V and Opinion 9.08. References Opinion 9.095. Noah, *Medicine's Epistemology: Mapping the Haphazard Diffusion of Knowledge in the Biomedical Community, 44 Ariz. L. Rev. 373, 404, 447, 448 (2002).*

Journal 2000 Discusses patent law and policy. Examines whether those who practice medicine should be excused from patent laws because of the conflict that medical procedure patents create with respect to the practice of medicine. Concludes that Congress should repeal section 287(c) of the Patent Act. Quotes Principle V and Opinions 9.08 and 9.09. Cites Opinion 8.03. References Opinion 10.01. Ho, *Patents, Patients, and Public Policy: An Incomplete Intersection at 35 USC § 287(c), 33 U.C. Davis L. Rev. 601, 603, 623, 624, 625, 631 (2000).*

Journal 2000 Discusses the issues affecting the patentability of surgical procedures. Notes the ethical considerations involved in patenting surgical procedures versus surgical devices. Suggests each patent regimen should strike a balance by weighing all the ethical factors considered important to society. Quotes Opinion 9.09. References Opinion 9.08 and Opinion 9.095. Martin, *Patentability of Methods of Medical Treatment: A Comparative Study, 82 J. Pat. & Trademark Off. Soc'y 381, 383-84, 388, 423 (2000).*

Journal 1999 Discusses congressional amendment of the US patent code, which relieved health care providers from liability for medical procedure patent infringement. Explores the debate surrounding medical procedure patents and concludes that the enforcability of such patents should be reevaluated. Quotes Opinions 9.08 and 9.09. Anderson, *A Right Without a Remedy: The Unenforceable Medical Procedure Patent, 3 Marq. Intell. Prop. L. Rev. 117, 132, 140 (1999).*

Journal 1999 Describes historical and ethical considerations regarding medical patents. Points out that patenting medical procedures adversely affects the reputation of physicians in the eyes of the public. Argues that new laws need to be enacted to prevent abuse of the medical patent system. Quotes Opinion 9.08. Packer, *Ethics and Medical Patents, 117 Arch. Ophthalmol. 824, 825 (1999).*

Journal 1998 Rejects arguments to ban or permit unrestricted patenting of medical and surgical procedures. Explores arguments for and against patenting of medical and surgical procedures. Proposes a compromise position. Quotes Opinions 9.08 and 9.095. Wear, Coles, Szczygiel, McEvoy, & Pegels, *Patenting Medical and Surgical Techniques: An Ethical-Legal Analysis, 23 J. Med. Phil. 75, 76, 87 (1998).*

Journal 1997 Explores the debate enveloping the patenting of medical procedures. Examines the beneficial and detrimental aspects of a ban on medical patents and pertinent ethical and economical factors. Suggests that allowing patents exacts too great a toll on society and science. Quotes Opinion 9.08. References Opinion 9.095. Judge, *Issues Surrounding the Patenting of Medical Procedures, 13 Santa Clara Computer & High Tech. L. J. 181, 202-03 (1997).*

Journal 1997 Examines the controversy surrounding the patenting of medical procedures. Concludes that patenting medical procedures has a negative effect on the physician-patient relationship and the medical profession. Quotes Opinion 9.095. References Opinions 9.08 and 9.09. Note, *Patenting Medical Procedures: A Search for a Compromise Between Ethics and Economics, 18 Cardozo L. Rev. 1527, 1544, 1547, 1554 (1997).*

Journal 1996 Examines the current status of medical procedure patents and discusses the statutory and case law requirements for obtaining a patent. Considers the ethical implications of patenting medical procedures. Argues against a legislative ban on such patents. Quotes Opinions 9.08, 9.09, and 9.095. Garris, *The Case for Patenting Medical Procedures, XXII Am. J. Law & Med. 85, 93, 94-95 (1996).*

Journal 1996 Explores the current rules for patenting medical procedures. Discusses the AMA's position that medical procedure patents are unethical. Concludes that a failure to grant patents will deter the development of new medical procedures. Erroneously quotes Opinion 9.08 (see Opinion 9.095). Lafferty, *Statutory and Ethical Barriers in the Patenting of Medical and Surgical Procedures, 29 J. Marshall L. Rev. 891, 912 (1996).*

Journal 1995 Explores the debates and commentaries regarding patenting medical instruments and processes. Concludes that current patent law fails to address the ethical concerns of physicians and their patients. Quotes Principles of Medical Ethics XI (1971) [now Principle VII] and Principle II (1971) [now Opinion 9.095] and Opinions 9.08 and 9.09. Reisman, *Physicians and Surgeons as Inventors: Reconciling Medical Process Patents and Medical Ethics, 10 High Tech. L. J. 355, 356, 368-70, 385 (1995).*

Journal 2011 Discusses the science surrounding gene patents, including ethical, business, and policy concerns, and examines the history of patent law relating to genes. Concludes with a discussion of *Association for Molecular Pathology v. U. S. Patent and Trademark Office* and the future of gene patents. Quotes Opinion 9.095. Liddle, *Gene Patents: The Controversy and the Law in the Wake of Myriad, 44 Suffolk U. L. Rev. 683, 686 (2011).*

Journal 2007 Discusses how a dissenting Supreme Court opinion in the case of *Metabolite Laboratories, Inc. v. Laboratory Corp. of America Holdings* will affect the scope of patentable material. Concludes that despite the court's holding that certiorari was improvidently granted, the dissent's espousal of a new standard of patentability is likely to

be extremely influential in future cases. References Opinion 9.095. Ho, *Lessons From Laboratory Corp. of America Holdings v. Metabolite Laboratories, Inc., 23 Santa Clara Computer & High Tech. L. J. 463, 482 (2007).*

Journal 2007 Argues that current US policy providing patent protection immunity to health care professionals violates the TRIPS agreement. Proposes a TRIPS-compliant compulsory licensing scheme to protect both economic and ethical interests in the patenting of medical procedures. References Opinion 9.095. Melvin, *An Unacceptable Exception: The Ramifications of Physician Immunity From Medical Procedure Patent Infringement Liability, 91 Minn. L. Rev. 1088, 1090 (2007).*

Journal 2007 Analyzes scientific, ethical, and legal issues raised in the exhumation and genetic analysis of historical figures. Concludes that biohistorical review boards should be created to generate guidelines for such research. Quotes Preamble and Opinion 2.08. Cites Opinions 2.079, 2.105, 5.05, 5.051, 5.075, 8.03, 8.031, 9.095, and 9.10. Paradise & Andrews, *Tales From the Crypt: Scientific, Ethical, and Legal Considerations for Biohistorical Analysis of Deceased Historical Figures, 26 Temp. J. Sci. Tech. & Envtl. L. 223, 287-88 (2007).*

Journal 2006 Examines competing interests arising in the granting of medical patents. Concludes that the law must restrict the granting of patents to the extent necessary to protect patient access to new procedures. Cites Opinion 9.095. Kesselheim & Mello, *Medical-Process Patents—Monopolizing the Delivery of Health Care, 355 New Eng. J. Med. 2036, 2036 (2006).*

Journal 2006 Examines the ethical use of patents. Proposes patent law reform to better serve societal interests. References Opinion 9.095. Washko, *Should Ethics Play a Special Role in Patent Law? 19 Geo. J. Legal Ethics 1027, 1029 (2006).*

Journal 2005 Examines the *Open Source Yoga Unity* lawsuit, raising the issue of whether Bikram Yoga can be copyrighted. Concludes that, by defining Bikram Yoga narrowly, it is subject to little or no copyright protection. Quotes Opinion 9.095. Susman, *Your Karma Ran Over My Dogma: Bikram Yoga and the (Im)Possibilities of Copyrighting Yoga, 25 Loy. L.A. Ent. L. Rev. 245, 272 (2005).*

Journal 2003 Discusses the US "patents first" policy and its impact on the field of biotechnology. Concludes it is poor policy to grant patents on morally controversial biotechnological subject matter before first examining whether the subject matter is patentable. Quotes Opinion 9.095. Bagley, *Patent First, Ask Questions Later: Morality and Biotechnology in Patent Law, 45 Wm. & Mary L. Rev. 469, 500 (2003).*

Journal 2003 Examines financial conflicts of interest that arise in the context of university-based human research. Concludes that federal regulations should replace traditional models of self-regulation to meaningfully protect human subjects. References Opinion 9.095. Jordan, *Financial Conflicts of Interest in Human Subjects Research: Proposals for a More Effective Regulatory Scheme*, 60 Wash. & Lee L. Rev. 15, 23 (2003).

Journal 2002 Examines various concerns regarding gene patents and discusses other policy alternatives. Concludes that policymakers are exploring alternatives to ensure that gene patents will benefit society. Quotes Opinion 2.08. Cites Opinion 9.095. Andrews, *The Gene Patent Dilemma: Balancing Commercial Incentives With Health Needs*, 2 Hous. J. Health L. & Pol'y 65, 74, 104 (2002).

Journal 2002 Evaluates the application of biomedical knowledge in clinical practice. Concludes that serious inadequacies exist in the current practice of evidence-based medicine. Quotes Principle V and Opinion 9.08. References Opinion 9.095. Noah, *Medicine's Epistemology: Mapping the Haphazard Diffusion of Knowledge in the Biomedical Community*, 44 Ariz. L. Rev. 373, 404, 447, 448 (2002).

Journal 1997 Considers the issues surrounding medical procedure patents. Reviews the adoption of federal legislation granting patent infringement immunity to physicians while performing medical or surgical procedures. Discusses

the medical community's position favoring immunity. Concludes that such a law sets a dangerous precedent. References Opinion 9.095. Lee, *35 USC § 287(c)—The Physician Immunity Statute*, 79 J. Pat. & Trademark Off. Soc'y 701, 702-04 (1997).

Journal 1997 Discusses federal patent legislation that protects physicians from liability for patent infringements. Describes legal and medical opinions on the matter. Notes that the legislation was passed in response to concerns regarding health care costs and patients' interests. Proposes that Congress reconsider the legislation. References Opinion 9.095. Note, *The New Patent Infringement Liability Exception for Medical Procedures*, 23 J. Legis. 265, 268 (1997).

Journal 1996 Discusses possible effects of a 1996 legislative enactment that was designed to limit the remedies for infringements on patented medical activities. Describes the legislative history of this enactment and notes the AMA's position against patenting of medical and surgical procedures. References Opinion 9.095. Mossinghoff, *Remedies Under Patents on Medical and Surgical Procedures*, 78 J. Pat. & Trademark Off. Soc'y 789, 790 (1996).

7.2.2 Release of Data from Unethical Experiments

Journal 2001 Focuses on the moral dilemmas raised by stem cell research. Concludes that problems arising as a result of use of embryonic stem cells may be avoided if adult

stem cells are used instead. Quotes Opinion 2.30. Orr & Hook, *Stem Cell Research: Magical Promise v. Moral Peril*, 2 Yale J. Health Pol'y, Law & Ethics 189, 197 (2001).

7.2.3 Patents and Dissemination of Research Products

Journal 2011 Discusses scientific and technological advancements in genetic research and the controversy surrounding patenting human genomic material. Concludes that although patent protection should be provided, modifications to the current system are necessary to ensure that genetic sequencing information is available to researchers to further advancement in health care. Cites Council on Ethical and Judicial Affairs Report 2-I-97 [now Opinion 2.105] and Report 4-I-01 [now Opinion 2.079]. Ratcliffe, *The Ethics of Genetic Patenting and the Subsequent Implications on the Future of Health Care*, 27 Touro L. Rev. 435, 438-39, 449 (2011).

Journal 2007 Analyzes scientific, ethical, and legal issues raised in the exhumation and genetic analysis of historical figures. Concludes that biohistorical review boards should be created to generate guidelines for such research. Quotes Preamble and Opinion 2.08. Cites Opinions 2.079, 2.105, 5.05, 5.051, 5.075, 8.03, 8.031, 9.095, and 9.10. Paradise & Andrews, *Tales From the Crypt: Scientific, Ethical, and Legal Considerations for Biohistorical Analysis of*

Deceased Historical Figures, 26 Temp. J. Sci. Tech. & Envtl. L. 223, 287-88 (2007).

Journal 2001 Examines whether DNA patents violate or threaten human dignity. Supports legislation banning patents on the whole human genome. Concludes that only patents that comprise complete commodification of human beings violate human dignity. References Opinion 2.105. Resnik, *DNA Patents and Human Dignity*, 29 J. L. Med. & Ethics 152, 158, 159 (2001).

Journal 2009 Discusses the judicial standard for reviewing physician noncompete covenants. Concludes courts should apply a strict standard to such covenants, rather than declare the covenants per se invalid. Quotes Principles IV and VII, Principles of Medical Ethics §5 (1957) [now Principle VI], Code of Medical Ethics Ch. II, Art. I §3 (1847) [now Opinion 5.02], Opinion 9.02, and Code of Medical Ethics Ch. II, Art. I §4 (1847) [now Opinion 9.09]. Cites Opinions 8.041, 8.115, 9.02, 9.06, 9.065, 9.067, 10.01, and 10.015. Koons, *Physician Employee Non-Compete Agreements on the Examining Table: The Need to Better Protect Patients'* *and the Public's Interests in Indiana, 6 Ind. Health L. Rev. 253, 272-77, 280-81 (2009).*

Journal 2009 Argues against the federal Physician Immunity Statute protecting physicians from infringement liability in certain situations involving patented medical procedures. Concludes the fundamental principles of the patent system can accommodate advances in biotechnology. Quotes Opinion 9.09. References Opinion 9.08. Rundle, *The Physician's Immunity Statute: A Botched Operation or a Model Procedure? 34 J. Corp. L. 943, 947 (2009).*

Journal 2000 Discusses patent law and policy. Examines whether those who practice medicine should be excused from patent laws because of the conflict that medical procedure patents create with respect to the practice of medicine. Concludes that Congress should repeal section 287(c) of the Patent Act. Quotes Principle V and Opinions 9.08 and 9.09. Cites Opinion 8.03. References Opinion 10.01. Ho, *Patents, Patients, and Public Policy: An Incomplete Intersection at 35 USC § 287(c), 33 U.C. Davis L. Rev. 601, 603, 623, 624, 625, 631 (2000).*

Journal 2000 Discusses the issues affecting the patentability of surgical procedures. Notes the ethical considerations involved in patenting surgical procedures versus surgical devices. Suggests each patent regimen should strike a balance by weighing all the ethical factors considered important to society. Quotes Opinion 9.09. References Opinion 9.08 and Opinion 9.095. Martin, *Patentability of Methods of Medical Treatment: A Comparative Study, 82 J. Pat. & Trademark Off. Soc'y 381, 383-84, 388, 423 (2000).*

Journal 1999 Discusses congressional amendment of the US patent code, which relieved health care providers from liability for medical procedure patent infringement. Explores the debate surrounding medical procedure patents and concludes that the enforcability of such patents should be reevaluated. Quotes Opinions 9.08 and 9.09. Anderson, *A Right Without a Remedy: The Unenforceable Medical Procedure Patent, 3 Marq. Intell. Prop. L. Rev. 117, 132, 140 (1999).*

Journal 1997 Examines the controversy surrounding the patenting of medical procedures. Concludes that patenting medical procedures has a negative effect on the physician-patient relationship and the medical profession. Quotes Opinion 9.095. References Opinions 9.08 and 9.09. Note, *Patenting Medical Procedures: A Search for a Compromise Between Ethics and Economics, 18 Cardozo L. Rev. 1527, 1544, 1547, 1554 (1997).*

Journal 1996 Examines the current status of medical procedure patents and discusses the statutory and case law requirements for obtaining a patent. Considers the ethical implications of patenting medical procedures. Argues against a legislative ban on such patents. Quotes Opinions 9.08, 9.09, and 9.095. Garris, *The Case for Patenting Medical Procedures, XXII Am. J. Law & Med. 85, 93, 94-95 (1996).*

Journal 1995 Explores the debates and commentaries regarding patenting medical instruments and processes. Concludes that current patent law fails to address the ethical concerns of physicians and their patients. Quotes Principles of Medical Ethics §10 (1971) [now Principle VII] and Principle II (1971) [now Opinion 9.095] and Opinions 9.08 and 9.09. Reisman, *Physicians and Surgeons as Inventors: Reconciling Medical Process Patents and Medical Ethics, 10 High Tech. L. J. 355, 356, 368-70, 385 (1995).*

Journal 1990 Explains how medical patents have developed into widely accepted legal instruments that receive broad respect from the courts. Questions the lack of Congressional expansion of patent protection in the field of biotechnology and suggests that Congress should begin expanding protection in this area. References Opinion 9.09. Noonan, *Patenting Medical Technology, 11 J. Legal Med. 263, 268 (1990).*

Journal 2011 Discusses the science surrounding gene patents, including ethical, business, and policy concerns, and examines the history of patent law relating to genes. Concludes with a discussion of *Association for Molecular Pathology v. U. S. Patent and Trademark Office* and the future of gene patents. Quotes Opinion 9.095. Liddle, *Gene Patents: The Controversy and the Law in the Wake of Myriad, 44 Suffolk U. L. Rev. 683, 686 (2011).*

Journal 2007 Discusses how a dissenting Supreme Court opinion in the case of *Metabolite Laboratories, Inc. v. Laboratory Corp. of America Holdings* will affect the scope of patentable material. Concludes that despite the court's holding that certiorari was improvidently granted, the dissent's espousal of a new standard of patentability is likely to be extremely influential in future cases. References Opinion 9.095. Ho, *Lessons From Laboratory Corp. of America Holdings v. Metabolite Laboratories, Inc., 23 Santa Clara Computer & High Tech. L. J. 463, 482 (2007).*

Journal 2007 Argues that current US policy providing patent protection immunity to health care professionals violates the TRIPS agreement. Proposes a TRIPS-compliant compulsory licensing scheme to protect both economic and ethical interests in the patenting of medical procedures. References Opinion 9.095. Melvin, *An Unacceptable Exception: The Ramifications of Physician Immunity From Medical Procedure Patent Infringement Liability, 91 Minn. L. Rev. 1088, 1090 (2007).*

Journal 2006 Examines competing interests arising in the granting of medical patents. Concludes that the law must restrict the granting of patents to the extent necessary to protect patient access to new procedures. Cites Opinion 9.095. Kesselheim & Mello, *Medical-Process Patents—Monopolizing the Delivery of Health Care, 355 New Eng. J. Med. 2036, 2036 (2006).*

Journal 2006 Examines the ethical use of patents. Proposes patent law reform to better serve societal interests. References Opinion 9.095. Washko, *Should Ethics Play a*

Special Role in Patent Law? 19 Geo. J. Legal Ethics 1027, 1029 (2006).

Journal 2005 Examines the *Open Source Yoga Unity* lawsuit, raising the issue of whether Bikram Yoga can be copyrighted. Concludes that, by defining Bikram Yoga narrowly, it is subject to little or no copyright protection. Quotes Opinion 9.095. Susman, *Your Karma Ran Over My Dogma: Bikram Yoga and the (Im)Possibilities of Copyrighting Yoga, 25 Loy. L.A. Ent. L. Rev. 245, 272 (2005).*

Journal 2003 Discusses the US "patents first" policy and its impact on the field of biotechnology. Concludes it is poor policy to grant patents on morally controversial biotechnological subject matter before first examining whether the subject matter is patentable. Quotes Opinion 9.095. Bagley, *Patent First, Ask Questions Later: Morality and Biotechnology in Patent Law, 45 Wm. & Mary L. Rev. 469, 500 (2003).*

Journal 2003 Examines financial conflicts of interest that arise in the context of university-based human research. Concludes that federal regulations should replace traditional models of self-regulation to meaningfully protect human subjects. References Opinion 9.095. Jordan, *Financial Conflicts of Interest in Human Subjects Research: Proposals for a More Effective Regulatory Scheme, 60 Wash. & Lee L. Rev. 15, 23 (2003).*

Journal 2002 Examines various concerns regarding gene patents and discusses other policy alternatives. Concludes that policymakers are exploring alternatives to ensure that gene patents will benefit society. Quotes Opinion 2.08. Cites Opinion 9.095. Andrews, *The Gene Patent Dilemma: Balancing Commercial Incentives With Health Needs, 2 Hous. J. Health L. & Pol'y 65, 74, 104 (2002).*

Journal 2002 Evaluates the application of biomedical knowledge in clinical practice. Concludes that serious inadequacies exist in the current practice of evidence-based medicine. Quotes Principle V and Opinion 9.08. References Opinion 9.095. Noah, *Medicine's Epistemology: Mapping the Haphazard Diffusion of Knowledge in the Biomedical Community, 44 Ariz. L. Rev. 373, 404, 447, 448 (2002).*

Journal 1998 Rejects arguments to ban or permit unrestricted patenting of medical and surgical procedures. Explores arguments for and against patenting of medical and surgical procedures. Proposes a compromise position. Quotes Opinions 9.08 and 9.095. Wear, Coles, Szczygiel,

McEvoy, & Pegels, *Patenting Medical and Surgical Techniques: An Ethical-Legal Analysis, 23 J. Med. Phil. 75, 76, 87 (1998).*

Journal 1997 Explores the debate enveloping the patenting of medical procedures. Examines the beneficial and detrimental aspects of a ban on medical patents and pertinent ethical and economical factors. Suggests that allowing patents exacts too great a toll on society and science. Quotes Opinion 9.08. References Opinion 9.095. Judge, *Issues Surrounding the Patenting of Medical Procedures, 13 Santa Clara Computer & High Tech. L. J. 181, 202-03 (1997).*

Journal 1997 Considers the issues surrounding medical procedure patents. Reviews the adoption of federal legislation granting patent infringement immunity to physicians while performing medical or surgical procedures. Discusses the medical community's position favoring immunity. Concludes that such a law sets a dangerous precedent. References Opinion 9.095. Lee, *35 USC § 287(c)—The Physician Immunity Statute, 79 J. Pat. & Trademark Off. Soc'y 701, 702-04 (1997).*

Journal 1997 Discusses federal patent legislation that protects physicians from liability for patent infringements. Describes legal and medical opinions on the matter. Notes that the legislation was passed in response to concerns regarding health care costs and patients' interests. Proposes that Congress reconsider the legislation. References Opinion 9.095. Note, *The New Patent Infringement Liability Exception for Medical Procedures, 23 J. Legis. 265, 268 (1997).*

Journal 1996 Explores the current rules for patenting medical procedures. Discusses the AMA's position that medical procedure patents are unethical. Concludes that a failure to grant patents will deter the development of new medical procedures. Erroneously quotes Opinion 9.08 (see Opinion 9.095). Lafferty, *Statutory and Ethical Barriers in the Patenting of Medical and Surgical Procedures, 29 J. Marshall L. Rev. 891, 912 (1996).*

Journal 1996 Discusses possible effects of a 1996 legislative enactment that was designed to limit the remedies for infringements on patented medical activities. Describes the legislative history of this enactment and notes the AMA's position against patenting of medical and surgical procedures. References Opinion 9.095. Mossinghoff, *Remedies Under Patents on Medical and Surgical Procedures, 78 J. Pat. & Trademark Off. Soc'y 789, 790 (1996).*

7.3.1 Ethical Use of Placebo Controls in Research

Journal 2004 Evaluates weaknesses in institutional review board (IRB) protection of human subjects. Concludes that one vehicle for enhancing human subjects protection is to hold IRBs legally accountable for negligent conduct. Cites Opinions 2.071, 2.075, and 8.0315. Noah, *Bioethical*

Malpractice: Risk and Responsibility in Human Research, 7 J. Health Care L. & Pol'y 175, 183, 235 (2004).

Journal 2003 Provides an update on the Declaration of Helsinki and the FDA's position on placebo-controlled medical research. Concludes that the FDA should reconsider its position in light of the principles articulated in the Declaration. Quotes Opinion 2.075. Michels & Rothman, *Update on Unethical Use of Placebos in Randomised Trials, 17 Bioethics 188, 200 (2003).*

Journal 2001 Reviews federal regulations and discusses challenges associated with developing guidelines relating to the use of placebos. Concludes that the use of placebo controls in human subjects research must be carefully regulated. Quotes Opinion 2.075. Hoffman, *The Use of Placebos*

in Clinical Trials: Responsible Research or Unethical Practice? 33 Conn. L. Rev. 449, 454-55, 496 (2001).

Journal 2010 Discusses the shortfalls and inadequacies of current informed consent protocols in the context of sham surgery–controlled trials. Concludes that investigating institutions should strengthen their informed consent protocols in this area. Cites Opinions 2.07 and 2.076. Bertram, *How Current Informed Consent Protocols Flunk the Sham Surgery Test: A New Frontier in Medicine and Ethics, 14 Quinnipiac Health L. J. 131, 133, 161-162 (2010).*

7.3.2 Research on Emergency Medical Interventions

Journal 2006 Discusses the evolution of health law in Virginia. Concludes that the area of health law continues to expand, develop, and be refined. Cites Opinions 3.03, 3.08, 5.01, 5.015, 5.02, 5.04, 5.055, 6.02, 6.021, 6.03, 6.04, 7.03, 7.04, 7.05, 8.054, 8.08, 8.081, 8.085, 8.115, 8.12, 8.14, 8.145, 8.19, and 9.045. Guanzon, *Health Care Law, 41 U. Rich. L. Rev. 179, 199 (2006).*

7.3.4 Maternal-Fetal Research

Journal 1991 Explores arguments for and against fetal tissue transplantation research, including arguments for and against the use of federal funds to support such research. Considers whether the donation model is appropriate for the transfer of fetal tissue, and whether a woman who chooses elective abortion is an appropriate donor. References Opinion 2.10. Childress, *Ethics, Public Policy, and Human Fetal Tissue Transplantation Research, Vol 1 Kennedy Inst. Ethics J. 93, 116 (June 1991).*

Journal 1991 Considers how the use of in vitro fertilization (IVF) has blurred the distinction between medical practice and research. Argues that medical-professional responsibility standards should be used to curtail the creation of life in vitro. Quotes Opinions 2.10 and 2.14. Comment, *Dangerous Relations: Doctors and Extracorporeal Embryos, The Need for New Limits to Medical Inquiry, 7 J. Contemp. Health L. & Pol'y 307, 309 (1991).*

7.3.5 Research Using Human Fetal Tissue

Journal 1991 Explores arguments for and against fetal tissue transplantation research, including arguments for and against the use of federal funds to support such research. Considers whether the donation model is appropriate for the transfer of fetal tissue, and whether a woman who chooses elective abortion is an appropriate donor. References Opinion 2.10. Childress, *Ethics, Public Policy, and Human Fetal Tissue Transplantation Research, Vol 1 Kennedy Inst. Ethics J. 93, 116 (June 1991).*

Journal 1991 Considers how the use of in vitro fertilization (IVF) has blurred the distinction between medical practice and research. Argues that medical-professional responsibility standards should be used to curtail the creation of life in vitro. Quotes Opinions 2.10 and 2.14. Comment, *Dangerous Relations: Doctors and Extracorporeal Embryos, The Need*

for New Limits to Medical Inquiry, 7 J. Contemp. Health L. & Pol'y 307, 309 (1991).

Journal 2002 Observes that changes in the health professions challenge certain assumptions about professional ethics. Concludes that these long-standing assumptions must be re-examined. Cites Opinion 2.161. References Opinion 8.13. Kelley, *The Meanings of Professional Life: Teaching Across the Health Professions, 27 J. Med. & Phil. 475, 485, 490, 491 (2002).*

Journal 1990 Presents an update on current medical research regarding Parkinson disease. Discusses the relevance of fetal tissue transplantation to this research. References Opinion 2.161. Joynt, *Neurology, 263 JAMA 2660 (1990).*

7.3.6 Research in Gene Therapy and Genetic Engineering

Journal 2006 Explores legal and ethical issues which may arise from prebirth genetic screening and enhancement. Concludes that courts will have to strongly weigh a woman's right to choose abortion against potential ethical problems. Quotes Opinion 2.11. McConnell, *Quality Control: The Implications of Negative Genetic Selection and Pre-Birth Genetic Enhancement*, 15 UCLA Women's L. J. 47, 61 (2006).

Journal 2000 Defines and describes human genetic enhancement. Explores the legal implications of this emerging technology as well as related societal concerns. Quotes Opinion 2.11. References Opinion 2.12. Mehlman, *The Law of Above Averages: Leveling the New Genetic Enhancement Playing Field*, 85 Iowa L. Rev. 517, 527-28, 559 (2000).

Journal 1999 Discusses regulatory concerns regarding genetic technology. Provides ideas on how society might regulate genetic enhancements. Argues that a variety of means of regulation need to be utilized to govern genetic technology. Quotes Opinion 2.11. Cites Opinion 9.065. References Opinion 2.138. Mehlman, *How Will We Regulate Genetic Enhancement?* 34 Wake Forest L. Rev. 671, 693-94, 695 (1999).

7.3.7 Safeguards in the Use of DNA Databanks

Journal 2011 Discusses scientific and technological advancements in genetic research and the controversy surrounding patenting human genomic material. Concludes that although patent protection should be provided, modifications to the current system are necessary to ensure that genetic sequencing information is available to researchers to further advancement in health care. Cites Council on Ethical and Judicial Affairs Report 2-I-97 [now Opinion 2.105] and Report 4-I-01 [now Opinion 2.079]. Ratcliffe, *The Ethics of Genetic Patenting and the Subsequent Implications on the Future of Health Care*, 27 Touro L. Rev. 435, 438-39, 449 (2011).

Journal 2007 Analyzes scientific, ethical, and legal issues raised in the exhumation and genetic analysis of historical figures. Concludes that biohistorical review boards should be created to generate guidelines for such research. Quotes Preamble and Opinion 2.08. Cites Opinions 2.079, 2.105, 5.05, 5.051, 5.075, 8.03, 8.031, 9.095, and 9.10. Paradise & Andrews, *Tales From the Crypt: Scientific, Ethical, and Legal Considerations for Biohistorical Analysis of Deceased Historical Figures*, 26 Temp. J. Sci. Tech. & Envtl. L. 223, 287-88 (2007).

7.3.9 Commercial Use of Human Biological Materials

S.D. Fla. 2003 Donors of tissue samples sought equitable and injunctive relief against a physician-researcher and affiliated hospitals doing research on Canavan disease. The researcher used the donations to obtain a gene patent and the hospitals restricted any activity related to the patent. District court dismissed all counts except the unjust enrichment claim. Court quoted Opinion 2.08 with respect to disclosure to patients of possible commercial application of research. *Greenberg v. Miami Children's Hospital Research Institute, Inc.*, 264 F. Supp. 2d 1064, 1070-71, n. 2.

Journal 2009 Discusses legislative changes and the increase in patentable material that led to the commercialization of scientific research. Concludes a mandatory disclosure regimen is necessary to preserve the interests of researchers and tissue donors in scientific research. Quotes Opinion 2.08. Overgaard, *Balancing the Interests of Researchers and Donors in the Commercial Scientific Research Marketplace*, 74 Brook. L. Rev. 1473, 1501, 1506 (2009).

Journal 2007 Discusses the evolution of informed consent doctrine. Concludes that, in context of research, informed consent exceptions should be substantially narrowed. Quotes Ch. I, Art. I, Sec. 4 (May 1847) [now Opinion 8.082] and Ch. I, Art. I, Sec. 1 (May 1847) [now Principles I and VIII]. References Opinions 2.08 and 8.08. Grimm, *Informed Consent for All! No Exceptions*, 37 N. M. L. Rev. 39, 39, 61 (2007).

Journal 2007 Analyzes scientific, ethical, and legal issues raised in the exhumation and genetic analysis of historical figures. Concludes that biohistorical review boards should be created to generate guidelines for such research. Quotes Preamble and Opinion 2.08. Cites Opinions 2.079, 2.105, 5.05, 5.051, 5.075, 8.03, 8.031, 9.095, and 9.10. Paradise & Andrews, *Tales From the Crypt: Scientific, Ethical, and Legal Considerations for Biohistorical Analysis of Deceased Historical Figures*, 26 Temp. J. Sci. Tech. & Envtl. L. 223, 287-88 (2007).

Journal 2006 Explores whether patients have a property interest in their own tissue. Concludes that courts must carefully consider evolving thought about interests of patients in their tissue samples. Cites Opinion 2.08. Andrews, *Two Perspectives: Rights of Donors: Who Owns Your Body? A Patient's Perspective on Washington University v. Catalona*, 34 J. L. Med. & Ethics 398, 404 (2006).

Journal 2006 Evaluates unjust enrichment claims against those patenting human genetic material. Concludes that opponents of the practice of patenting genetic material may bring such claims. Cites Opinion 2.08. Greenfield, *Greenberg v. Miami Children's Hospital: Unjust Enrichment and the Patenting of Human Genetic Material,* 15 Ann. Health L. 213, 248 (2006).

Journal 2005 Examines financial, ethical, moral, and legal issues surrounding the use of tissue samples stored in bio-banks. Concludes that a fiduciary duty should exist between health care providers and researchers who have established biobanks and individuals submitting tissue samples. Quotes Opinion 2.08. Andrews, *Harnessing the Benefits of Biobanks,* 33 J. L. Med. & Ethics 22, 25 (2005).

Journal 2004 Urges that Congress pass legislation authorizing the sale of human tissue for research purposes, but holding liable any researcher who wrongfully uses such tissue. Concludes this legislation would balance the interests of research subjects with those of the biotechnology industry. Cites Opinion 2.08. Gitter, *Ownership of Human Tissue: A Proposal for Federal Recognition of Human Research Participants' Property Rights in Their Biological Material,* 61 Wash. & Lee L. Rev. 257, 334 (2004).

Journal 2002 Examines various concerns regarding gene patents and discusses other policy alternatives. Concludes that policymakers are exploring alternatives to ensure that gene patents will benefit society. Quotes Opinion 2.08. Cites Opinion 9.095. Andrews, *The Gene Patent Dilemma: Balancing Commercial Incentives With Health Needs,* 2 Hous. J. Health L. & Pol'y 65, 74, 104 (2002).

Journal 1998 Discusses conflicts of interest in the physician-patient relationship arising out of use of financial incentives by managed care organizations. Considers how such conflicts are dealt with in the attorney-client relationship. Suggests that a financial incentive should be legally denounced if it unreasonably interferes with a physician's duty to properly care for and treat patients. Quotes Preamble, Fundamental Elements (1) [now Opinion 10.01], and Opinions 4.04, 5.01, 8.03, 8.13, and 9.06. Cites Fundamental Elements (4) [now Opinion 10.01] and Opinions 2.07, 2.08, and 2.132. Hall, *Third-Party Payor Conflicts of Interest in Managed Care: A Proposal for Regulation Based on the Model Rules of Professional Conduct,* 29 Seton Hall L. Rev. 95, 96, 107, 108, 109, 110, 111, 112, 134, 135, 136 (1998).

8 Physicians and the Health of the Community

8.1 Routine Universal Screening for HIV

Journal 2010 Examines published resources within the medical and legal fields that focus on confidentiality and evaluates those resources to determine if they help clarify confidentiality issues. Further, discusses differences between these professions that may be hindrances when serving the same patient or client. Concludes that, while both professions guard against disclosure of patient/client communications, they also allow for disclosure in certain instances such as imminent death, harm, or injury. References Principle IV and cites Opinions 2.02, 2.23, 2.24, and 5.05. Johns, *Multidisciplinary Practice and Ethics Part II—Lawyers, Doctors, and Confidentiality,* 6 NAELA J. 55, 57-65, 68 (2010).

Journal 2009 Examines the role of physicians during natural and man-made disasters. Concludes hospitals must make plans to define disaster response procedures that shift responsibility for survival from the physician to the community. Quotes Code of Ethics, Ch. III, Art. I §1 (1847) [now Opinion 9.067], Principle 5 (1957) [now Principle VI], Principle VI, and Opinions 2.23, 9.067, and 9.131. Cites Opinions 9.06, 9.067, and 9.12. Ahronheim, *Service by Health Care Providers in a Public Health Emergency: The Physician's Duty and the Law,* 12 J. Health Care L. & Pol'y 195, 209-11, 215, 225 (2009).

Journal 2007 Considers whether health care providers should initiate discussions of HIV testing for their patients. Concludes that adopting such a policy, with specialized informed consent, would help limit the spread of HIV. Quotes Opinion 2.23. Rajkumar, *A Human Rights Approach to Routine Provider-Initiated HIV Testing,* 7 Yale J. Health Pol'y L. & Ethics 319, 371 (2007).

Journal 2001 Compares the American system of patient confidentiality to the Austrian system. Discusses the debate between patients' rights and public safety. Concludes that the duty to warn third parties of dangerous patients should be discretionary instead of mandatory, except in cases of HIV seropositivity, which should involve mandatory disclosure to public health officials. Quotes Opinions 2.23, 5.05, and 5.06. Kenworthy, *The Austrian Psychotherapy Act: No Legal Duty to Warn,* 11 Ind. Int'l & Comp. L. Rev. 469, 480-81, 485, 490, 496 (2001).

Journal 2000 Examines the effect of HIV/AIDS on the relationship between the general public and health care professionals (HCPs). Discusses the importance of creating an environment in which HIV-positive patients do not fear disclosing their HIV status. Discusses policies and guidelines that address methods to prevent transmission of HIV from HCPs to patients. Quotes Opinion 2.23. References Opinions 9.13 and 9.131. Rediger, *Living in a World With HIV: Balancing Privacy, Privilege and the Right to Know Between Patients and Health Care Professionals*, 21 Hamline J. Pub. L. & Pol'y 443, 456-57, 461, 472 (2000).

Journal 1999 Explores the possibility of genetic testing in the managed care setting. Points out that genetic testing is not likely to reduce health care costs, but may improve health. Recommends ways in which genetic medicine can be practiced in the managed care context. Quotes Opinion 2.23. Rothstein & Hoffman, *Genetic Testing, Genetic Medicine, and Managed Care*, 34 Wake Forest L. Rev. 849, 883 (1999).

Journal 1999 Discusses whether health care professionals have the right to refuse to treat patients under common law and federal statutes and regulations. Explores the impact of the Americans with Disabilities Act and the US Supreme Court decision in *Bragdon v. Abbott* on the duties of health care professionals in the context of providing treatment to HIV-positive patients. Quotes Principle VI and Opinions 2.23 and 9.131. White, *Health Care Professionals and Treatment of HIV-Positive Patients*, 20 J. Legal Med. 67, 86 (1999).

Journal 1998 Compares the New York AIDS confidentiality statute with statutes that mandate testing for other communicable diseases. Discusses whether the legal response to AIDS will serve as a model for responses to undiscovered diseases. Suggests that the prohibition on involuntary HIV testing should be reconsidered. Cites Opinion 2.23. Fernandez, *Is AIDS Different?* 61 Alb. L. Rev. 1053 (1998).

Journal 1996 Discusses conflict between physicians' duty of confidentiality to patients and physicians' obligation to warn

third parties of foreseeable injuries. Examines physicians' current legal responsibility to breach confidentiality to prevent the spread of infectious diseases, including AIDS. Identifies guidelines for physicians. Cites Opinions 2.23 and 5.057. Comment, *Taking Tarasoff Where No One Has Gone Before: Looking at Duty to Warn Under the AIDS Crisis*, 15 St. Louis U. Pub. L. Rev. 471, 499 (1996).

Journal 1995 Observes that statutes criminalizing HIV transmission would pose a disincentive for testing and also infringe upon the patient's right to confidentiality because criminal prosecutions are a matter of public record. Concludes that legislatures must carefully consider such issues when drafting legislation to prevent the spread of HIV. Quotes Opinion 2.23. O'Toole, *HIV-Specific Crime Legislation: Targeting an Epidemic for Criminal Prosecution*, 10 J. L. & Health 183, 195, 199 (1995).

Journal 1990 Explores potential physician tort liability for failure to warn at-risk individuals of the danger of being infected by the physician's HIV-positive patient. Concludes that there is a legal duty requiring health care professionals to warn those persons foreseeably at risk of being infected by an HIV-positive patient. References Opinion 2.23. Labowitz, *Beyond Tarasoff: AIDS and the Obligation to Breach Confidentiality*, 9 St. Louis Univ. Pub. L. Rev. 495, 514 (1990).

Journal 1990 Considers the tension between confidentiality and the duty to warn in the context of AIDS and HIV. Considers the appropriateness of mandatory reporting and partner notification and proposes legal reforms in this area. References Opinion 2.23. Price, *Between Scylla and Charybdis: Charting a Course to Reconcile the Duty of Confidentiality and the Duty to Warn in the AIDS Context*, 94 Dickinson L. Rev. 435, 477 (1990).

8.2 Impaired Drivers and Their Physicians

Journal 2010 Examines published resources within the medical and legal fields that focus on confidentiality and evaluates those resources to determine if they help clarify confidentiality issues. Further, discusses differences between these professions that may be hindrances when serving the same patient or client. Concludes that, while both professions guard against disclosure of patient/client communications, they also allow for disclosure in certain instances such as imminent death, harm, or injury. References Principle IV and cites Opinions 2.02, 2.23, 2.24, and 5.05. Johns, *Multidisciplinary Practice and Ethics Part II—Lawyers, Doctors, and Confidentiality*, 6 NAELA J. 55, 57-65, 68 (2010).

Journal 2004 Considers third-party liability in situations where an elderly impaired driver negligently injures another. Discusses the impact on family members who occupy a special relationship with the driver. Concludes that a proper balance must be struck to encourage active family support.

Quotes Opinion 2.24. Martin, *Who Will Take the Keys From Grandpa?* 21 T. M. Cooley L. Rev. 257, 263, 264 (2004).

Journal 2002 Discusses issues regarding regulation of elderly drivers. Concludes that mandating physicians to report unfit elderly patients will protect the public and help resolve ethical and legal dilemmas. Quotes Opinions 1.02, 2.24, 5.05, and 10.01. Kane, *Driving Into the Sunset: A Proposal for Mandatory Reporting to the DMV by Physicians Treating Unsafe Elderly Drivers*, 25 U. Haw. L. Rev. 59, 59, 61, 62, 67, 69, 82, 83 (2002).

Journal 2002 Discusses malpractice liability in connection with treatment and diagnosis of dementia. Concludes that physicians must stay aware of new diagnostic and treatment developments in order to reduce risk. Cites Opinion 2.24. Kapp, *Legal Standards for the Medical Diagnosis and Treatment of Dementia*, 23 J. Legal Med. 359, 382 (2002).

Journal 2000 Explores physician involvement in the care of cognitively impaired elderly people who operate motor vehicles. Discusses conflicts that arise in fulfilling obligations to the patient, while upholding obligations to the welfare of the community. Cites Opinion 2.24. Berger & Rosner, *Ethical Challenges Posed by Dementia and Driving, 11 J. Clinical Ethics 304, 307, 308 (2000).*

8.3 Physicians' Responsibilities in Disaster Response and Preparedness

Journal 2010 Addresses whether health care workers should receive priority in treatment during an influenza epidemic. Using distributive justice principles and practical considerations, concludes that health care workers should not get priority treatment in such an epidemic and that medical utility should be the sole criterion in determining any treatment priority. Quotes Opinion 2.03. Cites Opinion 9.067. Rothstein, *Should Health Care Providers Get Treatment Priority in an Influenza Pandemic? 38 J. L. Med. & Ethics 412, 413, 415 (2010).*

Journal 2009 Examines the role of physicians during natural and man-made disasters. Concludes hospitals must make plans to define disaster response procedures that shift responsibility for survival from the physician to the community. Quotes Code of Ethics, Ch. III, Art. I §1 (1847) [now Opinion 9.067], Principle 5 (1957) [now Principle VI], Principle VI, and Opinions 2.23, 9.067, and 9.131. Cites Opinions 9.06, 9.067, and 9.12. Ahronheim, *Service by Health Care Providers in a Public Health Emergency: The Physician's Duty and the Law, 12 J. Health Care L. & Pol'y 195, 209-11, 215, 225 (2009).*

Journal 2009 Discusses the impact of pandemic influenza on customary legal standards of care imposed by state and federal regulatory authorities and the tort system. Concludes alternative standards of care should be developed in preparation for pandemic influenza to ensure health care providers are equipped to slow the spread of disease while caring for the sick. Quotes Opinion 9.067. Kinney, McCabe, Gilbert, & Shisler, *Altered Standards of Care for Health Care Providers in the Pandemic Influenza, 6 Ind. Health L. Rev. 1, 14 (2009).*

Journal 2009 Discusses the judicial standard for reviewing physician noncompete covenants. Concludes courts should apply a strict standard to such covenants, rather than declare the covenants per se invalid. Quotes Principles IV and VII, Principles of Medical Ethics §5 (1957) [now Principle VI], Code of Medical Ethics Ch. II, Art. I §3 (1847) [now Opinion 5.02], Opinion 9.02, and Code of Medical Ethics Ch. II, Art. I §4 (1847) [now Opinion 9.09]. Cites Opinions 8.041, 8.115, 9.02, 9.06, 9.065, 9.067, 10.01, and 10.015. Koons, *Physician Employee Non-Compete Agreements on the Examining Table: The Need to Better Protect Patients' and the Public's Interests in Indiana, 6 Ind. Health L. Rev. 253, 272-77, 280-81 (2009).*

Journal 2008 Examines the legal obligations of health care professionals during pandemics and discusses penalties imposed for refusing to do such work during a pandemic. Concludes policy makers should institute mechanisms to encourage professionals voluntarily to work during a pandemic. Quotes Opinions 9.067 and 9.131. Coleman, *Beyond the Call of Duty: Compelling Health Care Professionals to Work During an Influenza Pandemic, 94 Iowa L. Rev. 1, 12 (2008).*

Journal 2008 Examines the ethical reasons why physicians choose to provide treatment in disaster situations, even at great risk to themselves. Concludes that individual values play a substantial role in such decision making. Quotes Preamble, Opinion 9.131, and Ch. III, Art. 1, Sec. 1 (1847) [now Opinions 2.25 and 9.067]. Iserson, Heine, Larkin, Moskop, Baruch, & Aswegan, *Fight or Flight: The Ethics of Emergency Physician Disaster Response, 51 Annals of Emergency Med. 345, 346-47 (2008).*

Journal 2008 Discusses the duty of physicians to participate in pandemic care. Concludes that the extent of personal risk a physician is obligated to take has a limit, although the limit has yet to be clearly defined. Quotes Ch. III, Art. I, Sec. 1 (1847) [now Opinions 2.25 and 9.067]. Meerschaert, *Physicians' Duty to Participate in Pandemic Care, 300 JAMA 284, 284 (2008).*

Journal 2007 Examines physicians' duty to treat victims of highly infectious diseases during an epidemic. Concludes that no clear duty exists, and that if physicians are compelled to provide care by law they must be afforded sufficient due process to protect their property interests in their medical licenses. Quotes Ch. III, Art. I, Sec. I (May 1847) [now Opinions 2.25 and 9.067] and Opinion 9.131. References Principle 10 (1957) [now Principle VII]. Schwartz, *Doubtful Duty: Physicians' Legal Obligation to Treat During an Epidemic, 60 Stan. L. Rev. 657, 662, 663 (2007).*

Journal 2007 Speculates on the availability of funding for hospitals confronted with an infectious disease pandemic. Concludes that new legislation is required to ensure adequate funding for hospitals in such a situation. Quotes Ch. III, Art. I, Sec. 1 (May 1847) [now Opinions 2.25 and 9.067]. Williams, *Fluconomics: Preserving Our Hospital Infrastructure During and After a Pandemic, 7 Yale J. Health Pol'y L. & Ethics 99, 115 (2007).*

8.4 Ethical Use of Quarantine and Isolation

Journal 2008 Examines the ethical reasons why physicians choose to provide treatment in disaster situations, even at great risk to themselves. Concludes that individual values play a substantial role in such decision making. Quotes Preamble, Opinion 9.131, and Ch. III, Art. 1, Sec. 1 (May 1847) [now Opinions 2.25 and 9.067]. Iserson, Heine, Larkin, Moskop, Baruch, & Aswegan, *Fight or Flight: The Ethics of Emergency Physician Disaster Response, 51 Annals of Emergency Med. 345-353 (2008).*

Journal 2008 Discusses the duty of physicians to participate in pandemic care. Concludes that the extent of personal risk a physician is obligated to take has a limit, although the limit has yet to be clearly defined. Quotes Ch. III, Art. I, Sec. 1 (1847) [now Opinions 2.25 and 9.067]. Meerschaert, *Physicians' Duty to Participate in Pandemic Care, 300 JAMA 284, 284 (2008).*

Journal 2007 Discusses the role of job security and income reimbursement in ensuring voluntary compliance with quarantine orders in the US, and analyzes the adequacy of current laws to address such concerns. Concludes that existing statutes would be inadequate and proposes new model legislation. Cites Ch. III, Art. I, Sec. I (May 1847)

[now Opinion 2.25]. Rothstein & Talbott, *Job Security and Income Replacement for Individuals in Quarantine: The Need for Legislation, 10 J. Health Care L. & Pol'y 239, 239-40 (2007).*

Journal 2007 Examines physicians' duty to treat victims of highly infectious diseases during an epidemic. Concludes that no clear duty exists, and that if physicians are compelled to provide care by law they must be afforded sufficient due process to protect their property interests in their medical licenses. Quotes Ch. III, Art. I, Sec. I (May 1847) [now Opinions 2.25 and 9.067] and Opinion 9.131. References Principle 10 (1957) [now Principle VII]. Schwartz, *Doubtful Duty: Physicians' Legal Obligation to Treat During an Epidemic, 60 Stan. L. Rev. 657, 662, 663 (2007).*

Journal 2007 Speculates on the availability of funding for hospitals confronted with an infectious disease pandemic. Concludes that new legislation is required to ensure adequate funding for hospitals in such a situation. Quotes Ch. III, Art. I, Sec. 1 (May 1847) [now Opinions 2.25 and 9.067]. Williams, *Fluconomics: Preserving Our Hospital Infrastructure During and After a Pandemic, 7 Yale J. Health Pol'y L. & Ethics 99, 115 (2007).*

8.5 Disparities in Health Care

Journal 2006 Analyzes racial and ethnic disparities in health care. Concludes that greater political attention must be given to research in this area. References Opinion 9.121. Gamble & Stone, *U.S. Policy on Health Inequities: The Interplay of Politics and Research, 31 J. Health Pol. Pol'y & L. 93, 105-06 (2006).*

Journal 2006 Analyzes methods of measuring racial and ethnic disparities in health care. Concludes that calculating the disparity reduction profile and disparity index together provides a useful measure of change in disparity over time. References Opinion 9.121. Gibbs, Nsiah-Jefferson, McHugh, Trivedi, & Prothrow-Stith, *Reducing Racial and Ethnic Health Disparities: Exploring an Outcome-Oriented Agenda for Research and Policy, 31 J. Health Pol. Pol'y & L. 185, 216 (2006).*

Journal 2004 Examines how one-on-one social interactions may trigger racially biased conduct. Concludes that by affirmatively altering the nature of such interactions, discriminatory conduct may be thwarted. References Opinion 9.121. Wang, *Race as Proxy: Situational Racism and Self-fulfilling Stereotypes, 53 DePaul L. Rev. 1013, 1082-83 (2004).*

Journal 2003 Addresses physician bias in health care. Concludes that existing legal responses to biased medical decisions are inadequate and further development is needed. Quotes Opinions 9.121 and 9.122. Crossley, *Infected*

Judgment: Legal Responses to Physician Bias, 48 Vill. L. Rev. 195, 239, 297 (2003).

Journal 2003 Examines the history of medical research involving racial and ethnic minorities. Concludes that medical researchers must ensure the inclusion of racial and ethnic minorities in clinical trials whenever it is scientifically appropriate. References Opinion 9.121. Noah, *The Participation of Underrepresented Minorities in Clinical Research, 29 Am. J. Law & Med. 221, 223 (2003).*

Journal 2002 Considers how to evaluate the performance of Medicare managed care plans in serving ethnic minorities. Concludes that additional monitoring could help reduce existing disparities. References Opinion 9.121. Langwell & Moser, *Strategies for Medicare Health Plans Serving Racial and Ethnic Minorities, 23 Health Care Financing Rev. 131, 134, 146 (2002).*

Journal 2002 Examines how implicit cognitive biases of physicians may contribute to racial disparities in medical care. Considers legal safeguards that may address these disparities. Concludes that Congress must take affirmative steps to help remedy this problem. References Opinion 9.121. Shin, *Redressing Wounds: Finding a Legal Framework to Remedy Racial Disparities in Medical Care, 90 Cal. L. Rev. 2047, 2056, 2057, 2100 (2002).*

Journal 2001 Addresses racial and ethnic disparities in medical care. Concludes that the law plays a vital role in ending racial disparities in medical treatment through the enforcement of civil rights legislation. Quotes Opinion 9.121. Bowser, *Eliminating Racial and Ethnic Disparities in Medical Care, 30 Brief 24, 25 (Summer 2001).*

Journal 2001 Provides a comprehensive theoretical approach and policy recommendations to address racial profiling in health care. Concludes that medicine needs to rethink research and treatment in light of disparities based on race. Quotes Opinion 9.121. Bowser, *Racial Profiling in Health Care: An Institutional Analysis of Medical Treatment Disparities, 7 Mich. J. Race & L. 79, 119 (2001).*

Journal 2001 Explains the design and potential benefits of result-based compensation arrangements for health care. Concludes that a more reliable and efficient health care delivery system is fostered by such arrangements. Quotes Opinion 6.01. References Opinions 9.121 and 9.122. Hyman & Silver, *You Get What You Pay For: Result-Based Compensation for Health Care, 58 Wash. & Lee L. Rev. 1427, 1459, 1460, 1461, 1481-82 (2001).*

Journal 2001 Examines racial and ethnic inequalities in health care. Explains civil rights enforcement strategies and limitations. Concludes by proposing a comprehensive systematic approach, including regulatory and market-based incentives, to decrease racial and ethnic disparities in health care. References Opinion 9.121. Watson, *Race, Ethnicity and Quality of Care: Inequalities and Incentives, 27 Am. J. L. & Med. 203, 206 (2001).*

Journal 1997 Considers the use of race and gender to assess health care status and medical needs. Discusses the lack of consideration that Asian American women receive in the health care agenda. Proposes an examination of factors such as race, gender, and class status to provide a better understanding of the health needs of this group. References Opinions 9.121 and 9.122. Ikemoto, *The Fuzzy Logic of Race and Gender in the Mismeasure of Asian American Women's Health Needs, 65 U. Cin. L. Rev. 799, 800, 804, 810 (1997).*

Journal 1994 Observes that health care reform proposals present significant challenges to the role and ethics of attending physicians. Emphasizes that reform proposals must set forth the role envisioned for physicians and must articulate an acceptable ethical framework within which physicians may fulfill that role. Quotes Opinions 4.04, 9.121, and 9.122. Cites Opinions 2.03, 2.09, 5.01, and 8.03. Wolf, *Health Care Reform and the Future of Physician Ethics, 24 Hastings Center Rep. 28, 32, 40 (March/April 1994).*

Journal 1993 Presents findings by the Council on graduate medical education regarding access to health care. Recommends that more emphasis be placed on primary care, the physician workforce be redistributed to increase the number of physicians in rural and inner city areas, and that there be more racial and ethnic diversity in the medical profession. References Opinion 9.121. Rivo & Satcher, *Improving Access to Health Care Through Physician Workforce Reform, 270 JAMA 1074, 1075 (1993).*

Journal 1992 Discusses the impact of physicians' values on end-of-life decision making for patients. Examines how and why physician values may become dominant. References Opinions 2.20, 2.22, and 9.121. Orentlicher, *The Illusion of Patient Choice in End-of-Life Decisions, 267 JAMA 2101, 2102 (1992).*

Journal 1991 Describes the attributes of women who self-report pelvic inflammatory disease (PID). Presents the results of a study that examined these attributes, noting that risk factors were consistent with prior studies. References Opinion 9.121. Aral, Mosher, & Cates, *Self-reported Pelvic Inflammatory Disease in the United States, 1988, 266 JAMA 2570, 2573 (1991).*

Journal 1991 Compares the health conditions of blacks in South Africa with those in the US. Concludes that policy changes to address the health problems of South African blacks are also needed in this country. References Opinion 9.121. Brooks, Smith, & Anderson, *Medical Apartheid: An American Perspective, 266 JAMA 2746, 2748 (1991).*

Journal 2002 Analyzes gender disparities in the context of access to health care, insurance, treatment, and outcomes. Concludes that women are likely to encounter an unconscious bias in treatment or in the design of health care systems. References Opinion 9.122. Bobinski & Epps, *Women, Poverty, Access to Health Care, and the Perils of Symbolic Reform, 5 J. Gender, Race & Just. 233, 238 (2002).*

Journal 2001 Examines the woman-child stereotype and its connection to feminist goals. Concludes that the stereotype presents serious social and legal implications. References Opinion 9.122. Preston, *Baby Spice: Lost Between Feminine and Feminist, 9 Am. U. J. Gender Soc. Pol'y & L. 541, 590 (2001).*

Journal 2000 Describes mandatory prelitigation panels under the Utah Health Care Malpractice Act. Considers constitutional challenges to such panels. Concludes that prelitigation panels are an impediment to resolution of medical malpractice claims and should be eliminated. References Opinion 9.122. Brann, *Utah's Medical Malpractice Prelitigation Panel: Exploring State Constitutional Arguments Against a Nonbinding Inadmissible Procedure, 2000 Utah L. Rev. 359, 399-400 (2000).*

Journal 2000 Discusses racial disparities in health care. Supports development of national strategies to eliminate racial inequities in medical care. Concludes that strong political leadership and effective interdisciplinary research are needed to achieve this important goal. References Opinion 9.122. Williams & Rucker, *Understanding and Addressing Racial Disparities in Health Care, 21 Health Care Fin. Rev. 75, 88 (2000).*

Journal 1999 Discusses a study that evaluated the impact of gender differences on outcomes of hospitalized patients treated for infection. Concludes that gender may not be predictive of mortality. References Opinion 9.122. Crabtree,

Pelletier, Gleason, Pruett, & Sawyer, *Gender-Dependent Differences in Outcome After the Treatment of Infection in Hospitalized Patients*, 282 JAMA 2143, 2148 (1999).

Journal 1996 Considers the impact the doctrine of informed consent may have on the rate at which hysterectomy operations are performed. Discusses how stereotypes affect the quality of medical treatment women receive. Focuses on how informed consent may benefit the health and autonomy of women. References Opinion 9.122. Napoli, *The Doctrine of Informed Consent and Women: The Achievement of Equal Value and Equal Exercise of Autonomy*, 4 J. Gender & L. 335, 336 (1996).

Journal 1993 Discusses the underrepresentation of women in clinical trials and its medical relevance. Examines the extent to which women are underrepresented. Considers barriers to their participation and proposes ways to include women in clinical investigations. References Opinion 9.122. Bennett, *Inclusion of Women in Clinical Trials—Policies for Population Subgroups*, 329 New Eng. J. Med. 288, 289 (1993).

Journal 1993 Explains how the role of women in clinical trials has evolved historically. Examines specific current concerns related to women's involvement in clinical studies and how these concerns might be resolved. References Opinion 9.122. Merkatz, *Women in Clinical Trials: An Introduction*, 48 Food & Drug L. J. 161, 163 (1993).

Journal 1992 Investigates the exclusion of women and minorities from medical research study groups. Concludes that this problem illustrates the extent to which bias is still present in contemporary medicine and science. References Opinion 9.122. Dresser, *Wanted: Single, White Male for Medical Research*, 22 Hastings Center Rep. 24, 28 (Jan./Feb. 1992).

Journal 1992 Presents the results of a gender study analyzing the differences in quality of care for elderly patients hospitalized with one of four diseases. Concludes that study results are positive but notes that concerns regarding gender discrimination are not entirely eliminated. References Opinion 9.122. Pearson, Kahn, Harrison, Rubenstein, Rogers, Brook, & Keeler, *Differences in Quality of Care for Hospitalized Elderly Men and Women*, 268 JAMA 1883 (1992).

Journal 1992 Analyzes the impact of gender and age on hospital admissions for acute asthma attacks. Presents results of a study that looked at age and gender as factors affecting admissions and length of hospital stay. Concludes that biological distinctions between the sexes may play a role in the disease. References Opinion 9.122. Skobeloff, Spivey, St. Clair, & Schoffstall, *The Influence of Age and Sex on Asthma Admissions*, 268 JAMA 3437, 3439, 3440 (1992).

8.6 Promoting Patient Safety

7th Cir. 2011 Plaintiffs brought suit against physicians employed by federally funded health care facilities, alleging medical malpractice. Affirming, the court held that information conveyed by hospital to parents was not sufficient for parents to know there was malpractice-related cause to child's injuries and a reasonable person, when informed the child's injuries had been caused by infection that had been transmitted during birth, would not have searched for potential causes. The concurrence cites Opinion 8.12 in describing the physicians' responsibilities to the plaintiffs. *Arroyo v. United States*, 656 F.3d 663, 678.

Minn. 1970 Defendant-physician appealed order to answer interrogatories, claiming that a medical malpractice plaintiff is prohibited from compelling expert testimony from a defendant to prove a charge of malpractice without calling other medical witnesses. In holding that a defendant could be compelled to provide expert medical opinion in response to interrogatories, the court quoted Principle 1 (1957) [now Principle II and Opinion 8.12] for the proposition that physicians owe a duty of disclosure to their patients. *Anderson v. Florence*, 288 Minn. 351, 181 N.W.2d 873, 880, 880 n.7.

Journal 2011 Explains how the Padilla opinion provides guidance on scope far beyond its dialogue on clarity. Concludes that defense attorneys must advise noncitizen clients as specifically as research allows to adequately inform them about the immigration consequences of contemplated criminal dispositions. Cites Opinion 8.12. Nash, *Considering the Scope of Advisal Duties Under Padilla*, 33 Cardozo L. Rev. 549, 550 (2011).

Journal 2011 Examines the impact of the Patient Protection and Affordable Care Act on medical liability and the controversy over the need for federal medical liability reforms, including a damage cap. Concludes that further studies are needed regarding liability reforms and the Affordable Care Act. References Opinion 8.12. Nelson, Becker, & Morrisey, *Medical Liability and Health Care Reform*, 21 Health Matrix 443, 510 (2011).

Journal 2011 Discusses current research and initiatives regarding physician apologies and the possibility of amending the Federal Rules of Evidence to exclude admission of physician apologies. Concludes that physician apologies and general admissions of fault should be protected under Fed. R. Evid. 409. Quotes Opinion 8.12. Pearlmutter, *Physician Apologies and General Admissions of Fault: Amending the Federal Rules of Evidence*, 72 Ohio St. L. J. 687, 713 (2011).

Journal 2011 Analyzes opinion of Supreme Court of Ohio in *Ward v. Summa Health System* addressing statutory physician-patient privilege and whether it precludes discovery of relevant medical information from a physician regarding his or her own medical condition. Concludes that in holding that it does not court reached the proper result. Quotes Opinion 8.12. Searl, *Ward v. Summa Health System, 37 Ohio N.U. L. Rev. 879, 887-888 (2011).*

Journal 2011 Examines and analyzes medical apology programs. Argues that such programs allow for the manipulation of injured patients as a means to persuade them not to pursue monetary damages. Suggests changes in design for medical apology programs. Quotes Opinion 8.12. Teninbaum, *How Medical Apology Programs Harm Patients, 15 Chap. L. Rev. 307, 310 (2011).*

Journal 2009 Discusses the importance of disclosure for establishing trust in the physician-patient relationship and the infrequency of disclosure in the American health care industry. Concludes physicians should be required to disclose mistakes to their patients, and the law should impose tort liability on physicians who fail to disclose. Quotes Opinion 8.12. Bourne, *Medical Malpractice: Should Courts Force Doctors to Confess Their Own Negligence to Their Patients? 61 Ark. L. Rev. 621, 629 (2009).*

Journal 2009 Explores the jurisprudential foundation of the fiduciary duty physicians owe their patients and discusses the failure of physicians to disclose to patients errors and other emergent medical risks. Concludes law should recognize the physician's duty to disclose such risks by enforcing a cause of action for breach of that duty. Quotes Principles III and VIII and Opinions 8.12, 10.015, and 10.02. References Opinion 8.12. Hafemeister, *Lean on Me: A Physician's Fiduciary Duty to Disclose an Emergent Medical Risk to the Patient, 86 Wash. U. L. Rev. 1167, 1172-1173, 1178, 1182, 1185, 1188, 1209 (2009).*

Journal 2009 Discusses the absence of tort liability for medical malpractice in New Zealand, and the newly created patient right to health care services of an appropriate standard. Concludes New Zealand's statutory code and Health and Disability Commissioner Act allow for clear rulings without invoking tort law. Cites Opinion 8.12. Sladden & Graydon, *Liability for Medical Malpractice—Recent New Zealand Developments, 28 Med. & L. 301, 310 (2009).*

Journal 2008 Considers the utility of physician apologies for medical error and legal protection for physicians who apologize for mistakes. Concludes physicians must openly communicate with their patients and apologize for medical errors to strengthen the health care community. Quotes Opinions 8.08, 8.12, 10.01, and 10.015. References Opinion 8.12. Ebert, *Attorneys, Tell Your Clients to Say They're Sorry: Apologies in the Health Care Industry, 5 Ind. Health L. Rev. 337, 340-41, 344 (2008).*

Journal 2008 Explores the fiduciary relationship between physicians and patients, professional and ethical obligations of both physicians and lawyers, and the implications for conflict resolution in health care. Concludes physicians must put patient interests above their own and lawyers must work to discern clients' best interests and support client welfare.

Quotes Principle VIII and Opinions 8.12 and 10.015. Cites Principles I and II and Opinions 10.01 and 10.015. Scott, *Doctors as Advocates, Lawyers as Healers, 29 Hamline J. Pub. L. Pol'y, 331, 340-41, 347, 371 (2008).*

Journal 2007 Analyzes problems with the current medical malpractice system. Concludes that Hillary Clinton's proposed National Medical Error and Compensation (MEDiC) Act of 2005 would be effective in facilitating physician apologies, reducing incidence of medical errors, and improving resolution of malpractice disputes. Quotes Opinion 8.12. References Opinion 8.082. Geckeler, *The Clinton-Obama Approach to Medical Malpractice Reform: Reviving the Most Meaningful Features of Alternative Dispute Resolution, 8 Pepp. Disp. Resol. L. J. 171, 193 (2007).*

Journal 2007 Examines barriers to reporting of medical errors in professional journals. Concludes that legal protection should be provided for error reporting and that medical journals could serve as a suitable forum for disclosure. Quotes Opinion 8.12. Murphy, Stee, McEvoy, & Oshiro, *J. Reporting of Medical Errors, 131 Chest 890, 892 (2007).*

Journal 2007 Argues that issuance of apologies from physicians who commit medical errors will diminish the number of malpractice suits brought. Concludes that patients desire apologies in the case of medical errors and are less likely to sue when they are given. Cites Principles I, II, III, and IV and Opinion 8.12. Tabler, *Should Physicians Apologize for Medical Errors? 19 Health Lawyer 23, 23 (Jan. 2007).*

Journal 2006 Reviews the arguments made in Thomas Baker's book *The Medical Malpractice Myth.* Concludes that Baker's book provides the kind of useful dialogue which will lead to positive reform of the malpractice system. Quotes Opinion 8.12. Coombs, *The Medical Malpractice Myth, 27 J. Legal Med. 243, 249-50 (2006).*

Journal 2006 Discusses the evolution of health law in Virginia. Concludes that the area of health law continues to expand, develop, and be refined. Cites Opinions 3.03, 3.08, 5.01, 5.015, 5.02, 5.04, 5.055, 6.02, 6.021, 6.03, 6.04, 7.03, 7.04, 7.05, 8.054, 8.08, 8.081, 8.085, 8.115, 8.12, 8.14, 8.145, 8.19, and 9.045. Guanzon, *Health Care Law, 41 U. Rich. L. Rev. 179, 199 (2006).*

Journal 2006 Discusses tort liability for medical malpractice. Concludes that both physicians and attorneys should support a legal system which promotes patient safety. Quotes Opinions 8.12 and 10.015. Pegalis, *A Proposal to Use Common Ground That Exists Between the Medical and Legal Professions to Promote a Culture of Safety, 51 N. Y. L. Sch. L. Rev. 1057, 1070, 1073 (2006).*

Journal 2006 Reviews law and policy regulating the reporting of medical errors. Concludes that federal health programs will play a significant role in shaping future policies. Quotes Opinion 8.12. Sage, Zivin, & Chase, *Bridging the Relational-Regulatory Gap, 59 Vand. L. Rev. 1263, 1284 (2006).*

Journal 2006 Examines tort reform and the application of principles of restorative justice. Concludes that a "healing-centered framework" serves the best interest of patients and health care providers. Cites Opinion 8.12. Todres, *Toward Healing and Restoration for All: Reframing Medical Malpractice Reform, 39 Conn. L. Rev. 667, 728-29 (2006).*

Journal 2006 Discusses an attorney's role in advising health care professionals on disclosure of medical errors. Concludes attorneys should always encourage full disclosure to prevent harm to the patient. Quotes Opinion 8.12. Winslade & McKinney, *The Ethical Health Lawyer: To Tell or Not to Tell: Disclosing Medical Error, 34 J. L. Med. & Ethics 813, 814 (2006).*

Journal 2005 Considers tort liability reforms that focus on compensating injured patients fairly and quickly while increasing patient safety. Concludes that the current system is ineffective, and that nontort alternatives should be implemented to achieve these goals. Quotes Opinion 8.12. Bovbjerg & Tancredi, *Liability Reform Should Make Patients Safer: "Avoidable Classes of Events" Are a Key Improvement, 33 J. L. Med. & Ethics 478, 482 (2005).*

Journal 2005 Argues that abolishing or weakening the tort liability system will not improve the quality of health care, but may diminish it. Concludes that a systems-based approach coupled with a liability system that encourages high-quality care may improve health care delivery in the US. Quotes Opinion 8.12. References Opinion 6.01. Hyman & Silver, *The Poor State of Health Care Quality in the U.S.: Is Malpractice Liability Part of the Problem or Part of the Solution? 90 Cornell L. Rev. 893, 926, 965 (2005).*

Journal 2004 Argues that reduction of medical errors will reduce the number of medical malpractice lawsuits and insurance premiums while stabilizing health care access and costs. Concludes that short-term liability reform, open communication, and the integration of patients as partners in system improvement are necessary. References Opinion 8.12. Liang & Ren, *Medical Liability Insurance and Damage Caps: Getting Beyond Band Aids to Substantive Systems Treatment to Improve Quality and Safety in Healthcare, 30 Am. J. L. & Med. 501, 534 (2004).*

Journal 2002 Discusses therapeutic jurisprudence and the importance of trust in the structure of health care law. Concludes that understanding trust provides tools to formulate responses to new ethical, legal, and policy challenges. Quotes Principle Ch. I, Art. I, Sec. 4 (May 1847) [now Principle II and Opinion 8.12]. Hall, *Law, Medicine, and Trust, 55 Stan. L. Rev. 463, 471 (2002).*

Journal 2002 Advocates in favor of disclosure of information regarding a physician's clinical experience when obtaining informed consent. Concludes that the physician's experience is material and patients who inquire should be given this information. Quotes Principle Ch. I, Art. I, Sec. 4 (May 1847) [now Principle II and Opinion 8.12]. Iheukwumere, *Doctor, Are You Experienced? The Relevance of Disclosure of Physician Experience to a Valid*

Informed Consent, 18 J. Contemp. Health L. & Pol'y 373, 376-77 (2002).

Journal 2002 Examines various interpretations of JCAHO standards regarding informing patients about medical errors. Concludes that further clarification is needed regarding reportable events. Quotes Opinion 8.12. LeGros & Pinkall, *The New JCAHO Patient Safety Standards and the Disclosure of Unanticipated Outcomes, 35 J. Health L. 189, 203 (2002).*

Journal 2002 Analyzes the role of prognostication in physician-patient communication. Concludes that the patient-physician model of shared decision-making offers the best hope for reestablishing prognostication. Quotes Principles Ch. I, Art. I, Sec. 2 and 4 (1846) [now Principle IV and Opinions 8.12 and 10.01]. Cites Opinion 8.08. Rich, *Prognostication in Clinical Medicine: Prophecy or Professional Responsibility? 23 J. Legal Med. 297, 299, 318, 327 (2002).*

Journal 2001 Discusses whether the medical profession needs a policy on honesty. Reviews ethical codes and concludes they fail to offer physicians meaningful guidance about what constitutes "the truth" and when and how to disclose it. Quotes Principle II and Opinions 8.12 and 10.01. DeVita, *Honestly, Do We Need a Policy on Truth? 11 Kennedy Inst. Ethics J. 157, 158 (2001).*

Journal 2001 Examines the duty of physicians and medical students to disclose physician mistakes. Concludes that students develop professionally by recognizing personal ethical standards and determining how to manage conflicting priorities. Quotes Opinion 8.12. Wusthoff, *Medical Mistakes and Disclosure: The Role of the Medical Student, 286 JAMA 1080, 1080 (2001).*

Journal 2000 Examines the lost chance doctrine in medical malpractice cases. Reviews Texas law by evaluating the cases of *Kramer v. Lewisville Mem'l Hosp.* and *Park Place Hosp. v. Estate of Milo.* Examines the distinction between affirmative acts and omissions. Discusses the limitations and pitfalls of both cases. Quotes Opinion 8.12. Perdue & Binion, *A License to Kill: The Unintended (?) Consequence of Milo on Kramer, 41 S. Tex. L. Rev. 293, 309 (2000).*

Journal 1997 Compares past ethical opinions to current opinions and notes the differences. Comments on the forces that have changed medical ethics through the years. Notes differing theories on the future course of medical ethics. Quotes Fundamental Elements (Preamble) and Opinions 5.05, 5.057, 7.01, 8.12, 9.12, and 9.131. Cites Fundamental Elements (5) and Opinions 8.115 and 8.13. Buchanan, *Medical Ethics at the Millennium: A Brief Retrospective, 26 Colo. Law. 141, 142, 143, 144, 145 (1997).*

Journal 1996 Presents clinical problem-solving scenarios. Notes the AMA's instruction that physicians deal openly and honestly with patients. Considers the physician's role as educator and counselor. Opines that physicians must ensure that patients have the ability to make informed decisions. Quotes

Opinion 8.12. Sirmon & Kreisberg, *The Invisible Patient, 334 New Eng. J. Med. 908, 910, 911 (1996).*

Journal 1991 Discusses the manner in which a changing economy and an evolving health care system require society to expand its understanding of the physician-patient relationship. Concludes that open physician-patient discussion about available medical services and costs may become part of the standard of care. References Opinions 8.08 and 8.12. Morreim, *Economic Disclosure and Economic Advocacy: New Duties in the Medical Standard of Care, 12 J. Legal Med. 275, 306 (1991).*

Journal 1983 Discusses both moral and legal dilemmas in the use of placebos in treating patients. Concludes that, while arguments against placebo therapy are noble, a complete ban of placebo therapy is impractical and undesirable. Quotes Opinions 8.07 (1982) [now Opinion 8.08] and 8.11 (1982) [now Opinion 8.12]. Kapp, *Placebo Therapy and the Law: Prescribe With Care, 8 Am. J. Law & Med. 371, 391 (1983).*

Journal 2009 Argues it is inappropriate to create an evidentiary exclusion for medical apologies in an attempt to improve physician-patient communication. Concludes that the exclusion for medical apologies will allow lawyers to have greater involvement in the communications between physicians and patients, and will decrease the openness and efficacy of that communication. Quotes Opinion 8.121. Jesson & Knapp, *My Lawyer Told Me to Say I'm Sorry: Lawyers, Doctors, and Medical Apologies, 35 Wm. Mitchell L. Rev. 1410, 1420 (2009).*

Journal 2009 Explores the value of incident reports and their use for hospital quality assurance research. Discusses the relationship between incident reports and confidentiality statutes. Concludes incident reports should be used strictly as research aids in alerting hospitals to their own

shortcomings and that greater legal protection is needed for providers to freely report errors and improve care. Quotes Opinion 8.121. Mikk, *Making the Plaintiff's Bar Earn Its Keep: Rethinking the Hospital Incident Report, 53 N. Y. L. Sch. L. Rev. 133, 156 (2009).*

Journal 2008 Examines ethical issues related to broadcasting cardiothoracic surgeries for educational and media purposes. Concludes that seven ethical guidelines should be followed to ensure patient safety. Quotes Principle VIII and Opinion 8.121. Sade, *Broadcast of Surgical Procedures as a Teaching Instrument in Cardiothoracic Surgery, 86 Ann. Thorac. Surg. 357, 359 (2008).*

Journal 2006 Reviews the concept of therapeutic privilege. Concludes that the practice creates conflict between physician obligations under the concepts of autonomy and beneficence. Recommends that physicians maximize communication with patients by providing all pertinent information in the context of patient preferences. Cites Opinions 8.08, 8.081, 8.121, and 10.015. References Chap. I, Art. I, Sec. 4 (May 1847) [premise deleted from Code]. Bostick, Sade, McMahon, & Benjamin, *Report of the American Medical Association Council on Ethical and Judicial Affairs: Withholding Information From Patients: Rethinking the Propriety of "Therapeutic Privilege," 17 J. Clinical Ethics 302, 303 (Winter 2006).*

Journal 2006 Examines ethical dilemmas physicians may face as providers of pay-for-performance medical care. Concludes that this strategy offers a benefit to patients as long as physicians uphold stringent ethical standards and work together to ensure optimum patient care. Cites Principles I, V, VIII, and IX and Opinions 2.035, 2.095, 6.01, 8.021, 8.03, 8.0501, 8.053, 8.054, and 8.121. Bostick, Sade, & McMahon, *Report of the Council on Ethical and Judicial Affairs: Physician Pay-for-Performance Programs, 3 Ind. Health L. Rev. 429, 430, 431, 432-33, 434, 435, 436 (2006).*

8.8 Required Reporting of Adverse Events

Journal 2002 Challenges the general use of special informed consent disclosure rules in experimental therapy. Discusses the lack of a bright-line distinction between standard and experimental interventions. Concludes that focus should be placed on the distinctiveness of experimentation. Quotes Opinion 2.07. References Opinion 9.032. Noah, *Informed Consent and the Elusive Dichotomy Between Standard and Experimental Therapy, 28 Am. J. L. & Med. 361, 394, 395 (2002).*

Journal 2000 Describes possible solutions designed to improve postapproval regulation of prescription drugs so that fewer patients will suffer from adverse drug reactions. Concludes that the FDA along with physicians and clinical researchers should rethink the existing approach to monitoring of unexpected side effects. Quotes Principle V and Opinion 9.032. Cites Opinion 5.05. Noah, *Adverse*

Drug Reactions: Harnessing Experimental Data to Promote Patient Welfare, 49 Cath. U. L. Rev. 449, 477, 497-98 (2000).

Journal 2000 Evaluates the regulatory framework governing prescription drugs. Considers problems faced by elderly patients when taking FDA-approved medications. Concludes that, in order to optimize patient safety, the existing regulatory system must undergo important structural changes. Quotes Principle V and Opinion 9.032. Noah & Brushwood, *Adverse Drug Reactions in Elderly Patients: Alternative Approaches to Postmarket Surveillance, 33 J. Health L. 383, 400, 445 (2000).*

Journal 1999 Discusses the duty of manufacturers to discover potential adverse drug interactions with new drugs. Suggests that a manufacturer's duty to warn about adverse drug interactions may be the future subject of products liability lawsuits. References Opinion 9.032. McCormick, *Pharmaceutical Manufacturer's Duty to Warn of Adverse Drug Interactions, 66 Def. Couns. J. 59, 61 (1999).*

Journal 1993 Explains MedWatch, an FDA program designed to facilitate the reporting of adverse events

associated with the use of FDA-approved drugs and medical devices. Emphasizes that physicians are best able to provide such information. Quotes Opinion 9.032. Rheinstein, *MedWatch: The FDA Medical Products Reporting Program, 48 Am. Fam. Physician 636, 636 (1993).*

8.10 Preventing, Identifying, and Treating Violence and Abuse

Cal. App. 1982 Defendant was convicted of lewd act with a child and child molestation or annoyance, after licensed clinical psychologist reported defendant's admission of sexual conduct to authorities. The court held that the psychologist's testimony was properly admitted since a statute requiring the reporting of actual or suspected child abuse expressly made the psychotherapist-patient privilege inapplicable. The court quoted Principle 9 (1957) [now Principle IV and Opinions 2.02 and 5.05] in concluding the disclosure was not a breach of professional ethics. *People v. Stritzinger, 137 Cal. App. 3d 126, 186 Cal. Rptr. 750, 752 rev'd 34 Cal. 3d 505, 668 p.2d 738, 194 Cal. Rptr. 431 (1983).*

Md. Att'y Gen. 1977 Opinion addresses the obligation of a psychiatrist to report child abuse information obtained from a parent-patient. Referring to state statutes and to Principle 9 (1957) [now Principle IV and Opinions 2.02 and 5.05] the opinion concludes that the question of whether to disclose suspected child abuse is a matter left to the individual psychiatrist's professional and moral judgment. *Maryland Att'y Gen. Opinion, 62 Op. Att'y Gen. Md. 157, 160.*

Wis. Att'y Gen. 1987 Physicians may report cases of suspected child abuse or neglect when a patient discloses that he or she has abused a child in some manner. Where report is made in good faith, physicians are immune from any civil or criminal liability. Passing reference is made to Principle 9 (1957) [now Principle IV and Opinions 2.02 and 5.05] in support of this position. *Wisconsin Att'y Gen. Op. 10-87 (March 16, 1987) (LEXIS, States library, Wis. file).*

Journal 2010 Discusses futility disputes where a patient's surrogate wishes to prolong treatment that the physician deems medically ineffective, and the current lack of legal remedies to resolve them. Concludes that states need to establish fair, impartial, and patient-centered methods of resolving futility disputes including independent medical boards that would operate under procedural and substantive regulations. Quotes Opinions 2.02 and 2.035. References Opinions 2.17 and 2.20. Bassel, *Order at the End of Life: Establishing a Clear and Fair Mechanism for the Resolution of Futility Disputes, 63 Vand. L. Rev. 491, 494, 523 (2010).*

Journal 2010 Examines published resources within the medical and legal fields that focus on confidentiality and evaluates those resources to determine if they help clarify confidentiality issues. Further, discusses differences between these professions that may be hindrances when

serving the same patient or client. Concludes that, while both professions guard against disclosure of patient/client communications, they also allow for disclosure in certain instances such as imminent death, harm, or injury. References Principle IV and cites Opinions 2.02, 2.23, 2.24, and 5.05. Johns, *Multidisciplinary Practice and Ethics Part II—Lawyers, Doctors, and Confidentiality, 6 NAELA J. 55, 57-65, 68 (2010).*

Journal 2009 Examines the influence of HIV/AIDS on intimate partner violence and the current legal response to this violence. Concludes courts and legislatures must recognize the relationship between HIV/AIDS and domestic violence and take steps to allow victims to tell their stories in court. Cites Opinion 2.02. Stoever, *Stories Absent From the Courtroom: Responding to Domestic Violence in the Context of HIV and AIDS, 87 N. C. L. Rev. 1157, 1226 (2009).*

Journal 2008 Discusses the effect of *Crawford* and *Davis* on out-of-court statements made to medical personnel and the application of the Sixth Amendment Confrontation Clause to such statements. Concludes courts, when making a confrontation determination, must consider the intent of the declarant and the circumstances that influence the content of the declarant's statement. Quotes Opinion 9.07. Cites Opinion 2.02. Gordon, *Is There an Accuser in the House?: Evaluating Statements Made to Physicians and Other Medical Personnel in the Wake of Crawford v. Washington and Davis v. Washington, 38 N. M. L. Rev. 529, 529 (2008).*

Journal 2000 Examines physician value neutrality (PVN). Defines PVN as providing a foundation to suggest physicians must keep their values—religious, political, or otherwise—out of the patient-physician relationship. Concludes it is not clear how values can be removed from the patient-physician relationship without removing the very thing PVN supporters are trying to protect, the intrinsic value of persons. References Opinions 2.01, 2.02, 8.032, 8.05, 8.08, and 8.132. Beckwith & Peppin, *Physician Value Neutrality: A Critique, 28 J. L. Med. & Ethics 67, 72-73 (2000).*

Journal 2000 Examines public policies and medical practices intended to protect victims of domestic violence. Explores the possibility of liability for failure to act by health care professionals. Concludes that states need to develop public policy initiatives to address this and other related issues. References Opinion 2.02. Brown-Cranstoun,

Kringen v. Boslough and Saint Vincent Hospital: A New Trend for Healthcare Professionals Who Treat Victims of Domestic Violence? 33 J. Health L. 629, 649, 650 (2000).

Journal 2000 Discusses the physical health consequences of psychological intimate partner violence (IPV). Concludes that clinicians should screen for psychological, physical, and sexual IPV in order to minimize physical health consequences. References Opinion 2.02. Coker, Smith, Bethea, King, & McKeown, *Physical Health Consequences of Physical and Psychological Intimate Partner Violence, 9 Arch. Fam. Med. 451, 456, 457 (2000).*

Journal 2000 Describes the epidemiology of intimate partner violence. Explores medical, legal, and law enforcement responses to intimate partner violence. Urges further research relating to medical and legal issues associated with intimate partner violence as well as additional training of attorneys, health care providers, judges, and law enforcement personnel. References Opinion 2.02. Loue, *Intimate Partner Violence: Bridging the Gap Between Law and Science, 21 J. Legal Med. 1, 18 (2000).*

Journal 2000 Examines public reporting statutes and introduces the provisions of the Violence Against Women Act (VAWA). Compares VAWA and public reporting laws. Concludes that VAWA is superior legislation because it requires women to initiate their own claims against abusers. References Opinion 2.02. Vital, *Mandatory Reporting Statutes and the Violence Against Women Act: An Analytical Comparison, 10 Geo. Mason U. Civ. Rts. L. J. 171, 189 (2000).*

Journal 1999 Discusses the basis for holding professionals liable for failing to report abuse. Explains reasons why professionals should be held liable in tort when they fail to report abuse. Argues that imposing such liability will increase early detection and deter future abuse. References Opinion 2.02. Jones, *Kentucky Tort Liability for Failure to Report Family Violence, 26 N. Ky. L. Rev. 43, 58 (1999).*

Journal 1998 Emphasizes that physicians need to be aware of the signs of domestic violence. Points out that, because many victims seek medical treatment, physicians are in a key position to identify domestic violence. Argues that Florida should follow other states' examples and adopt a mandatory reporting act. References Opinion 2.02. Makar, *Domestic Violence: Why the Florida Legislature Must Do More to Protect the "Silent" Victims, 72 Fla. Bar J. 10, 16 (Nov. 1998).*

Journal 1998 Discusses proposed legislation in New York that would mandate physician reporting of domestic violence. Argues that mandatory reporting harms patients by threatening the physician-patient relationship. Suggests that victims of domestic violence may be less likely to

seek treatment or will be hesitant to speak freely with their physicians if reporting is mandatory. Cites Opinion 2.02. McFarlane, *Mandatory Reporting of Domestic Violence: An Inappropriate Response for New York Health Care Professionals, 17 Buff. Pub. Int. L. J. 1, 29 (1998).*

Journal 1998 Points out that most victims of elder abuse are socially isolated and thus few incidents of elder abuse are reported to authorities. Argues that current protections against elder abuse are inadequate. Suggests that the legal system and health professionals can make a difference in reducing elder abuse. Quotes Opinion 5.05. References Opinion 2.02. Moskowitz, *Saving Granny From the Wolf: Elder Abuse and Neglect—The Legal Framework, 31 Conn. L. Rev. 77, 116, 120, 121, 122 (1998).*

Journal 1997 Considers the best interests of children who are victims of domestic abuse. Advocates a rebuttable presumption against granting custody to a perpetrator. Concludes that courts should be educated about domestic violence. References Opinion 2.02. Comment, *Protecting Children Exposed to Domestic Violence in Contested Custody and Visitation Litigation, 6 B. U. Pub. Int. L. J. 501, 502, 505 (1997).*

Journal 1997 Reviews the historical treatment of domestic violence in tort law. Explores the difficulties victims of domestic violence suffer in pursuing traditional forms of relief. Considers this issue in the context of divorce proceedings. Offers practical guidance for achieving justice. References Opinion 2.02. Dalton, *Domestic Violence, Domestic Torts and Divorce: Constraints and Possibilities, 31 New. Eng. L. Rev. 319, 354 (1997).*

Journal 1996 Considers means of combating spousal abuse problems. Suggests various schemes of liability to increase aid to victims and reporting of problems. Observes that physicians may play an important role in eliminating spousal abuse. Concludes that imposition of civil liability on physicians for failure to report abuse will help remedy problems. References Opinion 2.02. Jones, *Battered Spouses' Damage Actions Against Non-Reporting Physicians, 45 DePaul L. Rev. 191 (1996).*

Journal 1994 Explores the ethical issues involved in a multidisciplinary team working with children in legal proceedings. Focuses on the relationships between professionals and the conflicts that arise regarding disclosure of confidential information and forced disclosure of nonprivileged information. Quotes Principles III and IV, Fundamental Elements (4), and Opinions 1.02 (1992) and 5.07 (1992) [now Opinion 5.05]. Cites Opinion 2.02. Glynn, *Multidisciplinary Representation of Children: Conflicts Over Disclosures of Client Communications, 27 J. Marshall L. Rev. 617, 625, 626, 630-32, 637, 639, 643 (1994).*

9 Professional Self-regulation

9.1.1 Romantic or Sexual Relationships with Patients

S.D. N.Y. 1999 Physician brought a 42 USC § 1983 claim seeking to enjoin the state board from revoking his license to practice medicine. The charges against the physician included allegations of engaging in sexual relations with patients. The board quoted Opinion 8.14 as a basis for its conclusion that engaging in sexual relations with patients is an ethical violation. The court held that, in order to enjoin the board, the physician had to show a substantial likelihood of success on the merits. Further, the court found that abstention was appropriate because the physician's case was pending administrative appeal. Finally, the court held that the statute that prohibited the stay of a license revocation pending appeal complied with due process. *Selkin v. State Board for Professional Medical Conduct, 63 F. Supp. 2d 397, 399-400.*

Cal. 1995 Patient sued ultrasound technician, who sexually assaulted her, and hospital for professional negligence, battery, and intentional and negligent infliction of emotional distress. In differentiating between the physician-patient relationship and the technician-patient relationship, the court cited AMA Council on Ethical and Judicial Affairs, Sexual Misconduct in the Practice of Medicine, 266 *JAMA* 2741 (1991) [now Opinion 8.14]. Finding that the technician's acts did not arise from any events or conditions of his employment, the court held that the hospital was not liable under respondeat superior. *Lisa M. v. Henry Mayo Newhall Memorial Hosp., 12 Cal. 4th 291, 907 P.2d 358, 48 Cal. Rptr. 2d 510, 517.*

Cal. App. 1992 Physician who had sexual relationship with patient brought a mandamus action challenging discipline imposed by medical board. The court concluded that a sexual relationship between physician and patient was alone an insufficient basis for discipline. An expert witness, referring to Opinion 8.14, testified that it is unethical for a physician to have a sexual relationship with a patient. However, focusing on the applicable state statute, the court found the relationship must affect the functions and duties of a physician to be a basis for discipline. *Gromis v. Medical Board, 8 Cal. App. 4th 589, 10 Cal. Rptr. 2d 452, 455 n.3, reh'g denied, 1992 Cal. App. LEXIS 1047, and review denied, 1992 Cal. LEXIS 5101.*

Ga. 2007 A physician who applied to the Georgia bar appealed a denial of his application by the Board to Determine Bar Fitness. The Georgia Supreme Court reviewed for abuse of discretion. In making its decision, the Board had considered that the physician had violated Opinion 8.14 by engaging in sexual relations with a patient and lost his medical license as a result. Based on this and other circumstances, the court held that the Board properly concluded the applicant lacked moral fitness. *In re Baska, 281 Ga. 676, 641 S.E.2d 533, 534.*

Md. App. 2003 Physician appealed decision upholding state board's order to revoke his medical license for unprofessional conduct. The physician engaged in consensual sexual relationships with several of his patients at places and times other than when medical care was given. Appeals court affirmed the board's ruling and held that the conduct occurred within the practice of medicine. Quotes Opinion 8.14. *Finucan v. Maryland State Board of Physicians Quality Assurance, 151 Md. App. 399, 827 A.2d 176, 181-82.*

Md. App. 1992 Patient's husband sought damages from defendant psychiatrist because of the sexual relationship initiated during treatment of the patient by the defendant. Although the court held that the plaintiff in this case could not recover damages in tort for disruption of a marriage, it cited favorably Opinion 8.14 (1989) for its declaration that "sexual misconduct in the practice of medicine" is unethical. *Homer v. Long, 90 Md. App. 1, 3 n.1, 599 A.2d 1193, 1193 n.1.*

Mass. 2005 Massachusetts Board of Registration in Medicine revoked the license of appellant physician for engaging in inappropriate sexual conduct with a patient. The administrative magistrate cited Opinion 8.14 in making the determination that a sexual relationship with a patient was professional misconduct. The court affirmed the board's ruling, finding that sufficient evidence existed to find professional misconduct by the appellant arising out of a sexual relationship with his patient. *Weinberg v. Board of Registration in Medicine, 443 Mass. 679, 824 N.E.2d 38, 42.*

Mass. App. 2003 Patient appealed summary judgment in suit against physician's estate for harm caused by their two-year consensual sexual affair. Once the affair began, the physician stopped treating the patient. The patient alleged malpractice, breach of fiduciary duty, intentional infliction of emotional distress, and unfair or deceptive practices. Appellate court upheld summary judgment. In analyzing the fiduciary duty claim, the court quoted Opinion 8.14. *Korper v. Weinstein, 57 Mass. App. 433, 783 N.E.2d 877, 881, n. 9.*

Mont. 2005 A psychiatrist had sexual relations with a patient. Following a hearing, the Montana Board of Medical Examiners revoked the psychiatrist's license, despite a recommendation by the hearing examiner for a 90-day suspension. With apparent reference to Opinion 8.14, one of the board members posited at the hearing that the psychiatrist had violated the code of medical ethics. The psychiatrist sought judicial review. The Supreme Court of Montana found that the board's decision was proper, that the penalty was consistent with findings of fact, and was not arbitrary or capricious. *Munn v. Montana Board of Medical Examiners, 329 Mont. 401, 124 P.3d 1123, 1126.*

N.Y. 2002 Surgical resident sexually assaulted patient while she was in recovery room. Patient sued hospital for negligence and vicarious liability. Trial court denied hospital's motion for summary judgment, but intermediate appellate court granted motion. New York Court of Appeals modified the ruling. It held that patient's vicarious liability claim failed because the misconduct was not in furtherance of hospital business or in the scope of the resident's employment. The court found, however, a sufficient basis for a negligence claim. References Opinion 8.14. *N.X. v. Cabrini Medical Center, 97 N.Y 2d 247, 765 N.E 2d 844, 847, n.2, 739 N.Y.S.2d 348.*

N.Y. Sup. 1998 Physician was convicted of sodomizing a patient and falsifying her records. He appealed in part on grounds that the prosecutor had introduced evidence regarding his sexual relationship with another patient in violation of a pretrial ruling. The court reversed the convictions and remanded the case for a new trial. The dissent cited Opinion 8.14, stating that the physician's sexual relationship with another patient violated ethical standards. Furthermore, the dissent argued that evidence of such a relationship was relevant to the case at hand. *People v. Griffin, 242 A.D.2d 70, 671 N.Y.S. 2d 34, 39.*

Ohio 1991 State medical board revoked license of physician who had consensual sexual relations with his patient. The court upheld the board's ruling that this violated Principles I, II, and IV. Dissenting judge, citing AMA Council on Ethical and Judicial Affairs, Sexual Misconduct in the Practice of Medicine, 266 *JAMA* 2741 [now Opinion 8.14], argued that until 1991, the AMA did not clearly deem sexual contact with a patient unethical. *Pons v. Ohio State Medical Bd., 66 Ohio St. 3d 619, 623, 625, 614 N.E.2d 748, 752, 753.*

Wash. App. 2006 A physician treated an elderly patient prior to her death. The patient's son-in-law later brought a malpractice suit alleging that the physician had sexual relations with his wife and that a sexual relationship existed between himself and the physician. In opposing a motion for summary judgment, the plaintiff filed an affidavit from a physician. With apparent reference to Opinion 8.14, the affidavit stated the defendant had violated the AMA Code of Medical Ethics and thereby, breached her duty of care. The trial court acknowledged that the AMA *Code* helped establish such a duty, but granted summary judgment. Plaintiff's claims were found to be deficient because he failed to set forth any facts that would prove the alleged sexual relationship with the physician. On appeal, the court affirmed. *Prestrud v. Blanco, 2006 WL 1633707, 2.*

Journal 2010 Explores how participation in online social networks may blur boundaries between personal and professional relationships for health care professionals and how such risks may be mitigated by use of network privacy and security settings. Suggests that health care institutions are likely to institute online social-networking policies for employees. Quotes Opinions 5.026, 5.027, 5.045, 5.046, 5.05, 5.059, 5.0591, 8.14, 9.08, and 9.123. Cites Opinions 5.026, 9.031, and 9.12. Terry, *Physicians and Patients Who "Friend" or "Tweet": Constructing a Legal Framework for Social Networking in a Highly Regulated Domain, 43 Ind. L. Rev. 285, 314-16, 319, 334-36, 338 (2010).*

Journal 2009 Discusses the willful blindness doctrine with respect to physicians charged with drug trafficking after prescribing to patients who resell drugs. Concludes there is a distinction between knowledge and willful blindness, and an actor who is morally justified in choosing to be blind should not be prosecuted under a statute requiring knowledge. Quotes Opinion 8.14. Hellman, *Prosecuting Doctors for Trusting Patients, 16 Geo. Mason L. Rev. 701, 712 (2009).*

Journal 2008 Argues that organ donation from a patient to his or her physician is unethical. Concludes that this practice would be exploitative to the patient and undermine public trust in the medical profession. Cites Opinions 8.14, 10.017, and 10.018. Steinberg & Pomfret, *A Novel Boundary Issue: Should a Patient Be an Organ Donor for Their Physician? 34 J. Med. Ethics 772, 772 (2008).*

Journal 2006 Discusses the evolution of health law in Virginia. Concludes that the area of health law continues to expand, develop, and be refined. Cites Opinions 3.03, 3.08, 5.01, 5.015, 5.02, 5.04, 5.055, 6.02, 6.021, 6.03, 6.04, 7.03, 7.04, 7.05, 8.054, 8.08, 8.081, 8.085, 8.115, 8.12, 8.14, 8.145, 8.19, and 9.045. Guanzon, *Health Care Law, 41 U. Rich. L. Rev. 179, 199 (2006).*

Journal 2006 Considers prisoners' rights to expression of sexuality and the state's legitimate interest in regulating that expression. Concludes that states should encourage healthy expressions of sexuality while protecting the goals of the Prison Rape Elimination Act. Cites Opinions 3.08, 8.14, 8.145, and 10.015. Smith, *Rethinking Prison Sex: Self-expression and Safety, 15 Colum. J. Gender & L. 185, 202 (2006).*

Journal 2004 Examines the relationship between administrative law and health law. Concludes that administrative law and health law will continue to be intertwined and that this relationship may provide benefits in the context of health care delivery. Cites Opinion 8.14. Jost, *Health Law and Administrative Law: A Marriage Most Convenient, 49 St. Louis U. L. J. 1, 20 (2004).*

Journal 2004 Analyzes various issues relating to the role of mental health professionals in capital punishment in light of Albert Bandura's model of "mechanisms of moral disengagement." Concludes that facilitating participation of mental health professionals in executions creates conflicts with the humanistic norms of the profession. Quotes Preamble and Opinions 1.01, 1.02, 2.06, 2.067, 2.20, 2.21, 2.211, and 8.14. Judges, *The Role of Mental Health Professionals in Capital Punishment: An Exercise in Moral Disengagement, 41 Hous. L. Rev. 515, 562, 568, 569, 570, 571-72, 581, 586, 588, 598 (2004).*

Journal 2003 Highlights the inadequacies of Washington tort law with respect to holding employers of sexually exploitative therapists accountable. Concludes that courts should premise employer liability on the foreseeability of transference. References Opinion 8.14. Allen, *The Foreseeability of Transference: Extending Employer Liability Under Washington Law for Therapist Sexual Exploitation of Patients, 78 Wash. L. Rev. 525, 531 (2003).*

Journal 2001 Explores changes in common law and statutory law that have promoted the marginalization of chastity. Considers rules governing the professions. Concludes with a legal agenda intended to help restore the social value of chastity. References Opinion 8.14. Rodes, *On Law and Chastity, 76 Notre Dame L. Rev. 643, 675 (2001).*

Journal 2000 Evaluates consensual sexual relationships between patients and physicians. Emphasis is placed on whether, and in what situation, a sexual relationship may constitute medical malpractice. Concludes that people should learn to take responsibility for their actions and that certain limitations should be placed on recovery for malpractice. References Opinion 8.14. Puglise, *"Calling Dr. Love": The* physician-patient *Sexual Relationship as Grounds for Medical Malpractice—Society Pays While the Doctor and Patient Play, 14 J. L. & Health 321, 324-25, 349 (2000).*

Journal 1999 Examines countertransference in professional relationships. Observes how the resulting power imbalance may give rise to the potential for sexual exploitation. Concludes by offering strategies for identifying and addressing emotional interference in the lawyer/client relationship. Cites Opinion 8.14. Silver, *Love, Hate, and Other Emotional Interference in the Lawyer/Client Relationship, 6 Clinical L. Rev. 259, 266 (1999).*

Journal 1998 Provides policy reasons why attorney-client sexual relations should be prohibited. Urges states to codify rules precluding such conduct during representation. Explains that such rules would pass constitutional scrutiny. Cites Opinion 8.14. Awad, *Attorney-Client Sexual Relations, 22 J. Legal. Prof. 131, 190 (1998).*

Journal 1998 Discusses types of discipline taken against physicians for sexual offenses. Points out that some physicians still may be permitted to practice medicine despite the commission of sexual misconduct. Proposes ways that might increase the chance that sex-related offenses will be reported. Quotes Opinion 8.14. Dehlendorf & Wolfe, *Physicians Disciplined for Sex-Related Offenses, 279 JAMA 1883 (1998).*

Journal 1997 Examines the balance needed between clinical objectivity and physician-patient bonding. Discusses personal boundaries and methods of coping with transgressions by both physicians and patients. Advocates a focus on communication with patients to allow physicians to maintain both an empathetic and objective relationship. References

Opinion 8.14. Farber, Novack, & O'Brien, *Love, Boundaries, and the* physician-patient *Relationship, 157 Arch. Intern. Med. 2291, 2292, 2293, 2294 (1997).*

Journal 1996 Discusses the ethical implications of sexual misconduct in the medical field. Examines the current civil and criminal tools used to curb physician-patient misconduct. Notes the inadequacy of physician reporting. Proposes a statutory approach to discipline physicians who abuse their fiduciary duties. Quotes Principle II. References Opinion 8.14. Note, *Sexual Conduct Within the* physician-patient *Relationship: A Statutory Framework for Disciplining This Breach of Fiduciary Duty, 1 Widener L. Symp. J. 501, 507 (1996).*

Journal 1994 Explores the negative consequences of physician-patient sexual relationships. Suggests that sexual contact be prohibited during the physician-patient relationship and for a period of time thereafter. Quotes Opinion 8.14. Appelbaum, Jorgenson, & Sutherland, *Sexual Relationships Between Physicians and Patients, 154 Arch. Intern. Med. 2561, 2561 (1994).*

Journal 1993 Examines the potential problems created by attorney-client sexual relations and the need for ethical guidelines. Examines ethical rules being debated in various states and proposes a model rule. References Opinion 8.14. Davis & Grimaldi, *Sexual Confusion: Attorney-Client Sex and the Need for a Clear Ethical Rule, 7 Notre Dame J. Law, Ethics, & Pub. Pol. 57, 61 (1993).*

Journal 1993 Discusses family privacy rights and considers the meaning of justice, self-respect, and the fundamental principles of physician ethics. Concludes that physicians have an ethical duty to intervene in domestic violence so long as such intervention does not breach confidentiality or violate patient autonomy. Quotes Principle IV and Opinion 5.05. References Opinions 8.14 and 9.131. Jecker, *Privacy Beliefs and the Violent Family: Extending the Ethical Argument for Physician Intervention, 269 JAMA 776, 778, 779 (1993).*

Journal 1993 Discusses the potential impact on health care practitioners of the AMA's prohibition against sexual relations between physicians and patients. Focuses on how the prohibition will influence disciplinary actions. Cites Opinion 8.14. Johnson, *Judicial Review of Disciplinary Action for Sexual Misconduct in the Practice of Medicine, 270 JAMA 1596 (1993).*

Journal 1993 Discusses potential problems caused by attorney-client sexual relations and examines various means to check such conduct. Proposes a new rule that would prohibit attorney-client sexual relations. References Opinion 8.14. Livingston, *When Libido Subverts Credo: Regulation of Attorney-Client Sexual Relations, 62 Fordham L. Rev. 5, 55 (1993).*

Journal 1993 Discusses the problems physicians may encounter by exposing the errant colleague, such as harm to the reporting physician's reputation and the fear of litigation. States that problems involving physician competency and unethical behavior should be investigated, and that physicians should take personal responsibility for reporting problems they observe. References Principle II and Opinions 8.14 and 9.031. Morreim, *Am I My Brother's Warden? Responding to the Unethical or Incompetent Colleague, 23 Hastings Center Rep. 19, 23 (May/June 1993).*

Journal 1993 Discusses the medical profession's ethical prohibition on physician-patient sexual contact. Concludes that legislatures and courts should give greater weight to the ethical code when defining standards of conduct for physician-patient sexual contact. Quotes Opinion 8.14. Note, physician-patient *Sexual Contact: The Battle Between the State and the Medical Profession, 50 Wash. & Lee L. Rev. 1725, 1725-26, 1734, 1752 (1993).*

Journal 1992 Discusses the problem of sex in the attorney-client relationship and compares this to that of the physician-patient. Proposes an explicit ban on sexual involvement between attorneys and their clients and advocates promulgation of a "bright line" rule. References Opinion 8.14. Goldberg, *Sex and the Attorney-Client Relationship: An Argument for a Prophylactic Rule, 26 Akron L. Rev. 45 (1992).*

Journal 1992 Examines the similarities and differences between the physician-patient and lawyer-client relationships regarding the problems associated with sexual relations. Advocates a rebuttable presumption that sexual contact between attorneys and clients is wrongful. Cites Opinion 8.14. Gutheil, Jorgenson, & Sutherland, *Prohibiting Lawyer-Client Sex, 20 Bull. Am. Acad. Psychiatry Law 365 (1992).*

Journal 1992 Finds that state medical boards increasingly rely upon psychiatric testimony in cases of alleged sexual abuse by physicians. Proposes that states adopt clear standards governing the admissibility of psychiatric testimony in administrative hearings. Quotes Opinion 8.14. Hyams, *Expert Psychiatric Evidence in Sexual Misconduct Cases Before State Medical Boards, XVIII Am. J. Law & Med. 171, 173, 174 (1992).*

9.1.2 Romantic or Sexual Relationships with Key Third Parties

Journal 2007 Addresses physician liability for an extramarital affair with a patient's spouse. Concludes that such an affair should be regarded as a breach of a fiduciary duty. Quotes Preamble, Principles I, II, and VIII, and Opinions 8.145, 9.04, 9.123, and 10.015. Demaine, *"Playing Doctor" With the Patient's Spouse: Alternative Conceptions of Health Professional Liability, 14 Va. J. Soc. Pol'y & L. 308, 325, 330-31, 331-32 (2007).*

Journal 2006 Discusses the evolution of health law in Virginia. Concludes that the area of health law continues to expand, develop, and be refined. Cites Opinions 3.03, 3.08, 5.01, 5.015, 5.02, 5.04, 5.055, 6.02, 6.021, 6.03, 6.04, 7.03, 7.04, 7.05, 8.054, 8.08, 8.081, 8.085, 8.115, 8.12, 8.14, 8.145, 8.19, and 9.045. Guanzon, *Health Care Law, 41 U. Rich. L. Rev. 179, 199 (2006).*

Journal 2006 Considers prisoners' rights to expression of sexuality and the state's legitimate interest in regulating that expression. Concludes that states should encourage healthy expressions of sexuality while protecting the goals of the Prison Rape Elimination Act. Cites Opinions 3.08, 8.14, 8.145, and 10.015. Smith, *Rethinking Prison Sex: Self-expression and Safety, 15 Colum. J. Gender & L. 185, 202 (2006).*

9.1.3 Sexual Harassment in the Practice of Medicine

Va. App. 2003 Physician appealed board of medicine's license probation order for unprofessional conduct. Board found the physician's pattern of inappropriate advances toward medical students violated medical ethical standards. Appellate court reversed, holding that the evidence was insufficient to support board's finding, since the ethical standards by which the physician should be adjudicated were not established by competent evidence. Quotes Opinions 3.08 and 9.05. *Goad v. Virginia Board of Medicine, 40 Va. App. 621, 580 S.E.2d 494, 498, n.7, 499, n.9.*

Journal 2006 Discusses the evolution of health law in Virginia. Concludes that the area of health law continues to expand, develop, and be refined. Cites Opinions 3.03, 3.08, 5.01, 5.015, 5.02, 5.04, 5.055, 6.02, 6.021, 6.03, 6.04, 7.03, 7.04, 7.05, 8.054, 8.08, 8.081, 8.085, 8.115, 8.12, 8.14, 8.145, 8.19, and 9.045. Guanzon, *Health Care Law, 41 U. Rich. L. Rev. 179, 199 (2006).*

Journal 2006 Considers prisoners' rights to expression of sexuality and the state's legitimate interest in regulating that expression. Concludes that states should encourage healthy expressions of sexuality while protecting the goals of the Prison Rape Elimination Act. Cites Opinions 3.08, 8.14, 8.145, and 10.015. Smith, *Rethinking Prison Sex: Self-expression and Safety, 15 Colum. J. Gender & L. 185, 202 (2006).*

9.2.1 Medical Student Involvement in Patient Care

Journal 2008 Discusses the problem of using patients for medical education purposes without patient consent. Concludes that new rules are needed to clarify when anesthetized, deceased, and conscious patients may be used for medical student training. Cites Opinion 8.087. Wilson, *"Unauthorized Practice": Regulating the Use of Anesthetized, Recently Deceased, and Conscious Patients in Medical Teaching, 44 Idaho L. Rev. 423, 424 (2008).*

Journal 2004 Discusses the practice of allowing medical students to perform pelvic examinations on female patients under anesthesia without obtaining consent. Concludes that physicians should obtain consent for this procedure as female patients have a right to control what is done to their body. Cites Opinion 8.087. Duncan, Luginbill, Richardson, & Wilson, *Using Tort Law to Secure Patient Dignity, 40 Trial 42, 46 (Oct. 2004).*

9.2.3 Performing Procedures on the Newly Deceased

Journal 2008 Argues preservation of individuals who die of uncontrolled cardiac death is authorized by the Uniform Anatomical Gift Act and does not violate the rights of family members. Concludes that organ donor population should be expanded to include individuals who die uncontrolled cardiac deaths to increase the number of organs available for transplant. Cites Opinions 2.157 and 8.181. Bonnie, Wright, & Dineen, *Legal Authority to Preserve Organs in Cases of Uncontrolled Cardiac Death: Preserving Family Choice, 36 J. L. Med. & Ethics 741, 743 (2008).*

Journal 2004 Questions whether newly dead patients may suffer any legal harm when resuscitation training procedures

are performed on them without consent. Concludes that performing these procedures without proper consent is illegal. Cites Opinion 8.181. Sperling, *Breaking Through the Silence: Illegality of Performing Resuscitation Procedures on the "Newly-Dead," 13 Ann. Health L. 393, 394, 396, 401, 425 (2004).*

Journal 2003 Analyzes the effect of Virginia law and court decisions on administrative law. Discusses one provision of law that incorporates the AMA's nonbinding ban on nonconsensual use of newly dead patients as training subjects. References Opinion 8.181. Kibler, *Administrative Law, 38 U. Rich. L. Rev. 39, 47 (2003).*

9.2.4 Disputes between Medical Supervisors and Trainees

Journal 1997 Discusses professionalism among attorneys. Emphasizes the need for individual accountability. Concludes that the rules of professional conduct should be modified to hold lawyers responsible for their actions. Quotes Opinion 9.055. Rice, *The Superior Orders Defense in Legal Ethics: Sending the Wrong Message to Young Lawyers, 32 Wake Forest L. Rev. 887, 908-09 (1997).*

Journal 1995 Examines the rights of health care professionals to refuse to participate in patient care on the basis of conscientious objection. Suggests steps that health care facilities may take when dealing with health care professionals who object to participating in patient care. Quotes Principles I and VI and Opinions 1.02, 2.035, and 9.055. Dellinger & Vickery, *When Staff Object to Participating in Care, 28 J. Health & Hospital Law 269, 272, 276 (1995).*

9.2.6 Continuing Medical Education

Journal 2000 Examines legal and ethical issues bearing upon pain management. Asserts that health care professionals have a legal and ethical duty to relieve pain and suffering of patients whenever possible. Suggests that this duty is legally enforceable. Quotes Principle V and Opinions 2.20 and 9.011. Rich, *A Prescription for the Pain: The Emerging Standard of Care for Pain Management, 26 Wm. Mitchell L. Rev. 1, 35-36, 85 (2000).*

Journal 2000 Examines issues relating to parental consent to circumcision. Identifies legal and ethical requirements for consent when medical professionals are treating adult patients. Analyzes the implications of those requirements for routine circumcision of infant males. Concludes that only

when the male is an adult and capable of making decisions can circumcision be ethically and legally performed. Quotes Opinion 8.08. References Opinions 8.03 and 9.011. Svoboda, Van Howe, & Dwyer, *Informed Consent for Neonatal Circumcision: An Ethical and Legal Conundrum, 17 J. Contemp. Health L. & Pol'y 61, 67, 73, 82 (2000).*

Journal 2000 Examines the practice of gift giving by the health care technology industry as incentives in the context of continuing medical education activities. Concludes that industry-wide standards must be developed governing interactions between physicians and representatives of health care technology industry companies. Cites Opinions 8.061 and 9.011. Tenery, *Interactions Between Physicians* *and the Health Care Technology Industry, 283 JAMA 391, 393 (2000).*

Journal 1992 Reviews concerns about commercial involvement in and funding of continuing medical education. Discusses CME requirements, accumulation of CME credits, and changes in standards governing commercial sponsorship. References Opinions 8.061 and 9.011. Wentz, Osteen,

& Cannon, *Continuing Medical Education: Unabated Debate, 268 JAMA 1118 (1992).*

Journal 1991 Discusses commercial support of continuing medical education. Explains ethical guidelines for accepting such assistance and how those guidelines have changed. References Opinions 8.061 and 9.011. Wentz, Osteen, & Gannon, *Refocusing Support and Direction, 266 JAMA 953 (1991).*

9.3.1 Physician Health and Wellness

Journal 1994 Discusses the issue of whom physicians must serve first: themselves, their patients, insurers, or society. Focuses on risks arising out of provider economic arrangements and risks arising out of other individual physician characteristics. Quotes Opinions 8.03 and 9.13. Cites Opinion 8.15. Bobinski, *Autonomy and Privacy: Protecting Patients From Their Physicians, 55 U. Pitt. L. Rev. 291, 302, 313 (1994).*

Md. 1993 Patients sued hospital and physician alleging that an operating surgeon has a duty to disclose his or her HIV-infected status. Quoting Opinions 9.13 and 9.131 (1992) for the proposition that a seropositive physician should not engage in activity that would create a risk of transmission of the disease to his or her patients, the court held that it could not say as a matter of law that an HIV-infected physician did not have a duty to warn patients of his condition or refrain from operating on them. *Faya v. Almaraz, 329 Md. 435, 449, 450, 620 A.2d 327, 334.*

Minn. App. 1993 Patients sued HIV-positive physician alleging negligent infliction of emotional distress. Trial court granted summary judgment holding that plaintiffs had failed to produce evidence sufficient to show "actual exposure" to the AIDS virus. The appellate court, in an unpublished opinion, held that the plaintiffs need only show that they were in the "zone of danger" of contracting HIV. The court referred to *Faya v. Almaraz, 329 Md. 435, 449, 620 A.2d 327, 334 (1993),* which had quoted Opinions 9.13 and 9.131 for the proposition that a physician who has an infectious disease should not engage in any activity that creates a risk of transmission of that disease to the patient. *K.A.C. v. Benson, 1993 Minn. App. LEXIS 1201.*

N.J. Super. 1991 Physician's estate sued hospital alleging that it violated state law against discrimination by restricting the physician's surgery privileges and requiring him to inform patients of his HIV-infected status before performing invasive procedures. The defendant hospital was also alleged to have breached its duty to maintain confidentiality of his seropositive diagnosis. The court held that the hospital had not discriminated against the physician since the hospital had relied on ethical and professional standards, including a report of the Council on Ethical and Judicial Affairs of the AMA dealing with the issue of AIDS [now Opinions 9.13 and 9.131]. However, the hospital was held to have

breached its fiduciary duty to maintain the confidentiality of the physician's medical records. Referring to *McIntosh v. Milano,* 168 N.J. Super. 466, 403 A.2d 500 (1979), which had quoted AMA Principles of Medical Ethics sec. 9 (1957) [now Principle IV and Opinion 5.05] in applying the "duty to warn" exception, the court noted that the disclosure in this case went far beyond the medical personnel directly involved in the treatment of the physician and those patients entitled to informed consent. *Estate of Behringer v. Medical Ctr., 249 N.J. Super. 597, 614, 633, 592 A.2d 1251, 1259, 1268.*

Journal 2000 Explores issues involving HIV-infected physicians and patients. Examines ethical and policy considerations and the Americans with Disabilities Act. Concludes that infected patients have the right to be treated, but infected physicians are not always afforded equal protection. Quotes Opinions 9.13 and 9.131. Halevy, *AIDS, Surgery, and the Americans with Disabilities Act, 135 Arch. Surg. 51, 52, 53 (2000).*

Journal 2000 Examines the effect of HIV/AIDS on the relationship between the general public and health care professionals (HCPs). Discusses the importance of creating an environment in which HIV-positive patients do not fear disclosing their HIV status. Discusses policies and guidelines that address methods to prevent transmission of HIV from HCPs to patients. Quotes Opinion 2.23. References Opinions 9.13 and 9.131. Rediger, *Living in a World With HIV: Balancing Privacy, Privilege and the Right to Know Between Patients and Health Care Professionals, 21 Hamline J. Pub. L. & Pol'y 443, 456-57, 461, 472 (2000).*

Journal 1997 Opines that physicians infected with HIV have an ethical and legal duty to disclose their status to patients before beginning invasive procedures. Suggests that the doctrine of informed consent and medical ethics guidelines require disclosure. Disagrees with public policy arguments favoring nondisclosure. References Opinions 9.13 and 9.131. Iheukwumere, *HIV-Positive Medical Practitioners: Legal and Ethical Obligations to Disclose, 71 St. John's L. Rev. 715, 732-34 (1997).*

Journal 1996 Discusses the doctrine of informed consent and its purpose. Posits that, due to patients' rights of self-determination, and the deadly nature of AIDS, physicians are morally and legally obligated to disclose their HIV status to patients where risk of transmission exists. Quotes Opinion 9.13. Note, *Torts: Defining the Duty Imposed on Physicians by the Doctrine of Informed Consent, 22 Wm. Mitchell L. Rev. 149, 160 (1996).*

Journal 1994 Examines the scope of a physician's duty to reveal HIV status to a patient before performing invasive procedures. Discusses applicable case law and advocates use of comprehensive and objective scientific data in evaluating potential liability in cases where physicians fail to disclose HIV status to patients. Quotes Opinions 9.13 and 9.131. Beane, *AIDS Crisis and the Health Care Community: Public Concerns Triggering Questionable Private Rights of Action for Emotional Harms and Legislative Response, 45 Mercer L. Rev. 633, 669 (1994).*

Journal 1994 Analyzes problems in proving emotional distress claims based on the fear of contracting AIDS, such as proof of exposure and injury, reasonableness of fear, and proof of negligence. Proposes that courts follow evidentiary and public policy standards developed in other phobia cases. Quotes Opinions 9.13 and 9.131. Comment, *AIDSphobia:*

Forcing Courts to Face New Areas of Compensation for Fear of a Deadly Disease, 39 Vill. L. Rev. 241, 277 (1994).

Journal 1994 Examines the responsibilities of real estate brokers to disclose a seller's AIDS status in light of a potential buyer's right to know all material facts affecting property value. Concludes that a seller's AIDS status is a material fact that a real estate broker must disclose. Quotes Opinions 9.13 and 9.131. Hartog, *The Psychological Impact of AIDS on Real Property and a Real Estate Broker's Duty to Disclose, 36 Ariz. L. Rev. 757, 772 (1994).*

Journal 1993 Provides an overview of the doctrine of informed consent and evaluates the disclosure obligations of HIV-positive health care professionals. Concludes that in developing coherent guidelines for informed consent in this context, the best approach is to have a public determination of what level of risk is tolerable. Cites Opinion 9.13. Nodzenski, *HIV-Infected Health Care Professionals and Informed Consent, 2 S. Cal. Interdisciplinary L. J. 299, 327 (1993).*

9.3.2 Physician Responsibilities to Impaired Colleagues

7th Cir. 2009 Plaintiff, a surgeon and resident of New Jersey, brought a defamation action against defendant, a surgeon and resident of New York, in federal district court in Illinois. The suit was based upon a letter sent by the defendant to a professional organization based in Chicago complaining about the plaintiff's testimony against the defendant in a malpractice action. The district judge dismissed the suit for improper venue and plaintiff appealed. The appeals court cited Opinion 9.031 in noting that a physician has a duty to notify the proper public or private authorities of unprofessional conduct by a fellow professional. The court held that New Jersey law governed the defamation action. *Kamelgard v. Macura, 585 F.3d 334, 338.*

D. Vt. 2004 Defendants filed a motion for summary judgment in physician's suit alleging, among other claims, defamation. The court granted the motion citing Opinion 9.031, holding that the AMA's Code of Medical Ethics required the defendants to report the plaintiff, given questions about his ability to practice medicine. *Agee v. Grunert, 349 F. Supp.2d 838, 843, 844.*

Ga. App. 1998 An emergency room physician sued another physician who examined a patient one day after the plaintiff, for libel and unfair business practices stemming from letters the second physician wrote regarding the emergency room physician's treatment of the patient. The court affirmed the trial court's grant of summary judgment on grounds that the concerns addressed in the letters were protected by a conditional privilege and that the plaintiff had not proved that the defendant wrote the letters with malice. The court quoted Opinion 9.031, as imposing a duty to report the plaintiff's

treatment of the patient. Furthermore, the court noted that according to the Opinion, the defendant was neither required to address the problem with the offending physician first, nor required to confine her concerns to peer review groups. *Dominy v. Shumpert, 235 Ga. App. 500, 510 S.E.2d 81, 85-86.*

Mich. App. 1968 Physician was properly dismissed from hospital staff for violating Principle 4 (1957) [now Principle II and Opinion 9.031] when on numerous occasions physician vilified other physicians, swore and screamed in the hospital, and quarreled with staff and hospital visitors. *Anderson v. Bd. of Trustees of Caro Community Hosp., 10 Mich. App. 348, 159 N.W.2d 347, 348-50.*

Journal 2010 Explores how participation in online social networks may blur boundaries between personal and professional relationships for health care professionals and how such risks may be mitigated by use of network privacy and security settings. Suggests that health care institutions are likely to institute online social-networking policies for employees. Quotes Opinions 5.026, 5.027, 5.045, 5.046, 5.05, 5.059, 5.0591, 8.14, 9.08, and 9.123. Cites Opinions 5.026, 9.031, and 9.12. Terry, *Physicians and Patients Who "Friend" or "Tweet": Constructing a Legal Framework for Social Networking in a Highly Regulated Domain, 43 Ind. L. Rev. 285, 314-16, 319, 334-36, 338 (2010).*

Journal 2004 Discusses application of the Americans with Disabilities Act in the professional disciplinary context. Concludes that medical and legal professionals who are unfit are being disciplined not because they are disabled, but primarily because of misconduct. Quotes Opinion 9.031.

Walker, *Protecting the Public: The Impact of the Americans with Disabilities Act on Licensure Considerations Involving Mentally Impaired Medical and Legal Professionals, 25 J. Legal Med. 441, 454 (2004).*

Journal 1993 Discusses the problems physicians may encounter by exposing an errant colleague, such as harm to the reporting physician's reputation and the fear of litigation.

States that problems involving physician competency and unethical behavior should be investigated, and that physicians should take personal responsibility for reporting problems they observe. References Principle II and Opinions 8.14 and 9.031. Morreim, *Am I My Brother's Warden? Responding to the Unethical or Incompetent Colleague, 23 Hastings Center Rep. 19, 23 (May/June 1993).*

9.4.1 Peer Review and Due Process

Ill. App. 1979 Physician sued professional association of orthopaedic surgeons after it denied his application for membership. Plaintiff claimed he was not fully informed of the basis of denial, received no notice or opportunity to attend the hearing in which his application was considered, and was neither allowed to hear adverse evidence nor present a defense. Since the association's bylaws required adherence to the Principles, including Opinion 6.18 (1977) [now Opinion 9.05], which demanded that due process be afforded a physician whose conduct is being reviewed, plaintiff alleged that the association had violated its own procedures in the application process. The court held that the applicant did not have a right to have his application considered according to the association's bylaws and could not obtain judicial review without a showing of economic necessity. *Treister v. American Academy of Orthopaedic Surgeons, 78 Ill. App. 3d 746, 396 N.E.2d 1225, 1228, 1232, 1238.*

Va. App. 2003 Physician appealed board of medicine's license probation order for unprofessional conduct. Board found the physician's pattern of inappropriate advances toward medical students violated medical ethical standards. Appellate court reversed, holding that the evidence was insufficient to support Board's finding, since the ethical standards by which the physician should be adjudicated were not established by competent evidence. Quotes Opinions 3.08 and 9.05. *Goad v. Virginia Board of Medicine, 40 Va. App. 621, 580 S.E.2d 494, 498, n.7, 499, n.9.*

Journal 2006 Considers licensing and disciplinary procedures of medical boards. Concludes that the standard of proof for a finding of unprofessional conduct should be heightened from a preponderance of the evidence to clear and convincing evidence. Cites Opinion 9.05. Spece & Marchalonis, *Sound Constitutional Analysis, Moral Principle, and Wise Policy Judgment Require a Clear and Convincing Evidence Standard of Proof in Physician Disciplinary Proceedings, 3 Ind. Health L. Rev. 107, 109 (2006).*

Journal 1984 Discusses litigation by physicians in situations where medical staff privileges have been denied, curtailed, or revoked. Offers an analysis of the relevant legal theories and practice considerations that form part of hospital privilege antitrust litigation but concludes that litigation based

on the Sherman Act—the predominant antitrust legislative scheme—in this context generally has been unsuccessful due to stringent requirements of proof. Cites Opinion 9.04 (1982) [now Opinion 9.05]. Tabor, *The Battle for Hospital Privileges, 251 JAMA 1602, 1602 (1984).*

Journal 1983 Describes special problems that may confront family physicians in the context of applying for hospital privileges. Offers a recommended approach to the application process which encourages physicians to document areas of residency training; become familiar with the hospital policies, guidelines, and procedures involved in applying for privileges; and solicit the support of staff physicians. Quotes Opinion 9.04 (1981) [now Opinion 9.05]. Pugno, *Hospital Privileges for Family Physicians: Rights, Rationale, and Resources, 17 J. Fam. Practice 77, 79 (1983).*

Journal 2011 Discusses the far-reaching effects of 2005 Illinois medical liability reform legislation. Explains how the 2010 Illinois Supreme Court decision in *Lebron v. Gottlieb* invalidated many beneficial aspects of this legislation. Quotes Opinion 10.015. Cites Opinion 9.10. Nelson, Swanson, & Buckley, *Lebron v. Gottlieb Memorial Hospital: Capping Medical Practice Reform in Illinois, 20 Annals Health L. 1, 7, 11 (Winter 2011).*

Journal 2007 Analyzes scientific, ethical, and legal issues raised in the exhumation and genetic analysis of historical figures. Concludes that biohistorical review boards should be created to generate guidelines for such research. Quotes Preamble and Opinion 2.08. Cites Opinions 2.079, 2.105, 5.05, 5.051, 5.075, 8.03, 8.031, 9.095, and 9.10. Paradise & Andrews, *Tales From the Crypt: Scientific, Ethical, and Legal Considerations for Biohistorical Analysis of Deceased Historical Figures, 26 Temp. J. Sci. Tech. & Envtl. L. 223, 287-88 (2007).*

Journal 2006 Discusses the efficacy of peer-review programs in preventing medical malpractice. Concludes that peer review is effective and that confidentiality of peer review must remain protected by law. Quotes Opinion 4.07. Cites Opinions 4.07 and 9.10. Moore, Pichert, Hickson, Federspiel, & Blackford, *Rethinking Peer Review: Detecting and Addressing Medical Malpractice Claims Risk, 59 Vand. L. Rev. 1175, 1144 (2006).*

9.4.2 Reporting Incompetent or Unethical Behavior by Colleagues

Cal. App. 1956 Physician-petitioner sought mandamus against local medical association whose bylaws provided for the expulsion of any member who violated the Principles. Petitioner had been expelled under the provision and the expulsion was affirmed by the AMA's Judicial Council. The initial grounds for expulsion was alleged violation of Principles Ch. III, Art. IV, Sec.4 (1947) [now Opinions 9.04 and 9.07], for disparaging statements regarding another physician in a report used in judicial proceedings. In holding that application of the provision to petitioner was contrary to public policy, the court noted that the physician's statements had been made at the request of a civil litigant and enjoyed a statutory testimonial privilege. Further, the court found that the AMA's right to formulate ethical principles did not extend to defining the duties of witnesses. Expulsion was also based on petitioner's critical comments about other physicians overheard by their patients in violation of Principles Ch. III, Art. IV, Sec.1 (1947) [now Principle II and Opinion 9.04]. The court found application of this Principle under the circumstances reasonable and not contrary to public policy. *Bernstein v. Alameda-Contra Costa Medical Ass'n, 139 Cal. App. 2d 241, 293 P.2d 862, 863, 863 nn.1, 2, 865 nn.4, 6, 866, 866 n.8, 867.*

Ohio 1980 A physician, charged with violating the state medical licensing statute by distributing controlled substances without a proper license and writing prescriptions for narcotics in the name of one person when they were intended for another, challenged the state medical board's decision to suspend his license and place him on two years' probation. Under the statute, a physician could be disciplined for various activities including violation of any provision of a code of ethics of a national professional organization such as the AMA. The board found in part that the physician's actions violated Principles 4 and 7 (1957) [now Principles II and III and Opinions 8.06 and 9.04]. The trial court reversed, holding that the board had insufficient evidence for its decision, and the court of appeals affirmed. On appeal, the Supreme Court held that expert testimony was not required at a hearing before a medical licensing board because they were experts and could determine for themselves whether the Principles had been violated. *Arlen v. State, 61 Ohio St. 2d 168, 399 N.E.2d 1251, 1252, 1253-54.*

Journal 2007 Addresses physician liability for an extramarital affair with a patient's spouse. Concludes that such an affair should be regarded as a breach of a fiduciary duty. Quotes Preamble, Principles I, II, and VIII, and Opinions 8.145, 9.04, 9.123, and 10.015. Demaine, *"Playing Doctor" With the Patient's Spouse: Alternative Conceptions of Health Professional Liability, 14 Va. J. Soc. Pol'y & L. 308, 325, 330-31, 331-32 (2007).*

Journal 2001 Examines issues relating to health care cost containment. Concludes that, if physicians are to meet the goals assigned to them in a cost-constrained health care system, then professional standards must be reevaluated and modified to afford meaningful guidance for clinical decision-making in the face of health care spending controls. Quotes Opinions 2.03, 2.09, 2.095, 8.032, and 9.04. Cites Opinions 8.02, 8.021, 8.051, and 8.13. Agrawal, *Resuscitating Professionalism: Self-regulation in the Medical Marketplace, 66 Mo. L. Rev. 341, 354, 355, 360, 361, 378, 388 (2001).*

Journal 1994 Discusses the role of professional societies in establishing ethical guidelines for physicians in the context of using medical innovations and new technologies. Observes that these standards must be supplemented by additional external measures or incentives in order to be most effective. Cites Opinions 1.01, 1.02, 8.061, 9.04, and 9.131. Orentlicher, *The Influence of a Professional Organization on Physician Behavior, 57 Alb. L. Rev. 583, 592, 593, 594, 595, 596 (1994).*

7th Cir. 2009 Plaintiff, a surgeon and resident of New Jersey, brought a defamation action against defendant, a surgeon and resident of New York, in federal district court in Illinois. The suit was based upon a letter sent by the defendant to a professional organization based in Chicago complaining about the plaintiff's testimony against the defendant in a malpractice action. The district judge dismissed the suit for improper venue and plaintiff appealed. The appeals court cited Opinion 9.031 in noting that a physician has a duty to notify the proper public or private authorities of unprofessional conduct by a fellow professional. The court held that New Jersey law governed the defamation action. *Kamelgard v. Macura, 585 F.3d 334, 338.*

D. Vt. 2004 Defendants filed a motion for summary judgment in physician's suit alleging, among other claims, defamation. The court granted the motion citing Opinion 9.031, holding that the AMA's Code of Medical Ethics required the defendants to report the plaintiff, given questions about his ability to practice medicine. *Agee v. Grunert, 349 F. Supp.2d 838, 843, 844.*

Ga. App. 1998 An emergency room physician sued another physician who examined a patient one day after the plaintiff, for libel and unfair business practices stemming from letters the second physician wrote regarding the emergency room physician's treatment of the patient. The court affirmed the trial court's grant of summary judgment on grounds that the concerns addressed in the letters were protected by a conditional privilege and that the plaintiff had not proved that the defendant wrote the letters with malice. The court quoted Opinion 9.031, as imposing a duty to report the plaintiff's treatment of the patient. Furthermore, the court noted that according to the Opinion, the defendant was neither required to address the problem with the offending physician first, nor required to confine her concerns to peer review groups. *Dominy v. Shumpert, 235 Ga. App. 500, 510 S.E.2d 81, 85-86.*

Mich. App. 1968 Physician was properly dismissed from hospital staff for violating Principle 4 (1957) [now Principle

II and Opinion 9.031] when on numerous occasions physician vilified other physicians, swore and screamed in the hospital, and quarreled with staff and hospital visitors. *Anderson v. Bd. of Trustees of Caro Community Hosp., 10 Mich. App. 348, 159 N.W.2d 347, 348-50.*

Journal 2010 Explores how participation in online social networks may blur boundaries between personal and professional relationships for health care professionals and how such risks may be mitigated by use of network privacy and security settings. Suggests that health care institutions are likely to institute online social-networking policies for employees. Quotes Opinions 5.026, 5.027, 5.045, 5.046, 5.05, 5.059, 5.0591, 8.14, 9.08, and 9.123. Cites Opinions 5.026, 9.031, and 9.12. Terry, *Physicians and Patients Who "Friend" or "Tweet": Constructing a Legal Framework for Social Networking in a Highly Regulated Domain, 43 Ind. L. Rev. 285, 314-16, 319, 334-36, 338 (2010).*

Journal 2004 Discusses application of the Americans with Disabilities Act in the professional disciplinary context. Concludes that medical and legal professionals who are unfit are being disciplined not because they are disabled, but primarily because of misconduct. Quotes Opinion 9.031. Walker, *Protecting the Public: The Impact of the Americans with Disabilities Act on Licensure Considerations Involving Mentally Impaired Medical and Legal Professionals, 25 J. Legal Med. 441, 454 (2004).*

Journal 1993 Discusses the problems physicians may encounter by exposing an errant colleague, such as harm to the reporting physician's reputation and the fear of litigation. States that problems involving physician competency and unethical behavior should be investigated, and that physicians should take personal responsibility for reporting problems they observe. References Principle II and Opinions 8.14 and 9.031. Morreim, *Am I My Brother's Warden? Responding to the Unethical or Incompetent Colleague, 23 Hastings Center Rep. 19, 23 (May/June 1993).*

9.4.3 Discipline and Medicine

Cal. App. 1956 Physician-petitioner sought mandamus against local medical association whose bylaws provided for the expulsion of any member who violated the Principles. Petitioner had been expelled under the provision and the expulsion was affirmed by the AMA's Judicial Council. The initial grounds for expulsion was alleged violation of Principles Ch. III, Art. IV, Sec.4 (1947) [now Opinions 9.04 and 9.07], for disparaging statements regarding another physician in a report used in judicial proceedings. In holding that application of the provision to petitioner was contrary to public policy, the court noted that the physician's statements had been made at the request of a civil litigant and enjoyed a statutory testimonial privilege. Further, the court found that the AMA's right to formulate ethical principles did not extend to defining the duties of witnesses. Expulsion was also based on petitioner's critical comments about other physicians overheard by their patients in violation of Principles Ch. III, Art. IV, Sec.1 (1947) [now Principle II and Opinion 9.04]. The court found application of this Principle under the circumstances reasonable and not contrary to public policy. *Bernstein v. Alameda-Contra Costa Medical Ass'n, 139 Cal. App. 2d 241, 293 P.2d 862, 863, 863 nn.1, 2, 865 nn.4, 6, 866, 866 n.8, 867.*

Ohio 1980 A physician, charged with violating the state medical licensing statute by distributing controlled substances without a proper license and writing prescriptions for narcotics in the name of one person when they were intended for another, challenged the state medical board's decision to suspend his license and place him on two years' probation. Under the statute, a physician could be disciplined for various activities including violation of any provision of a code of ethics of a national professional organization such as the AMA. The board found in part that the physician's

actions violated Principles 4 and 7 (1957) [now Principles II and III and Opinions 8.06 and 9.04]. The trial court reversed, holding that the board had insufficient evidence for its decision, and the court of appeals affirmed. On appeal, the Supreme Court held that expert testimony was not required at a hearing before a medical licensing board because they were experts and could determine for themselves whether the Principles had been violated. *Arlen v. State, 61 Ohio St. 2d 168, 399 N.E.2d 1251, 1252, 1253-54.*

Journal 2007 Addresses physician liability for an extramarital affair with a patient's spouse. Concludes that such an affair should be regarded as a breach of a fiduciary duty. Quotes Preamble, Principles I, II, and VIII, and Opinions 8.145, 9.04, 9.123, and 10.015. Demaine, *"Playing Doctor" With the Patient's Spouse: Alternative Conceptions of Health Professional Liability, 14 Va. J. Soc. Pol'y & L. 308, 325, 330-31, 331-32 (2007).*

Journal 2001 Examines issues relating to health care cost containment. Concludes that, if physicians are to meet the goals assigned to them in a cost-constrained health care system, then professional standards must be reevaluated and modified to afford meaningful guidance for clinical decision-making in the face of health care spending controls. Quotes Opinions 2.03, 2.09, 2.095, 8.032, and 9.04. Cites Opinions 8.02, 8.021, 8.051, and 8.13. Agrawal, *Resuscitating Professionalism: Self-regulation in the Medical Marketplace, 66 Mo. L. Rev. 341, 354, 355, 360, 361, 378, 388 (2001).*

Journal 1994 Discusses the role of professional societies in establishing ethical guidelines for physicians in the context of using medical innovations and new technologies. Observes that these standards must be supplemented by additional external measures or incentives in order to be most effective. Cites Opinions 1.01, 1.02, 8.061, 9.04, and 9.131. Orentlicher, *The Influence of a Professional*

Organization on Physician Behavior, 57 Alb. L. Rev. 583, 592, 593, 594, 595, 596 (1994).

9.4.4 Physicians with Disruptive Behavior

Journal 2010 Observes that miscommunicated, misunderstood, and forgotten information among physicians, nurses, and other hospital staff leads to serious patient injury. Concludes that to assess if a client's injury resulted from a miscommunication among hospital staff, attorneys must examine hospital policies and procedures, medical ethics, and communications technology in relation to information sharing. Quotes Opinions 3.02 and 9.045. Cohen, Dicecco, & Levin, *Failure to Communicate: When It Comes to Hospital Patient Care, Communication Between Doctor and Nurse Should Be Seamless. If It's Not, Patients Suffer. Here's How to Find Out if a Miscommunication Is at the Core of Your Client's Case, 46 Trial 38, 40-41 (May 2010).*

Journal 2009 Discusses the appropriateness of immunity in the institutional peer-review process in the context of a competitive market for physician services. Concludes that while the peer-review process performs an essential function for ensuring patient safety and quality care, reforms are needed to avoid abuses and ensure the process is conducted

effectively. Cites Opinion 9.045. Kinney, *Hospital Peer Review of Physicians: Does Statutory Immunity Increase Risk of Unwarranted Professional Injury? 13 Mich. St. U. J. Med. & L. 57, 78 (2009).*

Journal 2006 Analyzes dismissals of disruptive physicians from hospitals and the role of a whistleblower defense. Proposes hospitals should be granted a greater presumption of validity in dismissals made according to their bylaws. Quotes Opinion 9.045. Erwin, *Analyzing the Disruptive Physician: How State and Federal Courts Should Handle Whistleblower Cases Brought by Disruptive Physicians, 44 Duq. L. Rev. 275, 276 (2006).*

Journal 2006 Discusses the evolution of health law in Virginia. Concludes that the area of health law continues to expand, develop, and be refined. Cites Opinions 3.03, 3.08, 5.01, 5.015, 5.02, 5.04, 5.055, 6.02, 6.021, 6.03, 6.04, 7.03, 7.04, 7.05, 8.054, 8.08, 8.081, 8.085, 8.115, 8.12, 8.14, 8.145, 8.19, and 9.045. Guanzon, *Health Care Law, 41 U. Rich. L. Rev. 179, 199 (2006).*

9.5.2 Staff Privileges

Journal 2006 Discusses the efficacy of peer-review programs in preventing medical malpractice. Concludes that peer review is effective and that confidentiality of peer review must remain protected by law. Quotes Opinion 4.07. Cites Opinions 4.07 and 9.10. Moore, Pichert, Hickson, Federspiel, & Blackford, *Rethinking Peer Review: Detecting and Addressing Medical Malpractice Claims Risk, 59 Vand. L. Rev. 1175, 1144 (2006).*

Journal 1990 Presents current issues, policies, legislation, and judicial decisions regarding impaired physicians. Concludes by proposing enhanced confidentiality requirements in disciplinary proceedings and nationwide adoption of a uniform law in this area. Quotes Opinion 4.07. References Principle IV. Walzer, *Impaired Physicians: An Overview and Update of the Legal Issues, 11 J. Legal Med. 131, 174, 192 (1990).*

9.5.4 Civil Rights and Medical Professionals

Journal 1996 Examines possible legal avenues for addressing claims of employment discrimination based upon sexual orientation. Concludes that lesbians and gay men need greater employment protection and an explicit statutory

cause of action. Quotes Opinion 9.03. Gilmore, *Employment Protection for Lesbians and Gay Men, 6 L. & Sex. 83, 95 (1996).*

9.5.5 Gender Discrimination in Medicine

Journal 2000 Reports on a study conducted to evaluate issues relating to the advancement of women through the ranks of surgery and academic medicine. Concludes that

many of the obstacles women face in this context appear to be based upon subtle, even unconscious, societal attitudes and behaviors. References Opinion 9.035. Colletti,

Mulholland, & Sonnad, *Perceived Obstacles to Career Success for Women in Academic Surgery, 135 Arch. Surg. 972, 976 (2000).*

Journal 1996 Considers the pharmaceutical industry's failure to test products on female subjects. Comments on the potential for harm. Notes legal difficulties women experience when attempting to prove a drug was not adequately tested. Posits that litigation can affect the behavior of pharmaceutical companies. References Opinion 9.035. Comment, *Tort Reform to Ensure the Inclusion of Fertile Women in Early Phases of Commercial Drug Research, 3 U. Chi. L. Sch. Roundtable 355, 359 (1996).*

9.6.1 Advertising and Publicity

US 1977 Disciplinary sanctions were imposed by state bar against attorneys who violated state rule prohibiting advertising. After state court upheld sanctions, attorneys appealed to Supreme Court arguing that state rule violated federal antitrust laws and was unconstitutional. State bar argued that rule prohibiting advertising was justified to prevent adverse impact on the legal profession. In questioning this assertion, the Court referred to the position of the AMA announced in 235 *JAMA* 2328 (1976) and included in Opinions and Reports of the Judicial Council 6.00 (1977) [now Opinion 5.02], that the medical profession permits advertising by physicians. The Court held that the state may regulate some aspects of advertising, but that a blanket prohibition against advertising by attorneys was unconstitutional as a violation of the First Amendment. *Bates v. State Bar of Ariz., 433 US 350, 369-70 n.20.*

1st Cir. 1966 Physician sued electric shaver manufacturer for libel on basis of its use of reprints of an article quoting a study favorably mentioning manufacturer which allegedly falsely indicated that physician was one of the coauthors of the research study. Plaintiff asserted that he had agreed to participate in the research only if his name was not used in advertising claims since this would be a violation of established rules of ethics of the AMA, Opinions and Reports of the Judicial Council Sec. 5, Para. 29 (1965) [now Opinion 5.02]. These facts were considered sufficient to submit to the jury. *Sperry Rand Corp. v. Hill, 356 F.2d 181, 184, cert. denied, 384 US 973 (1966).*

2d Cir. 1980 Federal Trade Commission ordered AMA and others to cease, with some exceptions, imposing restraints on advertising and contract practice by physicians, as well as on business relations between physicians and laypersons. Commission found restraints violated 15 USC Sec. 45 (a)(1). See 94 FTC 701 (1979). AMA petitioned for judicial review of Commission's order. Court reviewed order, noting specific ethical pronouncements of AMA which Commission found improper, including the following: restrictions upon advertising and solicitation, Principle 5 (1957) and Opinions and Reports of the Judicial Council Sec. 5, Para. 11 (1971) [now Opinion 5.02]; restrictions on contract practice, Principle 6 (1957) and Opinions and Reports of the Judicial Council Sec. 6, Paras. 3, 4, and 5 (1971) [now Opinion 8.05]; and restrictions on business organizations and relations with laypersons, Opinions and Reports of the Judicial Council, Sec. 6, Paras. 14 and 15 (1971). The court rejected the AMA's argument that its ethical rules did not provide impetus for local and state medical societies to act against physicians violating its rules. Further, the court rejected the AMA's position that liability should be precluded because of revisions in the Opinions in 1977 and the Principles in 1980. Specifically, the court found that removal of the ban on patient solicitation and changes reflected in Principles II and IV (1980) did not render Commission's order moot. The order was therefore enforced with modifications. Dissenting judge, referring to 1980 revisions in Principles and to Opinions and Reports of the Judicial Council 4.05 and 6.00 (1977) [now Opinions 5.02 and 8.05], concluded order should not be enforced on grounds of mootness. *American Medical Ass'n v. FTC, 638 F.2d 443, 446, 446 n.1, 448, 449, 449 n.5, 450, 451, 455-57, aff'd, 455 US 676 (1982).*

D.C. Cir. 1980 Professional associations, including AMA, filed for judicial review of a Federal Trade Commission rule limiting the ability of states and professional associations to restrict advertising of eye exams as well as ophthalmic goods and services. Since the US Supreme Court had found certain restrictions on lawyer advertising unconstitutional while the case was pending, the court remanded the case for further consideration by the Commission. In its analysis of advertising in the eye care profession, the court quoted Principle 5 (1957) and the Opinions and Reports of the Judicial Council Sec. 10, Para. 4 (1971), which prohibited solicitation and advertising. However, the court also noted the intervening changes in the AMA's position regarding advertising, quoting the Opinions and Reports of the Judicial Council 6.00 (1977) [now Opinion 5.02], which permitted nondeceptive advertising. *American Optometric Ass'n v. F.T.C., 626 F.2d 896, 900-01, 913, 914, 914 n.11.*

E.D. Va. 1976 Health planning agency, which sought to compile directory of services and fees of community physicians, and consumer group interested in obtaining such information, challenged state statute which prohibited direct or indirect advertisement by physicians. In holding that the statute violated First Amendment rights, court noted that to protect the public from being misled as to medical quality, directory was designed in conformity with AMA advertising guidelines. Court quoted Judicial Council position published in 235 *JAMA* 2328 (1976), later included in Opinions and Reports of the Judicial Council 6.00 (1977) [now Opinion 5.02] to support analysis. *Health Sys. Agency v. Virginia*

State Bd. of Medicine, 424 F. Supp. 267, 274, 275 n.11, 276 Appendix B.

Cal. App. 1968 Plaintiff-physician sought dissolution of a medical partnership with defendant's decedent, and also sought a larger percentage of the partnership receipts based upon an alleged oral agreement. Defendant cross-claimed to enjoin plaintiff from taking physical control of the partnership offices and patient records. The trial court enjoined plaintiff from treating previous patients, requiring that he return all medical records and pay defendant all fees received from patients he had treated during the time of dispute. The appellate court reversed insofar as the injunction prohibited plaintiff from treating the patient who desired to continue to receive his services or prevented access to medical records essential for this purpose, citing Opinions and Reports of the Judicial Council Sec. 7, Para. 16, Sec. 5, Para. 21, and Sec. 9 (1966) [now Opinions 6.08, 5.02, and 5.05] to support view that patients may not be regarded as the subject of ownership. *Jones v. Fakehany, 261 Cal. App. 2d 298, 67 Cal. Rptr. 810, 815, 816 n.1.*

Fla. App. 1968 Physician sued to enjoin county medical association and telephone company from eliminating medical specialty headings in classified section of directory pursuant to guidelines issued by AMA's Judicial Council in June 1966 [now Opinion 5.02]. The court held that where medical association had no statutory authority to dictate directory listings, association's restrictions interfered with individual physicians' right to contract and deprived them of due process. *Dade County Medical Ass'n v. Samartino, 213 So. 2d 627, 629, n.2, 631.*

Mich. Att'y Gen. 1978 Opinion was requested from state attorney general as to constitutionality of blanket statutory prohibition of advertising by physicians and as to legality of expulsion of a member of a professional society for advertising that is otherwise proper. In finding the statutory restrictions unconstitutional, the opinion refers to the Judicial Council's advertising statement at 235 *JAMA* 2328 (1976) included as Opinion 6.00 (1977) [now Opinion 5.02]. *Michigan Att'y Gen. Opinion N. 5024, 1977-78 Att'y Gen. Op. 299, 303.*

N.Y. Sup. 1965 Physician sued publishing company to bar insertion of advertisement for baby and child care products in physician's book, seeking declaration that book contract was void to the extent that it allowed inclusion of such an advertisement. Physician asserted that the advertisement was contrary to public policy, citing Opinions and Reports of the Judicial Council Sec. 5, Para. 29 (1965) [now Opinion 5.02], which stated that a doctor should not lend his name to any product. In rejecting the physician's claim, the court was willing to give careful consideration to the AMA's view but concluded that it did not, in itself, constitute an expression of public policy. *Spock v. Pocket Books, Inc., 48 Misc. 2d 812, 266 N.Y.S.2d 77, 79.*

Journal 2009 Discusses the judicial standard for reviewing physician noncompete covenants. Concludes courts should apply a strict standard to such covenants, rather than declare the covenants per se invalid. Quotes Principles IV and VII, Principles of Medical Ethics §5 (1957) [now Principle VI], Code of Medical Ethics Ch. II, Art. I §3 (1847) [now Opinion 5.02], Opinion 9.02, and Code of Medical Ethics Ch. II, Art. I §4 (1847) [now Opinion 9.09]. Cites Opinions 8.041, 8.115, 9.02, 9.06, 9.065, 9.067, 10.01, and 10.015. Koons, *Physician Employee Non-Compete Agreements on the Examining Table: The Need to Better Protect Patients' and the Public's Interests in Indiana, 6 Ind. Health L. Rev. 253, 272-77, 280-81 (2009).*

Journal 2008 Questions what entity should be responsible for critically evaluating chiropractors. Concludes that chiropractic should be a self-regulated profession. Quotes Introduction (1847) [now Opinions 1.01 and 1.02]. References Ch. II, Art. I, Sec. 3 (1847) [now Opinion 5.02], and Ch. II, Art. IV, Sec. 1 (May 1847) [now Opinion 3.01]. Johnson, *Keeping a Critical Eye on Chiropractic, 31 J. of Manipulative and Physiological Therapeutics 559, 559 (2008).*

Journal 2007 Highlights inconsistencies in applying judicial deference to medical ethics. Concludes that courts should afford greater deference to established medical ethics standards. Quotes Principle I and Opinions 2.06 and Ch. II, Art. I, Sec. 3 (May 1847) [now Opinion 5.02]. Cites Opinions 4.01 and 7.05. Lerman, *Second Opinion: Inconsistent Deference to Medical Ethics in Death Penalty Jurisprudence, 95 Geo. L. J. 1941, 1945, 1974-75, 1976, 1977 (2007).*

Journal 2006 Discusses the evolution of health law in Virginia. Concludes that the area of health law continues to expand, develop, and be refined. Cites Opinions 3.03, 3.08, 5.01, 5.015, 5.02, 5.04, 5.055, 6.02, 6.021, 6.03, 6.04, 7.03, 7.04, 7.05, 8.054, 8.08, 8.081, 8.085, 8.115, 8.12, 8.14, 8.145, 8.19, and 9.045. Guanzon, *Health Care Law, 41 U. Rich. L. Rev. 179, 199 (2006).*

Journal 2001 Compares and contrasts certain ethical positions articulated by the legal and medical professions. Concludes that both professions generally agree on ethical principles, but sometimes differ in the manner of implementation. Quotes Principle II. Cites Opinion 5.02. Needell, *Legal Ethics in Medicine: Are Medical Ethics Different From Legal Ethics? 14 St. Thomas L. Rev. 31, 35, 50 (2001).*

Journal 1999 Explains modern jurisdictional analysis and how it applies in medical malpractice cases. Examines the impact of physician advertising, referrals, consultations, prescribing practices, and involvement in state programs on personal jurisdiction in medical malpractice cases. Cites Opinion 5.02. Booker, *Physicians, Malpractice, and State Lines: A Guide to Personal Jurisdiction in Medical Malpractice Lawsuits, 20 J. Legal Med. 385, 394 (1999).*

Journal 1990 Provides an overview of the recent developments in the area of physician advertising. Proposes alternative solutions to the practical and ethical problems raised. Quotes Opinion 5.02. Olson, *Physician Specialty Advertising: The Tendency to Deceive? 11 J. Legal Med. 351, 354 (1990).*

Journal 1984 Discusses the AMA policy on physician advertising and identifies several factors that may affect the decision to advertise. Among the important factors are variations in prominence of physician advertising from region to region and state to state, local attitudes of patients and physicians toward physician advertising, and acceptable forms of physician advertising. Quotes Opinion 5.01 (1984) [now Opinion 5.02]. Porter, *Physician Advertising—What Is Legal? What Is Ethical? What Is Acceptable? 80 Ohio State Med. J. 437, 437, 439 (1984)*.

9.6.2 Gifts to Physicians from Industry

Journal 2011 Compares how the US, France, and Japan oversee pharmaceutical industry–physician financial relationships. Concludes that reforms are needed in each nation, including an alternative to pharmaceutical industry funding for professional medical activities. References Opinion 8.061. Rodwin, *Reforming Pharmaceutical Industry-Physician Financial Relationships: Lessons From the United States, France, and Japan, 39 J. L. Med. & Ethics 662, 664 (2011)*.

Journal 2010 Examines manufacturer-physician consulting arrangements and discusses the evolution of fair market valuation. Proposes a set of standards for calculating fair market value for physician services to ensure compliance with legal requirements. Quotes Opinion 8.061. Eaton & Reid, *Mirror, Mirror on the Wall: Evaluating Fair Market Value for Manufacturer-Physician Consulting Arrangements, 65 Food & Drug L. J. 141, 147 (2010)*.

Journal 2010 Examines the economic basis of physician-industry relationships that result in conflicts of interest. Considers the measures taken by developed countries in response to such conflicts. Concludes by proposing an approach that comprehensively addresses problems caused by drug and device company marketing to physicians. Cites Opinion 8.061. Jost, *Confronting Conflict: Addressing Institutional Conflicts of Interest in Academic Medical Centers, 36 Am. J. L. & Med. 326, 336 (2010)*.

Journal 2010 Examines conflicts of interest experienced by academic medical centers between scientific integrity and corporate interests. Discusses approaches to ensure that academic medical centers effectively manage these conflicts. Proposes comprehensive policies to provide ways to identify, manage, and address institutional conflicts of interest in academic medical centers. Cites Opinion 8.061. Liang & Mackey, *Confronting Conflict: Addressing Institutional Conflicts of Interest in Academic Medical Centers, 36 Am. J. L. & Med. 136, 149 (2010)*.

Journal 2010 Discusses the importance of prescription medication, the factors that influence patient access to pharmaceuticals, and the potential for greater access to drugs with expiring patents. Concludes patent law reforms are unlikely to help patients afford medications in the near future, but that initiatives to concentrate the federal government's purchasing power could be effective in increasing access to pharmaceuticals. References Opinion 8.061. Tironi, *Pharmaceutical Pricing: A Review of Proposals to Improve Access and Affordability of Prescription Drugs, 19 Ann. Health L. 311, 360 (2010)*.

Journal 2009 Examines the effects of pharmaceutical marketing on physicians' fiduciary duty to place patients' interest first. Concludes that because of the fiduciary duty owed to patients, physicians have a legal obligation to avoid inappropriate exposure to pharmaceutical marketing. Quotes and cites Opinion 8.061. Hafemeister & Bryan, *Beware Those Bearing Gifts: Physicians' Fiduciary Duty to Avoid Pharmaceutical Marketing, 57 U. Kan. L. Rev. 491, 499, 512, 529 (2009)*.

Journal 2009 Discusses conflict of interest between cardio-thoracic surgeons and industry. Concludes that 13 ethical guidelines should be followed to avoid conflicts of interest. Cites Opinion 8.061. Mack & Sade, *Relations Between Cardiothoracic Surgeons and Industry, 87 Ann. Thorac. Surg. 1334, 1335 (2009)*.

Journal 2009 Examines the uses and prescribing patterns for antipsychotic medications, legal claims under which product liability suits may be brought, and the marketing techniques used by pharmaceutical companies in an effort to convince physicians to prescribe their drugs. Concludes pharmaceutical companies must be incentivized to provide physicians with more information about their drugs so they can make appropriate prescribing decisions. References Opinion 8.061. Mossman & Steinberg, *Promoting, Prescribing, and Pushing Pills: Understanding the Lessons of Anti-Psychotic Drug Litigation, 13 Mich. St. U. J. Med. & L. 263, 315-316 (2009)*.

Journal 2009 Explores the influence of pharmaceutical and medical device industry gift giving on physicians and discusses recent restrictions and prohibitions on gifting. Concludes that recent changes in industry gifting standards may not decrease overall spending on professional promotion and may not eliminate the benefit to industry. Quotes Opinion 8.061. Steinbrook, *Physician-Industry Relations—Will Fewer Gifts Make a Difference? 360 New Eng. J. Med. 557, 558 (2009)*.

Journal 2008 Discusses the pharmaceutical industry's practice of gifting to physicians and the failure of both parties to prevent corruption. Concludes state statutes are the most effective method to control prescription corruption. Quotes Opinion 8.061. Mehta, *Why Self-regulation Does Not Work: Resolving Prescription Corruption Caused by Excessive*

Gift-Giving by Pharmaceutical Manufacturers, 63 Food & Drug L. J. 799, 810-811 (2008).

Journal 2008 Examines expectations about hormone therapy and the controversy surrounding the treatment. Concludes patients and physicians must be more realistic in weighing hormone therapy's medical value while respecting patient choice. Apparent reference to Opinion 8.061. Schulkin, *Hormone Therapy, Dilemmas, Medical Decisions, 36 J. L. Med. & Ethics 73, 82 (2008).*

Journal 2008 Examines marketing practices commonly utilized by the pharmaceutical industry aimed at health care professionals and the legal, ethical, and legislative implications of such practices. Concludes health care providers and pharmaceutical vendors need to adopt policies to address legislative and regulatory changes, as well as the ethical issues stemming from their relationship. Quotes Opinion 8.061. Washlick & Welch, *Physician-Vendor Marketing and Financial Relationships Under Attack, 2 J. Health & Life Sci. L. 151, 164, 178-81 (2008).*

Journal 2007 Discusses liability of pharmaceutical companies for failure to provide package warnings with sample prescription drugs. Concludes that while the "learned intermediary" doctrine protects companies against tort liability, such protection should be eliminated. References Opinion 8.061. Poser, *Unlabeled Drug Samples and the Learned Intermediary: The Case for Drug Company Liability Without Preemption, 62 Food Drug L. J. 653, 667 (2007).*

Journal 2007 Analyzes the availability of data on pharmaceutical gifts to physicians in Vermont and Minnesota. Concludes that state laws requiring disclosure of industry gifts have not guaranteed easy access to this information. Cites Opinion 8.061. Ross, Lackner, Lurie, Gross, Wolfe, & Krumholz, *Pharmaceutical Company Payments to Physicians: Early Experiences With Disclosure Laws in Vermont and Minnesota, 297 JAMA 1216, 1216 (2007).*

Journal 2006 Discusses the dynamic of the patient-physician relationship. Concludes that truly shared decision-making is likely unattainable. References Opinion 8.061. Clayton, *The Web of Relations: Thinking About Physicians and Patients, 6 Yale J. Health Pol'y, L. & Ethics 465, 473 (2006).*

Journal 2006 Describes public dissatisfaction with self-regulation of pharmaceutical industry gifts to medical professionals, concluding that more regulatory restrictions may be needed. References Opinion 8.061. Dresser, *Pharmaceutical Company Gifts: From Voluntary Standards to Legal Demands, 36 Hastings Center Rep. 8, 9 (May/June 2006).*

Journal 2006 Considers regulation of pharmaceutical sales and marketing. Suggests that drug companies have an opportunity to modify their practices to better comply with new regulations. Quotes Opinion 8.061. Henderson & Cassady, *Drug Deals in 2006: Cutting Edge Legal and Regulatory*

Issues in the Pharmaceutical Industry, 15 Ann. Health L. 107, 131-32 (2006).

Journal 2006 Discusses increased regulation of gifts by pharmaceutical companies to physicians. Concludes that attorneys must be aware of the increased regulation in order to best advise their clients. Quotes Opinion 8.061. Rickard & Fehn, *Recent Developments in Regulation of Pharmaceutical Marketing Practices, 19 Health Lawyer 16, 17 (Dec. 2006).*

Journal 2005 Examines the pharmaceutical industry's influence on the shape and quality of medical education and practice. Concludes that the industry's influence on medical practitioners and the consequences of that influence on the American health care system are in transition. Quotes Opinion 8.061. Kapp, *Drug Companies, Dollars, and the Shaping of American Medical Practice, 29 S. Ill. U. L. J. 237, 249 (2005).*

Journal 2005 Conducted a survey to measure medical students' attitudes about interactions with drug companies. Concludes that future research should focus on ways to limit drug company influence so that decisions to prescribe medication are based upon the patient's best interest. Cites 8.061. Sierles, Brodkey, Cleary, McCurdy, Mintz, Frank, Lynn, Chao, Morgenstern, Shore, & Woodard, *Medical Students' Exposure to and Attitudes About Drug Company Interactions: A National Survey, 294 JAMA 1034, 1035 (2005).*

Journal 2004 Examines the intermediary doctrine and its effect on pharmaceutical manufacturer liability. Concludes that a balancing test must be employed in each instance to determine whether the physician or the pharmaceutical company is in the best position to warn the patient of dangers. References Opinion 8.061. Calabro, *Breaking the Shield of the Learned Intermediary Doctrine: Placing the Blame Where It Belongs, 25 Cardozo L. Rev. 2241, 2262, 2263 (2004).*

Journal 2004 Discusses the effect of federal fraud and abuse laws on the relationship between physicians and the pharmaceutical industry. Concludes that federal regulation of conflicts of interest created by physicians' relationships with pharmaceutical companies likely will increase. Cites Opinion 8.061. Studdert, Mello, & Brennan, *Financial Conflicts of Interest in Physicians' Relationships With the Pharmaceutical Industry—Self-regulation in the Shadow of Federal Prosecution, 351 New Eng. J. Med. 1891, 1900 (2004).*

Journal 2004 Describes financial conflicts of interest that may arise when physicians conduct clinical trials in the private practice setting. Concludes that safeguards must be put in place to protect patients, preserve the physician-patient relationship, and uphold the integrity of the research process. Cites Opinion 8.061. Williams, *Managing Physician Financial Conflicts of Interest in Clinical Trials Conducted in the Private Practice Setting, 59 Food & Drug L. J. 45, 67 (2004).*

Journal 2000 Compares the changes in physician roles in Japan and the US that exacerbate their conflicts of interest. Examines American physicians' dispensing practices and relations with pharmaceutical firms and hospital ownership. Concludes the US is reducing one of the main strengths it had in addressing physician conflicts: institutions of countervailing power and countervailing incentives. References Opinions 8.032 and 8.061, Rodwin & Okamoto, *Physicians' Conflicts of Interest in Japan and the United States: Lessons for the United States,* 25 J. Health Pol. Pol'y & L. 343, 355, 358 (2000).

Journal 2000 Examines the practice of gift giving by the health care technology industry as incentives in the context of continuing medical education activities. Concludes that industry-wide standards must be developed governing interactions between physicians and representatives of health care technology industry companies. Cites Opinions 8.061 and 9.011. Tenery, *Interactions Between Physicians and the Health Care Technology Industry,* 283 JAMA 391, 393 (2000).

Journal 2000 Examines data from several studies evaluating conflicts of interest triggered by gifts given to physicians by the pharmaceutical industry. Concludes that the efficacy of professional society guidelines to control such conflicts is questionable and there should be more systematic policies to address these concerns. References Opinion 8.061. Wazana, *Physicians and the Pharmaceutical Industry: Is a Gift Ever Just a Gift?* 283 JAMA 373, 380 (2000).

Journal 1999 Focuses on the purposes and broad applicability of the Medicare antikickback law. Describes how the law pertains to prescription drug and medical device manufacturers. Provides suggestions for antikickback law reform. Quotes Opinion 8.061. Bulleit & Krause, *Kickbacks, Courtesies, or Cost-Effectiveness? Application of the Medicare Antikickback Law to the Marketing and Promotional Practices of Drug and Medical Device Manufacturers,* 54 Food & Drug L. J. 279, 296 (1999).

Journal 1999 Discusses the impact *Daubert v. Merrell Dow Pharmaceuticals, Inc.* has had on scientific expert testimony. Explains that the scientific approach of dealing with bias may be inappropriate for maintaining scientific objectivity in litigation. Provides a strategy to deal with conflicts of interest in this context. Quotes Opinion 9.07. Cites Opinion 8.061. Patterson, *Conflicts of Interest in Scientific Expert Testimony,* 40 Wm. & Mary L. Rev. 1313, 1330, 1332, 1335, 1371 (1999).

Journal 1998 Discusses the conflict of interest posed by managed care organizations offering financial incentives to physicians. Explains that the duty to disclose and professionalism are not adequate protections against conflicts of interest. Suggests that financial incentives should be carefully circumscribed and that managed care organizations should focus primarily on quality of care. References Opinion 8.061. Emanuel & Goldman, *Protecting Patient Welfare in Managed Care: Six Safeguards,* 23 J. Health Pol. Pol'y & L. 635, 641 (1998).

Journal 1998 Examines the transition from paper medical records to electronic medical records. Identifies issues of confidentiality and privacy that arise as a result of the move to electronic medical records. Concludes that federal protection is needed to safeguard personal medical information. Quotes Principle IV and Opinions 5.07 and 5.075. Cites Opinion 8.061. Tsai, *Cheaper and Better: The Congressional Administrative Simplification Mandate Facilitates the Transition to Electronic Medical Records,* 19 J. Legal Med. 549, 570, 581 (1998).

Journal 1997 Discusses the process for marketing new drugs, medical devices, or biologics. Considers issues such as whether insurers or payers will cover these products, how much each will cost, and whether marketing programs comply with government regulations. References Opinion 8.061. Reiss, *Commentary on Payment and Reimbursement Issues Affecting the Marketing of Drugs, Medical Devices, and Biologics, With Emphasis on the Anti-Kickback Statute and Stark II,* 52 Food & Drug L. J. 99, 107 (1997).

Journal 1997 Explores the extent to which pharmaceutical drug samples are taken by physicians or other medical staff for personal use. Concludes that this practice is common and raises pertinent ethical issues. Quotes Opinion 8.061. Westfall, McCabe, & Nicholas, *Personal Use of Drug Samples by Physicians and Office Staff,* 278 JAMA 141, 142 (1997).

Journal 1994 Discusses the role of professional societies in establishing ethical guidelines for physicians in the context of using medical innovations and new technologies. Observes that these standards must be supplemented by additional external measures or incentives in order to be most effective. Cites Opinions 1.01, 1.02, 8.061, 9.04, and 9.131. Orentlicher, *The Influence of a Professional Organization on Physician Behavior,* 57 Alb. L. Rev. 583, 592, 593, 594, 595, 596 (1994).

Journal 1993 Examines how the Food and Drug Administration (FDA) regulates marketing of new medical devices and its authority to do so. Describes how these regulations differ from those governing drugs. References Opinion 8.061. Dennis, *Promotion of Devices: An Extension of FDA Drug Regulation or a New Frontier?* 48 Food & Drug L. J. 87 (1993).

Journal 1992 Surveys federal and state antikickback and antireferral statutes pertaining to drug and device marketing activities. Considers the effectiveness of regulatory safe harbors. Quotes Opinion 6.04 [now Opinion 8.06]. References Opinion 8.061. Kirschenbaum & Kuhlik, *Federal and State Laws Affecting Discounts, Rebates, and Other Marketing Practices for Drugs and Devices,* 47 Food & Drug L. J. 533, 560 (1992).

Journal 1992 Discusses the extent of the Food and Drug Administration's (FDA's) authority to regulate oral sales promotion of pharmaceuticals. Explores the debate over the extent of the FDA's power to regulate. References Opinion 8.061. Noah, *Death of a Salesman: To What Extent Can the FDA Regulate the Promotional Statements of Pharmaceutical Sales Representatives? 47 Food & Drug L. J. 309, 316 (1992).*

Journal 1992 Reviews concerns about commercial involvement in and funding of continuing medical education (CME). Discusses CME requirements, accumulation of CME credits, and changes in standards governing commercial sponsorship. References Opinions 8.061 and 9.011. Wentz, Osteen, & Cannon, *Continuing Medical Education: Unabated Debate, 268 JAMA 1118 (1992).*

Journal 1991 Examines legal, ethical, and economic concerns surrounding pharmaceutical company promotions. Concludes that pharmaceutical freebies can serve a positive role in health care if adequately regulated. Quotes Opinions 8.061 and 8.08. Note, *The Economic Wisdom of Regulating Pharmaceutical "Freebies," 1991 Duke L. J. 206, 216, 233, 234 (1991).*

Journal 1991 Discusses commercial support of continuing medical education. Explains ethical guidelines for accepting such assistance and how those guidelines have changed. References Opinions 8.061 and 9.011. Wentz, Osteen, & Gannon, *Refocusing Support and Direction, 266 JAMA 953 (1991).*

9.6.3 Incentives to Patients for Referrals

Journal 2010 Examines medical tourism and the referral-type fees foreign providers pay to brokers to bring patients from the United States. Concludes that while medical tourism is a viable option for uninsured or underinsured patients, disclosure of broker's fees would enhance competition and patient trust. Quotes Opinion 6.021. References Opinions 6.02 and 6.021. Spece, *Medical Tourism: Protecting Patients From Conflicts of Interest in Broker's Fees Paid by Foreign Providers, 6 J. Health & Biomedical L. 1, 3, 19 (2010).*

Journal 2006 Discusses the evolution of health law in Virginia. Concludes that the area of health law continues to expand, develop, and be refined. Cites Opinions 3.03, 3.08, 5.01, 5.015, 5.02, 5.04, 5.055, 6.02, 6.021, 6.03, 6.04, 7.03, 7.04, 7.05, 8.054, 8.08, 8.081, 8.085, 8.115, 8.12, 8.14, 8.145, 8.19, and 9.045. Guanzon, *Health Care Law, 41 U. Rich. L. Rev. 179, 199 (2006).*

9.6.4 Sale of Health-Related Products

Journal 2006 Reviews the regulation of dietary supplement manufacturing and labeling. Concludes that the FDA may have adequate authority to regulate dietary supplements. Quotes Opinion 8.063. Noah, *A Drug by Any Other Name. . . ? Paradoxes in Dietary Supplement Risk Regulation, 17 Stan. L. & Pol'y Rev. 165, 192 (2006).*

Journal 2002 Examines the ethical aspects of e-medicine. Concludes that, although e-medicine has benefits, physicians must understand its impact on the physician-patient relationship. Cites Opinions 8.062 and 8.063. Berg, *Ethics and E-Medicine, 46 St. Louis U. L. J. 61, 66 (2002).*

9.6.5 Sale of Non-Health-Related Products

N.Y. Sup. 2009 Physician moved to dismiss patient's claim for breach of fiduciary duty. Patient claimed that but for a physician-patient relationship with the physician, he would not have invested in the physician's new company. The court quoted Opinion 8.062 in determining that physician's conduct was objectionable, but nonetheless granted the motion to dismiss. *Otto v. Melman, 2009 WL 4348827, 4.*

Journal 2006 Discusses regulation of complementary and alternative medicine. Concludes that only minimal regulation of these practices is required. References

Principle 7 (1957) [now Opinion 8.06 and Opinion 8.062]. Lunstroth, *Voluntary Self-regulation of Complementary and Alternative Medicine Practitioners, 70 Alb. L. Rev. 209, 243 (2006).*

Journal 2002 Examines the ethical aspects of e-medicine. Concludes that, although e-medicine has benefits, physicians must understand its impact on the physician-patient relationship. Cites Opinions 8.062 and 8.063. Berg, *Ethics and E-Medicine, 46 St. Louis U. L. J. 61, 66 (2002)*

9.6.6 Prescribing and Dispensing Drugs and Devices

E.D. N.Y. 1975 Medical laboratories sought injunction against city's award of exclusive contracts for Medicaid services. The court granted a preliminary injunction and held that the laboratories had a substantial probability of success on the merits of the claim that Medicaid recipients would be deprived of statutory right of free choice of providers. In balancing the equities, the court also noted that the contracts would create an ethical dilemma for physicians who are required to provide patients with free choice of ancillary services under Opinions and Reports of the Judicial Council Sec. 1, Paras. 6 and 14 (1971) [now Opinions 8.03, 8.06, and 9.06]. *Bay Ridge Diagnostic Laboratory, Inc. v. Dumpson, 400 F. Supp. 1104, 1109-10.*

Cal. App. 1967 Physician-stockholders of publicly owned pharmaceutical corporations and physicians whose medical partnerships owned and operated pharmacies challenged statutory prohibition of physician membership, proprietory interest, and co-ownership of pharmacies. The court quoted Principles Ch. I, Sec. 6 (1947), and a 1960 Judicial Council rule, later included in Opinions and Reports of the Judicial Council Sec. 7, Para. 38 (1965) [now Opinions 8.03, 8.032, and 8.06], in its discussion of the potential conflict of interest created by such ownership. The court held that the statute prohibited physician partnerships from directly owning pharmacies but did not apply to an individual physician or a partnership of physicians who own stock in a corporation which owns and operates a pharmacy. *Magan Medical Clinic v. California State Bd. of Medical Examiners, 249 Cal. App. 2d 124, 57 Cal. Rptr. 256, 262.*

Minn. App. 1997 Patients brought suit against physician for prescribing a growth hormone drug while receiving kickbacks, in violation of the physician-patient fiduciary duty and the Minnesota Consumer Fraud Act. The distributor of the drug induced physicians to refer patients for the drug. The court cited Opinion 8.06 for the proposition that patients are entitled to receive medical opinions and referrals which are not motivated by physician gain. The court found, however, that the complaint sounded in medical malpractice and declined to allow a new cause of action based on breach of a fiduciary duty. Because the malpractice limitations had expired and the patients had failed to allege sufficient injury under the Consumer Fraud Act, the court affirmed dismissal with prejudice. *D.A.B v. Brown, 570 N.W. 2d 168, 170.*

Ohio 1980 A physician, charged with violating the state medical licensing statute by distributing controlled substances without a proper license and writing prescriptions for narcotics in the name of one person when they were intended for another, challenged the state medical board's decision to suspend his license and place him on two years' probation. Under the statute, a physician could be disciplined for various activities including violation of any provision of a code of ethics of a national professional organization such as the AMA. The board found in part that the physician's actions violated Principles 4 and 7 (1957) [now Principles II and III and Opinions 8.06 and 9.04]. The trial court

reversed, holding that the board had insufficient evidence for its decision, and the court of appeals affirmed. On appeal, the Supreme Court held that expert testimony was not required at a hearing before a medical licensing board because they were experts and could determine for themselves whether the Principles had been violated. *Arlen v. State, 61 Ohio St. 2d 168, 399 N.E.2d 1251, 1252, 1253-54.*

Mo. Att'y Gen. 1982 State attorney general, citing Opinion 8.06 (1982), concluded that a physician who requires a patient to accept drugs dispensed by the physician and refuses to provide the patient with a prescription for the patient's use elsewhere violates state antitrust law and has engaged in professional misconduct. A similar conclusion, again based in part on Opinion 8.06, was rendered regarding a physician who requires a patient to fill a prescription at a pharmacy in which the physician has a personal interest. *Missouri Att'y Gen. Op. No. 6 (July 8, 1982) (LEXIS, States library, Mo. file).*

Journal 2008 Analyzes off-label drug prescribing patterns, the limited market demand for post-approval clinical trials, and increased litigation targeted at financial relationships between physicians and pharmaceutical firms. Concludes issues in learning patterns in the medical profession and deficiencies in the production and dissemination of clinical knowledge must be addressed in the context of off-label prescribing. Cites Opinion 8.06. Johnson, *Polluting Medical Judgment? False Assumptions in the Pursuit of False Claims Regarding Off-Label Prescribing, 9 Minn. J. L. Sci. & Tech. 61, 103 (2009).*

Journal 2007 Explores regulation of the pharmacy benefit management industry. Concludes that current regulations are inadequate to prevent fraud and self-dealing, and that private sector regulation is the best solution. Cites Opinion 8.06. Garrett & Garis, *Leveling the Playing Field in the Pharmacy Benefit Management Industry, 42 Val. U. L. Rev. 33, 64 (2007).*

Journal 2006 Discusses the evolution of health law in Virginia. Concludes that the area of health law continues to expand, develop, and be refined. Cites Opinions 3.03, 3.08, 5.01, 5.015, 5.02, 5.04, 5.055, 6.02, 6.021, 6.03, 6.04 [now Opinion 8.06], 7.03, 7.04, 7.05, 8.054, 8.08, 8.081, 8.085, 8.115, 8.12, 8.14, 8.145, 8.19, and 9.045. Guanzon, *Health Care Law, 41 U. Rich. L. Rev. 179, 199 (2006).*

Journal 2006 Discusses regulation of complementary and alternative medicine. Concludes that only minimal regulation of these practices is required. References Principle 7 (1957) [now Opinion 8.06 and Opinion 8.062]. Lunstroth, *Voluntary Self-regulation of Complementary and Alternative Medicine Practitioners, 70 Alb. L. Rev. 209, 243 (2006).*

Journal 2002 Suggests a reconceptualization for bioethics that integrates an analysis of the history of moral change. Concludes that bioethical textbooks should include discussion about the history of bioethics and medical ethics. Quotes Opinion 2.20. References Opinions 6.02, 6.03, 6.04 [now Opinion 8.06], and 8.032. Baker, *Bioethics and History, 27 J. Med. & Phil. 447, 455, 469 (2002).*

Journal 2001 Explores how the *Pegram* case restricted the protection provided to HMOs by ERISA's state law pre-emption. Concludes that HMOs will be subject to increased litigation under two areas of state law—breach of statutory fiduciary duty and medical malpractice claims. Cites Opinion 8.06. McLean & Richards, *Managed Care Liability for Breach of Fiduciary Duty After Pegram v. Herdrich: The End of ERISA Preemption for State Law Liability for Medical Care Decision Making, 53 Fla. L. Rev. 1, 38 (2001).*

Journal 2001 Considers office dispensing of products within the dermatology practice. Examines related ethical issues. Concludes that the primary reasons patients buy products from their physicians are trust and knowledge, not convenience. Quotes Opinion 8.06. Ogbogu, Fleischer, Brodell, Bhalla, Draelos, & Feldman, *Physicians' and Patients' Perspectives on Office-Based Dispensing: The Central Role of the* physician-patient *Relationship, 137 Arch. Dermatol. 151, 151 (2001).*

Journal 2001 Explores the extent to which pediatricians should rely on their expertise when prescribing therapies and durable medical equipment for children with special health care needs. Emphasizes the importance of the pediatrician's role in this context and urges pediatricians to comply with pertinent AMA guidelines and relevant state and federal laws. Quotes Opinion 8.06. References Opinion 9.132. Sneed, May, & Stencel, *Physicians' Reliance on Specialists, Therapists, and Vendors When Prescribing Therapies and Durable Medical Equipment for Children With Special Health Care Needs, 107 Pediatrics 1283, 1287, 1288, 1289 (2001).*

Journal 1998 Discusses the physician's fiduciary duty to the patient. Explores the expansion of the "honest services" mail fraud statute to prosecute undisclosed fiduciary breaches. Concludes that the mail fraud statute may be used to prosecute physicians who fail to disclose financial incentives to their patients. Quotes Opinion 8.03. Cites Opinions 2.03 and 8.07 [now Opinion 8.06]. Jones, *Primum Non Nocere: The Expanding "Honest Services" Mail Fraud Statute and the* physician-patient *Fiduciary Relationship, 51 Vand. L. Rev. 139, 161, 164 (1998).*

Journal 1992 Surveys federal and state antikickback and antireferral statutes pertaining to drug and device marketing activities. Considers the effectiveness of regulatory safe harbors. Quotes Opinion 6.04 [now Opinion 8.06]. References Opinion 8.061. Kirschenbaum & Kuhlik, *Federal and State Laws Affecting Discounts, Rebates, and Other Marketing Practices for Drugs and Devices, 47 Food & Drug L. J. 533, 560 (1992).*

Journal 1991 Looks at the physician as a fiduciary and the law governing fiduciary relationships. Concludes that fiduciary concepts are a valuable basis for establishing ethical and legal guidelines for physician behavior. Quotes Opinions 2.19, 8.03 (1989) [now Opinion 8.032], and 8.06. Healey & Dowling, *Controlling Conflicts of Interest in the Doctor-Patient Relationship: Lessons From Moore v. Regents of the University of California, 42 Mercer L. Rev. 989, 997, 998 (1991).*

9.6.7 Direct-to-Consumer Advertisement of Prescription Drugs

Journal 2009 Reviews the history of pharmaceutical marketing, the creation of the FDA, and advertising regulation and laws. Concludes direct-to-consumer advertising has not fundamentally changed the relationship between pharmaceutical manufacturers and physicians, with physicians maintaining their essential role as the learned intermediary. Quotes Opinion 5.015. Schwartz, Silverman, Hulka, & Appel, *Marketing Pharmaceutical Products in the Twenty-First Century: An Analysis of the Continued Viability of Traditional Principles of Law in the Age of Direct-to-Consumer Advertising, 32 Harv. J. L. & Pub. Pol'y 333, 365 (2009).*

Journal 2007 Questions FDA restrictions prohibiting drug manufacturers from discussing off-label uses of their products. Concludes that such restrictions on speech violate the First Amendment under the *Central Hudson* test. References Opinion 5.015. Hall & Sobotka, *Inconsistent Government Policies: Why FDA Off-Label Regulation Cannot Survive First Amendment Review Under Greater New Orleans, 62 Food Drug L. J. 1, 31 (2007).*

Journal 2006 Discusses the evolution of health law in Virginia. Concludes that the area of health law continues to expand, develop, and be refined. Cites Opinions 3.03, 3.08, 5.01, 5.015, 5.02, 5.04, 5.055, 6.02, 6.021, 6.03, 6.04, 7.03, 7.04, 7.05, 8.054, 8.08, 8.081, 8.085, 8.115, 8.12, 8.14, 8.145, 8.19, and 9.045. Guanzon, *Health Care Law, 41 U. Rich. L. Rev. 179, 199 (2006).*

Journal 2004 Discusses whether the government may legally restrain direct-to-consumer advertising of genetic tests. Concludes that any such restraint on truthful and nonmisleading advertising in this context would be unconstitutional. References Opinion 5.015. Javitt, Stanley, & Hudson, *Direct-to-Consumer Genetic Tests, Government Oversight, and the First Amendment: What the Government Can (and Can't) Do to Protect the Public's Health, 57 Okla. L. Rev. 251, 280 (2004).*

Journal 2003 Discusses the pharmaceutical industry's direct-to-consumer (DTC) Internet advertising program. Concludes that reforms to Internet-based DTC advertising practices are necessary, with emphasis on the physician-patient relationship. References Opinion 5.015. Hall, *The Promise and Peril of Direct-to-Consumer Prescription Drug Promotion on the Internet, 7 DePaul J. Health Care L. 1, 35 (2003).*

Journal 2002 Examines the legal, ethical, and social implications of Internet direct-to-consumer advertising of

health products. Concludes that such advertising may be worthwhile, but privacy, product liability, and corporate responsibility issues must be addressed. References Opinion 5.015. Kao & Linden, *Direct-to-Consumer Advertising and the Internet: Informational Privacy, Product Liability and Organizational Responsibility, 46 St. Louis U. L. J. 157, 170 (2002).*

9.6.9 Physician Self-referral

C.D. Ill. 1992 A contractual agreement between a clinic and hospital providing undisclosed financial incentives for referrals constituted a "business" aspect of the medical profession and was not exempt from state's Consumer Fraud Act. Reference is made to Council on Ethical Judicial Affairs, Conflicts of Interest Physician Ownership of Medical Facilities, 267 *JAMA* 2366 (1992) [now Opinion 8.032], which mandates that a physician disclose his financial interest to his patient when making a referral. *Gadson v. Newman, 807 F. Supp. 1412, 1416.*

E.D. N.Y. 1975 Medical laboratories sought injunction against city's award of exclusive contracts for Medicaid services. The court granted a preliminary injunction and held that the laboratories had a substantial probability of success on the merits of the claim that Medicaid recipients would be deprived of statutory right of free choice of providers. In balancing the equities, the court also noted that the contracts would create an ethical dilemma for physicians who are required to provide patients with free choice of ancillary services under Opinions and Reports of the Judicial Council Sec. 1, Paras. 6 and 14 (1971) [now Opinions 8.032, 8.06, and 9.06]. *Bay Ridge Diagnostic Laboratory, Inc. v. Dumpson, 400 F. Supp. 1104, 1109-10.*

E.D. Va. 1995 Claimants sustained personal injuries when ships collided. In an admiralty action, court had to determine the extent of probable injuries sustained by the claimants. The court observed that a treating physician had referred one of the claimants for tests to a facility in which the physician had a substantial ownership interest. In finding that these tests and procedures were unnecessary and unreasonable, the court quoted Opinion 8.032. *In re Capt. Wool, Inc., 1995 US Dist. LEXIS 20128.*

Cal. App. 1967 Physician-stockholders of publicly owned pharmaceutical corporations and physicians whose medical partnerships owned and operated pharmacies challenged statutory prohibition of physician membership, proprietory interest, and co-ownership of pharmacies. The court quoted Principles Ch. I, Sec. 6 (1947), and a 1960 Judicial Council rule, later included in Opinions and Reports of the Judicial Council Sec. 7, Para. 38 (1965) [now Opinions 8.03, 8.032, and 8.06], in its discussion of the potential conflict of interest created by such ownership. The court held that the statute prohibited physician partnerships from directly owning pharmacies, but did not apply to an individual physician or

a partnership of physicians who own stock in a corporation which owns and operates a pharmacy. *Magan Medical Clinic v. California State Bd. of Medical Examiners, 249 Cal. App. 2d 124, 57 Cal. Rptr. 256, 262.*

Mass. Super. 1998 Plaintiff-surgeon filed suit against a medical group practice claiming that the defendants reduced referrals to him because he declined to join the group. Plaintiff claimed that the decline harmed his surgical practice. He alleged that the group's practice of taking 10% of members' income constituted unethical and illegal kickbacks. The court held that the decline in referrals was not connected to plaintiff not being a member of the group. The court also found that the plaintiff had not presented evidence that the decline in referrals harmed his practice. Finally, the court found that the fees paid by members of the group practice were gatekeeper fees rather than referral fees. The court quoted Opinion 6.02, in support of its decision that the defendants' fees did not constitute fee splitting. Further, the court referenced Opinion 8.032 concluding that a self-referral was not necessarily unethical if disclosed to the patient. *Boman v. Southeast Medical Services Group, 1998 WL 1182063, 11-12.*

Mich. Att'y Gen. 1977 State attorney general determined that, within limits, it was not illegal for physicians to refer patient specimens to clinical laboratories which they own or in which they have a financial interest. Opinion observes however that, under the Opinions and Reports of the Judicial Council Sec. 7, Paras. 21 and 22 (1972) [now Opinions 8.03 and 8.032], such referrals may be unethical. *Mich. Att'y Gen. Opinion No. 5229, 1977-78 Att'y Gen. Op. 234.*

Journal 2006 Discusses physician and attorney financial interests in ancillary businesses. Concludes that such interests are permissible, but that patients and clients should not be referred to any business in which the professional has an interest. Cites Opinion 8.032. Falit, *Ancillary Service and Self-referral Arrangements in the Medical and Legal Professions: Do Current Ethical, Legislative, and Regulatory Policies Adequately Serve the Interests of Patients and Clients? 58 S. C. L. Rev. 371, 373-74 (2006).*

Journal 2006 Reviews legislation and case law governing conscience clauses for medical professionals. Concludes that conscientious objections to providing care should be permitted only when based on accepted principles of medical ethics. Quotes Opinion 2.18 (1986) [now Opinion 2.20]. References Opinion 8.032. Swartz, *"Conscience Clauses" or "Unconscionable Clauses": Personal Beliefs Versus Professional Responsibilities, 6 Yale J. Health Pol'y, L. & Ethics 269, 317, 347 (2006).*

Journal 2005 Analyzes federal and state laws that address concerns associated with physician self-referral. Concludes that additional restrictions are needed to prohibit physicians from referring patients to publicly or privately funded facilities in which physicians have a financial interest. Quotes Opinion 8.032. Bethard, *Physician Self-referral: Beyond Stark II, 43 Brandeis L. J. 465, 468 (2005).*

Journal 2004 Discusses the practice of "economic credentialing," offering an overview of recent legal activity with respect to this controversial practice. Concludes that, despite certain areas of potential risk, it would appear that hospitals may utilize economic criteria when making credentialing decisions. Cites Opinion 8.032. Cohen, *An Examination of the Right of Hospitals to Engage in Economic Credentialing, 77 Temp. L. Rev. 705, 741 (2004).*

Journal 2004 Examines the practice of "self-referral" and various problems associated with regulation of this practice. Concludes that regulatory emphasis should focus on limiting conflicts of interest, particularly as they may arise when physician investors self-refer to specialty hospitals. Quotes Opinion 8.032. Kwiecinski, *Limiting Conflicts of Interest Arising From Physician Investment in Specialty Hospitals, 88 Marq. L. Rev. 413, 414, 428 (2004).*

Journal 2002 Suggests a reconceptualization for bioethics that integrates an analysis of the history of moral change. Concludes that bioethical textbooks should include discussion about the history of bioethics and medical ethics. Quotes Opinion 2.20. References Opinions 6.02, 6.03, 6.04 [now Opinion 8.06], and 8.032. Baker, *Bioethics and History, 27 J. Med. & Phil. 447, 455, 469 (2002).*

Journal 2001 Examines issues relating to health care cost containment. Concludes that, if physicians are to meet the goals assigned to them in a cost-constrained health care system, then professional standards must be reevaluated and modified to afford meaningful guidance for clinical decision-making in the face of health care spending controls. Quotes Opinions 2.03, 2.09, 2.095, 8.032, and 9.04. Cites Opinions 8.02, 8.021, 8.051, and 8.13. Agrawal, *Resuscitating Professionalism: Self-regulation in the Medical Marketplace, 66 Mo. L. Rev. 341, 354, 355, 360, 361, 378, 388 (2001).*

Journal 2001 Considers ethical aspects of physician conflicts of interest in the context of human subjects research. Focuses on conflicts that are associated with clinical trials of new drugs and devices. Concludes by discussing the impact of these conflicts of interest on trust in the physician-patient relationship. References Principle IV and Opinion 8.032. Miller, *Trusting Doctors: Tricky Business When It Comes to Clinical Research, 81 B. U. L. Rev. 423, 427-28 (2001).*

Journal 2000 Examines physician value neutrality (PVN). Defines PVN as providing a foundation to suggest physicians must keep their values—religious, political, or otherwise—out of the patient-physician relationship. Concludes it is not clear how values can be removed from the patient-physician relationship without removing the very thing PVN supporters are trying to protect, the intrinsic value of persons. References Opinions 2.01, 2.02, 8.032, 8.05, 8.08, and 8.132. Beckwith & Peppin, *Physician Value Neutrality: A Critique, 28 J. L. Med. & Ethics 67, 72-73 (2000).*

Journal 2000 Examines justice in health care by focusing on concepts of access and allocation. Presents four principles for the just allocation of health care resources: improving health; informing patients about the manner in which resources are allocated in the context of managed care; affording patients an opportunity to consent to such allocation of resources; and minimization of conflicts of interest. References Opinion 8.032. Emanuel, *Justice and Managed Care: Four Principles for the Just Allocation of Health Care Resources, 30 Hastings Center Rep. 8, 16 (May/June 2000).*

Journal 2000 Explores the legal, ethical, social, and economic considerations associated with use of new genetic techniques in the prediction and diagnosis of Alzheimer disease. Outlines the potential responsibilities and liabilities of physicians in connection with use of these techniques. References Opinions 2.132, 2.139, and 8.032. Kapp, *Physicians' Legal Duties Regarding the Use of Genetic Tests to Predict and Diagnose Alzheimer Disease, 21 J. Legal Med. 445, 456-57, 465-66 (2000).*

Journal 2000 Compares the changes in physician roles in Japan and the US that exacerbate their conflicts of interest. Examines American physicians' dispensing practices and relations with pharmaceutical firms and hospital ownership. Concludes the US is reducing one of the main strengths it had in addressing physician conflicts: institutions of countervailing power and countervailing incentives. References Opinions 8.032 and 8.061. Rodwin & Okamoto, *Physicians' Conflicts of Interest in Japan and the United States: Lessons for the United States, 25 J. Health Pol. Pol'y & L. 343, 355, 358 (2000).*

Journal 1999 Discusses issues surrounding ambulatory surgical centers. Focuses on self-referral laws, the federal antikickback statute, and tax issues. Outlines legal requirements pertaining to ambulatory surgical centers. Cites Opinion 8.032. DeMuro, *A Review of Key Legal Requirements Affecting Ambulatory Surgical Centers, 11 Health Law. 1, 7 (1999).*

Journal 1999 Explores the increased push toward mandatory disclosure laws regarding financial incentives imposed by managed care organizations. Discusses current laws and ethical guidelines. Emphasizes that efforts to mandate disclosure force physicians to focus on the effects of imposed incentives and the essence of the physician-patient relationship. References Opinions 8.032, 8.13, and 8.132. Miller &

Sage, *Disclosing Physician Financial Incentives, 281 JAMA 1424, 1425 (1999)*.

Journal 1999 Discusses the practice of physicians using nonpublic information to invest in stocks. Provides guidelines on insider trading laws for physicians. Observes that insider trading damages the public perception of the medical profession. References Opinion 8.032. Prentice, *Clinical Trial Results, Physicians, and Insider Trading, 20 J. Legal Med. 195, 221 (1999)*.

Journal 1999 Discusses the push to mandate disclosure in managed care programs. Explains the dangers of disclosing too much information. Provides objectives and goals for disclosure. Quotes Opinion 8.051. References Opinions 8.032 and 8.13. Sage, *Regulating Through Information: Disclosure Laws and American Health Care, 99 Colum. L. Rev. 1701, 1753, 1758, 1760 (1999)*.

Journal 1999 Explores the impact managed care organizations have had on health care. Explains that patients may not understand restrictions and incentives imposed by their managed care organizations when entering the program. Argues that such information should be disclosed at various times during the period of plan coverage. Cites Opinions 2.03, 8.03, 8.032, 8.051, 8.13, and 8.132. Wolf, *Toward a Systemic Theory of Informed Consent in Managed Care, 35 Hous. L. Rev. 1631, 1641, 1658, 1661, 1662, 1679 (1999)*.

Journal 1998 Discusses conflicts of interest in the physician-patient relationship arising out of use of financial incentives by managed care organizations. Considers how such conflicts are dealt with in the attorney-client relationship. Suggests that a financial incentive should be legally denounced if it unreasonably interferes with a physician's duty to properly care for and treat patients. Quotes Preamble, Fundamental Elements (1) [now Opinion 10.01] and Opinions 4.04, 5.01, 8.03, 8.13, and 9.06. Cites Fundamental Elements (4) [now Opinion 10.01], and Opinions 2.07, 2.08, and 2.132. Hall, *Third-Party Payor Conflicts of Interest in Managed Care: A Proposal for Regulation Based on the Model Rules of Professional Conduct, 29 Seton Hall L. Rev. 95, 96, 107, 108, 109, 110, 111, 112, 134, 135, 136 (1998)*.

Journal 1997 Discusses the quality of neurological care and the ethical conflicts that are created by the drive to contain costs. Focuses on quality management and cost-containment programs and the conflicts created when neurologists attempt to reconcile the interests of patients and society. References Opinions 8.032 and 8.13. Bernat, *Quality of Neurological Care: Balancing Cost Control and Ethics, 54 Arch. Neurol. 1341, 1343, 1345 (1997)*.

Journal 1995 Examines the metaphor of physicians as fiduciaries. Considers how the law holds physicians accountable in this regard. Quotes Preamble. Cites Opinion 8.03 (1986) [now Opinion 8.032]. Rodwin, *Strains in the Fiduciary Metaphor: Divided Physician Loyalties and Obligations in a Changing Health Care System, XXI Am. J. Law & Med. 241, 246, 250 (1995)*.

Journal 1993 Argues that legislative efforts to curb or prohibit physician investment and self-referral are misdirected.

Proposes a more effective solution to this problem: enforcement of existing laws. Quotes Opinion 8.032. Morreim, *Blessed Be the Tie That Binds? Antitrust Perils of Physician Investment and Self-referral, 14 J. Legal Med. 359, 367, 374, 377, 394, 409 (1993)*.

Journal 1993 Examines financial conflicts of interest involving physicians. Discusses ways to identify conflicts and possible remedies. References Opinion 8.032. Thompson, *Understanding Financial Conflicts of Interest, 329 New Eng. J. Med. 573 (1993)*.

Journal 1992 Discusses the safe harbor regulations under the Medicare and Medicaid Antikickback Statute, examines the Hanlester Network case, and describes the problem of physician self-referral. Concludes that a societal consensus is evolving against self-referral. References Opinion 8.032. Crane, *The Problem of Physician Self-referral Under the Medicare and Medicaid Antikickback Statute: The Hanlester Network Case and the Safe Harbor Regulation, 268 JAMA 85, 89, 90 (1992)*.

Journal 1992 Analyzes the Medicare Antifraud Statute and the safe harbor regulations in light of recent criticisms. Concludes that the antifraud statute is an appropriate way to deal with fraud, but that other steps also should be taken. References Opinion 8.032. Farley, *The Medicare Antifraud Statute and Safe Harbor Regulations: Suggestions for Change, 81 Georgetown L. J. 167, 184 (1992)*.

Journal 1992 Examines issues related to the responsibility of HIV-infected health care workers to protect patients from infection, including mandatory testing, disclosure to coworkers and supervisors, and the degree to which the practice of an HIV-infected health care worker should be modified. Concludes that courts likely will impose a requirement to disclose HIV-positive status to patients when there is a substantial risk of HIV transmission. Quotes Opinions 8.03 (1989) [now Opinion 8.032] and 8.07 (1989) [now Opinion 8.03]. References Opinion 9.131. Lieberman & Derse, *HIV-Positive Health Care Workers and the Obligation to Disclose: Do Patients Have a Right to Know? 13 J. Legal Med. 333, 353, 354 (1992)*.

Journal 1992 Examines a memorandum issued by the chief counsel of the Internal Revenue Service, which clearly identified certain transactions that could jeopardize the tax exempt status of hospitals. Concludes that the memorandum provides valuable guidance for hospitals in spite of its shortcomings. References Opinion 8.032. Mancino, *New GCM Suggests Rules for Ventures Between Nonprofit Hospitals and Doctors, 76 J. Taxation 164, 167 (1992)*.

Journal 1992 Analyzes the controversy over physician ownership of health care facilities. Considers a study of physician joint ventures in Florida and finds that current legislation prohibiting or restricting such arrangements is inadequate. Quotes Opinion 8.032. Mitchell & Scott, *Evidence on Complex Structures of Physician Joint Ventures, 9 Yale J. Regulation 489, 503 (1992)*.

Journal 1992 Discusses the problem of physician joint ventures and examines their prevalence in Florida. Concludes that these arrangements may cause physicians to prioritize economic incentives over patients' medical needs. References Opinion 8.032. Mitchell & Scott, *New Evidence of the Prevalence and Scope of Physician Joint Ventures, 268 JAMA 80, 84 (1992).*

Journal 1992 Examines the issue of physician joint ventures in the context of physical therapy and rehabilitation services. Finds that facility utilization, patient cost, and physician profits were higher at joint venture facilities. References Opinion 8.032. Mitchell & Scott, *Physician Ownership of Physical Therapy Services: Effects on Charges, Utilization, Profits, and Service Characteristics, 268 JAMA 2055, 2058 (1992).*

Journal 1992 Presents results of a study indicating that joint ventures in radiation therapy increase the use and cost of these services and reduce access to care in inner-city and rural areas. Concludes that physician joint ventures have negative consequences and proposes that carefully crafted legislation be enacted to ban such arrangements. Quotes Opinion 8.032. Mitchell & Sunshine, *Consequences of Physicians' Ownership of Health Care Facilities—Joint Ventures in Radiation Therapy, 327 New Eng. J. Med. 1497, 1500 (1992).*

Journal 1992 Examines the debate regarding physician self-referral. Argues in favor of the AMA's statement in general, but urges an even stronger and more comprehensive position in this context. References Opinion 8.032. Relman, *"Self-referral"—What's at Stake? 327 New Eng. J. Med. 1522, 1524 (1992).*

Journal 1992 Explores the problem of physician self-referral and overuse of physician-owned facilities. Concludes that in cases studied, physician ownership of a facility increased the use and cost of services. Quotes Opinion 8.032. Swedlow, Johnson, Smithline, & Milstein, *Increased Costs and Rates of Use in the California Workers' Compensation System as a Result of Self-referral by Physicians, 327 New Eng. J. Med. 1502 (1992).*

Journal 1991 Looks at the physician as a fiduciary and the law governing fiduciary relationships. Concludes that fiduciary concepts are a valuable basis for establishing ethical and legal guidelines for physician behavior. Quotes Opinions 2.19, 8.03 (1989) [now Opinion 8.032], and 8.06. Healey & Dowling, *Controlling Conflicts of Interest in the Doctor-Patient Relationship: Lessons From Moore v. Regents of the University of California, 42 Mercer L. Rev. 989, 997, 998 (1991).*

Journal 1991 Discusses the issue of HIV-infected surgeons in light of the New Jersey case decision in *Behringer v. Medical Center.* Considers future developments. References Opinions 8.032 and 9.131. Orentlicher, *HIV-Infected Surgeons: Behringer v. Medical Center, 266 JAMA 1134, 1136 (1991).*

Journal 1990 Discusses efforts of third-party payers to control health care expenditures for beneficiaries. Concludes that financial incentives to limit care and other cost-control techniques should be disclosed and that the rationale for such disclosure is compelling. Quotes Opinions 2.03, 2.09, and 8.03 [now Opinions 8.03 and 8.032]. Cites Opinions 2.19, 4.04, and 4.06. Hirshfeld, *Should Third Party Payors of Health Care Services Disclose Cost Control Mechanisms to Potential Beneficiaries? 14 Seton Hall Legis. J. 115, 130, 131, 144, 145, 146 (1990).*

Journal 1990 Examines various cost-control mechanisms utilized by prepaid health plans and other managed care programs and considers the impact of such mechanisms on clinical decision making. Emphasis is placed on the possible existence of conflicts of interest on the part of health care providers in this context. Quotes Opinions 8.03 [now Opinions 8.03 and 8.032] and 8.13 [now Opinion 8.132]. Hirshfeld, *Defining Full and Fair Disclosure in Managed Care Contracts, 60 The Citation 67, 70 (1990).*

Journal 1990 Balances the laissez-faire concerns of individual freedom and personal choice with the prohibitionists' desire to protect patients from poor quality care and unnecessary referrals. Concludes that civil remedies should be emphasized by extending the doctrines of bad faith and breach of contract into this arena. References Opinion 8.032. Morreim, *Physician Investment and Self-referral: Philosophical Analysis of a Contentious Debate, 15 J. Med. & Phil. 425, 428, 429, 430, 431 (1990).*

Journal 1985 Initially describes how existing doctrines protect the value of autonomy in the context of the physician-patient relationship, then examines various problems in the current protective scheme. Concludes by recommending the creation of an independent articulable protected interest in patient autonomy. Quotes Principles II and IV. Cites Opinions 4.04 (1984) [now Opinions 8.03 and 8.032] and 6.03 (1984) [now Opinion 6.02]. Shultz, *From Informed Consent to Patient Choice: A New Protected Interest, 95 Yale L. J. 219, 275 (1985).*

9.7.1 Medical Testimony

M.D. Pa. 1947 Motion for new trial in malpractice action following verdict for defendant-physicians. Patient had been treated surgically for tube-ovarian abscess, had profuse postoperative bleeding, and died of infection secondary to ruptured ectopic pregnancy. Plaintiff moved for a new trial on grounds that an officer of a local medical society persuaded plaintiff's expert not to testify. Although it denied the motion on other grounds, the court criticized the officer's conduct, noting that it was contrary to Principles Ch. 1, Sec. 7 (1947) [now Opinion 9.07], but refused to impute the impropriety to the defendants. *McHugh v. Audet, 72 F. Supp. 394, 404.*

Fed. Cl. 2010 Plaintiffs alleged that a vaccine administered by the defendant-physician caused injuries. In denying compensation to one of plaintiffs' experts, the court quotes Opinion 9.07 stating that physicians providing expert testimony should have recent and substantive experience in the area in question, and their testimony should reflect current scientific standards of care. The court found that a gene mutation in the plaintiff-patient more likely than not caused her injury and denied compensation. *Stone v. Secretary of the Department of Health and Human Services, 2010 WL 3790297, 8.*

Fed. Cl. 2007 Petitioners alleged their children's deafness was caused by vaccines. They sought compensation under the National Vaccine Injury Compensation Program. The court determined that petitioners' expert, a physician, lacked credibility and failed to present convincing evidence. The court questioned the expert's evidentiary presentation, his experience, and his education in the field. Citing Opinion 9.07, the court found that the physician went beyond his role as an expert and became an advocate for the family. The court held the petitioners were not entitled to compensation under the Program. *Hopkins v. Sec. of Dept. of Health and Human Services, 2007 WL 2454038, 6.*

Fed. Cl. 2006 Plaintiff filed suit under the National Childhood Vaccine Injury Act of 1986, claiming hepatitis B vaccination caused her transverse myelitis. Medical literature was inconclusive as to whether the vaccine could cause such injury. Medical experts testified for both parties and the court found in favor of plaintiff. Quoting Opinion 9.07, the court rebuked defendant's medical experts for their coercive efforts in threatening to undermine the reputation of plaintiff's expert witness. *Stevens v. Sec. of Dept. of Health and Human Services, 2006 WL 659525, 7-8.*

Fed. Cl. 2005 Petitioner filed suit under the National Vaccine Injury Compensation Program, alleging that his son suffered neurological injuries as a result of a tetanus toxoid vaccine. The court quoted Opinion 9.07 in determining that one of petitioner's expert witnesses gave testimony that departed from acceptable medical principles and was unsupported. The court concluded that the petitioner had not met the burden of proof and was not entitled to compensation. *Kelley v. Sec. of Dept. of Health and Human Services, 2005 WL 1125671, 7.*

Fed. Cl. 2004 Petitioner filed suit for injuries allegedly sustained after receiving a vaccination. The court found that petitioner had not shown by a preponderance of the evidence that she had suffered injury or that if she had, that the vaccination could cause the alleged injury. The court quoted Opinion 9.07 in holding that the petitioner did not present medical expert witnesses qualified to give testimony in the field of neurology. *Falksen v. Sec. of the Dept. of Health and Human Services, 2004 WL 785056, 10.*

Fed. Cl. 2003 Special master dismissed plaintiffs' allegation that, following a measles, mumps, rubella (MMR) vaccination, their infant son sustained acute encephalopathy. The special master, quoting Opinion 9.07, determined that plaintiffs' expert witness, a geneticist and obstetrician, was not qualified to testify about the effect of the MMR vaccine. *Weiss v. Sec. of the Dept. of Health and Human Services, 2003 U.S. Claims LEXIS 359 n.1.*

Cal. App. 1956 Physician-petitioner sought mandamus against local medical association whose bylaws provided for the expulsion of any member who violated the Principles. Petitioner had been expelled under the provision and the expulsion was affirmed by the AMA's Judicial Council. The initial grounds for expulsion was alleged violation of Principles, Ch. III, Art. IV, Sec. 4 (1947) [now Opinions 9.04 and 9.07], for disparaging statements regarding another physician in a report used in judicial proceedings. In holding that application of the provision to petitioner was contrary to public policy, the court noted that the physician's statements had been made at the request of a civil litigant and enjoyed a statutory testimonial privilege. Further, the court found that the AMA's right to formulate ethical principles did not extend to defining the duties of witnesses. Expulsion was also based on petitioner's critical comments about other physicians overheard by their patients in violation of Principles, Ch. III, Art. IV, Sec. 1 (1947) [now Principle II and Opinion 9.04]. The court found application of this Principle under the circumstances reasonable and not contrary to public policy. *Bernstein v. Alameda-Contra Costa Medical Ass'n, 139 Cal. App. 2d 241, 293 P.2d 862, 863, 863 nn.1, 2, 865 nn.4, 6, 866, 866 n.8, 867.*

N.J. 1995 Plaintiffs sued physician and manufacturer claiming that DPT shot administered to their daughter caused her to suffer seizures. Plaintiffs consulted pediatric neurologists, none of whom found a connection between the DPT vaccine and seizures. Court concluded that the videotaped depositions of two of the neurologists could be introduced by defendants because plaintiffs had waived all patient-physician privileges on this issue by bringing suit and because the neurologists did not examine the child in anticipation of litigation. The court cited Opinion 9.07 to support view that physicians have an obligation to assist in the administration of justice. *Stigliano v. Connaught Labs., Inc., 140 N. J. 305, 658 A.2d 715, 720-21.*

Wash. 1994 In a medical malpractice action against her former physician, plaintiff waived her physician-patient privilege with all physicians who had provided her care or treatment. In an ex parte interview, plaintiff's treating physician opined that defendant's conduct was not negligent. The defense listed the treating physician as an expert witness and plaintiff objected. The court concluded that waiver of the physician-patient privilege extends to all knowledge of the plaintiff's physicians. In holding that a patient cannot insist on physician confidentiality after bringing a civil proceeding, the court quoted Opinion 9.07. *Carson v. Fine, 123 Wash. 2d 206, 867 P.2d 610, 618.*

Journal 2010 Discusses the movement to adjudicate medical malpractice claims in special health courts. Concludes that the psychosocial development of physicians, combined with the position of authority granted to the medical industry within health courts, will result in an antipatient, pro–medical industry bias in medical malpractice claims within such courts. Cites Opinion 9.07. Farrow, *The Anti-Patient Psychology of Health Courts: Prescriptions From a Lawyer-Physician, 36 Am. J. L. & Med. 188, 219 (2010).*

Journal 2008 Discusses the effect of *Crawford* and *Davis* on out-of-court statements made to medical personnel and the application of the Sixth Amendment Confrontation Clause to such statements. Concludes courts, when making a confrontation determination, must consider the intent of the declarant and the circumstances that influence the content of the declarant's statement. Quotes Opinion 9.07. Cites Opinion 2.02. Gordon, *Is There an Accuser in the House? Evaluating Statements Made to Physicians and Other Medical Personnel in the Wake of Crawford v. Washington and Davis v. Washington, 38 N. M. L. Rev. 529, 529 (2008).*

Journal 2008 Discusses the importance of experts and sources of experts for low-income parties. Concludes aid is necessary for improving the quality of experts and for increasing access to experts for low-income parties. References Opinion 9.07. Wiseman, *Pro Bono Publico: The Growing Need for Expert Aid, 60 S. C. L. Rev. 493, 530 (2008).*

Journal 2007 Considers the benefits, in medical malpractice cases, of using a panel of expert judges as the trier of fact. Concludes that the risks of such a system outweigh the benefits. Quotes Opinion 9.07. Chow, *Health Courts: An Extreme Makeover of Medical Malpractice With Potentially Fatal Complications, 7 Yale J. Health Pol'y L. & Ethics 387, 399 (2007).*

Journal 2006 Reviews regulation of physician expert witnesses by the medical profession. Concludes that members of the profession are the proper authorities to police and discipline medical experts. Quotes Opinion 9.07. Turner, *Going After the "Hired Guns": Is Improper Expert Witness Testimony Unprofessional Conduct or the Negligent Practice of Medicine? 33 Pepp. L. Rev. 275, 304 (2006).*

Journal 2003 Uses public policy arguments to support a preponderance standard for medical license revocations in situations involving false testimony by a medical expert witness. Concludes that medical licensing boards can more effectively protect the public by using a preponderance standard. Quotes Principles II, III, and IV and Opinions 1.02 and 9.07. Widmer, *South Dakota Should Follow Public Policy and Switch to the Preponderance Standard for Medical License Revocation After In Re the Medical License of Dr. Reuben Setliff, M.D., 48 S. D. L. Rev. 388, 396-97, 402 (2003).*

Journal 2002 Examines the role and responsibilities of forensic bioethicists. Concludes that a professional code of conduct and other internal guidelines are needed to ensure professionalism in forensic bioethics. Quotes Opinion 9.07. Spielman, *Professionalism in Forensic Bioethics, 30 J. L. Med. & Ethics 420, 425, 427, 436 (2002).*

Journal 2000 Considers the rules governing expert testimony. Explores professional ethical standards affecting expert witnesses and concludes that codes of ethics have not succeeded in eliminating biased expert testimony. Recommends creation of an organization to assist courts in obtaining reliable expert witness testimony. Quotes Principle III and Opinion 6.01. Cites Principles I, II, and V and Opinions 1.02 and 9.07. Murphy, *Expert Witnesses at Trial: Where Are the Ethics? 14 Geo. J. Legal Ethics 217, 231-32 (2000).*

Journal 1999 Describes historical and present views regarding medical diagnosis. Discusses pressures physicians face that may affect the diagnostic process. Suggests that legal institutions can reduce these pressures, which will enhance the physician-patient therapeutic relationship. Quotes Principle II and Opinion 9.07. Noah, *Pigeonholing Illness: Medical Diagnosis as a Legal Construct, 50 Hastings L. J. 241, 301, 302 (1999).*

Journal 1999 Discusses the impact *Daubert v. Merrell Dow Pharmaceuticals, Inc.* has had on scientific expert testimony. Explains that the scientific approach of dealing with bias may be inappropriate for maintaining scientific objectivity in litigation. Provides a strategy to deal with conflicts of interest in this context. Quotes Opinion 9.07. Cites Opinion 8.061. Patterson, *Conflicts of Interest in Scientific Expert Testimony, 40 Wm. & Mary L. Rev. 1313, 1330, 1332, 1335, 1371 (1999).*

Journal 1999 Discusses the need for physicians to advocate on behalf of patients' rights in the context of health care delivery. Evaluates the nature and scope of the physician's role as advocate, noting that physicians cannot be expected to engage in attorney-like advocacy. Quotes Principles IV and VI, Fundamental Elements (2), (4), and (6) [now Opinion 10.01], Patient Responsibilities 5 [now Opinion 10.02], and Opinions 2.03, 2.07, 2.09, 2.16, 2.19, 3.06, 4.01, 4.04, 6.01, 7.02, 8.02, 8.03, 8.13, 8.132, 9.06, 9.07, and 9.131. Cites Opinions 5.05, 5.09, 7.01, 8.135, and 9.02. Sage, *Physicians as Advocates, 35 Hous. L. Rev. 1529, 1537, 1541, 1542, 1552-53, 1554, 1556, 1557, 1559, 1561-62, 1564, 1571, 1574, 1576, 1580 (1999).*

Journal 1998 Examines mechanisms of oversight for expert witness testimony by medical, legal, legislative, and regulatory agencies. Points out that the amount of malpractice litigation will increase the need for medical expert witnesses. Concludes that improvements in this context must uphold principles of due process and be acceptable to the medical and legal communities. Cites Opinions 6.01, 8.04, and 9.07. McAbee, *Improper Expert Medical Testimony: Existing and Proposed Mechanisms of Oversight, 19 J. Legal Med. 257, 265 (1998).*

Journal 1997 Reports on a study of physician attitudes regarding expert witnesses. Notes that a majority of physicians believe that medical expert testimony should be subject to peer review and, when appropriate, medical licensing board discipline. Quotes Principles II and VI and Opinion 9.07. Eitel, Hegeman, & Evans, *Medicine on Trial: Physicians' Attitudes About Expert Medical Witnesses, 18 J. Legal Med. 345, 355, 358 (1997).*

Journal 1997 Discusses the practice of ex parte communications between treating physicians and their patients' legal adversaries without informing the patient or obtaining consent. Examines harms that may occur in these situations. Argues that Oklahoma needs to prohibit treating physicians from communicating ex parte with their patients' legal adversaries. Quotes Opinions 5.05, 5.07, 5.08, 8.02, 8.03, and 9.07. Cites Opinion 7.02. McNaughton & McNaughton, *Divided Loyalty: The Dilemma of the Treating Physician Advocate, 22 Okla. City U. L. Rev. 1051, 1052, 1054, 1056, 1058, 1059, 1062 (1997).*

Journal 1994 Establishes guidelines for members of the American Academy of Pediatrics who are expert witnesses in medical liability cases. Emphasizes knowledge of the area of medicine involved, impartial testimony, evaluations based on generally accepted standards, and the duty to distinguish between malpractice and maloccurrence. Quotes Opinion 9.07. Cohn, Berger, Holzman, Lockhart, Reuben, Robertson, & Selbst, *Guidelines for Expert Witness Testimony in Medical Liability Cases, 94 Pediatrics 755, 756 (1994).*

Journal 1993 Discusses controversies surrounding how medical-legal consulting services and expert witnesses may be compensated. Examines relevant ethical guidelines in evaluating whether it is acceptable for a physician to be paid a flat fee for expert services rendered on behalf of a consulting business that receives a contingent fee. Quotes Opinion 9.07. Devlin, *Medical-Legal Consulting Services and Expert Witnesses: Payment Controversies, 9 Medical Practice Management 141 (Nov./Dec. 1993).*

Journal 1990 Considers the proper role of the expert witness in the realm of toxic tort litigation. Examines evidentiary rules regarding the admission of scientific evidence and considers various ways to solve testimonial problems. Quotes Opinion 9.07. Bernstein, *Out of the Frying Pan and Into the Fire: The Expert Witness Problem in Toxic Tort Litigation, 10 Rev. Litigation 117, 143 (1990).*

Journal 1990 Examines conflicting court decisions that have addressed the appropriateness of medical-legal consulting services and their use of contingent fee arrangements. Concludes by discussing the need for a less troublesome solution to the problems plaintiffs face in malpractice and personal injury cases. Quotes Opinion 6.01. Cites Opinions 6.12 (1989) [now Opinion 6.05] and 9.07. Dillon, *Contingent Fees and Medical-Legal Consulting Services: Economical or Unethical? 11 J. Legal Med. 93, 101, 111 (1990).*

9.7.2 Court-Initiated Medical Treatment in Criminal Cases

Wis. Sup. 2010 State petitioned for involuntary administration of psychotropic medication for defendant who was in custody after acquittal due to mental illness. Defendant argued that Wisconsin statute allowing for such treatment unconstitutionally violated his due process rights. The majority quotes Opinions 2.065 and 2.19 in finding the Wisconsin statute in question facially valid on procedural due process grounds. *State v. Wood, 323 Wis. 2d 321, 780 N.W.2d 63, 82-83.*

Journal 2011 Discusses the doctrine of informed consent and the influence of physician groups on the dissemination of information to patients. Concludes the doctrine of informed consent should be expanded by the courts, rather than continuing to allow professional societies to dictate provider guidelines for obtaining informed consent. Quotes Opinions 8.08, 10.01, and 10.015. References Opinion 2.065. Ginsberg, *Informed Consent: No Longer Just What the Doctor Ordered? The "Contributions" of Medical Associations and Courts to a More Patient Friendly Doctrine, 15 Mich. St. J. Med. & Law 17, 23, 24, 25, 26, 46 (2011).*

Journal 2008 Examines various types of neuroscience-based techniques used to prevent criminal behavior and the problems associated with such interventions. Concludes any treatments utilizing neuroscience in an effort to mitigate criminal behavior must be proven safe and effective prior to implementation. Quotes Opinion 2.065. Greely, *Neuroscience and Criminal Justice: Not Responsibility but Treatment, 56 U. Kan. L. Rev. 1103, 1131 (2008).*

Journal 2006 Examines the practice of chemically castrating repeat sex offenders. Concludes that chemical castration is cruel and unusual punishment which violates the Eighth Amendment. Cites Opinion 2.065. Stinneford, *Incapacitation Through Maiming: Chemical Castration, The Eighth Amendment, and the Denial of Human Dignity, 3 U. St. Thomas L. J. 559, 576 (2006).*

Journal 2004 Evaluates the constitutionality of involuntarily medicating mentally ill patients to restore competency for execution. Concludes that this practice should be held unconstitutional. Cites Opinion 2.06. References Opinion 2.065. Hensl, *Restored to Health to Be Put to Death: Reconciling the Legal and Ethical Dilemmas of Medicating to Execute in Singleton v. Norris, 49 Vill. L. Rev. 291, 324 (2004).*

9.7.3 Capital Punishment

U.S. 2008 Affirmed Kentucky Supreme Court decision that Kentucky's lethal injections protocol does not violate the Eighth Amendment's ban on cruel and unusual punishment. Alito, J., concurring, cited Opinion 2.06 and recognized (1) the ethical rules of the profession prohibiting physician participation in lethal injection executions and (2) that a modification of a lethal injection protocol is not "feasible" or "readily available" if it would require participation by persons whose professional ethics impede participation. *Baze v. Rees, 553 U.S. 35, 64 (2008) (Alito, J., concurring).*

6th Cir. 2009 Death row inmate intervened in action brought challenging Ohio's lethal injection protocol. Inmate argued the state's new one-drug protocol was inadequate regarding the competency, training, and supervision of execution personnel. In rejecting the argument that physicians should be required to oversee execution, the court noted Ohio statute permitting revocation of a physician's license for a violation of the Code of Ethics of the AMA. The court cited Opinion 2.06 prohibiting physician participation in executions. *Cooey v. Strickland, 589 F.3d 210, 227.*

6th Cir. 2007 A death row inmate challenged the method of execution under the Eighth Amendment. State officials moved to dismiss the complaint as untimely. The district court denied the motion. The Court of Appeals held that the state two-year statute of limitations applied and that, although the discovery rule extended the limitations period to the date when information about the execution procedure was available, plaintiff's claim was still untimely. The dissent argued that information about the execution procedure available to plaintiff was misleading. For example, the available information stated that a physician pronounces death. Quoting Opinion 2.06, the dissent noted this could constitute unethical conduct by a physician. *Cooey v. Strickland, 479 F.3d 412, 428.*

8th Cir. 2003 Prisoner convicted of capital felony murder was involuntarily medicated after a review panel held he was a danger to himself and others. Thereafter, the state set an execution date for prisoner because he was competent due to the medication. The Court of Appeals, en banc, affirmed lower court's denial of the prisoner's habeus corpus petition. Court found state had a duty to medicate the prisoner and that Eighth Amendment is not violated when a prisoner on death row regains competency as a result of involuntary medication. Dissenting judges, with apparent reference to Opinion 2.06, noted that the ethical standards of the AMA prohibit physicians from assisting in executions. *Singleton v. Norris, 319 F.3d 1018, 1036.*

D.D.C. 2001 District court found that the government was permitted to treat the defendant involuntarily with antipsychotic medication in order to render him nondangerous and mentally competent to stand trial. The court in making its decision that a pretrial detainee is not afforded the same prohibition against involuntary medication as a convicted defendant waiting to be executed apparently relied on Opinion 2.06. *United States v. Weston, 134 F. Supp. 2d 115, 126-27.*

E.D. Ky. 2007 Plaintiff, a death-row inmate, challenged the constitutionality of the state's method of execution. The state's execution protocol stipulated that if an IV could not be properly inserted, a request to postpone the execution should be made to the governor. Plaintiff sought to depose the state's governor (who was a physician) to determine what his response would be in such a situation and argued that because the governor was also a physician, he might issue medical advice. The court found this question irrelevant to the constitutional issue. Additionally, the court noted that, under the state's law, physicians must abide by the AMA Code of Medical Ethics and that Opinion 2.06 expressly prohibits supervising an execution. *Moore v. Rees, 2007 WL 1035013, 6.*

La. 1992 State's attempt to circumvent prohibition against execution of insane prisoners by forcibly medicating prisoner was held to be a violation of the prisoner's right to privacy and constituted cruel and unusual punishment. Noting that a physician's administration of medication in order to facilitate the prisoner's execution is contrary to the AMA's ethical code, in apparent reference to Opinion 2.06, the court held that involuntary administration of medication is not medical treatment but constitutes a part of capital punishment. *State v. Perry, 610 So. 2d 746, 753.*

N.C. 2009 Department of corrections and prison warden brought action against state medical board to enjoin board from taking any disciplinary action against physicians for participating in executions. The court cited the board's position statement prohibiting physician participation in executions, quoting Opinion 2.06. The court held the position statement was an invalid exercise of board's statutory powers. *North Carolina Department of Corrections v. North Carolina Medical Board, 363 N.C. 189, 675 S.E.2d 641, 644-65.*

S.C. 1993 State sought to reverse order vacating death sentence and imposing life imprisonment. The court stated that the critical issue inherent in the state's contention of error was whether the state could forcibly medicate a prisoner solely to make prisoner competent enough to execute. Citing Opinion 2.06, the court held that the AMA's position reinforces the prohibition against the state's use of medication solely to facilitate an insane prisoner's execution. *Singleton v. State, 437 S.E. 2d 53, 61.*

Tenn. App. 2004 Appeal from a district court order finding that Tennessee's three-drug lethal injection procedure does not constitute "cruel and unusual" punishment under the US or Tennessee constitutions or violate state professional practice statutes. The Court of Appeals of Tennessee, citing Opinion 2.06, concluded that the state legislature likely anticipated that licensed health care professionals would not participate in executions because such participation violates professional ethics codes. *Abdur'Rahman v. Bredesen, 2004 WL 2246227, n. 45.*

Va. Att'y Gen. 1994 Attorney General responded in the negative when asked whether a physician employed by the department of corrections may be disciplined by the board of medicine for participating in the execution of a prisoner where "participating" was defined as "attending or observing an execution, for making a determination that death has occurred, for issuing a certificate of death, or for performing any other function that applicable state statutes lawfully require to be performed by a physician in connection with an execution." Citing Opinion 2.06, the Attorney General noted that such ethical opinions are not legally conclusive and that if they conflict with a state statute, the statute controls. *Va. Att'y Gen. Op., 1994 Va. AG LEXIS 12.*

Journal 2011 Argues physicians should have the choice to participate in lethal injection executions. Concludes that although executions may proceed without physician involvement and the integrity and ethics of the medical profession must be protected, because executions performed without a physician have been mishandled, physician involvement is needed. Quotes Opinion 2.211. References Opinion 2.06. Nelson & Ashby, *Rethinking the Ethics of Physician Participation in Lethal Injection Execution, 41 Hastings Center Rep., 28, 29, 35 (May-June 2011).*

Journal 2010 Examines recent constitutional challenges to new guidelines for execution by lethal injection in Missouri under the Eighth Amendment's cruel and unusual punishment provisions. Concludes that, while the new Missouri guidelines were upheld as constitutional, legal challenges to the death penalty and lethal injections will continue. Cites Opinion 2.06. Maerz, *Death of the Challenge to Lethal Injection? Missouri's Protocol Deemed Constitutional Yet Again, 75 Mo. L. Rev. 1323, 1340-41 (2010).*

Journal 2010 Addresses whether states may forcibly administer antipsychotic drugs to insane death row inmates to restore their competence for execution. Concludes that execution after forcible medication with antipsychotic drugs violates both the Eighth and Fourteenth Amendments. Cites Opinion 2.06. Sewall, *Pushing Execution Over the Constitutional Line: Forcible Medication of Condemned Inmates and the Eighth and Fourteenth Amendments, 51 B.C. L. Rev. 1279, 1301 (2010).*

Journal 2010 Examines ethical implications of physician involvement in assessments of competence for execution. Concludes forensic psychiatrists should participate in such assessments to prevent executions of those lacking requisite competence. References Opinion 2.06. Weinstock, Leong, & Silva, *Competence to Be Executed: An Ethical Analysis Post Panetti, 28 Behav. Sci. Law 690, 691 (2010).*

Journal 2010 Discusses the right of prison inmates to refuse psychotropic medications and the evolution of medical, ethical, and legal guidelines for physicians in dealing with death row inmates. Concludes physicians need to strictly adhere to the medical-ethical guidelines that are in place

regarding death row inmates. Quotes Opinion 2.06. Zonana, *Physicians Must Honor Refusal of Treatment to Restore Competency by Non-Dangerous Inmates on Death Row, 38 J. L. Med. & Ethics 764, 766 (2010).*

Journal 2009 Examines opinions in *Baze v. Rees* from the US Supreme Court discussing the constitutionality of execution by lethal injection. Concludes the Supreme Court did not answer the medical ethics questions regarding lethal injection and urges physicians to remove themselves from the lethal injection procedure entirely. References Opinion 2.06. Annas, *Toxic Tinkering—Lethal-Injection Execution and the Constitution, 359 New Engl. J. Med. 1512, 1512 (2009).*

Journal 2009 Examines the ethical guidelines regarding physicians' participation in interrogations and statutory approaches aimed at eliminating such physician involvement. Concludes that to maintain the integrity of the medical profession, physician involvement in interrogations must be precluded by legislative action. Quotes Preamble and Opinions 2.067 and 2.068. Cites Opinions 2.06 and 2.068. Bahnassi, *Keeping Doctors Out of the Interrogation Room: A New Ethical Obligation That Requires the Backing of the Law, 19 Health Matrix 447, 449-51, 461, 464, 465-67, 469-70, 474-75 (2009).*

Journal 2009 Explores the Supreme Court's *Baze v. Rees* decision and the three-drug protocol for lethal injection. Discusses the necessity of judicial intervention to improve lethal injection protocols. Concludes courts should carefully consider their approach to challenges to lethal injection as an opportunity to prevent violation of Eighth Amendment rights. Quotes Preamble and Opinion 1.02. Cites Opinion 2.06. Berger, *Lethal Injection and the Problem of Constitutional Remedies, 27 Yale L. & Pol'y Rev. 259, 319, 320 (2009).*

Journal 2009 Examines the history of the anti–death penalty movement and analyzes recent Supreme Court decisions and their implications for protection of Eighth Amendment rights. Concludes America ultimately will abolish the death penalty as a violation of international law, consistent with its standing on other forms of cruel and degrading punishments. Cites Opinion 2.06. Bessler, *Revisiting Beccaria's Vision: The Enlightenment, America's Death Penalty, and the Abolition Movement, 4 NW J. L. & Soc. Pol'y 195, 299 (2009).*

Journal 2009 Examines historical and modern methods of execution and discusses the plurality, concurring, and dissenting opinions in *Baze v. Rees*. Concludes scientific testing and medical evidence should be used to conduct a thorough pain analysis of lethal injection to ensure the protocol comports with the Eighth Amendment. Quotes Opinion 2.06. Butler, *Baze v. Rees: Lethal Injection as a Constitutional Method of Execution, 86 Denv. U. L. Rev. 509, 530 (2009).*

Journal 2009 Discusses the development of the lethal injection method of execution and the lack of a constitutional standard for reviewing method-of-execution challenges. Concludes that states should strengthen their execution protocols in order to increase the likelihood of overcoming constitutional challenges. References Opinion 2.06. Heilman, *Contemplating "Cruel and Unusual": A Critical Analysis of Baze v. Rees in the Context of the Supreme Court's Eighth Amendment "Proportionality" Jurisprudence*, 58 Am. U. L. Rev. 633, 652 (2009).

Journal 2009 Argues that the trichemical combination used in lethal injection carries with it great risk of a needlessly painful execution. Concludes use of this execution method is inconsistent with the Eighth Amendment's Cruel and Unusual Punishment Clause. References Opinion 2.06. Hughes, *The Tri-Chemical Cocktail: Serene Brutality*, 72 Alb. L. Rev. 527, 540 (2009).

Journal 2009 Discusses US Supreme Court decisions shaping the law concerning capital punishment. Concludes that the October 2007 term produced opinions displaying conflicting views on the death penalty, but ultimately was important for those seeking to abolish the death penalty. Quotes Opinion 2.06. Klein, *An Analysis of the Death Penalty Jurisprudence of the October 2007 Supreme Court Term*, 25 Touro L. Rev. 625, 630 (2009).

Journal 2009 Describes death penalty cases in California wherein prosecutorial misconduct led to a reversal of either the sentence or the conviction. Concludes such misconduct is a systemic problem in California and clear distinctions are needed to help prosecutors avoid misconduct as they try death penalty cases. Cites Opinion 2.06. Minsker, *Prosecutorial Misconduct in Death Penalty Cases*, 45 Cal. W. L. Rev. 373, 400 (2009).

Journal 2009 Examines the element of pain present in lethal injection with respect to the Eighth Amendment prohibition on cruel and unusual punishment. Concludes use of the drug Pavulon causes paralysis and severe pain when administered and constitutes cruel and unusual punishment. Argues further that use of Pavulon in human executions should be eliminated. Quotes Opinion 2.06. Tapocsi, *Three Steps to Death: The Use of the Drug Pavulon in the Lethal Injection Protocol Utilized Today Violates the Eighth Amendment's Protection Against Cruel and Unusual Punishment*, 35 Ohio N. U. L. Rev. 425, 440 (2009).

Journal 2008 Discusses whether drug-induced competence warrants a finding of sanity in capital punishment cases, thereby qualifying an inmate for execution. Argues the practice of medicating mentally ill inmates to allow for their execution contradicts society's ethical and moral values and poses a question of constitutionality that should be addressed by the courts. Cites Opinion 2.06. Barua, *"Synthetic Sanity": A Way Around the Eighth Amendment?* 44 Crim. Law Bulletin 561, 574 (2008).

Journal 2008 Argues pain and punishment are inseparable components of the American justice system. Concludes lethal injection must include an element of pain and calls for renewed efforts to establish capital punishment protocols that conform to societal goals. Cites Opinion 2.06. Blecker,

Killing Them Softly: Meditations on a Painful Punishment of Death, 35 Fordham Urb. L. J. 969, 988 (2008).

Journal 2008 Analyzes the constitutionality of the three-drug lethal injection protocol and legal challenges to this method of execution. Concludes that because lethal injection is a complex and flawed procedure, the legislature should carefully evaluate current execution techniques to ensure humane punishment. Quotes Opinion 2.06. Gaitan, *Challenges Facing Society in the Implementation of the Death Penalty*, 35 Fordham Urb. L. J. 763, 767 (2008).

Journal 2008 Considers physician involvement in executions and the resulting ethical complications. Concludes the presence of physicians at executions compromises the physician's duties to society and to the medical profession. Quotes Opinion 2.06. Groner, *The Hippocratic Paradox: The Role of the Medical Profession in Capital Punishment in the United States*, 35 Fordham Urb. L. J. 883, 903-04 (2008).

Journal 2008 Discusses disciplinary safe harbor policies as a device for allowing physician participation in executions and examines several justifications relied upon by legislatures for such participation. Concludes the legal justifications of safe harbors are weak and that they may lead to a loss of confidence in the medical profession, and, if so, should not be adopted. Quotes Opinion 2.06. Sawicki, *Doctors, Discipline, and the Death Penalty: Professional Implications of Safe Harbor Policies*, 27 Yale L. & Pol'y Rev. 107, 121 (2008).

Journal 2007 Examines the role of the medical profession in participating in state-sanctioned lethal injection. Concludes that any participation is unethical because it causes harm and undermines trust. Cites Opinion 2.06. References Opinions 2.211 and 9.02. Black & Sade, *Lethal Injection and Physicians: State Law vs Medical Ethics*, 298 JAMA 2779, 2780, 2781 (2007).

Journal 2007 Examines flaws in lethal injection protocols across states. Concludes that a collaborative effort between legal and medical professionals is needed to revise protocols to meet basic constitutional requirements. Quotes Opinion 2.06. Denno, *The Lethal Injection Quandary: How Medicine Has Dismantled Death*, 76 Fordham L. Rev. 49, 80-81 (2007).

Journal 2007 Discusses challenges to the constitutionality of lethal injection made pursuant to 42 USC § 1983. Concludes that the Supreme Court must rule on the constitutionality of lethal injection to stem a flood of litigation in the lower federal courts. Quotes Opinion 2.06. Greer, *Legal Injection: The Supreme Court Enters the Lethal Injection Debate: Hill v. McDonough, 126 S. Ct. 2096 (2006)*, 30 Harv. J. L. & Pub. Pol'y 767, 774 (2007).

Journal 2007 Analyzes the impact of recent death penalty cases. Concludes that, in similar cases, the manner of execution may be challenged under 42 USC § 1983 and that a denial of the right to counsel of choice may result in an overturned conviction. Quotes Opinion 2.06. Klein, *Death*

Penalty and Right to Counsel Decisions in the October 2005 Term, 22 Touro L. Rev. 1003, 1012 (2007).

Journal 2007 Examines the constitutionality of lethal injection protocols. Concludes that current protocols are unconstitutional under the Eighth Amendment and suggests that, at minimum, the legislature should conduct a thorough investigation into humane methods of execution. Quotes Opinion 2.06. Kreitzberg & Richter, *But Can It Be Fixed? A Look at Constitutional Challenges to Lethal Injection Executions, 47 Santa Clara L. Rev. 445, 448, 449, 499, 502 (2007).*

Journal 2007 Highlights inconsistencies in applying judicial deference to medical ethics. Concludes that courts should afford greater deference to established medical ethics standards. Quotes Principle I and Opinions 2.06 and Ch. II, Art. I, Sec. 3 (May 1847) [now Opinion 5.02]. Cites Opinions 4.01 and 7.05. Lerman, *Second Opinion: Inconsistent Deference to Medical Ethics in Death Penalty Jurisprudence, 95 Geo. L. J. 1941, 1945, 1974-75, 1976, 1977 (2007).*

Journal 2007 Examines the potential for error in lethal injection procedures. Concludes that such procedures must be changed to ensure a painless execution and should cease to require participation of medical professionals. Quotes Opinion 2.06. Mottor, *Morales and Taylor: The Future of Lethal Injection, 6 Appalachian J. L. 287, 300-01 (2007).*

Journal 2007 Argues that there is a public right to know the identity of state executioners. Concludes that the state must be able to prove the qualification of the executioner, and that this is best accomplished by revealing their identity. Quotes Opinion 2.06. Roko, *Executioner Identities: Toward Recognizing a Right to Know Who Is Hiding Beneath the Hood, 75 Fordham L. Rev. 2791, 2799 (2007).*

Journal 2006 Discusses the ethical issue of incompetent inmates who face capital punishment. Formally recommends that all states adopt policy against execution of incompetent defendants. References Opinion 2.06. American Bar Association Task Force on Mental Disability and the Death Penalty (Igasaki et al), *Recommendation and Report on the Death Penalty and Persons With Mental Disabilities, 30 Mental & Physical Disability L. Rep. 668, 676 (2006).*

Journal 2006 Evaluates legal and ethical challenges to the use of the drug Pavulon in lethal injection executions. Concludes Pavulon should not be used because of the risk of cruel and unusual punishment. Cites Opinion 2.06. Ewart, *Use of the Drug Pavulon In Lethal Injections: Cruel and Unusual? 14 Wm. & Mary Bill of Rts. J. 1159, 1182 (2006).*

Journal 2006 Discusses mentally incompetent inmates and capital punishment. Proposes that, to be permissible, involuntary medication of death-row inmates must represent the best medically appropriate treatment. Quotes Principles I, III, and VIII and Opinion 2.06. Gabos, *The Perils of Singleton v. Norris: Ethics and Beyond, 32 Am. J. L. & Med. 117, 118, 125-26, 127 (2006).*

Journal 2006 Examines conflicts between physicians' personal and professional ethical obligations. Concludes that courts should give greater deference to professional moral guidelines. Quotes Opinion 2.06. Gottlieb, *Executions and Torture: The Consequences of Overriding Professional Ethics, 6 Yale J. Health Pol'y, L. & Ethics 351, 366, 367 (2006).*

Journal 2006 Examines the probability that lethal injection results in unnecessary suffering. Concludes that legislators should ban the practice until this can be disproven. Quotes Opinion 2.06. Wong, *Lethal Injection Protocols: The Failure of Litigation to Stop Suffering and the Case for Legislative Reform, 25 Temp. J. Sci. Tech. & Envtl. L. 263, 282 (2006).*

Journal 2005 Examines various justifications for postponing the execution of mentally ill prisoners on death row. Concludes that mistakes in postconviction adjudication should be minimized and that prisoners who lack genuine understanding of the nature of or purpose for their punishment should not be executed. References Opinion 2.06. Bonnie, *Mentally Ill Prisoners on Death Row: Unsolved Puzzles for Courts and Legislatures, 54 Cath. U. L. Rev. 1169, 1175 (2005).*

Journal 2005 Discusses the case of *Singleton v. Norris.* Concludes that a psychiatrist should not withhold necessary and appropriate treatment of a psychotic death-row inmate, even if it might restore competency for execution. Quotes Opinion 2.06. Cantor, *Of Pills and Needles: Involuntarily Medicating the Psychotic Inmate When Execution Looms, 2 Ind. Health L. Rev. 119, 154, 156, 164 (2005).*

Journal 2005 Considers legal issues raised by forcible medication of an inmate to restore competence prior to court-ordered execution. Concludes that the best solution is to delay execution until the inmate regains competency and it is no longer necessary to medicate. References Opinion 2.06. Kimbler, *Psychotic Journeys of the Green Mile, 22 T. M. Cooley L. Rev. 27, 48 (2005).*

Journal 2005 Examines the legal and ethical aspects of physician participation in capital punishment. Concludes that federal and state laws addressing this practice must be amended to harmonize the law with applicable principles of medical ethics. Quotes Opinion 2.06. Cites Opinion 2.21. References Opinion 2.01. Levy, *Conflict of Duty: Capital Punishment Regulations and AMA Medical Ethics, 26 J. Legal Med. 261, 268, 269, 270, 273 (2005).*

Journal 2005 Argues that the Eighth Circuit's ruling in *Singleton v. Norris* failed to consider the ethical standards of the medical community. Concludes that, as a result, physicians may be placed in an untenable position regarding treatment of mentally ill death-row inmates. Quotes Principle VIII and Opinions 1.02 and 2.06. Lloyd, *Primum Non Nocere: Singleton v. Norris and the Ethical Dilemma of Medicating the Condemned, 58 Ark. L. Rev. 225, 232, 233 (2005).*

Journal 2005 Argues that medicating a criminal defendant to restore competency is ethical, even in capital cases. Concludes that principles justifying administration of punishment in the legal system give rise to an ethical imperative for physicians to provide competence-restoring medical therapy. Quotes Principle III and Opinion 2.06. Mossman, *Is Prosecution "Medically Appropriate"? 31 New Eng. J. on Crim. & Civ. Confinement 15, 53-54, 59 (2005).*

Journal 2004 Discusses the history of restoring competency to execute and the Supreme Court's decision not to grant certiorari in *Singleton v. Norris*. Concludes that the Court must grant certiorari in a medicate-to-execute case and establish guidelines in this area. Quotes Opinion 2.06. Campbell, *Sell, Singleton, and Forcible Medication—Running Roughshod Over Liberty, 35 U. Tol. L. Rev. 691, 716 (2004).*

Journal 2004 Evaluates the constitutionality of involuntarily medicating mentally ill patients to restore competency for execution. Concludes that this practice should be held unconstitutional. Cites Opinion 2.06. References Opinion 2.065. Hensl, *Restored to Health to Be Put to Death: Reconciling the Legal and Ethical Dilemmas of Medicating to Execute in Singleton v. Norris, 49 Vill. L. Rev. 291, 324 (2004).*

Journal 2004 Analyzes various issues relating to the role of mental health professionals in capital punishment in light of Albert Bandura's model of "mechanisms of moral disengagement." Concludes that facilitating participation of mental health professionals in executions creates conflicts with the humanistic norms of the profession. Quotes Preamble and Opinions 1.01, 1.02, 2.06, 2.067, 2.20, 2.21, 2.211, and 8.14. Judges, *The Role of Mental Health Professionals in Capital Punishment: An Exercise in Moral Disengagement, 41 Hous. L. Rev. 515, 562, 568, 569, 570, 571-72, 581, 586, 588, 598 (2004).*

Journal 2004 Argues the existence of an international *jus cogens* norm against implementation of the death penalty. Concludes that this norm has developed in international law and may lead to abolition of the death penalty. Quotes Opinion 2.06. Sawyer, *The Death Penalty Is Dead Wrong: Jus Cogens Norms and the Evolving Standard of Decency, 22 Penn. St. Int'l L. Rev. 459, 477 (2004).*

Journal 2004 Analyzes the moral and ethical conflicts that are created by requiring health care professionals to involuntarily medicate death-row inmates to restore competency for execution. Concludes that it is cruel and unusual punishment to execute individuals who are forcibly medicated for this purpose. Quotes Opinion 2.06. Shaivitz, *Medicate-to-Execute: Current Trends in Death Penalty Jurisprudence and the Perils of Dual Loyalty, 7 J. Health Care L. & Pol'y 149, 167, 168 (2004).*

Journal 2003 Examines the manner in which psychiatrists participate in the criminal justice system. Concludes that, in some situations, this participation may violate principles of medical ethics. Cites Opinions 2.06 and 8.08.

Dolin, *A Healer or an Executioner? The Proper Role of a Psychiatrist in a Criminal Justice System, 17 J. L. & Health 169, 206, 213-14 (2003).*

Journal 2003 Discusses the inconsistent governmental regulation of drugs used in physician-assisted suicide (PAS) and lethal injections. Concludes that the FDA should regulate drugs used in lethal injections in the same manner it has attempted to regulate drugs used in PAS. Quotes Opinions 2.06 and 2.211. Miller, *A Death by Any Other Name: The Federal Government's Inconsistent Treatment of Drugs Used in Lethal Injections and Physician-Assisted Suicide, 17 J. L. & Health 217, 234-35 (2003).*

Journal 2003 Considers a legislative plan allowing voluntary, consensual organ donation by condemned prisoners. Concludes that, in view of the current organ shortage, the benefits of such a plan outweigh the concerns. Quotes Principle VII and Opinion 2.06. Perales, *Rethinking the Prohibition of Death Row Prisoners as Organ Donors: A Possible Lifeline to Those on Organ Donor Waiting Lists, 34 St. Mary's L. J. 687, 721, 725 (2003).*

Journal 2003 Discusses history of the death penalty in Colorado. Concludes that the trend is moving toward its abolition. Quotes Opinion 2.06. Radelet, *Capital Punishment in Colorado: 1859-1972, 74 U. Colo. L. Rev. 885, 940 (2003).*

Journal 2002 Addresses the problems arising out of legislative changes in methods of execution. Focuses on the change from electrocution to lethal injection. Concludes that, despite changes, executions are not necessarily more humane. Quotes Opinion 2.06. Denno, *When Legislatures Delegate Death: The Troubling Paradox Behind State Uses of Electrocution and Lethal Injection and What It Says About Us, 63 Ohio St. L. J. 63, 112-13 (2002).*

Journal 2002 Examines the standard for determining competency to be executed as applied to mentally ill death-row inmates. Favors commuting their sentences. Concludes a new standard that comports with the Eighth Amendment should be adopted. Quotes Opinion 2.06. Horstman, *Commuting Death Sentences of the Insane: A Solution for a Better, More Compassionate Society, 36 U. S. F. L. Rev. 823, 848 (2002).*

Journal 2002 Analyzes Arizona case law and other relevant law regarding medical treatment of individuals who are not competent to be executed. Concludes that the law should address this difficult problem in a more uniform manner. Cites Opinion 2.06. Levitt & Ryan, *Not Competent to Be Executed: Dilemmas Faced by Psychiatrists and Attorneys, 23 Am. J. Forensic Psych. 39, 47 (July 2002).*

Journal 2002 Examines medical professionalism. Considers how changes in health care give rise to physician frustration, which has served as an anchor for the Charter on Medical Professionalism. Quotes Opinion 2.06. Miles, *On a New Charter to Defend Medical Professionalism: Whose Profession Is It Anyway? 32 Hastings Center Rep. 46, 47 (May/June 2002).*

Journal 2001 Discusses the ethical, legal, and policy arguments affecting physician participation in capital punishment. Examines the tension created by conflicting state death penalty laws and medical practice acts. Concludes that an active role for physicians in lethal injection should be supported in an effort to reduce mishaps that may occur during executions. Quotes Opinion 2.06. Baum, *"To Comfort Always": Physician Participation in Executions, 5 N. Y. U. J. Legis. & Pub. Pol'y 47, 56-57 (2001).*

Journal 2001 Addresses the issue of whether death-row prisoners may be compelled to take psychotropic medications to render them mentally competent to be executed. Considers whether physicians should be required to violate principles of medical ethics in order to treat death-row inmates for this purpose. Quotes Opinion 2.06. Daugherty, *"Synthetic Sanity": The Ethics and Legality of Using Psychotropic Medications to Render Death Row Inmates Competent for Execution, 17 J. Contemp. H. L. & Pol'y 715, 730 (2001).*

Journal 2001 Discusses policies that consider physician participation in capital punishment to be unethical. Observes that such policies are without merit. Argues that such policies attempt to override the will of the people, their elected representatives, and the administration of justice. Concludes that these policies should be rescinded by state and national medical associations. Quotes Opinion 2.06. Keyes, *The Choice of Participation by Physicians in Capital Punishment, 22 Whittier L. Rev. 809, 810-11, 838 (2001).*

Journal 2000 Explores physicians' views regarding involvement in capital punishment. Concludes that, despite medical society policies, a majority of physicians believe participation in capital punishment is acceptable in certain circumstances. Quotes Opinion 2.06. Farber, Davis, Weiner, Jordan, Boyer, & Ubel, *Physicians' Attitudes About Involvement in Lethal Injection for Capital Punishment, 160 Arch. Intern. Med. 2912, 2912 (2000).*

Journal 2000 Explores issues and concerns associated with capital punishment. Discusses the controversy surrounding ways that physicians participate in capital punishment in this country. Concludes that capital punishment is not needed and cannot be fairly administered. Quotes Opinion 2.06. Martin, *Tessie Hutchinson and the American System of Capital Punishment, 59 Md. L. Rev. 553, 565 (2000).*

Journal 2000 Explores the history and legal rationale behind the prohibition against executing the insane. Considers relevant case law addressing the forced medication issue, especially as it relates to death-row inmates. Concludes the ultimate question should focus on what is in the prisoner's best interest. Cites Opinion 2.06. Miller-Rice, *The "Insane" Contradiction of Singleton v. Norris: Forced Medication in a Death Row Inmate's Medical Interest Which Happens to Facilitate His Execution, 22 U. Ark. Little Rock L. Rev. 659, 673 (2000).*

Journal 2000 Explores the debate regarding physician-assisted suicide. Concludes that autonomy should be

respected and that an individual's wishes for assisted suicide should be honored, unless the individual is misinformed or legally incompetent. Quotes Opinion 2.211. References Opinion 2.06. Urofsky, *Justifying Assisted Suicide: Comments on the Ongoing Debate, 14 Notre Dame J. L. Ethics & Pub. Pol'y 893, 918, 923 (2000).*

Journal 1999 Discusses the Uniform Declaration of Death Act and the dead-donor rule. Provides ethical justifications for sustaining current policies on non–heart-beating organ donation. Cites Opinions 2.06 and 2.162. DuBois, *Non–Heart-Beating Organ Donation: A Defense of the Required Determination of Death, 27 J. Law Med. & Ethics 126, 128 (1999).*

Journal 1998 Describes a survey regarding physician-assisted suicide given to members of the Group for the Advancement of Psychiatry. Discusses the results of the survey, noting that most surveyed psychiatrists oppose assisting patients to die. Cites Opinions 2.06 and 2.20. Kramer, Gruenberg, & Fidler, *Psychiatrists' Attitudes Toward Physician-Assisted Suicide: A Survey, 19 Am. J. Forensic Psychiatry 81, 87, 90 (1998).*

Journal 1998 Explains that a determination of mental capacity to consent must be made when a person requests physician-assisted suicide in a jurisdiction where such practice is legal. Explores the potential for liability in the context of making such a determination. Argues that standards regarding determination of mental capacity must be established by case law or legislation. Cites Opinion 2.211. References Opinion 2.06. Lipschitz, *Psychiatry and Consent for Physician-Assisted Suicide, 19 Am. J. Forensic Psychiatry 91, 103, 104 (1998).*

Journal 1997 Explores the Eighth Amendment prohibition against cruel and unusual punishment in the context of capital punishment. Discusses widely used methods of execution. Suggests that execution methods may be unconstitutionally excessive. Concludes the death penalty should not be imposed until methods are more humane. Quotes Opinion 2.06. Denno, *Getting to Death: Are Executions Constitutional? 82 Iowa L. Rev. 319, 385-86 (1997).*

Journal 1997 Describes capital punishment in the US. Considers ethical and moral issues implicated by physician participation. Opines that executions constitute harm and that physician participation contravenes professional ethical obligations. Quotes Opinion 2.06. Michalos, *Medical Ethics and the Executing Process in the United States of America, 16 Med. & Law 125, 131, 133 (1997).*

Journal 1996 Examines how execution practices affect crime deterrence. Explores trend toward private and more humane executions. Discusses similarity between lethal injection and medical procedures. Concludes that deterrence is not served by current execution practices and should not be advanced as support for the death penalty. Cites Opinion 2.06. Abernethy, *The Methodology of Death: Reexamining the Deterrence Rationale, 27 Colum. Hum. Rts. L. Rev. 379, 410-11 (1996).*

Journal 1996 Examines the death penalty statute in New York. Discusses statutory provisions and notes it is unethical for medical personnel to assist with executions. Concludes that the death penalty statute fails to deter crime and may be unconstitutional. Quotes Opinion 2.06. Acker, *When the Cheering Stopped: An Overview and Analysis of New York's Death Penalty Legislation, 17 Pace L. Rev. 41, 221-22 (1996).*

Journal 1996 Discusses the current shortage of available organs for transplant patients. Suggests several new methods for increasing the supply. Includes among these suggestions a proposal that inmates sentenced to death should be allowed to donate organs. Quotes Opinion 2.06. Coleman, *Brother, Can You Spare a Liver? Five Ways to Increase Organ Donation, 31 Val. U. L. Rev. 1, 30, 31 (1996).*

Journal 1996 Discusses the involvement of psychiatrists in capital punishment. Posits that physicians should not aid legal executions. Expresses support for the ethical resolutions of psychiatric and medical associations regarding this issue. Quotes Opinion 2.06. Freedman & Halpern, *The Erosion of Ethics and Morality in Medicine: Physician Participation in Legal Executions in the United States, 41 N. Y. L. Sch. L. Rev. 169, 174 (1996).*

Journal 1996 Proposes an alternative method of capital punishment to allow for organ donation by executed prisoners. Provides justifications for this proposal. Concludes that physicians should be able to ethically participate in this process. Quotes Principle VII. Cites Opinion 2.06. References Opinion 2.162 (1994) [subsequently amended]. Patton, *A Call for Common Sense: Organ Donation and the Executed Prisoner, 3 Va. J. Soc. Pol'y & L. 387, 404, 405, 407-10 (1996).*

Journal 1996 Considers physician participation in execution of capital offenders. Observes that this practice is unethical and contrary to the physician's role as a healer. Concludes that physicians should not participate in any aspect of executions. Quotes Opinion 2.06. Schoenholtz, Freedman, & Halpern, *The Legal Abuse of Physicians in Deaths in the United States: The Erosion of Ethics and Morality in Medicine, 42 Wayne L. Rev. 1505, 1542 (1996).*

Journal 1996 Discusses the role psychiatrists play in capital punishment. Notes that the ethical prohibition against physician participation in the process creates complications for psychiatrists. References Opinion 2.06. Zwirn, *Professionalism, Mental Disability, and the Death Penalty, 41 N. Y. L. Sch. L. Rev. 163, 165 (1996).*

Journal 1995 Summarizes the US Supreme Court's capital punishment jurisprudence. Explores the history and methodology of the New York Court of Appeals' constitutional adjudication of capital punishment issues and examines constitutional challenges to the death penalty in other states. Quotes Opinion 2.06. Falk & Cary, *Death-Defying Feats: State Constitutional Challenges to New York's Death Penalty, 4 J. L. & Pol'y 161, 233, 234 (1995).*

Journal 1995 Explores the relevance of historical account of capital punishment in New York to the contemporary debate regarding televised executions. Concludes that increased publicity may give both the public and the condemned more power over how executions are conducted. Cites Opinion 2.06. Madow, *Forbidden Spectacle: Executions, the Public and the Press in Nineteenth Century New York, 43 Buff. L. Rev. 461, 475 (1995).*

Journal 1994 Argues that assisted suicide is not an implicit right under the Fourteenth Amendment's liberty guarantee. Suggests that giving physicians the authority to determine the appropriateness of assisted suicide furthers no legitimate state interest. Cites Opinion 2.06. References Opinion 2.211. Marzen, *Out, Out Brief Candle: Constitutionally Prescribed Suicide for the Terminally Ill, 21 Hastings Const. L. Q. 799, 821 (1994).*

Journal 1994 Argues that physician aid-in-dying should be protected by the US Constitution and that patients should have a federal cause of action to challenge prohibitive state statutes. Considers how such a cause of action might affect public policy. Quotes Principles I and III. References Opinion 2.06. Note, *Toward a More Perfect Union: A Federal Cause of Action for Physician Aid-In-Dying, 27 U. Mich. J. L. Ref. 521, 538 (1994).*

Journal 1993 Considers whether criminal penalties should be imposed on a physician who assists in the suicide of a competent, nonterminal patient who requested such assistance. Presents the arguments for and against active euthanasia, with emphasis on the "slippery slope" argument. References Opinions 2.06 and 2.20. Persels, *Forcing the Issue of Physician-Assisted Suicide: Impact of the Kevorkian Case on the Euthanasia Debate, 14 J. Legal Med. 93, 115 (1993).*

Journal 1993 Explores the extent to which physicians may participate in capital punishment. Explains the policy behind prohibiting physicians from taking part in executions. Cites Opinion 2.06. Truog & Brennan, *Participation of Physicians in Capital Punishment, 329 New Eng. J. Med. 1346 (1993).*

Journal 1991 Considers ethical issues raised by the case of *Perry v. Louisiana*, where the state attempted to treat an insane death-row inmate in order to render him fit for execution. Explores various ethical questions involving mentally ill defendants/inmates and proposes increased discussion and reform of ethical guidelines. Quotes Opinion 2.06. Note, *Perry v. Louisiana: Medical Ethics on Death Row—Is Judicial Intervention Warranted? 4 Georgetown J. Legal Ethics 707, 714 (1991).*

Journal 1987 Concludes that a policy or practice of active voluntary euthanasia is not desirable, linking a moral prohibition against active voluntary euthanasia to the moral prohibition against physicians actively participating in capital punishment. In place of any practice of active voluntary euthanasia, recommends increased use of hospices, greater emphasis on training physicians to care for the dying patient, and further research aimed at producing symptomatic relief in dying patients. Cites Opinions 2.06, 8.10 (1986) [now Opinion 8.11], and 9.06. Shewmon, *Active Voluntary Euthanasia: A Needless Pandora's Box, 3 Issues in Law and Med. 219, 220, 222, 243 (1987).*

Journal 1987 Focuses on the decision of the US Supreme Court in *Ford v. Wainwright,* wherein the Court ruled that the Eighth Amendment forbids the execution of a condemned inmate who has become insane. Noting that physicians should not ethically participate in a legally authorized execution, except to make a determination or certification of death, concludes that participation by mental health professionals in assessing competency for execution is incompatible with the general ethics of the profession. Cites Opinion 2.06. Wallace, *Incompetency for Execution: The Supreme Court Challenges the Ethical Standards of the Mental Health Professions, 8 J. Legal Med. 265, 267 (1987).*

Journal 1986 Observes that the AMA policy on capital punishment expressly forbids psychiatrists from making determinations of competency for execution. Compares the psychiatrist's determination of competency for execution to the behavior of Nazi physicians, and condemns as inherently dishonest any therapy not grounded in the patient's best interests. References Principle I and Opinion 2.06. Sargent, *Treating the Condemned to Death, 16 Hastings Center Rep. 5, 5 (Dec. 1986).*

Journal 1983 Focuses on the medical-ethical dilemma inherent in the application of medical technology to bring about death and observes that medical professional organizations have done little to solve the dilemma. Concludes that there is a need for federal legislation preempting the multiplicity of state-sanctioned methods to reduce the potential of abuse of civil and human rights. References 1980 AMA Policy Statement [now Opinion 2.06]. Finks, *Lethal Injection: An Uneasy Alliance of Law and Medicine, 4 J. Legal Med. 383, 392, 394 (1983).*

9.7.4 Physician Participation in Interrogation

Journal 2011 Examines the participation of medical personnel in torture of Guantanamo detainees and violations of international and domestic law that occurred as a result. Concludes that the government should take certain steps to address such violations, including civil remedies for victims of torture. Cites Opinions 2.067 and 2.068. Brennan, *Torture of Guantanamo Detainees With the Complicity of Medical Health Personnel: The Case for Accountability and Providing a Forum for Redress for These International Wrongs, 45 U.S.F. L. Rev. 1005, 1045 (2011).*

Journal 2009 Examines the ethical guidelines regarding physicians' participation in interrogations and statutory approaches aimed at eliminating such physician involvement. Concludes that to maintain the integrity of the medical profession, physician involvement in interrogations must be precluded by legislative action. Quotes Preamble and Opinions 2.067 and 2.068. Cites Opinions 2.06 and 2.068, Bahnassi, *Keeping Doctors Out of the Interrogation Room: A New Ethical Obligation that Requires the Backing of the Law, 19 Health Matrix 447, 449-51, 461, 464, 465-67, 469-70, 474-75 (2009).*

Journal 2009 Asserts that military psychiatrists should not participate in interrogations. Concludes that the US military should revise its policies to conform to the ethical standards of the medical profession. Cites Opinion 2.068. Heyman, *Military Medical Ethics, 395 New Eng. J. Med. 2728, 2729 (2009).*

Journal 2009 Proposes revisions to the Declaration of Tokyo regarding physician participation in the practice of torture. Concludes that physicians have a duty to be proactive in preventing torture. Cites Opinion 2.067. References Opinion 2.068. Miles & Freedman, *Medical Ethics and Torture: Revising the Declaration of Tokyo, 373 Lancet 344, 344-45 (2009).*

Journal 2007 Discusses physician involvement in abuse of enemy combatants detained by the US. Concludes that the AMA will continue to advocate for ethical treatment of detainees. Cites Opinions 2.067 and 2.068. Langston, *Ethical Treatment of Military Detainees, 370 Lancet 1999, 1999 (2007).*

Journal 2007 Considers how health care professionals should respond to interrogation and detention policies used in Guantanamo Bay. Concludes that while individuals face pressure to comply with military orders, they should adhere to principles of medical ethics. Quotes Opinion 2.068. Marks, *Doctors as Pawns? Law and Medical Ethics at Guantanamo Bay, 37 Seton Hall L. Rev. 711, 725 (2007).*

Journal 2007 Describes ethical issues surrounding physician participation in the interrogation of military detainees. Concludes medical professionals are required to put the well-being of the detainee ahead of other "dual-loyalty" considerations. Quotes Opinion 2.068. Miles, *Medical Ethics and the Interrogation of Guantanamo 063, 7 Am. J. Bioethics 5, 9 (April 2007).*

Journal 2006 Analyzes liability of the US government and private contractors for acts of torture committed at Abu Ghraib. Concludes that human rights law should be further developed to provide for liability analogous to tort law. References Opinion 2.068. Garfield, *Bridging a Gap in Human Rights Law: Prisoner of War Abuse as "War Tort," 37 Geo. J. Int'l L. 725, 743 (2006).*

9.7.5 Torture

W.D. Mich. 2006 Plaintiffs, state prisoners, filed a class action alleging that inadequate medical care violated the Eighth Amendment. Quoting Opinion 2.067, plaintiff's medical expert testified that prison conditions should be classified as torture and that it was unethical for any physician to support or fail to oppose such conditions. Upon further findings of inadequate care, the court held the practices violated the Eighth Amendment, granted a preliminary injunction, and ordered other relief. *Hadix v. Caruso, 461 F.Supp. 2d 574, 581, 596.*

Journal 2011 Examines the participation of medical personnel in torture of Guantanamo detainees and violations of international and domestic law that occurred as a result. Concludes that the government should take certain steps to address such violations, including civil remedies for victims of torture. Cites Opinions 2.067 and 2.068. Brennan, *Torture of Guantanamo Detainees With the Complicity of Medical Health Personnel: The Case for Accountability and Providing a Forum for Redress for These International Wrongs, 45 U.S.F. L. Rev. 1005, 1045 (2011).*

Journal 2009 Examines the ethical guidelines regarding physicians' participation in interrogations and statutory approaches aimed at eliminating such physician involvement. Concludes that to maintain the integrity of the medical profession, physician involvement in interrogations must be precluded by legislative action. Quotes Preamble and Opinions 2.067 and 2.068. Cites Opinions 2.06 and 2.068, Bahnassi, *Keeping Doctors Out of the Interrogation Room: A New Ethical Obligation That Requires the Backing of the Law, 19 Health Matrix 447, 449-51, 461, 464, 465-67, 469-70, 474-75 (2009).*

Journal 2009 Proposes revisions to the Declaration of Tokyo regarding physician participation in the practice of torture. Concludes that physicians have a duty to be proactive in preventing torture. Cites Opinion 2.067. References Opinion 2.068. Miles & Freedman, *Medical Ethics and Torture: Revising the Declaration of Tokyo, 373 Lancet 344, 344-45 (2009).*

Journal 2007 Discusses physician involvement in abuse of enemy combatants detained by the US. Concludes that the AMA will continue to advocate for ethical treatment of detainees. Cites Opinions 2.067 and 2.068. Langston, *Ethical Treatment of Military Detainees, 370 Lancet 1999, 1999 (2007).*

Journal 2007 Discusses the responsibilities of health care professionals compelled by the US government to participate in torture and other unethical practices against detainees. Concludes that health care professionals must adhere to the Geneva Conventions and uphold the ethical practice of medicine. Quotes Opinion 2.067. Rubenstein, *First, Do No Harm: Health Professionals and Guantanamo, 37 Seton Hall L. Rev. 733, 738 (2007).*

Journal 2006 Examines conflicting loyalties of military medical personnel, which lead to militarily sanctioned human rights abuses. Concludes that immediate reform is necessary to prevent abuses and proposes an increase in education, supervision, and sanctioning. Quotes Opinion 2.067. Clark, *Medical Ethics at Guantanamo Bay and Abu Ghraib: The Problem of Dual Loyalty, 34 J. L. Med. & Ethics 570, 573 (2006).*

Journal 2006 Reviews the policy of the US government regarding the use of torture. Concludes that all forms of torture must be prohibited. Quotes Opinion 2.067. Goldstone, *Symposium: "Torture and the War on Terror": Combating Terrorism: Zero Tolerance for Torture, 37 Case W. Res. J. Int'l L. 343, 346 (2006).*

Journal 2005 Examines ethical guidelines for health personnel created by the Department of Defense in response to recent allegations of abuse and torture by US forces. Concludes that the guidelines allow physicians to participate in interrogation practices that contravene international ethical principles. Cites Opinion 1.02. References Opinion 2.067. Rubenstein, Pross, Davidoff, & Iacopino, *Coercive US Interrogation Policies: A Challenge to Medical Ethics, 294 JAMA 1544 (2005).*

Journal 2004 Analyzes various issues relating to the role of mental health professionals in capital punishment in light of Albert Bandura's model of "mechanisms of moral disengagement." Concludes that facilitating participation of mental health professionals in executions creates conflicts with the humanistic norms of the profession. Quotes Preamble and Opinions 1.01, 1.02, 2.06, 2.067, 2.20, 2.21, 2.211, and 8.14. Judges, *The Role of Mental Health Professionals in Capital Punishment: An Exercise in Moral Disengagement, 41 Hous. L. Rev. 515, 562, 568, 569, 570, 571-72, 581, 586, 588, 598 (2004).*

10 Interprofessional Relationships

10.1 Ethics Guidance for Physicians in Nonclinical Roles

Journal 2010 Reviews a book with case studies of controversial issues of bioethics, health law, and human rights. Concludes that, while in many areas bioethics relates to human rights issues, human rights issues not directly involving the conduct of health professionals or human health are not within the scope of expertise of bioethicist. Quotes Opinion 8.02. Rothstein, *Worst Case Bioethics: Death, Disaster, and Public Health*, 31 *J. Legal Med.* 331, 333 (2010).

Journal 2001 Examines issues relating to health care cost containment. Concludes that, if physicians are to meet the goals assigned to them in a cost-constrained health care system, then professional standards must be reevaluated and modified to afford meaningful guidance for clinical decision-making in the face of health care spending controls. Quotes Opinions 2.03, 2.09, 2.095, 8.032, and 9.04. Cites Opinions 8.02, 8.021, 8.051, and 8.13. Agrawal, *Resuscitating Professionalism: Self-regulation in the Medical Marketplace*, 66 *Mo. L. Rev.* 341, 354, 355, 360, 361, 378, 388 (2001).

Journal 2001 Discusses the prohibition on nonlawyer ownership of legal service providers. Considers how ethical rules and standards governing physicians have been directed toward preserving independent judgment. Concludes that ethical conflicts created by abandoning the prohibition on nonlawyer ownership of legal service providers may be managed by following the medical ethics model. Quotes Principle VI and Opinions 2.03, 2.09, 8.02, 8.021, 8.03, 8.05, 8.051, 8.054, 8.13,

and 8.132. Harris & Foran, *The Ethics of Middle-Class Access to Legal Services and What We Can Learn From the Medical Profession's Shift to a Corporate Paradigm*, 70 *Fordham L. Rev.* 775, 817, 821, 822, 823, 824 (2001).

Journal 1999 Discusses the need for physicians to advocate on behalf of patients' rights in the context of health care delivery. Evaluates the nature and scope of the physician's role as advocate, noting that physicians cannot be expected to engage in attorney-like advocacy. Quotes Principles IV and VI, Fundamental Elements (2), (4), and (6) [now Opinion 10.01], Patient Responsibilities 5 [now Opinion 10.02], and Opinions 2.03, 2.07, 2.09, 2.16, 2.19, 3.06, 4.01, 4.04, 6.01, 7.02, 8.02, 8.03, 8.13, 8.132, 9.06, 9.07, and 9.131. Cites Opinions 5.05, 5.09, 7.01, 8.135, and 9.02. Sage, *Physicians as Advocates*, 35 *Hous. L. Rev.* 1529, 1537, 1541, 1542, 1552-53, 1554, 1556, 1557, 1559, 1561-62, 1564, 1571, 1574, 1576, 1580 (1999).

Journal 1997 Discusses the practice of ex parte communications between treating physicians and their patients' legal adversaries without informing the patient or obtaining consent. Examines harms that may occur in these situations. Argues that Oklahoma needs to prohibit treating physicians from communicating ex parte with their patients' legal adversaries. Quotes Opinions 5.05, 5.07, 5.08, 8.02, 8.03, and 9.07. Cites Opinion 7.02. McNaughton & McNaughton, *Divided Loyalty: The Dilemma of the Treating Physician Advocate*, 22 *Okla. City U. L. Rev.* 1051, 1052, 1054, 1056, 1058, 1059, 1062 (1997).

10.1.1 Ethical Obligations of Medical Directors

Journal 2006 Examines ethical dilemmas physicians may face as providers of pay-for-performance medical care. Concludes that this strategy offers a benefit to patients as long as physicians uphold stringent ethical standards and work together to ensure optimum patient care. Cites Principles I, V, VIII, and IX and Opinions 2.035, 2.095, 6.01, 8.021, 8.03, 8.0501, 8.053, 8.054, and 8.121. Bostick, Sade, & McMahon, *Report of the Council on Ethical and Judicial Affairs: Physician Pay-for-Performance Programs*, 3 *Ind. Health L. Rev.* 429, 430, 431, 432-33, 434, 435, 436 (2006).

Journal 2001 Examines issues relating to health care cost containment. Concludes that, if physicians are to meet the goals assigned to them in a cost-constrained health care system, then professional standards must be reevaluated and modified to afford meaningful guidance for clinical decision-making in the face of health care spending controls. Quotes Opinions 2.03, 2.09, 2.095, 8.032, and

9.04. Cites Opinions 8.02, 8.021, 8.051, and 8.13. Agrawal, *Resuscitating Professionalism: Self-regulation in the Medical Marketplace*, 66 *Mo. L. Rev.* 341, 354, 355, 360, 361, 378, 388 (2001).

Journal 2001 Discusses the prohibition on nonlawyer ownership of legal service providers. Considers how ethical rules and standards governing physicians have been directed toward preserving independent judgment. Concludes that ethical conflicts created by abandoning the prohibition on nonlawyer ownership of legal service providers may be managed by following the medical ethics model. Quotes Principle VI and Opinions 2.03, 2.09, 8.02, 8.021, 8.03, 8.05, 8.051, 8.054, 8.13, and 8.132. Harris & Foran, *The Ethics of Middle-Class Access to Legal Services and What We Can Learn From the Medical Profession's Shift to a Corporate Paradigm*, 70 *Fordham L. Rev.* 775, 817, 821, 822, 823, 824 (2001).

10.4 Nurses

Journal 2010 Observes that miscommunicated, misunderstood, and forgotten information among physicians, nurses, and other hospital staff leads to serious patient injury. Concludes that to assess if a client's injury resulted from a miscommunication among hospital staff, attorneys must examine hospital policies and procedures, medical ethics, and communications technology in relation to information

sharing. Quotes Opinions 3.02 and 9.045. Cohen, Dicecco, & Levin, *Failure to Communicate: When It Comes to Hospital Patient Care, Communication Between Doctor and Nurse Should Be Seamless. If It's Not, Patients Suffer. Here's How to Find Out if a Miscommunication Is at the Core of Your Client's Case, 46 Trial 38, 40-41 (May 2010).*

10.5 Allied Health Professionals

Journal 2008 Questions whether it is ethical for ophthalmologists to teach surgery to optometrists. Concludes that the welfare of the patient must be the primary consideration in making this determination. Quotes Opinion 3.03. Packer, Parke II, & Pellegrino, *Should Ophthalmologists Teach Surgery to Optometrists? 126 Arch. Ophthalmol. 1458, 1458 (2008).*

Journal 2006 Discusses the evolution of health law in Virginia. Concludes that the area of health law continues to expand, develop, and be refined. Cites Opinions 3.03, 3.08, 5.01, 5.015, 5.02, 5.04, 5.055, 6.02, 6.021, 6.03, 6.04, 7.03, 7.04, 7.05, 8.054, 8.08, 8.081, 8.085, 8.115, 8.12, 8.14, 8.145, 8.19, and 9.045. Guanzon, *Health Care Law, 41 U. Rich. L. Rev. 179, 199 (2006).*

10.7 Ethics Committees in Health Care Institutions

Journal 2009 Examines the decision-making function of health care ethics committees (HECs) and their role in the adjudication of treatment disputes. Concludes the adjudicatory authority of HECs should be relocated to a multi-institutional HEC to prevent a single institution's HEC from having control in the adjudication of its own dispute. Quotes Opinions 9.11 and 9.115. Cites Opinion 9.115. Pope, *Multi-Institutional Healthcare Ethics Committees: The Procedurally Fair Internal Dispute Resolution Mechanism, 31 Campbell L. Rev. 257, 276, 300, 312 (2009).*

Journal 2007 Discusses patients' right to refuse medical treatment and the corresponding duties of health care professionals. Concludes that detailed, carefully prepared advance directives are necessary to fulfill patients' wishes. Quotes Ch. II (1940) [now Opinions 8.08 and 8.082] and Opinions 2.035, 2.037, 2.20, 2.225, 8.081, and 10.015. Cites Opinions 9.11 and 9.115. Stamatakis, *Beyond Advance Directives: Personal Autonomy and the Right to Refuse Life-Sustaining Medical Treatment, 47 N. H. B. J. 20, 29-30 (2007).*

Journal 2005 Discusses ethical issues that arise when attorneys serve on hospital ethics committees or as ethics

consultants. Concludes that, despite certain potential hazards, attorneys may fairly participate in these important roles. Quotes Opinion 9.11. McQuire, Majumder, & Cheney, *The Ethical Health Lawyer, 33 J. L. Med. & Ethics 603, 604 (2005).*

Journal 2004 Compares formal and informal education in ethics for medical and law students. Concludes that law students would benefit from additional informal ethics education strategies while medical students would benefit from additional formal approaches. Cites Opinion 9.11. References Preamble. Egan, Parsi, & Ramirez, *Comparing Ethics Education in Medicine and Law: Combining the Best of Both Worlds, 13 Annals Health L. 303, 316, 323 (2004).*

Journal 2002 Discusses the role of clinical ethicists and their potential legal liability as a result of participating in case consultations. Concludes that clinical ethicists can limit their liability by acting primarily as mediators or facilitators. Quotes Opinion 9.11. Sontag, *Are Clinical Ethics Consultants in Danger? An Analysis of the Potential Legal Liability of Individual Clinical Ethicists, 151 U. Pa. L. Rev. 667, 679 (2002).*

10.7.1 Ethics Consultations

Journal 2009 Examines the decision-making function of health care ethics committees (HECs) and their role in the adjudication of treatment disputes. Concludes the adjudicatory authority of HECs should be relocated to a multi-institutional HEC to prevent a single institution's HEC

from having control in the adjudication of its own dispute. Quotes Opinions 9.11 and 9.115. Cites Opinion 9.115. Pope, *Multi-Institutional Healthcare Ethics Committees: The Procedurally Fair Internal Dispute Resolution Mechanism, 31 Campbell L. Rev. 257, 276, 300, 312 (2009).*

Journal 2007 Discusses patients' right to refuse medical treatment and the corresponding duties of health care professionals. Concludes that detailed, carefully prepared advance directives are necessary to fulfill patients' wishes. Quotes Ch. II (1940) [now Opinions 8.08 and 8.082] and Opinions 2.035, 2.037, 2.20, 2.225, 8.081, and 10.015. Cites Opinions 9.11 and 9.115. Stamatakis, *Beyond Advance Directives: Personal Autonomy and the Right to Refuse Life-Sustaining Medical Treatment, 47 N. H. B. J. 20, 29-30 (2007).*

Journal 2006 Examines US and UK terminal illness jurisprudence. Proposes new legislation should be drafted to allow for palliative care when curative treatments are no longer appropriate. Cites Opinions 2.037 and 9.115. Feldhammer, *Medical Torture: End of Life Decision-Making in the United Kingdom and United States, 14 Cardozo J. Int'l & Comp. L. 511, 514-15, 532 (2006).*

11 Financing and Delivery of Health Care

11.1.1 Defining Basic Health Care

Journal 2011 Analyzes the ability of Medicaid patients to access subspecialty care in Connecticut based on a questionnaire directed towards physicians. Concludes reform in Medicaid reimbursement, changes in licensing requirements, new rules for participation in Medicaid, and greater regulation of community service could help equalize Medicaid patients' access to subspecialty care. Quotes Opinions 2.095 and 9.065. Grewal, Sofair, Guevara, & Manthous, *Medicaid Patients' Access to Subspecialty Care in Connecticut, 75 Conn. Med. 489, 490 (2011).*

Journal 2006 Examines ethical dilemmas physicians may face as providers of pay-for-performance medical care. Concludes that this strategy offers a benefit to patients as long as physicians uphold stringent ethical standards and work together to ensure optimum patient care. Cites Principles I, V, VIII, and IX and Opinions 2.035, 2.095, 6.01, 8.021, 8.03, 8.0501, 8.053, 8.054, and 8.121. Bostick, Sade, & McMahon, *Report of the Council on Ethical and Judicial Affairs: Physician Pay-for-Performance Programs, 3 Ind. Health L. Rev. 429, 430, 431, 432-33, 434, 435, 436 (2006).*

Journal 2004 Analyzes the constitutions of countries throughout the world, focusing on language that pertains to health care. Concludes that, although a majority of constitutions have such language, this fact is not highly related to each nation's allocation of resources to health and health care. References Opinion 2.095. Kinney & Clark, *Provisions for Health and Health Care in the Constitutions of the Countries of the World, 37 Cornell Int'l L. J. 285, 289 (2004).*

Journal 2001 Examines issues relating to health care cost containment. Concludes that, if physicians are to meet the goals assigned to them in a cost-constrained health care system, then professional standards must be reevaluated

and modified to afford meaningful guidance for clinical decision-making in the face of health care spending controls. Quotes Opinions 2.03, 2.09, 2.095, 8.032, and 9.04. Cites Opinions 8.02, 8.021, 8.051, and 8.13. Agrawal, *Resuscitating Professionalism: Self-regulation in the Medical Marketplace, 66 Mo. L. Rev. 341, 354, 355, 360, 361, 378, 388 (2001).*

Journal 1996 Considers challenges to the psychiatrist-patient relationship that are triggered by managed care cost-containment methodologies. Offers guidance to psychiatrists for addressing these challenges. References Opinions 2.095, 8.13, and 8.132. Hoge, *APA Resource Document: I. The Professional Responsibilities of Psychiatrists in Evolving Health Care Systems, 24 Bull. Am. Acad. Psychiatry Law 393, 405 (1996).*

Journal 1994 Considers how greater patient autonomy has led to situations in which medical care may be viewed as futile. Suggests that the law has intruded too far into this area of medicine. Quotes Opinion 2.035. Cites Opinions 2.03, 2.095, 2.17, 2.19, 2.20, and 2.22. Cultice, *Medical Futility: When Is Enough, Enough? 27 J. Health & Hosp. Law 225, 230, 256 (1994).*

Journal 1994 Considers how patients with insufficient financial resources place physicians in a conflict-of-interest situation with respect to patient needs and the financial interests of the physician, other patients, and society. Suggests that rules of contract and malpractice law do not provide satisfactory guidelines to resolve these conflicts. Cites Opinions 2.09 and 2.095. Mehlman & Massey, *The Patient-Physician Relationship and the Allocation of Scarce Resources: A Law and Economics Approach, 4 Kennedy Inst. Ethics J. 291, 292 (1994).*

11.1.3 Allocating Limited Health Care Resources

Journal 2010 Examines recent health care reform proposals and their failure to address many issues, including health disparities. Concludes that access to health care should be treated as a human right to reform the health care system to harmonize with core values. Cites Opinion 2.03. McClellan, *Health Disparities, Health Care Reform, Morality, and the Law: "Keep Your Government Hands Off of My Medicare," 82 Temp. L. Rev 1141, 1151, 1154-55 (2010).*

Journal 2010 Addresses whether health care workers should receive priority in treatment during an influenza epidemic. Using distributive justice principles and practical considerations, concludes that health care workers should not get priority treatment in such an epidemic and that medical utility should be the sole criterion in determining any treatment priority. Quotes Opinion 2.03. Cites Opinion 9.067. Rothstein, *Should Health Care Providers Get Treatment Priority in an Influenza Pandemic? 38 J. L. Med. & Ethics 412, 413, 415 (2010).*

Journal 2009 Proposes a novel method of predicting risk of liver transplant for any donor/recipient pair. Concludes that considering the age of the donor, together with the sickness of the recipient, provides the best prediction of outcome. Cites Opinion 2.03. Halldorson, Bakthavatsalam, Fix, Reyes, & Perkins, *D-MELD, a Simple Predictor of Post Liver Transplant Mortality for Optimization of Donor/Recipient Matching, 9 Am. J. of Transplantation 318, 324 (2009).*

Journal 2008 Argues that as a matter of public health, physicians must control antibiotic administration to combat antibiotic resistance. Concludes that despite limited incentives for antibiotic conservation, physicians must acknowledge their important role in mitigating the public health threat of antibiotic resistance. Quotes Principles VII and VIII and Opinions 2.09 and 10.015. Cites Opinion 2.03. Saver, *In Tepid Defense of Population Health: Physicians and Antibiotic Resistance, 34 Am. J. L. & Med. 431, 457 (2008).*

Journal 2006 Examines the public reaction to the Terri Schiavo case. Concludes that public fears were misplaced and that all persons benefited from the decision. Quotes Opinions 2.03, 2.035, and 2.17. Cites Opinion 2.22. Cerminara, *Musings on the Need to Convince Some People With Disabilities That End-of-Life Decision-Making Advocates Are Not Out to Get Them, 37 Loy. U. Chi. L. J. 343, 347 (2006).*

Journal 2006 Reviews policy surrounding medical futility in the US and UK. Concludes that communication and collaboration with patients and their families is the best solution for addressing decisions about futile care. Quotes Opinion 2.035. Cites Opinion 2.03. Rowland, *Communicating Past the Conflict: Solving the Medical Futility Controversy With Process-Based Approaches, 14 U. Miami Int'l & Comp. L. Rev. 271, 278-79 (2006).*

Journal 2003 Discusses the practice of gainsharing and argues that providing physicians and hospitals with certain financial incentives to reduce health costs may be of value in health care reform. Concludes with suggestions for how best to proceed in this difficult context. Quotes Opinions 2.03, 2.09, 4.04, and 8.03. References Opinion 8.13. Saver, *Squandering the Gain: Gainsharing and the Continuing Dilemma of Physician Financial Incentives, 98 Nw. U. L. Rev. 145, 219, 221, 222 (2003).*

Journal 2002 Examines whether managed care organizations should be obligated to disclose physician financial incentives that may limit patient care. Concludes that mandatory disclosure is in the best interest of patients and physicians. Quotes Opinions 2.03 and 8.13. Talesh, *Breaking the Learned Helplessness of Patients: Why MCOs Should Be Required to Disclose Financial Incentives, 26 Law & Psychol. Rev. 49, 60-61, 63 (2002).*

Journal 2001 Examines issues relating to health care cost containment. Concludes that, if physicians are to meet the goals assigned to them in a cost-constrained health care system, then professional standards must be reevaluated and modified to afford meaningful guidance for clinical decision-making in the face of health care spending controls. Quotes Opinions 2.03, 2.09, 2.095, 8.032, and 9.04. Cites Opinions 8.02, 8.021, 8.051, and 8.13. Agrawal, *Resuscitating Professionalism: Self-regulation in the Medical Marketplace, 66 Mo. L. Rev. 341, 354, 355, 360, 361, 378, 388 (2001).*

Journal 2001 Discusses the prohibition on nonlawyer ownership of legal service providers. Considers how ethical rules and standards governing physicians have been directed toward preserving independent judgment. Concludes that ethical conflicts created by abandoning the prohibition on nonlawyer ownership of legal service providers may be managed by following the medical ethics model. Quotes Principle VI and Opinions 2.03, 2.09, 8.02, 8.021, 8.03, 8.05, 8.051, 8.054, 8.13, and 8.132. Harris & Foran, *The Ethics of Middle-Class Access to Legal Services and What We Can Learn From the Medical Profession's Shift to a Corporate Paradigm, 70 Fordham L. Rev. 775, 817, 821, 822, 823, 824 (2001).*

Journal 2000 Considers how social and political values shape normative understandings of health and disease. Concludes that the challenge for developing universal canonical accounts of health and disease arises out of moral diversity. Quotes Opinion 2.03. Cherry, *Polymorphic Medical Ontologies: Fashioning Concepts of Disease, 25 J. Med. & Phil. 519, 532 (2000).*

Journal 1999 Analyzes federal regulations regarding allocation of organs for transplantation. Explores the political background and controversy surrounding allocation of human organs. Cites Opinion 2.03. McMullen, *Equitable Allocation of Human Organs: An Examination of the New Federal Regulation, 20 J. Legal Med. 405, 412 (1999).*

Journal 1999 Points out that several states do not allow patients to designate their physicians as health care proxies.

Observes that such restrictions inhibit patient autonomy. Provides justification in support of permitting appointments of physicians as proxies. Cites Opinion 2.03. Rai, Siegler, & Lantos, *The Physician as a Health Care Proxy, 29 Hastings Center Rep. 14, 19 (Sep./Oct. 1999)*.

Journal 1999 Discusses the need for physicians to advocate on behalf of patients' rights in the context of health care delivery. Evaluates the nature and scope of the physician's role as advocate, noting that physicians cannot be expected to engage in attorney-like advocacy. Quotes Principles IV and VI, Fundamental Elements (2), (4), and (6) [now Opinion 10.01], Patient Responsibilities 5 [now Opinion 10.02], and Opinions 2.03, 2.07, 2.09, 2.16, 2.19, 3.06, 4.01, 4.04, 6.01, 7.02, 8.02, 8.03, 8.13, 8.132, 9.06, 9.07, and 9.131. Cites Opinions 5.05, 5.09, 7.01, 8.135, and 9.02. Sage, *Physicians as Advocates, 35 Hous. L. Rev. 1529, 1537, 1541, 1542, 1552-53, 1554, 1556, 1557, 1559, 1561-62, 1564, 1571, 1574, 1576, 1580 (1999)*.

Journal 1999 Explores the impact managed care organizations have had on health care. Explains that patients may not understand restrictions and incentives imposed by their managed care organizations when entering the program. Argues that such information should be disclosed at various times during the period of plan coverage. Cites Opinions 2.03, 8.03, 8.032, 8.051, 8.13, and 8.132. Wolf, *Toward a Systemic Theory of Informed Consent in Managed Care, 35 Hous. L. Rev. 1631, 1641, 1658, 1661, 1662, 1679 (1999)*.

Journal 1998 Discusses the physician's fiduciary duty to the patient. Explores the expansion of the "honest services" mail fraud statute to prosecute undisclosed fiduciary breaches. Concludes that the mail fraud statute may be used to prosecute physicians who fail to disclose financial incentives to their patients. Quotes Opinion 8.03. Cites Opinions 2.03 and 8.07 [now Opinion 8.06]. Jones, *Primum Non Nocere: The Expanding "Honest Services" Mail Fraud Statute and the* physician-patient *Fiduciary Relationship, 51 Vand. L. Rev. 139, 161, 164 (1998)*.

Journal 1997 Posits that cost-containment schemes in managed care systems have eroded the fiduciary duty physicians owe patients. Notes that MCOs are prohibiting patients from trusting and relying on physicians. Concludes that patients must seek quality assurance from sources other than their physicians. Quotes Opinions 2.03, 2.09, and 8.13. Jacobi, *Patients at a Loss: Protecting Health Care Consumers Through Data Driven Quality Assurance, 45 U. Kan. L. Rev. 705, 720, 721, 759 (1997)*.

Journal 1996 Examines the role of physicians in managed health care. Posits that the new system of managed care is beneficial because it combines high performance with affordable outcomes. Concludes that outcome-based payment systems, with tort reform, will maximize results. Quotes Opinion 2.03 (1984) [subsequently amended]. Furrow, *Incentivizing Medical Practice: What (if Anything) Happens to Professionalism? 1 Widener L. Symp. J. 1, 9 (1996)*.

Journal 1996 Discusses the trend toward conserving resources expended on health care by withholding services absent a showing of necessity. Claims that the high standard of care physicians owe patients is jeopardized by medical treatment decisions based on coverage concerns. Concludes that the legal structure regarding health care plans should be changed. Quotes Preamble, Principles I, II, III, IV, V, VI, and VII, and Opinion 2.03. Hirshfeld & Thomason, *Medical Necessity Determinations: The Need for a New Legal Structure, 6 Health Matrix 3, 8-9 (1996)*.

Journal 1996 Considers whether the Oregon Health Plan discriminates on the basis of race by excluding coverage for obesity, which disproportionately affects African American women. Discusses discrimination in federally funded health care programs and the purpose of Title VI. Quotes Opinion 2.03. Jurevic, *Disparate Impact Under Title VI: Discrimination, By Any Other Name, Will Still Have the Same Impact, 15 St. Louis U. Pub. L. Rev. 237, 253 (1996)*.

Journal 1996 Discusses conflicts of interest between health care professionals and patients created by managed health care and the drive toward reduction of costs. Suggests that a multidisciplinary group of health professionals could act as patient advocates to help protect their interests. Quotes Opinion 2.03. Mehlman, *Medical Advocates: A Call for a New Profession, 1 Widener L. Symp. J. 299, 314 (1996)*.

Journal 1996 Considers the change from traditional medical care systems to managed care, noting the conflicts of interest this creates between physicians' ethical obligations and financial concerns. Discusses these issues in the context of managed behavioral health care. Suggests community-based care and social supports as a solution. Quotes Opinions 2.03 and 4.04. Petrila, *Ethics, Money, and the Problem of Coercion in Managed Behavioral Health Care, 40 St. Louis U. L. J. 359, 377 (1996)*.

Journal 1994 Considers how greater patient autonomy has led to situations in which medical care may be viewed as futile. Suggests that the law has intruded too far into this area of medicine. Quotes Opinion 2.035. Cites Opinions 2.03, 2.095, 2.17, 2.19, 2.20, and 2.22. Cultice, *Medical Futility: When Is Enough, Enough? 27 J. Health & Hosp. Law 225, 230, 256 (1994)*.

Journal 1994 Discusses the practice of physician rationing and how the principles of beneficence and autonomy are consistent with the practice. Explores the objection to using financial incentives, commonly adopted by health maintenance organizations (HMOs), to promote rationing and concludes that rationing should be allowed in some circumstances. Quotes Opinion 2.03. Hall, *Rationing Health Care at the Bedside, 69 N. Y. U. L. Rev. 693, 704 (1994)*.

Journal 1994 Observes that health care reform proposals present significant challenges to the role and ethics of attending physicians. Emphasizes that reform proposals must set forth the role envisioned for physicians and must articulate an acceptable ethical framework within which physicians may fulfill that role. Quotes Opinions 4.04, 9.121, and 9.122. Cites Opinions 2.03, 2.09, 5.01, and 8.03. Wolf, *Health Care Reform and the Future of Physician Ethics*, 24 Hastings Center Rep. 28, 32, 40 (March/April 1994).

Journal 1992 Discusses two California cases focusing on the liability of physicians and third-party payers when medically necessary care is denied. Concludes that physicians also may be obligated to advocate patient interests in attempting to secure payment from third parties when appropriate. Quotes Opinion 2.03. Comment, *Who's in Charge: The Doctor or the Dollar? Assessing the Relative Liability of Third Party Payors and Doctors After Wickline and Wilson*, 18 J. Contemp. L. 285, 301, 302 (1992).

Journal 1992 Examines the major health care rationing issues facing the US including increasing costs and decreasing access. Concludes that the standard of care should not be changed and that rationing should be a separate enterprise undertaken pursuant to explicit criteria. Quotes Opinions 2.03, 2.09, and 4.04. Hirshfeld, *Should Ethical and Legal Standards for Physicians Be Changed to Accommodate New Models for Rationing Health Care?* 140 Univ. Pa. L. Rev. 1809, 1816 (1992).

Journal 1991 Focuses on the denial of insurance benefits for experimental medical procedures, and explains the de novo review process under ERISA. Concludes that there is need for a structure that will permit greater objectivity in the context of data collection as well as judicial determination. Cites Opinions 2.03 and 2.09. Note, *Denial of Coverage for "Experimental" Medical Procedures: The Problem of De Novo Review Under ERISA*, 79 Kentucky L. J. 801, 824 (1990-91).

Journal 1990 Discusses economic considerations in clinical decision-making, with emphasis on the standard of care. Concludes that organized medicine has made valuable contributions through development of practice parameters that offer guidance in the exercise of clinical judgment. Cites Opinions 2.03 and 2.09. Hirshfeld, *Economic Considerations in Treatment Decisions and the Standard of Care in Medical Malpractice Litigation*, 264 JAMA 2004, 2007 (1990).

Journal 1990 Discusses efforts of third-party payers to control health care expenditures for beneficiaries. Concludes that financial incentives to limit care and other cost-control techniques should be disclosed and that the rationale for such disclosure is compelling. Quotes Opinions 2.03, 2.09, and 8.03. Cites Opinions 2.19, 4.04, and 4.06. Hirshfeld, *Should Third Party Payors of Health Care Services Disclose Cost Control Mechanisms to Potential Beneficiaries?* 14 Seton Hall Legis. J. 115, 130, 131, 144, 145, 146 (1990).

Journal 1988 Discusses various circumstances that have led to proposals for the rationing of health care by hospitals and other providers in order to contain health care costs. Because of the impact such proposals may have on older persons, focus is placed on the Age Discrimination Act of 1975 and its likely effect on the use of age as a criterion for rationing in the context of heart transplantation. Quotes Opinion 2.02 (1982) [now Opinion 2.03]. Silver, *From Baby Doe to Grandpa Doe: The Impact of the Federal Age Discrimination Act on the Hidden Rationing of Medical Care*, 37 Catholic Univ. L. Rev. 993, 1013 (1988).

Journal 1985 Notes that considerations of cost and availability of advanced medical technology raise troublesome ethical and legal issues. In addressing these issues, examines potential mechanisms for rationing expensive lifesaving medical treatment, concluding that the cost of rationing probably exceeds the benefits. Quotes Opinion 2.02 (1982) [now Opinion 2.03]. Mehlman, *Rationing Expensive Lifesaving Medical Treatments*, 1985 Wisconsin L. Rev. 239, 250, 260 (1985).

11.1.4 Financial Barriers to Health Care Access

Journal 2008 Argues waiver of patient coinsurance costs creates unfair competition among physicians and has negative economic consequences for those paying providers. Suggests close monitoring of waivers will reduce inflation of health care charges, diminish interference with the health plan insurer–network provider relationship, and discourage overutilization of medical services. Quotes Opinion 6.12. Cites Opinion 6.13. Bernstein & Seybert, *Everyone Pays the Price When Healthcare Providers Waive Patients' Co-insurance Obligations*, 21 Health Law. 20, 22 (Dec. 2008).

Journal 2008 Reviews current physician practices of collecting money from indebted patients. Concludes that physicians should continue to refrain from aggressive debt collection. Quotes Opinions 6.08 and 6.12. Hall & Schneider, *The Professional Ethics of Billing and Collections*, 300 JAMA 1806, 1807 (2008).

Journal 2005 Discusses legal and ethical problems associated with patient surcharges. Concludes that surcharges are necessary to combat rising malpractice insurance premiums and a declining payment environment. Cites Principle IX and Opinion 6.12. Landfair, *Transforming Physicians Into Business Savvy Entrepreneurs: Patient Surcharges Charge Onto the Scene of Physician Reimbursement*, 43 Duq. L. Rev. 257, 268, 269 (2005).

Journal 2000 Examines civil and criminal liability in connection with the practice of professional courtesy fee waivers and discounts. Discusses conflicts between the long-standing traditional practice of professional courtesy and a prudent and ethical course under current law. Quotes Opinion 6.12. Cites Opinion 6.13. Schmidt, *Professional Courtesy Discounts Under Siege—Part II*, 29 Colo. Law. 59, 62 (Jan. 2000).

Journal 2011 Analyzes the ability of Medicaid patients to access subspecialty care in Connecticut based on a questionnaire directed towards physicians. Concludes reform in Medicaid reimbursement, changes in licensing requirements, new rules for participation in Medicaid, and greater regulation of community service could help equalize Medicaid patients' access to subspecialty care. Quotes Opinions 2.095 and 9.065. Grewal, Sofair, Guevara, & Manthous, *Medicaid Patients' Access to Subspecialty Care in Connecticut, 75 Conn. Med. 489, 490 (2011)*.

Journal 2011 Examines the medical-legal partnership (MLP) and its impact on legal services, health care delivery, and public policy. Concludes MLPs provide a unique opportunity to reach vulnerable populations and build advocacy capacity among all health care professionals by addressing health concerns with legal solutions as part of regular care. Quotes Opinion 9.065. Tames, Cotter, Melendez, Scudder, & Colvin, *Medical-Legal Partnership: Evolution or Revolution, 45 Clearinghouse Rev. 124, 127 (2011)*.

Journal 2009 Discusses the judicial standard for reviewing physician noncompete covenants. Concludes courts should apply a strict standard to such covenants, rather than declare the covenants per se invalid. Quotes Principles IV and VII, Principles of Medical Ethics §5 (1957) [now Principle VI], Code of Medical Ethics Ch. II, Art. I §3 (1847) [now Opinion 5.02], Opinion 9.02, and Code of Medical Ethics Ch. II, Art. I §4 (1847) [now Opinion 9.09]. Cites Opinions 8.041, 8.115, 9.02, 9.06, 9.065, 9.067, 10.01, and 10.015. Koons, *Physician Employee Non-Compete Agreements on the Examining Table: The Need to Better Protect Patients' and the Public's Interests in Indiana, 6 Ind. Health L. Rev. 253, 272-77, 280-81 (2009)*.

Journal 2008 Explores interdisciplinary training for law and medical students to advance broad social goals. Concludes partnerships in legal and medical education are useful for training effective practitioners in both fields and for increasing cooperation between physicians and lawyers to better serve the community. Quotes Opinion 9.065. Tyler, *Allies Not Adversaries: Teaching Collaboration to the Next Generation of Doctors and Lawyers to Address Social Inequality, 11 J. Health Care L. & Pol'y 249, 259-60 (2008)*.

Journal 2007 Reviews the legal and ethical problems surrounding concierge medical practice. Concludes that concierge medicine should remain restricted to a small class of wealthy individuals. Cites Opinions 8.05, 8.055, 8.115, 9.06, and 9.065. Carnahan, *Concierge Medicine: Legal and Ethical Issues, 35 J. L. Med. & Ethics 211, 212-13 (2007)*.

Journal 2007 Reviews Deborah Rhode's analysis of pro bono obligations of lawyers from her book, *Pro Bono in Principle and in Practice: Public Service and the Professions*. Concludes that a mandatory pro bono requirement is a better solution than an incentive-based system. Quotes Opinion 10.01. References Opinion 9.065. Lininger,

From Park Place to Community Chest: Rethinking Lawyers' Monopoly, 101 Nw. U. L. Rev. 1343, 1349 (2007).

Journal 2006 Explores the legal and ethical issues surrounding concierge medicine. Concludes that concierge medicine is best restricted to a small class of wealthy individuals. Quotes Principle IX and Opinion 8.055. Cites Principle VI and Opinions 8.055, 8.11, 8.115, 9.065, and 10.05. Carnahan, *Law, Medicine, and Wealth: Does Concierge Medicine Promote Health Care Choice, or Is It a Barrier to Access? 17 Stan. L. & Pol'y Rev. 121, 149-50, 151, 152, 153-54 (2006)*.

Journal 2006 Evaluates hospital-based charity health care programs. Concludes that improvements to these programs will benefit both patients and business for the hospital. References Opinion 9.065. Elliott, *The Charity Care Crisis—Where Does the Money Go? 8 J. Health Care Compliance. 11, 13 (September/October 2006)*.

Journal 2006 Evaluates legal implications of consumer-driven health care. Concludes that a system of consumer-driven health care is feasible and offers many benefits to patients. Quotes Opinions 8.055 and 9.065. Hall, *Paying for What You Get and Getting What You Pay For: Legal Responses to Consumer-Driven Health Care, 69 Law & Contemp. Prob. 159, 165 (2006)*.

Journal 2006 Discusses the role of EMTALA in mandating care for the uninsured. Concludes EMTALA is inadequate and Congress should take steps toward establishing a program for universal health care. Quotes Principle IX, Ch. II, Art. V, Sec. 9 (May 1847) [now Opinion 9.065], and Ch. III, Art. I, Sec. 3 (May 1847) [now Opinion 9.065]. Hermer, *The Scapegoat: EMTALA and Emergency Department Overcrowding, 14 J. L. & Pol'y 695, 713-14 (2006)*.

Journal 2005 Argues that it is in the best interest of the public to ensure that all have access to the legal system. Concludes that government funding must be available in Wyoming to increase the availability of legal services to those in need. References Opinion 9.065. Burman, *Wyoming Attorneys' Pro Bono "Obligation," 5 Wyo. L. Rev. 421, 428 (2005)*.

Journal 2005 Discusses ethical, legal, and policy issues associated with treatment and research involving patients who are in a persistent vegetative or minimally conscious state. Concludes that patients in these states are at risk for therapeutic failures until physicians can more accurately determine which patients will benefit from treatment and accurately convey such information to families or surrogates. Quotes Principles VII and IX and Opinions 8.031, 8.0315, 9.065, 10.01, and 10.015. Tovino & Winslade, *A Primer on the Law and Ethics of Treatment, Research, and Public Policy in the Context of Severe Traumatic Brain Injury, 14 Ann. Health L. 1, 18, 38, 39, 40, 41 (2005)*.

Journal 2000 Discusses and evaluates different systems for addressing consumer concerns about managed health care. Asserts that current legal systems for identifying and resolving consumer concerns are not understood by most consumers and are not accessible by many, especially the uninsured. Concludes that several immediate steps are realistic for moving toward reform. Cites Principle VI. References Opinions 8.13 and 9.065. Kinney, *Tapping and Resolving Consumer Concerns About Health Care, 26 Am. J. Law & Med. 335, 337, 375 (2000).*

Journal 2000 Evaluates recent Texas legislation that affords immunity to health care professionals who provide free health care services to the poor. Concludes that such legislation creates a dual standard of care, requiring indigent patients to forfeit their legal rights in exchange for health care. Quotes Opinion 10.01. References Opinion 9.065. Pulido, *Immunity of Volunteer Health Care Providers in Texas: Bartering Legal Rights for Free Medical Care, 2 Scholar: St. Mary's L. Rev. Minority Issues 323, 330 (2000).*

Journal 1999 Discusses regulatory concerns regarding genetic technology. Provides ideas on how society might regulate genetic enhancements. Argues that a variety of means of regulation need to be utilized to govern genetic technology. Quotes Opinion 2.11. Cites Opinion 9.065. References Opinion 2.138. Mehlman, *How Will We Regulate*

Genetic Enhancement? 34 Wake Forest L. Rev. 671, 693-94, 695 (1999).

Journal 1997 Considers the current approach to health care in the US. Examines financing mechanisms, and suggests that reform could be effected through a decentralized, community-based approach. Proposes use of volunteer systems in which medical personnel would care for certain patients free of charge or at reduced rates. Quotes Fundamental Elements (6) [now Opinion 10.01]. References Opinion 9.065. Solomon & Asaro, *Community-Based Health Care: A Legal and Policy Analysis, 24 Fordham Urb. L. J. 235, 276-77 (1997).*

Journal 1996 Describes the problem of lack of access to medical care by the indigent. Recognizes the commitment of the medical profession to providing care for indigent patients. Observes that state initiatives that provide physicians tort immunity in exchange for volunteer service can improve access to care by the indigent. Quotes Fundamental Elements (6) [now Opinion 10.01]. References Opinion 9.065. Comment, *Statutory Immunity for Volunteer Physicians: A Vehicle for Reaffirmation of the Doctor's Beneficent Duties—Absent the Rights Talk, 1 Widener L. Symp. J. 425, 448, 449 (1996).*

11.2.1 Professionalism in Health Care Systems

D. N. J. 1999 Patient sued her managed care organization alleging that she suffered injuries due to failure to obtain timely approval for a nonmember physician to perform her back surgery. The plaintiff apparently relied on Opinion 8.13 to show that the defendant had a duty to advocate for her in seeking prompt approval for her surgery. The court, however, stated that the plaintiff's reference to the Opinion failed to establish such a duty because the Code of Medical Ethics does not have the force of law. *Pryzbowski v. US Health Care, Inc., 64 F. Supp. 2d 361, 370.*

S.D.N.Y. 1997 Employee brought suit against a health maintenance organization (HMO) under contract with her employer to provide health benefits. The suit alleged various theories of liability ranging from breach of implied contract to breach of fiduciary duties. Employee sought redress pursuant to the civil enforcement provisions of the Employee Retirement Income Security Act of 1974. The court granted HMO's motion to dismiss all claims except for the breach of fiduciary duty stemming from HMO's alleged policy of restricting the disclosure of noncovered treatments. The court quoted report of AMA Council on Ethical and Judicial Affairs [now Opinion 8.13] in holding that physicians have an ethical duty to fully disclose treatment options to patients regardless of whether treatment occurs in a managed care environment. *Weiss v. Cigna Healthcare, Inc., 972 F. Supp. 748, 751-52.*

Mass. Super. 2004 Defendants filed a motion for partial summary judgment in an action alleging they were liable

for not disclosing their financial interests in an experimental program that the decedent participated in. The court denied the defendants' motion, referencing Opinion 8.13 in stating physicians should disclose financial incentives and restrictions placed on them by their HMO. *Darke v. Estate of Isner, 2004 WL 1325635, 3.*

Ohio Att'y Gen. 1999 State attorney general concluded that physicians who render opinions regarding the necessity of medical services for health insuring corporations are not engaged in the practice of medicine. Additionally, physicians who render opinions regarding medical necessity for appeals of adverse determinations do not fall under the regulatory, investigatory, or enforcement authority of the Ohio State Medical Board. Quoting Opinions 8.03, 8.11, and 8.13, the attorney general stated that physicians have an ethical duty to provide appropriate treatment for patients. *Ohio Att'y Gen. Op. No. 99-044, 1999 WL 692623.*

Journal 2006 Examines the process of physician deselection and the protections afforded to physicians. Concludes that physicians should be able to make a legal challenge to a dismissal made without cause. Quotes Opinion 8.13. Coppolo, *Not Just a Minimum Income Policy for Physicians: The Need for Good Faith and Fair Dealing in Physician Deselection Disputes, 48 Wm. and Mary L. Rev. 677, 686 (2006).*

Journal 2006 Examines external review systems used for adjudication of disputes between patients and managed care organizations. Concludes that external review systems do not satisfy constitutional due process requirements. Quotes Opinions and Reports of the Judicial Council Sec. 6, Para. 4 (1969) [now Opinion 8.05]. References Opinion 8.13. Hunter, *Managed Process, Due Care: Structures of Accountability in Health Care, 6 Yale J. Health Pol'y L. & Ethics 93, 107, 113 (2006).*

Journal 2006 Argues for an alternative framework by which health ethics, policy, and law can address equitable distribution of health care. Concludes that a new paradigm would lead to a more efficient and compassionate system. References Opinions 2.22 and 8.13. Ruger, *Health, Capability, and Justice: Toward a New Paradigm of Health Ethics, Policy and Law, 15 Cornell J. L. & Pub. Pol'y 403, 425, 465 (2006).*

Journal 2006 Considers the role of informed consent and patient autonomy as a central tenet of bioethics. Concludes that the field should focus most strongly on serving the practical needs and desires of patients. References Opinion 8.13. Schneider, *After Autonomy, 41 Wake Forest L. Rev. 411, 429-30 (2006).*

Journal 2006 Critiques the Uniform Health-Care Decisions Act. Concludes that the Act poses dangers to disabled patients, and proposes safeguards against such dangers. References Opinion 8.13. Stith, *The Semblance of Autonomy: Treatment of Persons With Disabilities Under the Uniform Health-Care Decisions Act, 22 Issues L. & Med. 39, 63-64 (2006).*

Journal 2005 Argues that in *Aetna v. Davila/Cigna v. Calad*, the Supreme Court missed an opportunity to overturn unjust ERISA policies. Concludes that the principle of complete ERISA preemption as articulated in these consolidated cases is unsatisfactory because it violates the separation of powers doctrine. Quotes Principle VIII. Cites Opinions 8.054, 8.13, 8.135, 9.123, 10.01, and 10.015. Nelson, *AETNA v. DAVILA/CIGNA v. CALAD: A Missed Opportunity, 31 Wm. Mitchell L. Rev. 843, 847, 849, 850, 880 (2005).*

Journal 2003 Reviews state laws designed to protect physicians acting as patient advocates in managed care organizations. Concludes that federal and state law must make it easier for physicians to challenge denials of or delays in patient care. Quotes Opinions 8.054, 8.13, and 10.01. Fentiman, *Patient Advocacy and Termination From Managed Care Organizations: Do State Laws Protecting Health Care Professional Advocacy Make Any Difference? 82 Neb. L. Rev. 508, 515-16, 517-18 (2003).*

Journal 2002 Observes that changes in the health professions challenge certain assumptions about professional ethics. Concludes that these long-standing assumptions must be re-examined. Cites Opinion 2.161. References Opinion 8.13. Kelley, *The Meanings of Professional Life: Teaching Across the Health Professions, 27 J. Med. & Phil. 475, 485, 490, 491 (2002).*

Journal 2002 Considers whether physicians should be required to disclose information regarding financial incentives received from patients' HMOs. Concludes that physicians should not be required to disclose these incentives. References Opinion 8.13. Reuland, *Health Maintenance Organizations and Physician Financial Incentive Plans: Should Physician Disclosure Be Mandatory? 27 Iowa J. Corp. L. 293, 312 (2002).*

Journal 2002 Examines whether managed care organizations should be obligated to disclose physician financial incentives that may limit patient care. Concludes that mandatory disclosure is in the best interest of patients and physicians. Quotes Opinions 2.03 and 8.13. Talesh, *Breaking the Learned Helplessness of Patients: Why MCOs Should Be Required to Disclose Financial Incentives, 26 Law & Psychol. Rev. 49, 60-61, 63 (2002).*

Journal 2001 Examines issues relating to health care cost containment. Concludes that, if physicians are to meet the goals assigned to them in a cost-constrained health care system, then professional standards must be reevaluated and modified to afford meaningful guidance for clinical decision-making in the face of health care spending controls. Quotes Opinions 2.03, 2.09, 2.095, 8.032, and 9.04. Cites Opinions 8.02, 8.021, 8.051, and 8.13. Agrawal, *Resuscitating Professionalism: Self-regulation in the Medical Marketplace, 66 Mo. L. Rev. 341, 354, 355, 360, 361, 378, 388 (2001).*

Journal 2001 Examines the doctrine of informed consent with respect to nontraditional issues, such as a physician's duty to disclose personal information. Concludes there must be a balance that will accommodate the needs of both the patient and the physician. References Opinion 8.13. Hanson, *Informed Consent and the Scope of a Physician's Duty of Disclosure, 77 N. D. L. Rev. 71, 89, 91 (2001).*

Journal 2001 Discusses the prohibition on nonlawyer ownership of legal service providers. Considers how ethical rules and standards governing physicians have been directed toward preserving independent judgment. Concludes that ethical conflicts created by abandoning the prohibition on nonlawyer ownership of legal service providers may be managed by following the medical ethics model. Quotes Principle VI and Opinions 2.03, 2.09, 8.02, 8.021, 8.03, 8.05, 8.051, 8.054, 8.13, and 8.132. Harris & Foran, *The Ethics of Middle-Class Access to Legal Services and What We Can Learn From the Medical Profession's Shift to a Corporate Paradigm, 70 Fordham L. Rev. 775, 817, 821, 822, 823, 824 (2001).*

Journal 2000 Discusses and evaluates different systems for addressing consumer concerns about managed health care. Asserts that current legal systems for identifying and resolving consumer concerns are not understood by most consumers and are not accessible by many, especially the uninsured. Concludes that several immediate steps are realistic for moving toward reform. Cites Principle VI. References Opinions 8.13 and 9.065. Kinney, *Tapping and*

Resolving Consumer Concerns About Health Care, 26 Am. J. Law & Med. 335, 337, 375 (2000).

Journal 2000 Reviews the case of *Corporate Health Insurance, Inc. v. Texas Dept. of Insurance* and discusses its impact on HMO liability in Texas. Considers the conflicts of interest managed care imposes upon physicians. Concludes that, without national amendments to the scope of ERISA, HMOs are not compelled to provide quality health care. References Opinion 8.13. Lockhart, *The Safest Care Is to Deny Care: Implications of Corporate Health Insurance, Inc. v. Texas Department of Insurance on HMO Liability in Texas, 41 S. Tex. L. Rev. 621, 628, 634 (2000).*

Journal 2000 Describes the fiduciary aspects of the physician-patient relationship. Explores the conflicts that may occur between physicians and pregnant women in the health care setting. Proposes legal strategies to address these conflicts. Quotes Opinions 8.08 and 10.01. References Opinion 8.13. Oberman, *Mothers and Doctors' Orders: Unmasking the Doctor's Fiduciary Role in Maternal-Fetal Conflicts, 94 Nw. U. L. Rev. 451, 456, 462, 493 (2000).*

Journal 1999 Describes the gag clause debate in managed care and analyzes the types of incentives that might limit physician-patient communication. Concludes that, to protect patient access to information about treatment options and their health plans, antigag legislation must be coupled with a thorough examination of the extent to which financial incentives will be permitted to impact managed health care delivery. Quotes Opinion 8.13. Krause, *The Brief Life of the Gag Clause: Why Antigag Clause Legislation Isn't Enough, 67 Tenn. L. Rev. 1, 4, 43 (1999).*

Journal 1999 Describes the development of managed care organizations. Examines professional associations' statements regarding managed care organizations. Argues that physicians and managed care organizations should be viewed as economically disciplined, moral cofiduciaries for patients. References Opinion 8.13. McCullough, *A Basic Concept in the Clinical Ethics of Managed Care: Physicians and Institutions as Economically Disciplined Moral Co-Fiduciaries of Populations of Patients, 24 J. Med. Phil. 77, 82-83, 87, 89, 91, 96 (1999).*

Journal 1999 Explores the increased push toward mandatory disclosure laws regarding financial incentives imposed by managed care organizations. Discusses current laws and ethical guidelines. Emphasizes that efforts to mandate disclosure force physicians to focus on the effects of imposed incentives and the essence of the physician-patient relationship. References Opinions 8.032, 8.13, and 8.132. Miller & Sage, *Disclosing Physician Financial Incentives, 281 JAMA 1424, 1425 (1999).*

Journal 1999 Discusses the need for physicians to advocate on behalf of patients' rights in the context of health care delivery. Evaluates the nature and scope of the physician's role as advocate, noting that physicians cannot be expected to engage in attorney-like advocacy. Quotes Principles IV and VI, Fundamental Elements (2), (4), and (6) [now Opinion

10.01], Patient Responsibilities 5 [now Opinion 10.02], and Opinions 2.03, 2.07, 2.09, 2.16, 2.19, 3.06, 4.01, 4.04, 6.01, 7.02, 8.02, 8.03, 8.13, 8.132, 9.06, 9.07, and 9.131. Cites Opinions 5.05, 5.09, 7.01, 8.135, and 9.02. Sage, *Physicians as Advocates, 35 Hous. L. Rev. 1529, 1537, 1541, 1542, 1552-53, 1554, 1556, 1557, 1559, 1561-62, 1564, 1571, 1574, 1576, 1580 (1999).*

Journal 1999 Discusses the push to mandate disclosure in managed care programs. Explains the dangers of disclosing too much information. Provides objectives and goals for disclosure. Quotes Opinion 8.051. References Opinions 8.032 and 8.13. Sage, *Regulating Through Information: Disclosure Laws and American Health Care, 99 Colum. L. Rev. 1701, 1753, 1758, 1760 (1999).*

Journal 1999 Argues that the benefits of managed care organizations are outweighed by the resulting changes in the physician's role as advocate. Characterizes the traditional notion of physician advocacy. States that recent changes in the law regarding communication in managed care organizations have shifted the matter more toward patient self-advocacy. Quotes Opinion 8.13. Spielman, *Managed Care Regulation and the Physician-Advocate, 47 Drake L. Rev. 713, 717, 719 (1999).*

Journal 1999 Discusses financial incentives offered to physicians by managed care organizations. Argues that evidence of financial incentives should be admissible in medical malpractice cases. Quotes Opinion 8.13. References Opinion 8.132. Sugarman & Yarashus, *Admissibility of Managed Care Financial Incentives in Medical Malpractice Cases, 34 Tort & Ins. L. J. 735, 743, 746, 759 (1999).*

Journal 1999 Explores the impact managed care organizations have had on health care. Explains that patients may not understand restrictions and incentives imposed by their managed care organizations when entering the program. Argues that such information should be disclosed at various times during the period of plan coverage. Cites Opinions 2.03, 8.03, 8.032, 8.051, 8.13, and 8.132. Wolf, *Toward a Systemic Theory of Informed Consent in Managed Care, 35 Hous. L. Rev. 1631, 1641, 1658, 1661, 1662, 1679 (1999).*

Journal 1998 Analyzes Hall's book *Making Medical Spending Decisions: The Law, Ethics and Economics of Rationing Mechanisms.* Discusses cost-based rationing for medical services and physician bedside rationing. Concludes that patients should be informed in advance when their physician may receive financial incentives for withholding care. Quotes Opinion 8.13. Agrawal, *Chicago Hope Meets the Chicago School, 96 Mich. L. Rev. 1793, 1804 (1998).*

Journal 1998 Discusses changes in the health care system. Explains why patients need more power in the managed care system. Suggests that patients should use class action suits as a method to assert power over managed care organizations. References Opinions 8.13 and 8.132. Cerminara, *The Class Action Suit as a Method of Patient Empowerment in the Managed Care Setting, 24 Am. J. Law & Med. 7, 16, 17, 23 (1998).*

Journal 1998 Discusses conflicts of interest in the physician-patient relationship arising out of use of financial incentives by managed care organizations. Considers how such conflicts are dealt with in the attorney-client relationship. Suggests that a financial incentive should be legally denounced if it unreasonably interferes with a physician's duty to properly care for and treat patients. Quotes Preamble, Fundamental Elements (1) [now Opinion 10.01], and Opinions 4.04, 5.01, 8.03, 8.13, and 9.06. Cites Fundamental Elements (4) [now Opinion 10.01] and Opinions 2.07, 2.08, and 2.132. Hall, *Third-Party Payor Conflicts of Interest in Managed Care: A Proposal for Regulation Based on the Model Rules of Professional Conduct,* 29 Seton Hall L. Rev. 95, 96, 107, 108, 109, 110, 111, 112, 134, 135, 136 (1998).

Journal 1998 Asserts that managed care organizations assume fiduciary obligations by exercising discretionary control over the administration of an ERISA plan. Argues that ERISA requires managed care organizations and physicians to disclose financial incentives intended to influence physician decision-making. References Opinions 8.13 and 8.132. Johnson, *ERISA Doctor in the House? The Duty to Disclose Physician Incentives to Limit Health Care,* 82 Minn. L. Rev. 1631, 1639, 1649, 1655 (1998).

Journal 1998 Discusses changes in the health care system. Analyzes conflicts of interest arising from the practice of capitation. Argues that physicians should refuse to sign contracts with health care plans offering incentives that may present a temptation to undertreat patients. References Opinion 8.13. Kassirer, *Managing Care—Should We Adopt a New Ethic?* 339 New Eng. J. Med. 397 (1998).

Journal 1998 Expresses concern about the impact of managed care cost-containment practices on the physician-patient relationship. Advocates the need for disclosure of information about these practices to patients. Evaluates and recommends a Maryland law that requires such disclosure. Cites Opinion 8.13. Khanna, Silverman, & Schwartz, *Disclosure of Operating Practices by Managed-Care Organizations to Consumers of Healthcare: Obligations of Informed Consent,* 9 J. Clinical Ethics 291, 293, 296 (1998).

Journal 1998 Discusses quality and safety concerns arising under managed care systems. Explores benefits and detriments of the proposed patients' bill of rights. Advocates legislation to provide safeguards from cost-containment mechanisms utilized by managed care programs. Quotes Opinion 8.13. Misocky, *The Patients' Bill of Rights: Managed Care Under Siege,* 15 J. Contemp. Health L. & Pol'y 57, 73 (1998).

Journal 1998 Explores clinical freedom and the Hippocratic Oath. Discusses issues of patient trust and confidence. Suggests that a sense of confidence will not be present if managerial priorities are dominant factors in resource allocation. References Opinion 8.13. Newdick, *Public Health Ethics and Clinical Freedom,* 14 J. Contemp. Health L. & Pol'y 335, 336, 339, 356, 359, 361 (1998).

Journal 1998 Discusses communication conflicts between physicians and managed care organizations. Describes legal responses to gag provisions imposed by managed care organizations. Assesses the impact of gag practices on physician-patient communication. Quotes Opinion 8.13. Spielman, *After the Gag Episode: Physician Communication in Managed Care Organizations,* 22 Seton Hall Legis. J. 437, 453, 461, 463 (1998).

Journal 1998 Argues that health maintenance organizations (HMOs) do not have an incentive to act reasonably because they are not held accountable under tort law. Points out that the duty to act reasonably is imposed on most of society in order to deter negligence. Advocates imposing the same duty on HMOs. References Opinion 8.13. Wertheimer, *Ockham's Scalpel: A Return to a Reasonableness Standard,* 43 Vill. L. Rev. 321, 327 (1998).

Journal 1997 Discusses the quality of neurological care and the ethical conflicts that are created by the drive to contain costs. Focuses on quality management and cost-containment programs and the conflicts created when neurologists attempt to reconcile the interests of patients and society. References Opinions 8.032 and 8.13. Bernat, *Quality of Neurological Care: Balancing Cost Control and Ethics,* 54 Arch. Neurol. 1341, 1343, 1345 (1997).

Journal 1997 Compares past ethical opinions to current opinions and notes the differences. Comments on the forces that have changed medical ethics through the years. Notes differing theories on the future course of medical ethics. Quotes Fundamental Elements (Preamble) and Opinions 5.05, 5.057, 7.01, 8.12, 9.12, and 9.131. Cites Fundamental Elements (5) and Opinions 8.115 and 8.13. Buchanan, *Medical Ethics at the Millennium: A Brief Retrospective,* 26 Colo. Law. 141, 142, 143, 144, 145 (1997).

Journal 1997 Examines the use of gag clauses in the managed care setting. Explores the conflict of interest between physicians' loyalty to HMOs and their duty to patients. Questions whether patients can give informed consent based on inadequate information. Emphasizes the need for more comprehensive regulation. Quotes Opinion 8.13. Comment, *Physician Gag Clauses—The Hypocrisy of the Hippocratic Oath,* 21 So. Ill. U. L. J. 313, 318, 320 (1997).

Journal 1997 Reviews the conflict between the economics of managed care and physicians' ethical obligations to patients. Questions whether a patient may give informed consent to treatment without knowledge of all available alternatives. Offers a proposal for disclosure of managed care cost-containment mechanisms and incentives to patients. Quotes Opinion 8.13. Hall, *A Theory of Economic Informed Consent,* 31 Ga. L. Rev. 511, 521, 524-25 (1997).

Journal 1997 Posits that cost-containment schemes in managed care systems have eroded the fiduciary duty physicians owe patients. Notes that managed care organizations (MCOs) are prohibiting patients from trusting and relying on physicians. Concludes that patients must seek quality assurance from sources other than their physicians. Quotes

Opinions 2.03, 2.09, and 8.13. Jacobi, *Patients at a Loss: Protecting Health Care Consumers Through Data Driven Quality Assurance, 45 U. Kan. L. Rev. 705, 720, 721, 759 (1997).*

Journal 1997 Explores the responsibilities imposed on physicians by managed care and capitation. Notes that physicians are called on to act as gatekeepers, controlling access to specialty services and tests. Considers whether primary care physicians in capitated groups are satisfied with the quality of care they provide. References Opinion 8.13. Kerr, Hays, Mittman, Siu, Leake, & Brook, *Primary Care Physicians' Satisfaction With Quality of Care in California Capitated Medical Groups, 278 JAMA 308, 312 (1997).*

Journal 1997 Discusses the practice of physician deselection by managed care organizations. Suggests that deselection harms the physician-patient relationship and creates a conflict of interest. Argues that solutions to deselection should consider effects on the patient rather than on the physician. Quotes Principle III. Cites Principle I and Opinions 8.05 and 8.13. Liner, *Physician Deselection: The Dynamics of a New Threat to the* physician-patient *Relationship, 23 Am. J. Law & Med. 511, 513, 527 (1997).*

Journal 1997 Examines national health care reform and managed care. Notes that state regulatory policies in this context evidence common concerns. Suggests ways in which the government can promote patient and physician rights. References Opinion 8.13. Miller, *Managed Care Regulation: In the Laboratory of the States, 278 JAMA 1102, 1104, 1108-09 (1997).*

Journal 1997 Discusses physician frustration with managed care plans caused by gag clauses and cost-containment mechanisms. Reviews the development of managed care organizations and federal attempts at limiting the use of gag clauses. Concludes that gag clauses are inherently flawed and compromise quality health care. Quotes Principles II and V, Fundamental Elements (1), and Opinion 8.13. Note, *Physicians, Bound and Gagged: Federal Attempts to Combat Managed Care's Use of Gag Clauses, 21 Seton Hall Legis. J. 567, 601-02 (1997).*

Journal 1997 Describes gag provisions in managed care contracts. Explains the context in which gag provisions may undermine the physician-patient relationship, as well as the conflicts of interest they may create. Proposes legislation to address these problems. Quotes Opinion 8.13. Note, *Stop Gagging Physicians! 7 Health Matrix 187, 193, 200, 208-09 (1997).*

Journal 1997 Examines the need for change in interpretation of state laws under the saving clause of the Employment Retirement Income Security Act. Discusses any willing provider laws and concludes that they should receive saving clause protection. References Opinion 8.13. Pittman, *Any Willing Provider Laws and ERISA's Saving Clause: A New Solution for an Old Problem, 64 Tenn. L. Rev. 409, 416 (1997).*

Journal 1997 Discusses the need for balance between business ethics and medical ethics in the context of managed care. Explores two models for integrating ethics and managed care. Proposes the adoption of a collective responsibility model to improve quality of care. Quotes Principles I, II, III, IV, and V. Cites Preamble. References Opinion 8.13. Regan, *Regulating the Business of Medicine: Models for Integrating Ethics and Managed Care, 30 Colum. J. L. & Soc. Probs. 635, 651, 656, 657 (1997).*

Journal 1997 Examines utilization review in the managed care context. Discusses a survey of third-party utilization review firms, noting practices that advance and undermine adherence to important professional norms. Quotes Opinion 9.031. References Opinion 8.13. Schlesinger, Gray, & Perreira, *Medical Professionalism Under Managed Care: The Pros and Cons of Utilization Review, 16 Health Affairs 106, 119, 120, 124 (1997).*

Journal 1996 Discusses the use of practice guidelines to improve medical care quality and to aid in decreasing health care costs. Evaluates pertinent ethical considerations. Concludes that, when used appropriately, guidelines have clinical value. References Opinion 8.13. Berger & Rosner, *The Ethics of Practice Guidelines, 156 Arch. Intern. Med. 2051, 2053, 2056 (1996).*

Journal 1996 Considers the economic implications for physicians brought about by the change from traditional fee-for-service care to capitation. Discusses capitation payments in the American health care system. Alludes to pertinent ethical issues. References Opinion 8.13. Bodenheimer & Grumbach, *Capitation or Decapitation: Keeping Your Head in Changing Times, 276 JAMA 1025, 1031 (1996).*

Journal 1996 Examines the business of health care and the ethical implications of managed care. Describes incentives that affect the delivery of health care. Suggests that a redistribution of excess revenues would help both patients and nonprofit hospitals coexist with managed care. Quotes Opinion 8.13. Bond, *Diverse and Perverse Incentives in Managed Care: Where Will the Pendulum Stop? 1 Widener L. Symp. J. 141, 151, 154 (1996).*

Journal 1996 Discusses the trend toward health care reform. Focuses on benefits and problems posed by managed mental health care. Posits that the moral problems of managed mental health care, including quality concerns, are curable. Concludes that managed mental health care may prove superior to fee-for-service care. References Opinion 8.13. Boyle, *Managed Care in Mental Health: A Cure, or a Cure Worse Than the Disease? 40 St. Louis U. L. J. 437, 448 (1996).*

Journal 1996 Discusses the threat managed health care poses to patients and physicians. Explores direct incentives given to physicians by managed care organizations and the impact these incentives have on physician behavior. Proposes possible methods for dealing with the problems that such incentives create. References Opinion 8.13. Greely, *Direct Financial Incentives in Managed Care: Unanswered Questions, 6 Health Matrix 53, 81 (1996).*

Journal 1996 Discusses the change from fee-for-service health care financing to managed care. Notes that cost-containment mechanisms modify physicians' behaviors and patients' access to health care. Emphasizes that physicians must remain committed to following ethical guidelines. References Opinion 8.13. Hammes & Webster, *Professional Ethics and Managed Care in Dermatology, 132 Arch. Dermatol. 1070, 1072, 1073 (1996).*

Journal 1996 Discusses workers' compensation and the medical care provided to injured employees. Examines the effect of managed care on workers' compensation. Advocates focusing on prevention of injuries and quality of care. References Opinion 8.13. Hashimoto, *The Future Role of Managed Care and Capitation in Workers' Compensation, XXII Am. J. Law & Med. 233, 258, 259 (1996).*

Journal 1996 Considers challenges to the psychiatrist-patient relationship that are triggered by managed care cost-containment methodologies. Offers guidance to psychiatrists for addressing these challenges. References Opinions 2.095, 8.13, and 8.132. Hoge, *APA Resource Document: I. The Professional Responsibilities of Psychiatrists in Evolving Health Care Systems, 24 Bull. Am. Acad. Psychiatry Law 393, 405 (1996).*

Journal 1996 Discusses the problems managed care raises within the framework of the physician-patient relationship. Considers issues specific to psychiatry. Advocates legal regulation to improve upon and bring structural change to managed care systems. Cites Opinion 8.13. Hoge, *APA Resource Document: II. Regulatory Guidelines for Protecting the Interests of Psychiatric Patients in Emerging Health Care Systems, 24 Bull. Am. Acad. Psychiatry Law 407, 412, 418 (1996).*

Journal 1996 Considers procedural issues relative to patient protection in the context of capitated health care plans. Examines regulations governing capitated health plans and consumer protection issues. Offers suggestions regarding policy making, rate setting, dispute resolution, and judicial review. References Opinion 8.13. Kinney, *Procedural Protections for Patients in Capitated Health Plans, XXII Am. J. Law & Med. 301, 319-20 (1996).*

Journal 1996 Explains the conflict between managed care, which focuses on controlling costs, and traditional health care values, which focus on patient autonomy. Proposes a solution to this conflict requiring that patients incur certain economic consequences in obtaining health care and that managed care organizations disclose resource management techniques. References Opinion 8.13. Morreim, *Diverse and Perverse Incentives of Managed Care: Bringing Patients Into Alignment, 1 Widener L. Symp. J. 89, 129 (1996).*

Journal 1996 Discusses efforts to reduce health care costs. Considers whether personal financial incentives given to physicians decrease level of care given to patients. Suggests that, while financial incentives may create ethical concerns, they serve an important function by containing costs.

Concludes that efforts to eliminate them completely are misguided. References Opinion 8.13. Orentlicher, *Paying Physicians More to Do Less: Financial Incentives to Limit Care, 30 U. Rich. L. Rev. 155, 167 (1996).*

Cal. App. 2002 State agency appealed a writ of mandamus requiring it to approve managed care plan's proposed amendment to discontinue coverage of sexual dysfunction prescription drugs. Agency based its authority to disapprove on a statute empowering it to regulate health plan prescription drug coverage. California Court of Appeals affirmed. The court held that the agency exceeded its statutory authority. References Opinion 8.135 regarding managed care drug formulary systems. *Kaiser Foundation Health Plan, Inc. v. Zingale, 99 Cal. App. 4th 1018, 121 Cal. Rptr. 2d 741, 746.*

Journal 2006 Discusses preemption of lawsuits against managed care organizations by the Employee Retirement Income Security Act of 1974 (ERISA). Proposes a "bifurcated legal regime" to decrease the protective scope of ERISA. Quotes Opinions 8.053 and 8.135. Madison, *ERISA and Liability for Provision of Medical Information, 84 N. C. L. Rev. 471, 540 (2006).*

Journal 2000 Describes the American formulary system and the economic efficiencies that can be realized when physicians comply. Describes how the formulary system fits into and underlies health care electronic data interchange. Concludes that congressional action is needed to fully extend the formulary system to Medicaid programs in all 50 states. References Opinion 8.135. Buckles, *Electronic Formulary Management and Medicaid: Maximizing Economic Efficiency and Quality of Care in the Age of Electronic Prescribing, 11 U. Fla. J. L. & Pub. Pol'y 179, 182-83 (2000).*

1st Cir. 1984 Plaintiff-physicians sued defendant-insurer, alleging defendant's ban on balance billing practice violated antitrust law. That practice required defendant to pay the physicians treating defendant's insureds only if the physicians agreed not to make any additional charges to the insureds. In holding that defendant's billing practice did not violate antitrust law, the court noted in passing a 1954 law journal article that cited, with an incorrect reference, Principles Ch. III, Art. VI, Sec. 3 (1947) in arguing that selling services to third parties might interfere with the absolute ethical obligation that a doctor owes to the patient. The specific concept treated by this Principle is no longer directly treated although Opinion 8.05 reflects similar concerns. *Kartell v. Blue Shield of Mass., Inc., 749 F.2d 922, 926, cert. denied, 471 US 1029 (1985).*

2d Cir. 1980 Federal Trade Commission ordered AMA and others to cease, with some exceptions, imposing restraints on advertising and contract practice by physicians, as well as on business relations between physicians and laypersons. Commission found restraints violated 15 USC § 45(a)(1). See 94 FTC 701 (1979). AMA petitioned for judicial review of Commission's order. Court reviewed order, noting specific ethical pronouncements of AMA which Commission found improper, including the following: restrictions upon advertising and solicitation, Principle 5 (1957) and Opinions and Reports of the Judicial Council Sec. 5, Para. 11 (1971) [now Opinion 5.02]; restrictions on contract practice, Principle 6 (1957) and Opinions and Reports of the Judicial Council Sec. 6, Paras. 3, 4, and 5 (1971) [now Opinion 8.05]; and restrictions on business organizations and relations with laypersons, Opinions and Reports of the Judicial Council Sec. 6, Paras. 14 and 15 (1971). Court rejected AMA's argument that its ethical rules did not provide impetus for local and state medical societies to act against physicians violating its rules. Further, court rejected AMA's position that liability should be precluded because of revisions in the Opinions in 1977 and the Principles in 1980. Specifically, the court found that removal of the ban on patient solicitation and changes reflected in Principles II and IV (1980) did not render Commission's order moot. The order was therefore enforced with modifications. Dissenting judge, referring to 1980 revisions in Principles and to Opinions and Reports of the Judicial Council 4.05 and 6.00 (1977) [now Opinions 5.02 and 8.05], concluded order should not be enforced on grounds of mootness. *American Medical Ass'n v. FTC, 638 F.2d 443, 446, 446 n.1, 448, 449, 449 n.5, 450, 451, 455-57, aff'd, 455 US 676 (1982).*

7th Cir. 1984 Plaintiff brought medical malpractice suit against several physicians appointed to the Veterans Administration Department of Medicine and Surgery. The court held that strict control test for determining whether defendants ought to be considered employees or independent contractors under the Federal Tort Claims Act was not appropriate because the ethical obligation of a physician to a patient, evidenced by Principle 6 (1957) [now Opinions 8.03 and 8.05], required that independent judgment be exercised, preventing a physician from being strictly controlled by the Veterans Administration. *Quilico v. Kaplan, 749 F.2d 480, 483-84.*

10th Cir. 1983 Pursuant to the Federal Tort Claims Act, plaintiff sued the federal government for the negligence of a neurosurgeon, allegedly an employee of a Veteran's Administration (VA) hospital. Plaintiff argued that applying the traditional control test to determine a physician's employment status was inappropriate because physicians are bound by Principle 6 (1957) [now Opinions 8.03 and 8.05] requiring them to have free and complete exercise of [their] medical judgment and skill. However, the court did not reach the merits of that argument because the contractual agreement between the neurosurgeon and the VA hospital was outside the parameters of an employer-employee relationship with the government, thus precluding plaintiff's claim. *Lurch v. United States, 719 F.2d 333, 337, cert. denied, 466 US 927 (1984).*

D.C. Cir. 1942 Medical associations appealed conviction on charges of conspiracy to restrain trade or commerce where associations attempted to prevent competition by elimination of prepaid, low-cost medical and hospital care. Principles Ch. III, Art. VI, Secs. 2 and 3 [now Opinion 8.05] limiting

contract practice had been used as a basis to discipline members of medical association employed by prepaid medical organization. The court held that the associations were subject to the Sherman Antitrust Act and that the evidence sustained the conviction. *American Medical Ass'n v. United States, 130 F.2d 233, 238-239 n.23, aff'd, 317 US 519 (1943).*

N.D. Ill. 2008 Administrator of the estate of patient filed suit under the Federal Tort Claims Act and state wrongful death act after patient died as a result of a mistake during surgery at Veteran's Administration hospital. Defendant physician moved to dismiss on the grounds that, as a federal employee, she was exempt from personal liability for services performed within the scope of her employment at the VA. The court cited earlier case quoting Principle 6 (1957) [now Opinions 8.03 and 8.05] and determining that, because physicians are free to choose whom to serve, they are not federal employees and the strict control test may not be appropriate. Finding issues of fact to resolve, the court denied the defendant's motion for summary judgment. *Monroe v. United States, 2008 U.S. Dist. LEXIS 22455, 9.*

Miss. 2003 Patient's estate appealed summary judgment in favor of physician and hospital in wrongful death action. Supreme Court affirmed, holding that physician was a state employee and that purchase of liability insurance did not waive immunity. In examining physician's status, the court found that the exercise of professional judgment and discretion are not determinative of employment status. Quotes Principle 6 (1957) [now Opinions 8.03 and 8.05]. *Corey v. Skelton, 834 So.2d 681, 685.*

Miss. 2002 Plaintiff in malpractice action appealed grant of summary judgment in favor of neurosurgeon who allegedly performed a thoracic diskectomy on the wrong disk. A resident performed the patient's physical and wrote the majority of the chart notes. The Mississippi Supreme Court affirmed the lower court. The court held that as a state employee the physician was immune from liability and that his exercise of professional judgment in treating patients did not change his status and insurance did not waive immunity. Quotes Principle 6 (1957) [now Opinions 8.03 and 8.05]. *Clayton v. Harkey, 826 So.2d 1283, 1287.*

Miss. 2001 Patient filed suit asserting that a physician was negligent in performing surgery. The trial court granted the physician's summary judgment motion and held that the physician, employed by a state university medical center, was immune under state law. Finding genuine issues of fact, the state Supreme Court reversed and remanded the case for further proceedings. In a separate opinion, one justice quoted Principle 6 (1957) [now Opinions 8.03 and 8.05], in evaluating the degree of control exercised by the state over the physician. This justice, stressing that the physician exercised discretion in treating the patient independent of the state's control, found no basis to hold the physician an employee for immunity purposes. *Conley v. Warren, 797 So. 2d 881, 886.*

Miss. 2000 Beneficiaries of patient's estate appealed summary judgment in malpractice action for a physician on sovereign immunity grounds. The court reversed and remanded the case finding issues of fact to be resolved at trial. The majority set out a five-part test to determine the employment status of a physician working at a state health care facility, including the degree of control and direction exercised by the state over the physician. In a separate opinion one justice quoted Principle 6 (1957) [now Opinions 8.03 and 8.05], stating that, "A physician should not dispose of his services under terms or conditions which tend to interfere with or impair the free and complete exercise of his medical judgment and skill. . . ." This justice reasoned that the physician could not claim the state controlled his medical discretion or treatment of patients and thus was clearly not an employee entitled to immunity. *Miller v. Meeks, 762 So. 2d 302, 314.*

Miss. 2000 Patient brought a medical malpractice action against physicians after receiving treatment at a state university medical center. The jury returned a verdict against the physicians. The Mississippi Supreme Court reversed, finding that the physicians were immune from liability as state employees. In determining the status of the physicians, the court noted that the physicians retained a considerable amount of professional discretion in treating the patient, quoting Principle 6 (1957) [now Opinions 8.03 and 8.05]. However, this alone was not determinative, and in the court's view the physicians were state employees. *Sullivan v. Washington, 768 So. 2d 881, 885.*

Miss. App. 2003 Patient brought malpractice action against physicians working at a state university teaching hospital. Patient argued that the physicians were independent contractors and sovereign immunity did not apply. Appellate court, citing the Mississippi Supreme Court's decision in *Miller v. Mecks*, 762 So.2d 302 (Miss. 2000), affirmed the trial court and held that sovereign immunity applied because the physicians were state employees. Quotes Principle 6 (1957) [now Opinions 8.03 and 8.05]. *Brown v. Warren, 858 So.2d 168, 175 (2003).*

Wash. 1951 Plaintiff, a charitable, not-for-profit medical corporation, offered prepaid health care services to members and their families. Suit was filed against county medical society and others for damages and injunction for defendants' alleged efforts to monopolize prepaid medical care in area and unlawfully restrain competition by plaintiff and its physicians. Defendants alleged as affirmative defense that their efforts were designed to curb unethical prepaid contract practice by plaintiff. Court examined at length AMA's position regarding contract practice including Principles Ch. III, Art. VI, Secs. 3 and 4 (1947) [now Principle VI and Opinions 8.05 and 9.06] concluding nothing in plaintiff's practice violated the AMA's ethical guidelines. Further, quoting Principles Ch. III, Art. III, Sec. 1 (1947) [now Opinion 8.04] dealing with consultations, court noted that defendants' efforts impeded plaintiff's physicians from obtaining consultations. Court concluded defendants' actions constituted unlawful, monopolistic behavior and issued an injunction, although it declined to award damages. *Group Health Coop. v. King County Medical Soc'y, 39 Wash. 2d 586, 237 P.2d 737, 744, 750-51, 759-60.*

Journal 2007 Reviews the legal and ethical problems surrounding concierge medical practice. Concludes that concierge medicine should remain restricted to a small class of wealthy individuals. Cites Opinions 8.05, 8.055, 8.115, 9.06, and 9.065. Carnahan, *Concierge Medicine: Legal and Ethical Issues, 35 J. L. Med. & Ethics 211, 212-13 (2007).*

Journal 2004 Discusses the concept of medical necessity and its effect on the health care system. Concludes that issues regarding medical necessity must be dealt with to achieve meaningful health care reform. Quotes Opinion 8.05. Blanchard, *"Medical Necessity" Determinations—A Continuing Healthcare Policy Problem, 37 J. Health L. 599, 620 (2004).*

Journal 2000 Examines physician value neutrality (PVN). Defines PVN as providing a foundation to suggest physicians must keep their values—religious, political, or otherwise—out of the patient-physician relationship. Concludes it is not clear how values can be removed from the patient-physician relationship without removing the very thing PVN supporters are trying to protect, the intrinsic value of persons. References Opinions 2.01, 2.02, 8.032, 8.05, 8.08, and 8.132. Beckwith & Peppin, *Physician Value Neutrality: A Critique, 28 J. L. Med. & Ethics 67, 72-73 (2000).*

1st. Cir. 2008 Trial court granted summary judgment for orthopedic surgeon in suit brought against manufacturer of orthopedic implant devices for breach of contract and violations of state consumer protection statutes. On appeal, the surgeon submitted an affidavit from a medical ethics expert that cited Opinion 8.0501, declaring that the payment of kickbacks from a medical device manufacturer to a physician is unethical. The appeals court held that the manufacturer breached the contract by halting royalty payments to the physician. *Jasty v. Wright Medical Technology, Inc., 528 F.3d 28, 38, n. 12.*

Journal 2010 Examines legal and ethical issues confronting medical-legal partnerships, as well as the benefits and challenges of such partnerships. Concludes that as long as critical professional obligations are recognized and ethical boundaries are maintained, medical and legal professionals can collaborate without compromising professional duties or ethical goals. Quotes Opinion 8.0501. Boumil, Freitas, & Freitas, *Multidisciplinary Representation of Patients: The Potential for Ethical Issues and Professional Duty Conflicts in the Medical-Legal Partnership Model, 13 J. Health Care L. & Pol'y 107, 124 (2010).*

Journal 2006 Examines ethical dilemmas physicians may face as providers of pay-for-performance medical care. Concludes that this strategy offers a benefit to patients as long as physicians uphold stringent ethical standards and work together to ensure optimum patient care. Cites Principles I, V, VIII, and IX and Opinions 2.035, 2.095, 6.01,

8.021, 8.03, 8.0501, 8.053, 8.054, and 8.121. Bostick, Sade, & McMahon, *Report of the Council on Ethical and Judicial Affairs: Physician Pay-for-Performance Programs, 3 Ind. Health L. Rev. 429, 430, 431, 432-33, 434, 435, 436 (2006).*

Journal 2003 Discusses conflicts of interest caused when managed care organizations provide financial incentives to physicians. Concludes that the focus of managed care is not well-suited for the doctor-patient relationship. Quotes Opinion 8.03. Cites Principle VII. References Opinion 8.051. Hall, *Bargaining With Hippocrates: Managed Care and the Doctor-Patient Relationship, 54 S. C. L. Rev. 689, 696, 735 (2003).*

Journal 2008 Explores the tension experienced by health care professionals who provide care and compete in a market economy. Concludes if health care professions continue commercializing, providers must strive to maintain ethical standards and appropriate professional-patient relationships. Quotes Opinion 8.054. Peltier & Guisti, *Commerce and Care: The Irreconcilable Tension Between Selling and Caring, 39 McGeorge L. Rev. 785, 794 (2008).*

Journal 2006 Discusses the evolution of health law in Virginia. Concludes that the area of health law continues to expand, develop, and be refined. Cites Opinions 3.03, 3.08, 5.01, 5.015, 5.02, 5.04, 5.055, 6.02, 6.021, 6.03, 6.04, 7.03, 7.04, 7.05, 8.054, 8.08, 8.081, 8.085, 8.115, 8.12, 8.14, 8.145, 8.19, and 9.045. Guanzon, *Health Care Law, 41 U. Rich. L. Rev. 179, 199 (2006).*

Journal 2002 Examines how managed care has adversely affected information disclosure in the physician-patient relationship. Concludes that, unless courts expand applicability of principles of informed consent, patient self-determination and autonomy will continue to be undermined. Quotes Principle VIII and Opinions 8.03, 8.053, 8.054, and 8.08. Morris, *Dissing Disclosure: Just What the Doctor Ordered, 44 Ariz. L. Rev. 313, 344, 349, 362, 363, 366 (2002).*

Journal 2006 Scrutinizes the benefits of pay-for-performance financial incentives. Concludes that such incentives will not alleviate the need for health insurance. Cites Opinion 6.01. References Opinion 8.056. Sage & Kalyan, *Horses or Unicorns: Can Paying for Performance Make Quality Competition Routine? 31 J. Health Pol. Pol'y & L. 531, 531-32, 554 (2006).*

11.2.2 Conflicts of Interest in Patient Care

Journal 2003 Discusses the practice of gainsharing and argues that providing physicians and hospitals with certain financial incentives to reduce health costs may be of value in health care reform. Concludes with suggestions for how best to proceed in this difficult context. Quotes Opinions 2.03, 2.09, 4.04, and 8.03. References Opinion 8.13. Saver, *Squandering the Gain: Gainsharing and the Continuing Dilemma of Physician Financial Incentives, 98 Nw. U. L. Rev. 145, 219, 221, 222 (2003).*

Journal 1999 Discusses the need for physicians to advocate on behalf of patients' rights in the context of health care delivery. Evaluates the nature and scope of the physician's role as advocate, noting that physicians cannot be expected to engage in attorney-like advocacy. Quotes Principles IV and VI, Fundamental Elements (2), (4), and (6) [now Opinion 10.01], Patient Responsibilities 5 [now Opinion 10.02], and Opinions 2.03, 2.07, 2.09, 2.16, 2.19, 3.06, 4.01, 4.04, 6.01, 7.02, 8.02, 8.03, 8.13, 8.132, 9.06, 9.07, and 9.131. Cites Opinions 5.05, 5.09, 7.01, 8.135, and 9.02. Sage, *Physicians as Advocates, 35 Hous. L. Rev. 1529, 1537, 1541, 1542, 1552-53, 1554, 1556, 1557, 1559, 1561-62, 1564, 1571, 1574, 1576, 1580 (1999).*

Journal 1998 Discusses conflicts of interest in the physician-patient relationship arising out of use of financial incentives by managed care organizations. Considers how such conflicts are dealt with in the attorney-client relationship. Suggests that a financial incentive should be legally denounced if it unreasonably interferes with a physician's duty to properly care for and treat patients. Quotes Preamble,

Fundamental Elements (1) [now Opinion 10.01] and Opinions 4.04, 5.01, 8.03, 8.13, and 9.06. Cites Fundamental Elements (4) [now Opinion 10.01], and Opinions 2.07, 2.08, and 2.132. Hall, *Third-Party Payor Conflicts of Interest in Managed Care: A Proposal for Regulation Based on the Model Rules of Professional Conduct, 29 Seton Hall L. Rev. 95, 96, 107, 108, 109, 110, 111, 112, 134, 135, 136 (1998).*

Journal 1996 Considers the change from traditional medical care systems to managed care, noting the conflicts of interest this creates between physicians' ethical obligations and financial concerns. Discusses these issues in the context of managed behavioral health care. Suggests community-based care and social supports as a solution. Quotes Opinions 2.03 and 4.04. Petrila, *Ethics, Money, and the Problem of Coercion in Managed Behavioral Health Care, 40 St. Louis U. L. J. 359, 377 (1996).*

Journal 1994 Observes that health care reform proposals present significant challenges to the role and ethics of attending physicians. Emphasizes that reform proposals must set forth the role envisioned for physicians and must articulate an acceptable ethical framework within which physicians may fulfill that role. Quotes Opinions 4.04, 9.121, and 9.122. Cites Opinions 2.03, 2.09, 5.01, and 8.03. Wolf, *Health Care Reform and the Future of Physician Ethics, 24 Hastings Center Rep. 28, 32, 40 (March/April 1994).*

Journal 1993 Discusses the problem of physicians withholding needed medical treatment from HIV-infected infants. Concludes that current law should be expanded to eliminate this discrimination. Quotes Opinions 2.09, 2.17, 2.20, 2.22, 4.04, and 8.03. Crossley, *Of Diagnoses and Discrimination: Discriminatory Nontreatment of Infants With HIV Infection, 93 Columbia L. Rev. 1581, 1620, 1621 (1993).*

Journal 1992 Examines the major health care rationing issues facing the US including increasing costs and decreasing access. Concludes that the standard of care should not be changed and that rationing should be a separate enterprise undertaken pursuant to explicit criteria. Quotes Opinions 2.03, 2.09, and 4.04. Hirshfeld, *Should Ethical and Legal Standards for Physicians Be Changed to Accommodate New Models for Rationing Health Care? 140 Univ. Pa. L. Rev. 1809, 1816 (1992).*

Journal 1990 Discusses efforts of third-party payers to control health care expenditures for beneficiaries. Concludes that financial incentives to limit care and other cost-control techniques should be disclosed and that the rationale for such disclosure is compelling. Quotes Opinions 2.03, 2.09, and 8.03. Cites Opinions 2.19, 4.04, and 4.06. Hirshfeld, *Should Third Party Payors of Health Care Services Disclose Cost Control Mechanisms to Potential Beneficiaries? 14 Seton Hall Legis. J. 115, 130, 131, 144, 145, 146 (1990).*

7th Cir. 1984 Plaintiff brought medical malpractice suit against several physicians appointed to the Veterans Administration Department of Medicine and Surgery. The court held that strict control test for determining whether defendants ought to be considered employees or independent contractors under the Federal Tort Claims Act was not appropriate because the ethical obligation of a physician to a patient, evidenced by Principle 6 (1957) [now Opinions 8.03 and 8.05], required that independent judgment be exercised, preventing a physician from being strictly controlled by the Veterans Administration. *Quilico v. Kaplan, 749 F.2d 480, 483-84.*

10th Cir. 1983 Pursuant to the Federal Tort Claims Act, plaintiff sued the federal government for the negligence of a neurosurgeon, allegedly an employee of a Veteran's Administration (VA) hospital. Plaintiff argued that applying the traditional control test to determine a physician's employment status was inappropriate because physicians are bound by Principle 6 (1957) [now Opinions 8.03 and 8.05] requiring them to have free and complete exercise of medical judgment and skill. However, the court did not reach the merits of that argument because the contractual agreement between the neurosurgeon and the VA hospital was outside the parameters of an employer-employee relationship with the government, thus precluding plaintiff's claim. *Lurch v. United States, 719 F.2d 333, 337, cert. denied, 466 US 927 (1984).*

N.D. Ill. 2010 Sister of deceased patient brought adversary proceeding against bankrupt physician to except from discharge debt stemming from physician's alleged breach of fiduciary duties. The bankruptcy court quotes Opinions 7.01 and 8.03 in finding that a fiduciary duty was established by

nature of the physician-patient relationship that continued after patient's death. *In re Odeh, 431 B.R. 807, 814.*

N.D. Ill. 2008 Administrator of the estate of patient filed suit under the Federal Tort Claims Act and state wrongful death act after patient died as a result of a mistake during surgery at Veteran's Administration (VA) hospital. Defendant physician moved to dismiss on the grounds that, as a federal employee, she was exempt from personal liability for services performed within the scope of her employment at the VA. The court cited earlier case quoting Principle 6 (1957) [now Opinions 8.03 and 8.05] and determining that, because physicians are free to choose whom to serve, they are not federal employees and the strict control test may not be appropriate. Finding issues of fact to resolve, the court denied the defendant's motion for summary judgment. *Monroe v. United States, 2008 U.S. Dist. LEXIS 22455, 9.*

Army Crim. App. 2004 Appellant, in a general court martial hearing, was found guilty of unpremeditated murder. The Court of Appeals for the Armed Forces set aside and remanded the judgment to the Army Court of Criminal Appeals to determine whether there was a conflict of interest in allowing mental health providers who had a prior psychotherapist-patient relationship with the appellant to serve on his sanity board. The court determined there was no conflict of interest. In making this determination, the court quoted Opinion 10.015 and cited Opinion 8.03 to analyze the aspects of the physician-patient relationship. *United States v. Best, 59 M.J. 886, 891 n. 8.*

Cal. App. 1967 Physician-stockholders of publicly owned pharmaceutical corporations and physicians whose medical partnerships owned and operated pharmacies challenged statutory prohibition of physician membership, proprietory interest, and co-ownership of pharmacies. The court quoted Principles Ch. I, Sec. 6 (1947), and a 1960 Judicial Council rule, later included in Opinions and Reports of the Judicial Council Sec. 7, Para. 38 (1965) [now Opinions 8.03, 8.032, and 8.06], in its discussion of the potential conflict of interest created by such ownership. The court held that the statute prohibited physician partnerships from directly owning pharmacies but did not apply to an individual physician or a partnership of physicians who own stock in a corporation which owns and operates a pharmacy. *Magan Medical Clinic v. California State Bd. of Medical Examiners, 249 Cal. App. 2d 124, 57 Cal. Rptr. 256, 262.*

Mich. Att'y Gen. 1977 State attorney general determined that, within limits, it was not illegal for physicians to refer patient specimens to clinical laboratories which they own or in which they have a financial interest. Opinion observes, however, that, under the Opinions and Reports of the Judicial Council Sec. 7, Paras. 21 and 22 (1972) [now Opinions 8.03 and 8.032], such referrals may be unethical. *Mich. Att'y Gen. Opinion No. 5229, 1977-78 Att'y Gen. Op. 234.*

Miss. 2003 Patient's estate appealed summary judgment in favor of physician and hospital in wrongful death action. Supreme Court affirmed, holding that physician was a state employee and that purchase of liability insurance did not waive immunity. In examining physician's status, the court found that the exercise of professional judgment and discretion are not determinative of employment status. Quotes Principle 6 (1957) [now Opinions 8.03 and 8.05]. *Corey v. Skelton, 834 So.2d 681, 685.*

Miss. 2002 Plaintiff in malpractice action appealed grant of summary judgment in favor of neurosurgeon who allegedly performed a thoracic diskectomy on the wrong disk. A resident performed the patient's physical and wrote the majority of the chart notes. The Mississippi Supreme Court affirmed the lower court. The court held that as a state employee the physician was immune from liability and that his exercise of professional judgment in treating patients did not change his status and insurance did not waive immunity. Quotes Principle 6 (1957) [now Opinions 8.03 and 8.05]. *Clayton v. Harkey, 826 So.2d 1283, 1287.*

Miss. 2001 Patient filed suit asserting that a physician was negligent in performing surgery. The trial court granted the physician's summary judgment motion and held that the physician, employed by a state university medical center, was immune under state law. Finding genuine issues of fact, the state Supreme Court reversed and remanded the case for further proceedings. In a separate opinion, one justice quoted Principle 6 (1957) [now Opinions 8.03 and 8.05], in evaluating the degree of control exercised by the state over the physician. This justice, stressing that the physician exercised discretion in treating the patient independent of the state's control, found no basis to hold the physician an employee for immunity purposes. *Conley v. Warren, 797 So. 2d 881, 886.*

Miss. 2000 Beneficiaries of patient's estate appealed summary judgment in malpractice action for a physician on sovereign immunity grounds. The court reversed and remanded the case finding issues of fact to be resolved at trial. The majority set out a five-part test to determine the employment status of a physician working at a state health care facility, including the degree of control and direction exercised by the state over the physician. In a separate opinion one justice quoted Principle 6 (1957) [now Opinions 8.03 and 8.05], stating that, "A physician should not dispose of his services under terms or conditions which tend to interfere with or impair the free and complete exercise of his medical judgment and skill. . . ." This justice reasoned that the physician could not claim the state controlled his medical discretion or treatment of patients and thus was clearly not an employee entitled to immunity. *Miller v. Meeks, 762 So. 2d 302, 314.*

Miss. 2000 Patient brought a medical malpractice action against physicians after receiving treatment at a state university medical center. The jury returned a verdict against the physicians. The Mississippi Supreme Court reversed, finding that the physicians were immune from liability as state employees. In determining the status of the physicians, the court noted that the physicians retained a considerable amount of professional discretion in treating the patient, quoting Principle 6 (1957) [now Opinions 8.03 and 8.05]. However, this alone was not determinative, and in the court's view the physicians were state employees. *Sullivan v. Washington, 768 So. 2d 881, 885.*

Miss. App. 2003 Patient brought malpractice action against physicians working at a state university teaching hospital. Patient argued that the physicians were independent contractors and sovereign immunity did not apply. Appellate court, citing the Mississippi Supreme Court's decision in *Miller v. Mecks*, 762 So.2d 302 (Miss. 2000), affirmed the trial court and held that sovereign immunity applied because the physicians were state employees. Quotes Principle 6 (1957) [now Opinions 8.03 and 8.05]. *Brown v. Warren, 858 So.2d 168, 175 (2003).*

Ohio Att'y Gen. 1999 State attorney general concluded that physicians who render opinions regarding the necessity of medical services for health insuring corporations are not engaged in the practice of medicine. Additionally, physicians who render opinions regarding medical necessity for appeals of adverse determinations do not fall under the regulatory, investigatory, or enforcement authority of the Ohio State Medical Board. Quoting Opinions 8.03, 8.11, and 8.13, the attorney general stated that physicians have an ethical duty to provide appropriate treatment for patients. *Ohio Att'y Gen. Op. No. 99-044, 1999 WL 692623.*

Journal 2009 Explores the nature of the physician-patient relationship and the impact of increased availability of medical information on patient autonomy and physician responsibility to exercise independent judgment. Concludes physicians must treat patients in accordance with their fiduciary obligation to use their own judgment when confronted with a patient demanding unnecessary medical services. Quotes Preamble, Principles I and VIII, and Opinions 2.035, 8.03, and 10.015. Hafemeister, *The Fiduciary Obligation of Physicians to "Just Say No" if an "Informed" Patient Demands Services That Are Not Medically Indicated, 39 Seton Hall L. Rev. 335, 372, 373, 374 (2009).*

Journal 2007 Analyzes scientific, ethical, and legal issues raised in the exhumation and genetic analysis of historical figures. Concludes that biohistorical review boards should be created to generate guidelines for such research. Quotes Preamble and Opinion 2.08. Cites Opinions 2.079, 2.105, 5.05, 5.051, 5.075, 8.03, 8.031, 9.095, and 9.10. Paradise & Andrews, *Tales From the Crypt: Scientific, Ethical, and Legal Considerations for Biohistorical Analysis of Deceased Historical Figures, 26 Temp. J. Sci. Tech. & Envtl. L. 223, 287-88 (2007).*

Journal 2006 Examines ethical dilemmas physicians may face as providers of pay-for-performance medical care. Concludes that this strategy offers a benefit to patients as long as physicians uphold stringent ethical standards and work together to ensure optimum patient care. Cites

Principles I, V, VIII, and IX and Opinions 2.035, 2.095, 6.01, 8.021, 8.03, 8.0501, 8.053, 8.054, and 8.121. Bostick, Sade, & McMahon, *Report of the Council on Ethical and Judicial Affairs: Physician Pay-for-Performance Programs, 3 Ind. Health L. Rev. 429, 430, 431, 432-33, 434, 435, 436 (2006).*

Journal 2006 Discusses the prevalence and cause of physicians' failure to provide proper care. Concludes that patients should be able to sue their physicians for breach of fiduciary duty. Quotes Principle VIII and Opinion 8.03. Mehlman, *Dishonest Medical Mistakes, 59 Vand. L. Rev. 1137, 1144 (2006).*

Journal 2003 Discusses conflicts of interest caused when managed care organizations provide financial incentives to physicians. Concludes that the focus of managed care is not well-suited for the doctor-patient relationship. Quotes Opinion 8.03. Cites Principle VII. References Opinion 8.051. Hall, *Bargaining With Hippocrates: Managed Care and the Doctor-Patient Relationship, 54 S. C. L. Rev. 689, 696, 735 (2003).*

Journal 2002 Examines how managed care has adversely affected information disclosure in the physician-patient relationship. Concludes that, unless courts expand applicability of principles of informed consent, patient self-determination and autonomy will continue to be undermined. Quotes Principle VIII and Opinions 8.03, 8.053, 8.054, and 8.08. Morris, *Dissing Disclosure: Just What the Doctor Ordered, 44 Ariz. L. Rev. 313, 344, 349, 362, 363, 366 (2002).*

Journal 2001 Considers conflicts of interest in clinical research and other types of medical practice. Compares the way in which doctors and lawyers address conflicts of interest in professional practice. Concludes that physicians are unaware of the need to create a meaningful conflict-of-interest doctrine for medical practice. Quotes Preamble, Principle IV, and Opinions 2.07, 8.03, 8.031, and 10.01. Moore, *What Doctors Can Learn From Lawyers About Conflicts of Interest, 81 B. U. L. Rev. 445, 447, 449-50 (2001).*

Journal 2001 Examines financial conflict of interest issues that arise in the context of clinical research. Concludes that open communication among stakeholders is necessary to resolve these issues. Quotes Opinions 8.03 and 8.031. Rose, *Financial Conflicts of Interest: How Are We Managing? 8 Wid. L. Symp. J. 1, 24 (2001).*

Journal 2000 Discusses patent law and policy. Examines whether those who practice medicine should be excused from patent laws because of the conflict that medical procedure patents create with respect to the practice of medicine. Concludes that Congress should repeal section 287(c) of the Patent Act. Quotes Principle V and Opinions 9.08 and 9.09. Cites Opinion 8.03. References Opinion 10.01. Ho, *Patents, Patients, and Public Policy: An Incomplete Intersection at 35 USC § 287(c), 33 U. C. Davis L. Rev. 601, 603, 623, 624, 625, 631 (2000).*

Journal 2000 Examines issues relating to parental consent to circumcision. Identifies legal and ethical requirements for consent when medical professionals are treating adult patients. Analyzes the implications of those requirements for routine circumcision of infant males. Concludes that only when the male is an adult and capable of making decisions can circumcision be ethically and legally performed. Quotes Opinion 8.08. References Opinions 8.03 and 9.011. Svoboda, Van Howe, & Dwyer, *Informed Consent for Neonatal Circumcision: An Ethical and Legal Conundrum, 17 J. Contemp. Health L. & Pol'y 61, 67, 73, 82 (2000).*

Journal 1999 Asserts that patient autonomy is closely linked to patient-doctor discourse. Proposes a constitutional framework for evaluating how governmental regulations may interfere with such discourse. Concludes by emphasizing the importance of protecting the quality of doctor-patient discourse. Quotes Preamble and Opinion 8.03. Gatter, *Protecting Patient-Doctor Discourse: Informed Consent and Deliberative Autonomy, 78 Or. L. Rev. 941, 956 (1999).*

Journal 1999 Explores ethical and legal issues surrounding physician incentives in managed care. Concludes that successful ERISA claims for breach of fiduciary duty will hold managed care organizations accountable for controlling medical costs. Quotes Opinion 8.03. Marsh, *Sacrificing Patients for Profits: Physician Incentives to Limit Care and ERISA Fiduciary Duty, 77 Wash. U. L. Q. 1323, 1332 (1999).*

Journal 1999 Explores the impact managed care organizations have had on health care. Explains that patients may not understand restrictions and incentives imposed by their managed care organizations when entering the program. Argues that such information should be disclosed at various times during the period of plan coverage. Cites Opinions 2.03, 8.03, 8.032, 8.051, 8.13, and 8.132. Wolf, *Toward a Systemic Theory of Informed Consent in Managed Care, 35 Hous. L. Rev. 1631, 1641, 1658, 1661, 1662, 1679 (1999).*

Journal 1998 Discusses the physician's fiduciary duty to the patient. Explores the expansion of the "honest services" mail fraud statute to prosecute undisclosed fiduciary breaches. Concludes that the mail fraud statute may be used to prosecute physicians who fail to disclose financial incentives to their patients. Quotes Opinion 8.03. Cites Opinions 2.03 and 8.07 [now Opinion 8.06]. Jones, *Primum Non Nocere: The Expanding "Honest Services" Mail Fraud Statute and the Physician-Patient Fiduciary Relationship, 51 Vand. L. Rev. 139, 161, 164 (1998).*

Journal 1998 Explores aspects of trust in physician-patient relations. Discusses the transformation of the health care system and the need for regulation. Points out that too much involvement by politicians and legislators will put the health care system at risk. References Opinions 6.02 and 8.03. Mechanic, *The Functions and Limitations of Trust in the Provision of Medical Care, 23 J. Health Pol. Pol'y & Law 661, 667 (1998).*

Journal 1997 Discusses physician-patient trust in the managed care environment. Explores options for enhancing trustworthiness in this context. Quotes Opinion 8.03. Gray, *Trust and Trustworthy Care in the Managed Care Era, 16 Health Affairs 34, 38, 47-48 (1997).*

Journal 1997 Discusses the practice of ex parte communications between treating physicians and their patients' legal adversaries without informing the patient or obtaining consent. Examines harms that may occur in these situations. Argues that Oklahoma needs to prohibit treating physicians from communicating ex parte with their patients' legal adversaries. Quotes Opinions 5.05, 5.07, 5.08, 8.02, 8.03, and 9.07. Cites Opinion 7.02. McNaughton & McNaughton, *Divided Loyalty: The Dilemma of the Treating Physician Advocate, 22 Okla. City U. L. Rev. 1051, 1052, 1054, 1056, 1058, 1059, 1062 (1997).*

Journal 1995 Addresses presidential disability, its past impact on American government, and possible solutions to potential problems. Proposes enhancement of the role of the President's physician. Quotes Opinion 8.03. Cites Opinions 5.04 and 5.05. Abrams, *The Vulnerable President and the Twenty-Fifth Amendment, With Observations on Guidelines, a Health Commission, and the Role of the President's Physician, 30 Wake Forest L. Rev. 453, 466, 471 (1995).*

Journal 1994 Discusses the issue of whom physicians must serve first: themselves, their patients, insurers, or society. Focuses on risks arising out of provider economic arrangements and risks arising out of other individual physician characteristics. Quotes Opinions 8.03 and 9.13. Cites Opinion 8.15. Bobinski, *Autonomy and Privacy: Protecting Patients From Their Physicians, 55 U. Pitt. L. Rev. 291, 302, 313 (1994).*

Journal 1992 Examines issues related to the responsibility of HIV-infected health care workers to protect patients from infection, including mandatory testing, disclosure to coworkers and supervisors, and the degree to which the practice of an HIV-infected health care worker should be modified. Concludes that courts likely will impose a requirement to disclose HIV-positive status to patients when there is a substantial risk of HIV transmission. Quotes Opinions 8.03 (1989) [now Opinion 8.032] and 8.07 (1989) [now Opinion 8.03]. References Opinion 9.131. Lieberman & Derse, *HIV-Positive Health Care Workers and the Obligation to Disclose: Do Patients Have a Right to Know? 13 J. Legal Med. 333, 353, 354 (1992).*

Journal 1990 Explains how the federal Medicare and Medicaid Anti-Fraud and Abuse statute limits the ability of physicians to adapt investment and referral strategies to an increasingly competitive health care marketplace. Proposes giving regulatory power over physician investments back to the states, which are more able to recognize and exempt beneficial arrangements from otherwise restrictive statutory schemes. Cites Opinion 8.03. Comment, *Regulating Physician Investment and Referral Behavior in the Competitive Health Care Marketplace of the '90s—An Argument for Decentralization, 65 Wash. L. Rev. 657, 658 (1990).*

Journal 1990 Examines various cost-control mechanisms utilized by prepaid health plans and other managed care programs and considers the impact of such mechanisms on clinical decision making. Emphasis is placed on the possible existence of conflicts of interest on the part of health care providers in this context. Quotes Opinions 8.03 [now Opinions 8.03 and 8.032] and 8.13 [now Opinion 8.132]. Hirshfeld, *Defining Full and Fair Disclosure in Managed Care Contracts, 60 The Citation 67, 70 (1990).*

Journal 1990 Discusses efforts of third-party payers to control health care expenditures for beneficiaries. Concludes that financial incentives to limit care and other cost-control techniques should be disclosed and that the rationale for such disclosure is compelling. Quotes Opinions 2.03, 2.09, and 8.03. Cites Opinions 2.19, 4.04, and 4.06. Hirshfeld, *Should Third Party Payors of Health Care Services Disclose Cost Control Mechanisms to Potential Beneficiaries? 14 Seton Hall Legis. J. 115, 130, 131, 144, 145, 146 (1990).*

Journal 1989 Analyzes the Medicare and Medicaid Patient and Program Protection Act of 1987 and discusses the complexity of fraud and abuse issues that confront hospitals and health care providers who undertake financially attractive business arrangements. Concludes that the 1987 Act, along with its implementing regulations, can offer meaningful guidance in an area of uncertainty for the health care industry. Quotes Opinion 4.05 (1986) [now Opinion 8.03]. Comment, *Curing the Health Care Industry: Government Response to Medicare Fraud and Abuse, 5 J. Contemp. Health L. & Pol'y 175, 189 (1989).*

Journal 1985 Initially describes how existing doctrines protect the value of autonomy in the context of the physician-patient relationship, then examines various problems in the current protective scheme. Concludes by recommending the creation of an independent articulable protected interest in patient autonomy. Quotes Principles II and IV. Cites Opinions 4.04 (1984) [now Opinions 8.03 and 8.032] and 6.03 (1984) [now Opinion 6.02]. Shultz, *From Informed Consent to Patient Choice: A New Protected Interest, 95 Yale L. J. 219, 275 (1985).*

Ill. App. 1999 Administrator of estate brought suit against physician and health maintenance organization (HMO). The suit alleged medical negligence and breach of a fiduciary duty to deceased for the physician's failure to disclose contract with the HMO that created incentives to minimize diagnostic tests and specialist referrals. The court quoted Opinion 8.132, stating that, while a violation of professional ethics does not in itself establish a breach of the legal standard of care, it is relevant in determining whether such a breach occurred. *Neade v. Portes, 303 Ill.App.3d 799, 710 N.E. 2d 418, 427.*

Journal 2002 Explores how courts have attempted to provide relief when managed care organizations cause harm. Concludes that the judiciary has evidenced respect for the legislative process in this context. Quotes Opinion 8.132. Spector, *Managed Healthcare Liability Issues, 32 Cumb. L. Rev. 311, 335-36 (2002).*

Journal 2001 Discusses the prohibition on nonlawyer ownership of legal service providers. Considers how ethical rules and standards governing physicians have been directed toward preserving independent judgment. Concludes that ethical conflicts created by abandoning the prohibition on nonlawyer ownership of legal service providers may be managed by following the medical ethics model. Quotes Principle VI and Opinions 2.03, 2.09, 8.02, 8.021, 8.03, 8.05, 8.051, 8.054, 8.13, and 8.132. Harris & Foran, *The Ethics of Middle-Class Access to Legal Services and What We Can Learn From the Medical Profession's Shift to a Corporate Paradigm, 70 Fordham L. Rev. 775, 817, 821, 822, 823, 824 (2001).*

Journal 2001 Examines the changing duties of health care providers to disclose managed care financial incentives to patients. Concludes that managed care organizations, not physicians, should be obligated to make such disclosures. Quotes Opinion 8.132. Kurfirst, *The Duty to Disclose HMO Physician Incentives, 13 (3) Health Law 18, 18, 22 (2001).*

Journal 2001 Examines patient attitudes toward physician compensation models. Concludes that most wealthier, well-educated, Caucasian patients are the least satisfied with capitation. References Opinion 8.132. Pereira & Pearson, *Patient Attitudes Toward Physician Financial Incentives, 161 Arch. Intern. Med. 1313, 1316, 1317 (2001).*

Journal 2001 Examines the concept of fiduciary duty in the managed care context. Considers potential liability of health plans and providers for breach of this duty. Reviews the US Supreme Court decision in *Pegram v. Herdrich.* Concludes that *Pegram* left many unanswered questions concerning ERISA's fiduciary requirements for health plans and providers. Quotes Opinion 8.132. Rosoff, *Breach of Fiduciary Duty Lawsuits Against MCOs, 22 J. Legal Med. 55, 65 (2001).*

Journal 2000 Examines physician value neutrality (PVN). Defines PVN as providing a foundation to suggest physicians must keep their values—religious, political, or otherwise—out of the patient-physician relationship. Concludes it is not clear how values can be removed from the patient-physician relationship without removing the very thing PVN supporters are trying to protect, the intrinsic value of persons. References Opinions 2.01, 2.02, 8.032, 8.05, 8.08, and 8.132. Beckwith & Peppin, *Physician Value Neutrality: A Critique, 28 J. L. Med. & Ethics 67, 72-73 (2000).*

Journal 2000 Examines the fiduciary nature of the physician-patient relationship. Explores crucial policy implications of the *Neade v. Portes* decision. Concludes that policy makers, not courts, should address whether physician

involvement in managed care plans fundamentally implies a profit motive. Quotes Opinion 8.132. Potter, *Failure to Disclose HMO Incentives and the Breach of Fiduciary Duty: Is a New Cause of Action Against Physicians the Best Solution? 34 USF. L. Rev. 733, 753 (2000).*

Journal 1999 Considers the viability of a legal cause of action for negligent referral in the physician-patient relationship. Examines differences between the legal and medical professions and discusses variations in the applicable standards of care. Cites Opinion 8.132. Martin, *Legal Malpractice: Negligent Referral as a Cause of Action, 29 Cumb. L. Rev. 679, 686 (1999).*

Journal 1999 Explores the increased push toward mandatory disclosure laws regarding financial incentives imposed by managed care organizations. Discusses current laws and ethical guidelines. Emphasizes that efforts to mandate disclosure force physicians to focus on the effects of imposed incentives and the essence of the physician-patient relationship. References Opinions 8.032, 8.13, and 8.132. Miller & Sage, *Disclosing Physician Financial Incentives, 281 JAMA 1424, 1425 (1999).*

Journal 1999 Discusses financial incentives offered to physicians by managed care organizations. Argues that evidence of financial incentives should be admissible in medical malpractice cases. Quotes Opinion 8.13. References Opinion 8.132. Sugarman & Yarashus, *Admissibility of Managed Care Financial Incentives in Medical Malpractice Cases, 34 Tort & Ins. L. J. 735, 743, 746, 759 (1999).*

Journal 1998 Discusses changes in the health care system. Explains why patients need more power in the managed care system. Suggests that patients should use class action suits as a method to assert power over managed care organizations. References Opinions 8.13 and 8.132. Cerminara, *The Class Action Suit as a Method of Patient Empowerment in the Managed Care Setting, 24 Am. J. Law & Med. 7, 16, 17, 23 (1998).*

Journal 1998 Asserts that managed care organizations assume fiduciary obligations by exercising discretionary control over the administration of an ERISA plan. Argues that ERISA requires managed care organizations and physicians to disclose financial incentives intended to influence physician decision-making. References Opinions 8.13 and 8.132. Johnson, *ERISA Doctor in the House? The Duty to Disclose Physician Incentives to Limit Health Care, 82 Minn. L. Rev. 1631, 1639, 1649, 1655 (1998).*

Journal 1996 Considers challenges to the psychiatrist-patient relationship that are triggered by managed care cost-containment methodologies. Offers guidance to psychiatrists for addressing these challenges. References Opinions 2.095, 8.13, and 8.132. Hoge, *APA Resource Document: I. The Professional Responsibilities of Psychiatrists in Evolving Health Care Systems, 24 Bull. Am. Acad. Psychiatry Law 393, 405 (1996).*

11.2.3 Contracts to Deliver Health Care Services

1st Cir. 1984 Plaintiff-physicians sued defendant-insurer, alleging defendant's ban on balance billing practice violated antitrust law. That practice required defendant to pay the physicians treating defendant's insureds only if the physicians agreed not to make any additional charges to the insureds. In holding that defendant's billing practice did not violate antitrust law, the court noted in passing a 1954 law journal article that cited, with an incorrect reference, Principles Ch. III, Art. VI, Sec. 3 (1947) in arguing that selling services to third parties might interfere with the absolute ethical obligation that a doctor owes to the patient. The specific concept treated by this Principle is no longer directly treated although Opinion 8.05 reflects similar concerns. *Kartell v. Blue Shield of Mass., Inc., 749 F.2d 922, 926, cert. denied, 471 US 1029 (1985).*

2d Cir. 1980 Federal Trade Commission ordered AMA and others to cease, with some exceptions, imposing restraints on advertising and contract practice by physicians, as well as on business relations between physicians and laypersons. Commission found restraints violated 15 USC § 45(a)(1). See 94 FTC 701 (1979). AMA petitioned for judicial review of Commission's order. Court reviewed order, noting specific ethical pronouncements of AMA which Commission found improper, including the following: restrictions upon advertising and solicitation, Principle 5 (1957) and Opinions and Reports of the Judicial Council Sec. 5, Para. 11 (1971) [now Opinion 5.02]; restrictions on contract practice, Principle 6 (1957) and Opinions and Reports of the Judicial Council Sec. 6, Paras. 3, 4, and 5 (1971) [now Opinion 8.05]; and restrictions on business organizations and relations with laypersons, Opinions and Reports of the Judicial Council Sec. 6, Paras. 14 and 15 (1971). Court rejected AMA's argument that its ethical rules did not provide impetus for local and state medical societies to act against physicians violating its rules. Further, court rejected AMA's position that liability should be precluded because of revisions in the Opinions in 1977 and the Principles in 1980. Specifically, the court found that removal of the ban on patient solicitation and changes reflected in Principles II and IV (1980) did not render Commission's order moot. The order was therefore enforced with modifications. Dissenting judge, referring to 1980 revisions in Principles and to Opinions and Reports of the Judicial Council 4.05 and 6.00 (1977) [now Opinions 5.02 and 8.05], concluded order should not be enforced on grounds of mootness. *American Medical Ass'n v. FTC, 638 F.2d 443, 446, 446 n.1, 448, 449, 449 n.5, 450, 451, 455-57, aff'd, 455 US 676 (1982).*

7th Cir. 1984 Plaintiff brought medical malpractice suit against several physicians appointed to the Veterans Administration Department of Medicine and Surgery. The court held that strict control test for determining whether defendants ought to be considered employees or independent contractors under the Federal Tort Claims Act was not appropriate because the ethical obligation of a physician to a patient, evidenced by Principle 6 (1957) [now Opinions 8.03

and 8.05], required that independent judgment be exercised, preventing a physician from being strictly controlled by the Veterans Administration. *Quilico v. Kaplan, 749 F.2d 480, 483-84.*

10th Cir. 1983 Pursuant to the Federal Tort Claims Act, plaintiff sued the federal government for the negligence of a neurosurgeon, allegedly an employee of a Veteran's Administration (VA) hospital. Plaintiff argued that applying the traditional control test to determine a physician's employment status was inappropriate because physicians are bound by Principle 6 (1957) [now Opinions 8.03 and 8.05] requiring them to have free and complete exercise of [their] medical judgment and skill. However, the court did not reach the merits of that argument because the contractual agreement between the neurosurgeon and the VA hospital was outside the parameters of an employer-employee relationship with the government, thus precluding plaintiff's claim. *Lurch v. United States, 719 F.2d 333, 337, cert. denied, 466 US 927 (1984).*

D.C. Cir. 1942 Medical associations appealed conviction on charges of conspiracy to restrain trade or commerce where associations attempted to prevent competition by elimination of prepaid, low-cost medical and hospital care. Principles Ch. III, Art. VI, Secs. 2 and 3 [now Opinion 8.05] limiting contract practice had been used as a basis to discipline members of medical association employed by prepaid medical organization. The court held that the associations were subject to the Sherman Antitrust Act and that the evidence sustained the conviction. *American Medical Ass'n v. United States, 130 F.2d 233, 238-239 n.23, aff'd, 317 US 519 (1943).*

N.D. Ill. 2008 Administrator of the estate of patient filed suit under the Federal Tort Claims Act and state wrongful death act after patient died as a result of a mistake during surgery at Veteran's Administration hospital. Defendant physician moved to dismiss on the grounds that, as a federal employee, she was exempt from personal liability for services performed within the scope of her employment at the VA. The court cited earlier case quoting Principle 6 (1957) [now Opinions 8.03 and 8.05] and determining that, because physicians are free to choose whom to serve, they are not federal employees and the strict control test may not be appropriate. Finding issues of fact to resolve, the court denied the defendant's motion for summary judgment. *Monroe v. United States, 2008 U.S. Dist. LEXIS 22455, 9.*

Miss. 2003 Patient's estate appealed summary judgment in favor of physician and hospital in wrongful death action. Supreme Court affirmed, holding that physician was a state employee and that purchase of liability insurance did not waive immunity. In examining physician's status, the court found that the exercise of professional judgment and discretion are not determinative of employment status. Quotes Principle 6 (1957) [now Opinions 8.03 and 8.05]. *Corey v. Skelton, 834 So.2d 681, 685.*

Miss. 2002 Plaintiff in malpractice action appealed grant of summary judgment in favor of neurosurgeon who allegedly performed a thoracic diskectomy on the wrong disk. A resident performed the patient's physical and wrote the majority of the chart notes. The Mississippi Supreme Court affirmed the lower court. The court held that as a state employee the physician was immune from liability and that his exercise of professional judgment in treating patients did not change his status and insurance did not waive immunity. Quotes Principle 6 (1957) [now Opinions 8.03 and 8.05]. *Clayton v. Harkey, 826 So.2d 1283, 1287.*

Miss. 2001 Patient filed suit asserting that a physician was negligent in performing surgery. The trial court granted the physician's summary judgment motion and held that the physician, employed by a state university medical center, was immune under state law. Finding genuine issues of fact, the state Supreme Court reversed and remanded the case for further proceedings. In a separate opinion, one justice quoted Principle 6 (1957) [now Opinions 8.03 and 8.05], in evaluating the degree of control exercised by the state over the physician. This justice, stressing that the physician exercised discretion in treating the patient independent of the state's control, found no basis to hold the physician an employee for immunity purposes. *Conley v. Warren, 797 So. 2d 881, 886.*

Miss. 2000 Beneficiaries of patient's estate appealed summary judgment in malpractice action for a physician on sovereign immunity grounds. The court reversed and remanded the case finding issues of fact to be resolved at trial. The majority set out a five-part test to determine the employment status of a physician working at a state health care facility, including the degree of control and direction exercised by the state over the physician. In a separate opinion one justice quoted Principle 6 (1957) [now Opinions 8.03 and 8.05], stating that, "A physician should not dispose of his services under terms or conditions which tend to interfere with or impair the free and complete exercise of his medical judgment and skill. . . ." This justice reasoned that the physician could not claim the state controlled his medical discretion or treatment of patients and thus was clearly not an employee entitled to immunity. *Miller v. Meeks, 762 So. 2d 302, 314.*

Miss. 2000 Patient brought a medical malpractice action against physicians after receiving treatment at a state university medical center. The jury returned a verdict against the physicians. The Mississippi Supreme Court reversed, finding that the physicians were immune from liability as state employees. In determining the status of the physicians, the court noted that the physicians retained a considerable amount of professional discretion in treating the patient, quoting Principle 6 (1957) [now Opinions 8.03 and 8.05]. However, this alone was not determinative, and in the court's view the physicians were state employees. *Sullivan v. Washington, 768 So. 2d 881, 885.*

Miss. App. 2003 Patient brought malpractice action against physicians working at a state university teaching hospital.

Patient argued that the physicians were independent contractors and sovereign immunity did not apply. Appellate court, citing the Mississippi Supreme Court's decision in *Miller v. Mecks*, 762 So.2d 302 (Miss. 2000), affirmed the trial court and held that sovereign immunity applied because the physicians were state employees. Quotes Principle 6 (1957) [now Opinions 8.03 and 8.05]. *Brown v. Warren, 858 So.2d 168, 175 (2003).*

Wash. 1951 Plaintiff, a charitable, not-for-profit medical corporation, offered prepaid health care services to members and their families. Suit was filed against county medical society and others for damages and injunction for defendants' alleged efforts to monopolize prepaid medical care in area and unlawfully restrain competition by plaintiff and its physicians. Defendants alleged as affirmative defense that their efforts were designed to curb unethical prepaid contract practice by plaintiff. Court examined at length AMA's position regarding contract practice including Principles Ch. III, Art. VI, Secs. 3 and 4 (1947) [now Principle VI and Opinions 8.05 and 9.06] concluding nothing in plaintiff's practice violated the AMA's ethical guidelines. Further, quoting Principles Ch. III, Art. III, Sec. 1 (1947) [now Opinion 8.04] dealing with consultations, court noted that defendants' efforts impeded plaintiff's physicians from obtaining consultations. Court concluded defendants' actions constituted unlawful, monopolistic behavior and issued an injunction, although it declined to award damages. *Group Health Coop. v. King County Medical Soc'y, 39 Wash. 2d 586, 237 P.2d 737, 744, 750-51, 759-60.*

Journal 2007 Reviews the legal and ethical problems surrounding concierge medical practice. Concludes that concierge medicine should remain restricted to a small class of wealthy individuals. Cites Opinions 8.05, 8.055, 8.115, 9.06, and 9.065. Carnahan, *Concierge Medicine: Legal and Ethical Issues, 35 J. L. Med. & Ethics 211, 212-13 (2007).*

Journal 2006 Examines external review systems used for adjudication of disputes between patients and managed care organizations. Concludes that external review systems do not satisfy constitutional due process requirements. Quotes Opinions and Reports of the Judicial Council Sec. 6, Para. 4 (1969) [now Opinion 8.05]. References Opinion 8.13. Hunter, *Managed Process, Due Care: Structures of Accountability in Health Care, 6 Yale J. Health Pol'y L. & Ethics 93, 107, 113 (2006).*

Journal 2004 Discusses the concept of medical necessity and its effect on the health care system. Concludes that issues regarding medical necessity must be dealt with to achieve meaningful health care reform. Quotes Opinion 8.05. Blanchard, *"Medical Necessity" Determinations—A Continuing Healthcare Policy Problem, 37 J. Health L. 599, 620 (2004).*

Journal 2001 Discusses the prohibition on nonlawyer ownership of legal service providers. Considers how ethical rules and standards governing physicians have been directed toward preserving independent judgment. Concludes that ethical conflicts created by abandoning the prohibition on nonlawyer ownership of legal service providers may be managed by following the medical ethics model. Quotes Principle VI and Opinions 2.03, 2.09, 8.02, 8.021, 8.03, 8.05, 8.051, 8.054, 8.13, and 8.132. Harris & Foran, *The Ethics of Middle-Class Access to Legal Services and What We Can Learn From the Medical Profession's Shift to a Corporate Paradigm, 70 Fordham L. Rev. 775, 817, 821, 822, 823, 824 (2001).*

Journal 2000 Examines physician value neutrality (PVN). Defines PVN as providing a foundation to suggest physicians must keep their values—religious, political, or otherwise—out of the patient-physician relationship. Concludes it is not clear how values can be removed from the patient-physician relationship without removing the very thing PVN supporters are trying to protect, the intrinsic value of persons. References Opinions 2.01, 2.02, 8.032, 8.05, 8.08, and 8.132. Beckwith & Peppin, *Physician Value Neutrality: A Critique, 28 J. L. Med. & Ethics 67, 72-73 (2000).*

Journal 1997 Discusses the practice of physician deselection by managed care organizations. Suggests that deselection harms the physician-patient relationship and creates a conflict of interest. Argues that solutions to deselection should consider effects on the patient rather than on the physician. Quotes Principle III. Cites Principle I and Opinions 8.05 and 8.13. Liner, *Physician Deselection: The Dynamics of a New Threat to the physician-patient Relationship, 23 Am. J. Law & Med. 511, 513, 527 (1997).*

1st. Cir. 2008 Trial court granted summary judgment for orthopedic surgeon in suit brought against manufacturer of orthopedic implant devices for breach of contract and violations of state consumer protection statutes. On appeal, the surgeon submitted an affidavit from a medical ethics expert that cited Opinion 8.0501, declaring that the payment of kickbacks from a medical device manufacturer to a physician is unethical. The appeals court held that the manufacturer breached the contract by halting royalty payments to the physician. *Jasty v. Wright Medical Technology, Inc., 528 F.3d 28, 38, n. 12.*

Journal 2010 Examines legal and ethical issues confronting medical-legal partnerships, as well as the benefits and challenges of such partnerships. Concludes that as long as critical professional obligations are recognized and ethical boundaries are maintained, medical and legal professionals can collaborate without compromising professional duties or ethical goals. Quotes Opinion 8.0501. Boumil, Freitas, & Freitas, *Multidisciplinary Representation of Patients: The Potential for Ethical Issues and Professional Duty Conflicts in the Medical-Legal Partnership Model, 13 J. Health Care L. & Pol'y 107, 124 (2010).*

Journal 2006 Examines ethical dilemmas physicians may face as providers of pay-for-performance medical care. Concludes that this strategy offers a benefit to patients as long as physicians uphold stringent ethical standards and work together to ensure optimum patient care. Cites

Principles I, V, VIII, and IX and Opinions 2.035, 2.095, 6.01, 8.021, 8.03, 8.0501, 8.053, 8.054, and 8.121. Bostick, Sade, & McMahon, *Report of the Council on Ethical and Judicial Affairs: Physician Pay-for-Performance Programs, 3 Ind. Health L. Rev. 429, 430, 431, 432-33, 434, 435, 436 (2006).*

Journal 1990 Discusses efforts of third-party payers to control health care expenditures for beneficiaries. Concludes that financial incentives to limit care and other cost-control techniques should be disclosed and that the rationale for such disclosure is compelling. Quotes Opinions 2.03, 2.09, and 8.03. Cites Opinions 2.19, 4.04, and 4.06. Hirshfeld, *Should Third Party Payors of Health Care Services Disclose Cost Control Mechanisms to Potential Beneficiaries? 14 Seton Hall Legis. J. 115, 130, 131, 144, 145, 146 (1990).*

S.D. Fla. 2001 Insured patients under health care plans sued managed care companies alleging improper nondisclosure of policies and procedures imposing restrictions on physicians' judgment as to appropriate medical treatment. The insureds sued under both the Racketeer Influenced and Corrupt Organizations Act (RICO) and the Employee Retirement Income Security Act (ERISA). The court, with one exception, dismissed without prejudice both the RICO and ERISA claims. Among the plaintiffs' arguments was that the defendants had included "gag clauses" in their physician contracts in violation of Opinion 8.053. *In Re Managed Care Litigation, 150 F.Supp.2d 1330, 1335.*

Journal 2006 Discusses preemption of lawsuits against managed care organizations by the Employee Retirement Income Security Act of 1974 (ERISA). Proposes a "bifurcated legal regime" to decrease the protective scope of ERISA. Quotes Opinions 8.053 and 8.135. Madison, *ERISA and Liability for Provision of Medical Information, 84 N. C. L. Rev. 471, 540 (2006).*

Journal 2002 Examines how managed care has adversely affected information disclosure in the physician-patient relationship. Concludes that, unless courts expand applicability of principles of informed consent, patient self-determination and autonomy will continue to be undermined. Quotes Principle VIII and Opinions 8.03, 8.053, 8.054, and 8.08. Morris, *Dissing Disclosure: Just What the Doctor Ordered, 44 Ariz. L. Rev. 313, 344, 349, 362, 363, 366 (2002).*

Journal 2008 Explores the tension experienced by health care professionals who provide care and compete in a market economy. Concludes if health care professions continue commercializing, providers must strive to maintain ethical standards and appropriate professional-patient relationships. Quotes Opinion 8.054. Peltier & Guisti, *Commerce and Care: The Irreconcilable Tension Between Selling and Caring, 39 McGeorge L. Rev. 785, 794 (2008).*

Journal 2006 Discusses the evolution of health law in Virginia. Concludes that the area of health law continues to expand, develop, and be refined. Cites Opinions 3.03, 3.08, 5.01, 5.015, 5.02, 5.04, 5.055, 6.02, 6.021, 6.03, 6.04, 7.03, 7.04, 7.05, 8.054, 8.08, 8.081, 8.085, 8.115, 8.12, 8.14, 8.145,

8.19, and 9.045. Guanzon, *Health Care Law, 41 U. Rich. L. Rev. 179, 199 (2006).*

Journal 2005 Argues that in *Aetna v. Davila/Cigna v. Calad*, the Supreme Court missed an opportunity to overturn unjust ERISA policies. Concludes that the principle of complete ERISA preemption as articulated in these consolidated cases is unsatisfactory because it violates the separation of powers doctrine. Quotes Principle VIII. Cites Opinions 8.054, 8.13, 8.135, 9.123, 10.01, and 10.015. Nelson, *AETNA v. DAVILA/CIGNA v. CALAD: A Missed Opportunity, 31 Wm. Mitchell L. Rev. 843, 847, 849, 850, 880 (2005).*

Journal 2003 Reviews state laws designed to protect physicians acting as patient advocates in managed care organizations. Concludes that federal and state law must make it easier for physicians to challenge denials of or delays in patient care. Quotes Opinions 8.054, 8.13, and 10.01. Fentiman, *Patient Advocacy and Termination From Managed Care Organizations. Do State Laws Protecting Health Care Professional Advocacy Make Any Difference? 82 Neb. L. Rev. 508, 515-16, 517-18 (2003).*

Journal 2002 Examines how managed care has adversely affected information disclosure in the physician-patient relationship. Concludes that, unless courts expand applicability of principles of informed consent, patient self-determination and autonomy will continue to be undermined. Quotes Principle VIII and Opinions 8.03, 8.053, 8.054, and 8.08. Morris, *Dissing Disclosure: Just What the Doctor Ordered, 44 Ariz. L. Rev. 313, 344, 349, 362, 363, 366 (2002).*

Journal 2006 Scrutinizes the benefits of pay-for-performance financial incentives. Concludes that such incentives will not alleviate the need for health insurance. Cites Opinion 6.01. References Opinion 8.056. Sage & Kalyan, *Horses or Unicorns: Can Paying for Performance Make Quality Competition Routine? 31 J. Health Pol. Pol'y & L. 531, 531-32, 554 (2006).*

D. N. J. 1999 Patient sued her managed care organization alleging that she suffered injuries due to failure to obtain timely approval for a nonmember physician to perform her back surgery. The plaintiff apparently relied on Opinion 8.13 to show that the defendant had a duty to advocate for her in seeking prompt approval for her surgery. The court, however, stated that the plaintiff's reference to the Opinion failed to establish such a duty because the Code of Medical Ethics does not have the force of law. *Pryzbowski v. US Health Care, Inc., 64 F. Supp. 2d 361, 370.*

S.D.N.Y. 1997 Employee brought suit against a health maintenance organization (HMO) under contract with her employer to provide health benefits. The suit alleged various theories of liability ranging from breach of implied contract to breach of fiduciary duties. Employee sought redress pursuant to the civil enforcement provisions of the Employee Retirement Income Security Act of 1974. The court granted HMO's motion to dismiss all claims except for the breach of fiduciary duty stemming from HMO's alleged policy of

restricting the disclosure of noncovered treatments. The court quoted report of AMA Council on Ethical and Judicial Affairs [now Opinion 8.13] in holding that physicians have an ethical duty to fully disclose treatment options to patients regardless of whether treatment occurs in a managed care environment. *Weiss v. Cigna Healthcare, Inc., 972 F. Supp. 748, 751-52.*

Mass. Super. 2004 Defendants filed a motion for partial summary judgment in an action alleging they were liable for not disclosing their financial interests in an experimental program that the decedent participated in. The court denied the defendants' motion, referencing Opinion 8.13 in stating physicians should disclose financial incentives and restrictions placed on them by their HMO. *Darke v. Estate of Isner, 2004 WL 1325635, 3.*

Ohio Att'y Gen. 1999 State attorney general concluded that physicians who render opinions regarding the necessity of medical services for health insuring corporations are not engaged in the practice of medicine. Additionally, physicians who render opinions regarding medical necessity for appeals of adverse determinations do not fall under the regulatory, investigatory, or enforcement authority of the Ohio State Medical Board. Quoting Opinions 8.03, 8.11, and 8.13, the attorney general stated that physicians have an ethical duty to provide appropriate treatment for patients. *Ohio Att'y Gen. Op. No. 99-044, 1999 WL 692623.*

Journal 2006 Examines the process of physician deselection and the protections afforded to physicians. Concludes that physicians should be able to make a legal challenge to a dismissal made without cause. Quotes Opinion 8.13. Coppolo, *Not Just a Minimum Income Policy for Physicians: The Need for Good Faith and Fair Dealing in Physician Deselection Disputes, 48 Wm. and Mary L. Rev. 677, 686 (2006).*

Journal 2006 Argues for an alternative framework by which health ethics, policy, and law can address equitable distribution of health care. Concludes that a new paradigm would lead to a more efficient and compassionate system. References Opinions 2.22 and 8.13. Ruger, *Health, Capability, and Justice: Toward a New Paradigm of Health Ethics, Policy and Law, 15 Cornell J. L. & Pub. Pol'y 403, 425, 465 (2006).*

Journal 2006 Considers the role of informed consent and patient autonomy as a central tenet of bioethics. Concludes that the field should focus most strongly on serving the practical needs and desires of patients. References Opinion 8.13. Schneider, *After Autonomy, 41 Wake Forest L. Rev. 411, 429-30 (2006).*

Journal 2006 Critiques the Uniform Health-Care Decisions Act. Concludes that the Act poses dangers to disabled patients, and proposes safeguards against such dangers. References Opinion 8.13. Stith, *The Semblance of Autonomy: Treatment of Persons With Disabilities Under the Uniform Health-Care Decisions Act, 22 Issues L. & Med. 39, 63-64 (2006).*

Journal 2002 Observes that changes in the health professions challenge certain assumptions about professional ethics. Concludes that these long-standing assumptions must be re-examined. Cites Opinion 2.161. References Opinion 8.13. Kelley, *The Meanings of Professional Life: Teaching Across the Health Professions,* 27 *J. Med. & Phil.* 475, 485, 490, 491 (2002).

Journal 2002 Considers whether physicians should be required to disclose information regarding financial incentives received from patients' HMOs. Concludes that physicians should not be required to disclose these incentives. References Opinion 8.13. Reuland, *Health Maintenance Organizations and Physician Financial Incentive Plans: Should Physician Disclosure Be Mandatory?* 27 *Iowa J. Corp. L.* 293, 312 (2002).

Journal 2002 Examines whether managed care organizations should be obligated to disclose physician financial incentives that may limit patient care. Concludes that mandatory disclosure is in the best interest of patients and physicians. Quotes Opinions 2.03 and 8.13. Talesh, *Breaking the Learned Helplessness of Patients: Why MCOs Should Be Required to Disclose Financial Incentives,* 26 *Law & Psychol. Rev.* 49, 60-61, 63 (2002).

Journal 2001 Examines issues relating to health care cost containment. Concludes that, if physicians are to meet the goals assigned to them in a cost-constrained health care system, then professional standards must be reevaluated and modified to afford meaningful guidance for clinical decision-making in the face of health care spending controls. Quotes Opinions 2.03, 2.09, 2.095, 8.032, and 9.04. Cites Opinions 8.02, 8.021, 8.051, and 8.13. Agrawal, *Resuscitating Professionalism: Self-regulation in the Medical Marketplace,* 66 *Mo. L. Rev.* 341, 354, 355, 360, 361, 378, 388 (2001).

Journal 2001 Examines the doctrine of informed consent with respect to nontraditional issues, such as a physician's duty to disclose personal information. Concludes there must be a balance that will accommodate the needs of both the patient and the physician. References Opinion 8.13. Hanson, *Informed Consent and the Scope of a Physician's Duty of Disclosure,* 77 *N. D. L. Rev.* 71, 89, 91 (2001).

Journal 2000 Discusses and evaluates different systems for addressing consumer concerns about managed health care. Asserts that current legal systems for identifying and resolving consumer concerns are not understood by most consumers and are not accessible by many, especially the uninsured. Concludes that several immediate steps are realistic for moving toward reform. Cites Principle VI. References Opinions 8.13 and 9.065. Kinney, *Tapping and Resolving Consumer Concerns About Health Care,* 26 *Am. J. Law & Med.* 335, 337, 375 (2000).

Journal 2000 Reviews the case of *Corporate Health Insurance, Inc. v. Texas Dept. of Insurance* and discusses its impact on HMO liability in Texas. Considers the conflicts of interest managed care imposes upon physicians. Concludes

that, without national amendments to the scope of ERISA, HMOs are not compelled to provide quality health care. References Opinion 8.13. Lockhart, *The Safest Care Is to Deny Care: Implications of Corporate Health Insurance, Inc. v. Texas Department of Insurance on HMO Liability in Texas,* 41 *S. Tex. L. Rev.* 621, 628, 634 (2000).

Journal 2000 Describes the fiduciary aspects of the physician-patient relationship. Explores the conflicts that may occur between physicians and pregnant women in the health care setting. Proposes legal strategies to address these conflicts. Quotes Opinions 8.08 and 10.01. References Opinion 8.13. Oberman, *Mothers and Doctors' Orders: Unmasking the Doctor's Fiduciary Role in Maternal-Fetal Conflicts,* 94 *Nw. U. L. Rev.* 451, 456, 462, 493 (2000).

Journal 1999 Describes the gag clause debate in managed care and analyzes the types of incentives that might limit physician-patient communication. Concludes that, to protect patient access to information about treatment options and their health plans, antigag legislation must be coupled with a thorough examination of the extent to which financial incentives will be permitted to impact managed health care delivery. Quotes Opinion 8.13. Krause, *The Brief Life of the Gag Clause: Why Antigag Clause Legislation Isn't Enough,* 67 *Tenn. L. Rev.* 1, 4, 43 (1999).

Journal 1999 Describes the development of managed care organizations. Examines professional associations' statements regarding managed care organizations. Argues that physicians and managed care organizations should be viewed as economically disciplined, moral cofiduciaries for patients. References Opinion 8.13. McCullough, *A Basic Concept in the Clinical Ethics of Managed Care: Physicians and Institutions as Economically Disciplined Moral Co-Fiduciaries of Populations of Patients,* 24 *J. Med. Phil.* 77, 82-83, 87, 89, 91, 96 (1999).

Journal 1999 Explores the increased push toward mandatory disclosure laws regarding financial incentives imposed by managed care organizations. Discusses current laws and ethical guidelines. Emphasizes that efforts to mandate disclosure force physicians to focus on the effects of imposed incentives and the essence of the physician-patient relationship. References Opinions 8.032, 8.13, and 8.132. Miller & Sage, *Disclosing Physician Financial Incentives,* 281 *JAMA* 1424, 1425 (1999).

Journal 1999 Discusses the need for physicians to advocate on behalf of patients' rights in the context of health care delivery. Evaluates the nature and scope of the physician's role as advocate, noting that physicians cannot be expected to engage in attorney-like advocacy. Quotes Principles IV and VI, Fundamental Elements (2), (4), and (6) [now Opinion 10.01], Patient Responsibilities 5 [now Opinion 10.02], and Opinions 2.03, 2.07, 2.09, 2.16, 2.19, 3.06, 4.01, 4.04, 6.01, 7.02, 8.02, 8.03, 8.13, 8.132, 9.06, 9.07, and 9.131. Cites Opinions 5.05, 5.09, 7.01, 8.135, and 9.02. Sage, *Physicians as Advocates,* 35 *Hous. L. Rev.* 1529, 1537, 1541, 1542,

1552-53, 1554, 1556, 1557, 1559, 1561-62, 1564, 1571, 1574, 1576, 1580 (1999).

Journal 1999 Discusses the push to mandate disclosure in managed care programs. Explains the dangers of disclosing too much information. Provides objectives and goals for disclosure. Quotes Opinion 8.051. References Opinions 8.032 and 8.13. Sage, *Regulating Through Information: Disclosure Laws and American Health Care, 99 Colum. L. Rev. 1701, 1753, 1758, 1760 (1999).*

Journal 1999 Argues that the benefits of managed care organizations are outweighed by the resulting changes in the physician's role as advocate. Characterizes the traditional notion of physician advocacy. States that recent changes in the law regarding communication in managed care organizations have shifted the matter more toward patient self-advocacy. Quotes Opinion 8.13. Spielman, *Managed Care Regulation and the Physician-Advocate, 47 Drake L. Rev. 713, 717, 719 (1999).*

Journal 1999 Discusses financial incentives offered to physicians by managed care organizations. Argues that evidence of financial incentives should be admissible in medical malpractice cases. Quotes Opinion 8.13. References Opinion 8.132. Sugarman & Yarashus, *Admissibility of Managed Care Financial Incentives in Medical Malpractice Cases, 34 Tort & Ins. L. J. 735, 743, 746, 759 (1999).*

Journal 1999 Explores the impact managed care organizations have had on health care. Explains that patients may not understand restrictions and incentives imposed by their managed care organizations when entering the program. Argues that such information should be disclosed at various times during the period of plan coverage. Cites Opinions 2.03, 8.03, 8.032, 8.051, 8.13, and 8.132. Wolf, *Toward a Systemic Theory of Informed Consent in Managed Care, 35 Hous. L. Rev. 1631, 1641, 1658, 1661, 1662, 1679 (1999).*

Journal 1998 Analyzes Hall's book *Making Medical Spending Decisions: The Law, Ethics and Economics of Rationing Mechanisms.* Discusses cost-based rationing for medical services and physician bedside rationing. Concludes that patients should be informed in advance when their physician may receive financial incentives for withholding care. Quotes Opinion 8.13. Agrawal, *Chicago Hope Meets the Chicago School, 96 Mich. L. Rev. 1793, 1804 (1998).*

Journal 1998 Discusses changes in the health care system. Explains why patients need more power in the managed care system. Suggests that patients should use class action suits as a method to assert power over managed care organizations. References Opinions 8.13 and 8.132. Cerminara, *The Class Action Suit as a Method of Patient Empowerment in the Managed Care Setting, 24 Am. J. Law & Med. 7, 16, 17, 23 (1998).*

Journal 1998 Discusses conflicts of interest in the physician-patient relationship arising out of use of financial incentives by managed care organizations. Considers how such conflicts are dealt with in the attorney-client

relationship. Suggests that a financial incentive should be legally denounced if it unreasonably interferes with a physician's duty to properly care for and treat patients. Quotes Preamble, Fundamental Elements (1) [now Opinion 10.01], and Opinions 4.04, 5.01, 8.03, 8.13, and 9.06. Cites Fundamental Elements (4) [now Opinion 10.01] and Opinions 2.07, 2.08, and 2.132. Hall, *Third-Party Payor Conflicts of Interest in Managed Care: A Proposal for Regulation Based on the Model Rules of Professional Conduct, 29 Seton Hall L. Rev. 95, 96, 107, 108, 109, 110, 111, 112, 134, 135, 136 (1998).*

Journal 1998 Asserts that managed care organizations assume fiduciary obligations by exercising discretionary control over the administration of an ERISA plan. Argues that ERISA requires managed care organizations and physicians to disclose financial incentives intended to influence physician decision-making. References Opinions 8.13 and 8.132. Johnson, *ERISA Doctor in the House? The Duty to Disclose Physician Incentives to Limit Health Care, 82 Minn. L. Rev. 1631, 1639, 1649, 1655 (1998).*

Journal 1998 Discusses changes in the health care system. Analyzes conflicts of interest arising from the practice of capitation. Argues that physicians should refuse to sign contracts with health care plans offering incentives that may present a temptation to undertreat patients. References Opinion 8.13. Kassirer, *Managing Care—Should We Adopt a New Ethic? 339 New Eng. J. Med. 397 (1998).*

Journal 1998 Expresses concern about the impact of managed care cost-containment practices on the physician-patient relationship. Advocates the need for disclosure of information about these practices to patients. Evaluates and recommends a Maryland law that requires such disclosure. Cites Opinion 8.13. Khanna, Silverman, & Schwartz, *Disclosure of Operating Practices by Managed-Care Organizations to Consumers of Healthcare: Obligations of Informed Consent, 9 J. Clinical Ethics 291, 293, 296 (1998).*

Journal 1998 Discusses quality and safety concerns arising under managed care systems. Explores benefits and detriments of the proposed patients' bill of rights. Advocates legislation to provide safeguards from cost-containment mechanisms utilized by managed care programs. Quotes Opinion 8.13. Misocky, *The Patients' Bill of Rights: Managed Care Under Siege, 15 J. Contemp. Health L. & Pol'y 57, 73 (1998).*

Journal 1998 Explores clinical freedom and the Hippocratic Oath. Discusses issues of patient trust and confidence. Suggests that a sense of confidence will not be present if managerial priorities are dominant factors in resource allocation. References Opinion 8.13. Newdick, *Public Health Ethics and Clinical Freedom, 14 J. Contemp. Health L. & Pol'y 335, 336, 339, 356, 359, 361 (1998).*

Journal 1998 Discusses communication conflicts between physicians and managed care organizations. Describes legal responses to gag provisions imposed by managed care organizations. Assesses the impact of gag practices on physician-patient communication. Quotes Opinion 8.13. Spielman, *After the Gag Episode: Physician Communication in Managed Care Organizations, 22 Seton Hall Legis. J. 437, 453, 461, 463 (1998).*

Journal 1998 Argues that health maintenance organizations (HMOs) do not have an incentive to act reasonably because they are not held accountable under tort law. Points out that the duty to act reasonably is imposed on most of society in order to deter negligence. Advocates imposing the same duty on HMOs. References Opinion 8.13. Wertheimer, *Ockham's Scalpel: A Return to a Reasonableness Standard, 43 Vill. L. Rev. 321, 327 (1998).*

Journal 1997 Discusses the quality of neurological care and the ethical conflicts that are created by the drive to contain costs. Focuses on quality management and cost-containment programs and the conflicts created when neurologists attempt to reconcile the interests of patients and society. References Opinions 8.032 and 8.13. Bernat, *Quality of Neurological Care: Balancing Cost Control and Ethics, 54 Arch. Neurol. 1341, 1343, 1345 (1997).*

Journal 1997 Compares past ethical opinions to current opinions and notes the differences. Comments on the forces that have changed medical ethics through the years. Notes differing theories on the future course of medical ethics. Quotes Fundamental Elements (Preamble) and Opinions 5.05, 5.057, 7.01, 8.12, 9.12, and 9.131. Cites Fundamental Elements (5) and Opinions 8.115 and 8.13. Buchanan, *Medical Ethics at the Millennium: A Brief Retrospective, 26 Colo. Law. 141, 142, 143, 144, 145 (1997).*

Journal 1997 Examines the use of gag clauses in the managed care setting. Explores the conflict of interest between physicians' loyalty to HMOs and their duty to patients. Questions whether patients can give informed consent based on inadequate information. Emphasizes the need for more comprehensive regulation. Quotes Opinion 8.13. Comment, *Physician Gag Clauses—The Hypocrisy of the Hippocratic Oath, 21 So. Ill. U. L. J. 313, 318, 320 (1997).*

Journal 1997 Reviews the conflict between the economics of managed care and physicians' ethical obligations to patients. Questions whether a patient may give informed consent to treatment without knowledge of all available alternatives. Offers a proposal for disclosure of managed care cost-containment mechanisms and incentives to patients. Quotes Opinion 8.13. Hall, *A Theory of Economic Informed Consent, 31 Ga. L. Rev. 511, 521, 524-25 (1997).*

Journal 1997 Posits that cost-containment schemes in managed care systems have eroded the fiduciary duty physicians owe patients. Notes that managed care organizations (MCOs) are prohibiting patients from trusting and relying on physicians. Concludes that patients must seek quality assurance from sources other than their physicians. Quotes Opinions 2.03, 2.09, and 8.13. Jacobi, *Patients at a Loss: Protecting Health Care Consumers Through Data Driven Quality Assurance, 45 U. Kan. L. Rev. 705, 720, 721, 759 (1997).*

Journal 1997 Explores the responsibilities imposed on physicians by managed care and capitation. Notes that physicians are called on to act as gatekeepers, controlling access to specialty services and tests. Considers whether primary care physicians in capitated groups are satisfied with the quality of care they provide. References Opinion 8.13. Kerr, Hays, Mittman, Siu, Leake, & Brook, *Primary Care Physicians' Satisfaction With Quality of Care in California Capitated Medical Groups, 278 JAMA 308, 312 (1997).*

Journal 1997 Examines national health care reform and managed care. Notes that state regulatory policies in this context evidence common concerns. Suggests ways in which the government can promote patient and physician rights. References Opinion 8.13. Miller, *Managed Care Regulation: In the Laboratory of the States, 278 JAMA 1102, 1104, 1108-09 (1997).*

Journal 1997 Discusses physician frustration with managed care plans caused by gag clauses and cost-containment mechanisms. Reviews the development of managed care organizations and federal attempts at limiting the use of gag clauses. Concludes that gag clauses are inherently flawed and compromise quality health care. Quotes Principles II and V, Fundamental Elements (1), and Opinion 8.13. Note, *Physicians, Bound and Gagged: Federal Attempts to Combat Managed Care's Use of Gag Clauses, 21 Seton Hall Legis. J. 567, 601-02 (1997).*

Journal 1997 Describes gag provisions in managed care contracts. Explains the context in which gag provisions may undermine the physician-patient relationship, as well as the conflicts of interest they may create. Proposes legislation to address these problems. Quotes Opinion 8.13. Note, *Stop Gagging Physicians! 7 Health Matrix 187, 193, 200, 208-09 (1997).*

Journal 1997 Examines the need for change in interpretation of state laws under the saving clause of the Employment Retirement Income Security Act. Discusses any willing provider laws and concludes that they should receive saving clause protection. References Opinion 8.13. Pittman, *Any Willing Provider Laws and ERISA's Saving Clause: A New Solution for an Old Problem, 64 Tenn. L. Rev. 409, 416 (1997).*

Journal 1997 Discusses the need for balance between business ethics and medical ethics in the context of managed care. Explores two models for integrating ethics and managed care. Proposes the adoption of a collective responsibility model to improve quality of care. Quotes Principles I, II, III, IV, and V. Cites Preamble. References Opinion 8.13. Regan, *Regulating the Business of Medicine: Models for Integrating Ethics and Managed Care, 30 Colum. J. L. & Soc. Probs. 635, 651, 656, 657 (1997).*

Journal 1997 Examines utilization review in the managed care context. Discusses a survey of third-party utilization review firms, noting practices that advance and undermine adherence to important professional norms. Quotes Opinion 9.031. References Opinion 8.13. Schlesinger, Gray,

& Perreira, *Medical Professionalism Under Managed Care: The Pros and Cons of Utilization Review, 16 Health Affairs 106, 119, 120, 124 (1997).*

Journal 1996 Discusses the use of practice guidelines to improve medical care quality and to aid in decreasing health care costs. Evaluates pertinent ethical considerations. Concludes that, when used appropriately, guidelines have clinical value. References Opinion 8.13. Berger & Rosner, *The Ethics of Practice Guidelines, 156 Arch. Intern. Med. 2051, 2053, 2056 (1996).*

Journal 1996 Considers the economic implications for physicians brought about by the change from traditional fee-for-service care to capitation. Discusses capitation payments in the American health care system. Alludes to pertinent ethical issues. References Opinion 8.13. Bodenheimer & Grumbach, *Capitation or Decapitation: Keeping Your Head in Changing Times, 276 JAMA 1025, 1031 (1996).*

Journal 1996 Examines the business of health care and the ethical implications of managed care. Describes incentives that affect the delivery of health care. Suggests that a redistribution of excess revenues would help both patients and nonprofit hospitals coexist with managed care. Quotes Opinion 8.13. Bond, *Diverse and Perverse Incentives in Managed Care: Where Will the Pendulum Stop? 1 Widener L. Symp. J. 141, 151, 154 (1996).*

Journal 1996 Discusses the trend toward health care reform. Focuses on benefits and problems posed by managed mental health care. Posits that the moral problems of managed mental health care, including quality concerns, are curable. Concludes that managed mental health care may prove superior to fee-for-service care. References Opinion 8.13. Boyle, *Managed Care in Mental Health: A Cure, or a Cure Worse Than the Disease? 40 St. Louis U. L. J. 437, 448 (1996).*

Journal 1996 Discusses the threat managed health care poses to patients and physicians. Explores direct incentives given to physicians by managed care organizations and the impact these incentives have on physician behavior. Proposes possible methods for dealing with the problems that such incentives create. References Opinion 8.13. Greely, *Direct Financial Incentives in Managed Care: Unanswered Questions, 6 Health Matrix 53, 81 (1996).*

Journal 1996 Discusses the change from fee-for-service health care financing to managed care. Notes that cost-containment mechanisms modify physicians' behaviors and patients' access to health care. Emphasizes that physicians must remain committed to following ethical guidelines. References Opinion 8.13. Hammes & Webster, *Professional Ethics and Managed Care in Dermatology, 132 Arch. Dermatol. 1070, 1072, 1073 (1996).*

Journal 1996 Discusses workers' compensation and the medical care provided to injured employees. Examines the effect of managed care on workers' compensation. Advocates focusing on prevention of injuries and quality of care. References Opinion 8.13. Hashimoto, *The Future Role of Managed Care and Capitation in Workers' Compensation, XXII Am. J. Law & Med. 233, 258, 259 (1996).*

Journal 1996 Considers challenges to the psychiatrist-patient relationship that are triggered by managed care cost-containment methodologies. Offers guidance to psychiatrists for addressing these challenges. References Opinions 2.095, 8.13, and 8.132. Hoge, *APA Resource Document: I. The Professional Responsibilities of Psychiatrists in Evolving Health Care Systems, 24 Bull. Am. Acad. Psychiatry Law 393, 405 (1996).*

Journal 1996 Discusses the problems managed care raises within the framework of the physician-patient relationship. Considers issues specific to psychiatry. Advocates legal regulation to improve upon and bring structural change to managed care systems. Cites Opinion 8.13. Hoge, *APA Resource Document: II. Regulatory Guidelines for Protecting the Interests of Psychiatric Patients in Emerging Health Care Systems, 24 Bull. Am. Acad. Psychiatry Law 407, 412, 418 (1996).*

Journal 1996 Considers procedural issues relative to patient protection in the context of capitated health care plans. Examines regulations governing capitated health plans and consumer protection issues. Offers suggestions regarding policy making, rate setting, dispute resolution, and judicial review. References Opinion 8.13. Kinney, *Procedural Protections for Patients in Capitated Health Plans, XXII Am. J. Law & Med. 301, 319-20 (1996).*

Journal 1996 Explains the conflict between managed care, which focuses on controlling costs, and traditional health care values, which focus on patient autonomy. Proposes a solution to this conflict requiring that patients incur certain economic consequences in obtaining health care and that managed care organizations disclose resource management techniques. References Opinion 8.13. Morreim, *Diverse and Perverse Incentives of Managed Care: Bringing Patients Into Alignment, 1 Widener L. Symp. J. 89, 129 (1996).*

Journal 1996 Discusses efforts to reduce health care costs. Considers whether personal financial incentives given to physicians decrease level of care given to patients. Suggests that, while financial incentives may create ethical concerns, they serve an important function by containing costs. Concludes that efforts to eliminate them completely are misguided. References Opinion 8.13. Orentlicher, *Paying Physicians More to Do Less: Financial Incentives to Limit Care, 30 U. Rich. L. Rev. 155, 167 (1996).*

11.2.3.1 Restrictive Covenants

N.D. Ill. 1996 A corporation which provided hair transplants brought suit against a physician group under contract to provide medical services to the corporation. The complaint alleged that the defendants had breached the contract in bad faith by attempting to start their own company, by hiring staff members away, and by threatening to enforce noncompetition covenants in their contracts should any physicians attempt to remain with the corporation. The court referred to Opinion 9.02 as explicitly discouraging the use of restrictive covenants in contracts with physicians. Additionally, with apparent reference to Opinion 7.03, the court noted that defendants had not sent notices advising patients of the departure of physicians from the corporation, or of the departing physicians' new practice locations. *Cleveland Hair Clinic, Inc. v. Puig,* 968 F. Supp. 1227, 1246.

Ariz. 1999 Medical practice sought to enforce a restrictive covenant with defendant-physician. The trial court denied the plaintiff's request for a preliminary injunction and found that the restrictive covenant was unenforceable. The Arizona Supreme Court held that covenants not to compete between physicians will be strictly construed for reasonableness. Under this analysis, the court found that the restrictive covenant was unreasonable, overbroad, and unenforceable. The court quoted Opinions 9.02 and 9.06, recognizing that the AMA discourages restrictive covenants and supports free choice and competition. *Valley Medical Specialists v. Farber,* 194 Ariz. 363, 982 P.2d 1277, 1282.

Ariz. App. 1989 Plaintiff, an orthopaedic surgeon formerly employed by defendant, appealed a lower court's grant of a preliminary injunction which enforced the restrictive covenant in plaintiff's employment contract with defendant. Plaintiff asserted that Opinion 9.02 discouraged the use of such restrictive covenants and thus the covenant at issue should be declared per se unenforceable. The appellate court declined to make that declaration, noting that not all restrictive covenants are contrary to public policy and that the lower court had appropriately modified the terms of the covenant. *Phoenix Orthopaedic Surgeons, Ltd. v. Peairs,* 164 Ariz. 54, 60, 790 P.2d 752, 758.

Ga. 1988 Following termination of employment contract between the employer, a provider of psychiatric services, and a physician, the employer filed suit seeking an injunction to enforce a covenant not to compete. Supreme Court, without opinion, upheld trial court's order granting an injunction. Dissenting judge, quoting Opinion 9.02 (1986) reasoned that restrictive covenants in such physician employment agreements are "illegal per se as against public policy irrespective of whether the covenant is reasonable." *Shankman v. Coastal Psychiatric Assocs.,* 258 Ga. 294, 295, 368 S.E.2d 753, 754 (dissent).

Ill. 2006 Physicians appealed a grant of preliminary injunction enforcing restrictive covenants in their employment contracts. Quoting Opinions 9.02, 9.06, and 10.01 and referencing Opinion 8.115, the Illinois Supreme Court gave

thorough consideration to the AMA's position on restrictive covenants. While acknowledging the ethical problems associated with such contracts, the court found the covenants reasonable in scope. The decision to ban restrictive covenants, the court reasoned, was best left to the legislature. *Mohanty v. St. John Heart Clinic, S.C.,* 225 Ill.2d 52, 866 N.E.2d 85, 94, 106-07, 107-08.

Ill. App. 2002 Ophthalmologist terminated employment contract with an eye clinic and intentionally practiced in an area prohibited by a noncompetition clause in the contract. The Illinois Appellate Court, while noting that under Opinion 9.02 (1986) noncompetition agreements are "discouraged," held that such agreements are enforceable in the medical profession in Illinois. *Prairie Eye Center v. Butler,* 329 Ill. App. 3d 293, 768 N.E.2d 414, 420.

Ill. App. 2000 Physician challenged trial court's decision upholding noncompete clause in the physician's employment contract with a health care provider. The appellate court reversed the decision, quoting Opinions 9.02 (1986) and 9.06 (1982). The court stated that the AMA disfavors the use of any restrictive employment or partnership agreements among physicians and emphasized the fact that such agreements are not in the public interest. The court also noted that patients might suffer if such agreements are upheld. *Carter-Shields v. Alton Health Institute,* 317 Ill. App. 3d 260, 739 N.E.2d 569, 576-77, *vacated* 201 Ill. 2d 441, 777 N.E.2d 948 (2002).

Ind. 2008 Professional corporation brought suit against a podiatrist it formerly employed to enforce noncompetition restriction of employment contract. The court quoted Opinion 9.02 with respect to the enforceability of such covenants. The court held that noncompetition agreements between a physician and a medical group are not per se void as against public policy and are enforceable so long as they are reasonable. *Cent. Ind. Podiatry, P.C. v. Krueger,* 882 N.E.2d 723, 728, n. 4.

Ind. App. 1987 Medical corporation sued physician who was former employee at will pursuant to covenant not to compete in employment contract seeking an injunction or liquidated damages. Court upheld covenant against physician's claim that enforcement was inappropriate where he had been terminated without good cause. Concurring judge, citing Opinion 9.02 (1986), expressed view that such covenants should be unenforceable as against public policy. *Gomez v. Chua Medical Corp.,* 510 N.E.2d 191, 197.

Kan. 2005 Appellee surgeons sought a restraining order and injunction prohibiting enforcement of covenants not to compete in their employment contracts on the grounds that Opinion 9.02 prohibits such covenants, making them void as against public policy. The Kansas Supreme Court held that neither Opinion 9.02 nor Kansas case law makes restrictive covenants unenforceable per se. Restrictive covenants are unenforceable only if they are excessive in geographic scope and duration or fail to make reasonable accommodations for the patient's choice of physician. *Idbeis v. Wichita Surgical Specialists, 279 Kan. 755, 112 P.2d 81, 87, 88.*

Kan. App. 1985 Members of a medical partnership sought an injunction to enforce a covenant not to compete against defendant-physician, a former partner. Defendant asserted that the covenant was void as against public policy relying on Opinion 9.02 (1984). The court however ruled that the covenant was reasonable as defined by precedent and that it was bound to follow this precedent as opposed to the AMA's position regarding such covenants. Defendant further argued enforcement of the covenant was precluded because the partnership had violated ethical norms, apparently referring to Opinions 6.03 and 6.04 (1984) [now Opinions 6.02 and 6.03], which were part of partnership contract. The court held defendant was estopped from complaining about the partnership's actions due to his own conduct. *Axtell Clinic v. Cranston, No. 56,745 (Kan. Ct. App. June 20, 1985) (LEXIS, States Library, Ka. file).*

Mich. App. 2006 Physician signed an employment contract with a restrictive covenant and liquidated damages provision. When the physician resigned and violated the covenant, the employer brought an action seeking payment of liquidated damages. The physician counterclaimed, alleging the restrictive covenant was unreasonable and void on both statutory and public policy grounds. On appeal, the physician argued that the covenant was unreasonable in light of Opinion 9.02. The appeals court reasoned that the employer had a valid interest in retaining patients in the area and that the covenant was not unreasonable. *St. Clair Medical, P.C. v. Borgiel, 270 Mich.App. 260, 715 N.W.2d 914, 920-21.*

Minn. 1983 Dispute arose between physician and clinic concerning covenant not to compete contained in employment contract entered into by physician after commencement of employment. Physician challenged enforceability of covenant due to lack of consideration to support it. The court agreed with physician and denied enforcement. In so ruling court did not reach issue of whether such covenants, in the context of medical practice, are against public policy. The court however noted that under Opinion 9.01 (1982) [now Opinion 9.02] the AMA discourages such restrictive covenants. *Freeman v. Duluth Clinic, 334 N.W.2d 626, 631.*

N.J. 2005 Appellant hospital filed suit in superior court to enforce a covenant not to compete against respondent, a neurosurgeon. The court refused to enforce the covenant and found for the respondent. On appeal, the appellate division reversed. It found that Opinion 9.02 and case law support the conclusion that restrictive covenants are unenforceable only when they are unreasonable in scope and duration or do not make reasonable accommodations for the patient's choice of physician. Quoting Opinion 9.02, the Supreme Court of New Jersey agreed that physician restrictive covenants are not unenforceable per se, but reversed the appellate division because the geographic restriction of the covenant was injurious to the public. *Community Hosp. Group Inc. v. More, 183 N.J. 36, 869 A.2d 884, 896.*

N.J. 1978 Plaintiff and defendant, both physicians, had entered into an employment contract which included in its terms a restrictive covenant provision. When defendant failed to abide by the covenant upon termination of the employment contract, plaintiff sued to enforce the covenant. In affirming the lower court's decision to enforce the restrictive covenant, the appellate court quoted Opinion 4.63 (1977) [now Opinion 9.02] and stated that, although it hesitated to give weight to the rules of private organizations, even if it followed the Opinion the decision to uphold the covenant would be proper. *Karlin v. Weinberg, 77 N.J. 408, 390 A.2d 1161, 1168 n.6.*

N.J. Super. 2004 Respondent physician appealed dismissal of complaint, arguing that restrictive covenants are void per se as a matter of public policy and that the court should not follow prior case law. The trial court quoted Opinion 9.02 and compared it to the previous opinion on restrictive covenants to determine that the AMA is currently more hostile toward restrictive covenants than it had been previously. The court noted that it must apply precedent and enforce the restrictive covenant. If any change is to be made in the law, it must be made by the New Jersey Supreme Court. The appeals court agreed and affirmed. *Pierson v. Med. Health Ctrs., 2004 WL 1416265, 3.*

N.J. Super. 2003 Hospital filed suit to enforce a covenant not to compete against respondent neurosurgeon. The court refused to enforce the covenant and found for the respondent. In reversing, the appellate division found the respondent's argument that the restrictive covenant should be unenforceable based on Opinion 9.02 unpersuasive. The appellate division stated that AMA ethical standards and case law support the conclusion that restrictive covenants are unenforceable only when they are unreasonable in scope and duration or do not make reasonable accommodations for the patient's choice of physician. *Community Hosp. Group Inc. v. More, 365 N.J. Super. 84, 838 A.2d 472, 488.*

N.J. Super. 1977 Plaintiff, a dermatologist who had previously employed defendant-dermatologist, sued to enforce a postemployment restrictive covenant signed by defendant. In holding the covenant enforceable, the court noted Opinion 4.63 (1977) [now Opinion 9.02], which at the time stated there was "no ethical proscription" against entering into a restrictive covenant if its terms are reasonable. Note that Opinion 9.02 now "discourages" such restrictive agreements. *Karlin v. Weinberg, 148 N.J. Super. 243, 372 A.2d 616, 618, aff'd, 77 N.J. 408, 390 A.2d 1161 (1978).*

N.Y. Sup. 2007 Plaintiff, an otolaryngologist, signed an employment contract with defendant, which included a covenant not to compete, restricting practice within 30 miles of defendant's offices for a period of three years. Plaintiff resigned and defendant sought enforcement. Citing Opinion 9.02, plaintiff argued that the contract was unreasonable in scope and unnecessary to protect any legitimate business interest of defendant. The court disagreed, noting that Opinion 9.02 merely discourages such agreements and does not prohibit them. The noncompete agreement was held reasonable, in both temporal and geographic scope, to protect the legitimate business interests of defendant's goodwill and patient base. Although it was overbroad in prohibiting the general practice of medicine, partial enforcement was appropriate to prohibit practice of otolaryngology. *Awwad v. Capital Region Otolaryngology Head & Neck Group, 2007 N.Y. Misc. LEXIS 8593, 19.*

N.Y. Sup. 2005 Plaintiff health center moved for an injunction to stop defendant physician and former employee from opening up a pediatric practice within 10 miles of the health center. The court, citing Opinion 9.02, stated that the AMA does not hold that restrictive covenants are unethical and unenforceable per se and that court should not utilize the AMA's position to impose an outright ban on physician restrictive covenants. The court found that the plaintiff had not shown that the defendant would use unfair means to compete, and therefore the plaintiff was not entitled to the protection of the restrictive covenant. *Oak Orchard Cmty. Health Ctr. v. Blasco, 8 Misc. 3d 927, 800 N.Y.S.2d. 277, 281, n. 3.*

N.C. App. 2006 Physicians entered an employment contract that included a noncompetition clause, as well as a clause stating the contract would be void if it did not comply with the AMA Code of Medical Ethics. In an action challenging the enforceability of the noncompete agreement, the physicians argued the provision violated Opinion 9.02 and was void under either the contractual terms or on public policy grounds. The court concluded the noncompete agreement was not per se against public policy and that the clause requiring compliance with the AMA Code was intended solely to address concerns regarding physician autonomy. *Calhoun v. WHA Medical Clinic, PLLC, 178 N.C.App. 585, 632 S.E.2d 563, 568.*

Ohio App. 1991 Medical corporation sought an injunction to enforce a covenant not to compete against defendant-physician. The lower court granted summary judgment based on a referee's report which concluded that, under Principle VI and Opinions 6.11, 9.02, and 9.06 (1989), restrictive covenants were per se unenforceable as a matter of public policy. While recognizing a strong public interest in allowing open access to health care, the appellate court in reversing held that Opinion 9.02, which applied specifically to restrictive covenants, only "discouraged" such covenants. *Ohio Urology, Inc. v. Poll, 72 Ohio. App. 446, 450, 451, 594 N.E.2d 1027, 1030, 1031.*

Tenn. 2005 Respondent, a private medical practice, filed suit to enforce a noncompetition covenant contained in a physician's employment contract. The trial court found that the covenant was enforceable, and the court of appeals affirmed. The Tennessee Supreme Court reversed. Quoting Opinions 9.02 and 9.06 it found that such covenants are not enforceable because they violate public policy. *Murfreesboro Med. Clinic v. Udom, 166 S.W.3d 674, 679, 684, 685.*

Journal 2010 Discusses the background and policies of traditional noncompete agreements and evaluates the arguments underlying the use of restrictive covenants in the health care field. Concludes that enforcing physician noncompete clauses ultimately hurts patients, and that courts should create an exception regarding such clauses similar to that for attorney noncompete clauses. Quotes Opinion 9.06. Cites Opinion 9.02. Klimkina, *Are Noncompete Contracts Between Physicians Bad Medicine? Advocating in the Affirmative by Drawing a Public Policy Parallel to the Legal Profession, 98 Ky. L. J. 131, 147-148 (2010).*

Journal 2009 Discusses the judicial standard for reviewing physician noncompete covenants. Concludes courts should apply a strict standard to such covenants, rather than declare the covenants per se invalid. Quotes Principles IV and VII, Principles of Medical Ethics §5 (1957) [now Principle VI], Code of Medical Ethics Ch. II, Art. I §3 (1847) [now Opinion 5.02], Opinion 9.02, and Code of Medical Ethics Ch. II, Art. I §4 (1847) [now Opinion 9.09]. Cites Opinions 8.041, 8.115, 9.02, 9.06, 9.065, 9.067, 10.01, and 10.015. Koons, *Physician Employee Non-Compete Agreements on the Examining Table: The Need to Better Protect Patients' and the Public's Interests in Indiana, 6 Ind. Health L. Rev. 253, 272-77, 280-81 (2009).*

Journal 2009 Examines the economic impact of specialty hospitals on general hospitals and discusses efforts of general hospitals to remove competition. Concludes that specialty hospitals are not responsible for ensuring the economic viability of general hospitals and that general hospitals should focus on bolstering their own resources, rather than on eliminating competition from specialty hospitals. Quotes Opinion 9.02. Steinbuch, *Placing Profits Above Hippocrates: The Hypocrisy of General Service Hospitals, 31 U. Ark. Little Rock L. Rev. 505, 512 (2009).*

Journal 2008 Examines for-profit medical specialty groups and their impact on competition for specialty services. Concludes for-profit medical groups must not be allowed to eliminate competition to garner higher profits until a market for affordable health care services is established. Cites Opinion 9.02. Kinney, *The Corporate Transformation of Medical Specialty Care: The Exemplary Case of Neonatology, 36 J. L. Med. & Ethics 790, 791 (2008).*

Journal 2008 Discusses covenants not to compete and Kentucky cases dealing with physician noncompetition agreements. Concludes Kentucky should enact legislation permitting reasonable noncompetition agreements ancillary to sale of practice contracts to increase patient choice of physician. Quotes Principle VIII and Opinion 9.02. Naiser, *Physician Noncompetition Agreements in Kentucky: The Past Discounting of Public Interests and a Proposed Solution, 47 U. Louisville L. Rev. 195, 195, 200 (2008).*

Journal 2007 Examines the role of the medical profession in participating in state-sanctioned lethal injection. Concludes that any participation is unethical because it causes harm and undermines trust. Cites Opinion 2.06. References Opinions 2.211 and 9.02. Black & Sade, *Lethal*

Injection and Physicians: State Law vs Medical Ethics, 298 JAMA 2779, 2780, 2781 (2007).

Journal 2007 Discusses the enforceability of medical noncompete agreements in Michigan. Concludes that such agreements are likely enforceable, but may be invalidated based on local availability of medical services. Quotes Opinion 9.02. Quick, *Contract Law: Physician, Meet Thy Covenant: Noncompete Agreements in the Medical Profession, 86 Mich. Bar J. 22, 23 (2007).*

Journal 2006 Explores the use of "no-hire" clauses in the field of health care. Concludes that enforcement of such clauses should be determined on the basis of reasonableness. Cites Opinion 9.02. Basanta, *"No-Hire" Clauses in Healthcare Sector Contracts: Their Use and Enforceability, 39 J. Health L. 451, 453 (2006).*

Journal 2006 Reviews the Tennessee Supreme Court decision banning physician covenants not to compete. Concludes the policy decisions discussed by the court are vital in deciding if and when to enforce covenants not to compete. References Opinion 9.02. Belville, *Most Covenants Not to Compete Against Physicians Are No Longer Enforceable in Tennessee, 7 Transactions 419, 434 (2006).*

Journal 2006 Discusses the Tennessee Supreme Court decision prohibiting physician noncompete agreements. Suggests the court should have adopted a standard of reasonableness for noncompete agreements. Quotes Opinion 9.02. Cites Opinion 9.06. Carr, *Contracts—Murfreesboro Medical Clinic, P.A. v. Udom: Physician Noncompete Agreements Go Under the Knife: The Tennessee Supreme Court Rejects Physician Noncompete Agreements, 36 U. Mem. L. Rev. 1115, 1128, 1131 (2006).*

Journal 2006 Examines physician restrictive covenants. Concludes that under the current balancing test, courts should give considerable weight to the public interest in preserving the physician-patient relationship. Quotes Opinions 9.02 and 9.06. Cites Opinions 6.11, 8.11, 8.115, and 9.06. Malloy, *Physician Restrictive Covenants: The Neglect of Incumbent Patient Interests, 41 Wake Forest L. Rev. 189, 207-08, 217, 218 (2006).*

Journal 2006 Discusses noncompete agreements in surgeon employment contracts. Concludes that covenants not to compete should be unenforceable per se against surgeons. Quotes Opinions 9.02 and 9.06. Wyatt, *Buy Out or Get Out: Why Covenants Not to Compete in Surgeon Employment Contracts Are Truly Bad Medicine, 45 Washburn L. J. 715, 720 (2006).*

Journal 2005 Discusses the ban of physician noncompetition covenants by the Tennessee Supreme Court. Concludes that new contractual terms will need to be drafted to balance employer and employee interests in the medical profession. Quotes Opinion 9.06. References Opinion 9.02. Schuler, *Knock Out? Supreme Court Deals a Blow to Non-Competes for Docs, but This Fight Is Not Over, 41 Tenn. B.J. 16, 19 (Dec. 2005).*

Journal 2003 Discusses conflicting Illinois case law regarding medical restrictive covenants. Concludes the Illinois Supreme Court should validate medical restrictive covenants that protect a business interest. Quotes Opinion 9.02. Gimbel & Zaremski, *Medical Restrictive Covenants in Illinois: At the Crossroads of Carter-Shields and Prairie Eye Center, 12 Annals Health L. 1, 12 (2003).*

Journal 2003 Highlights the legal and ethical concerns surrounding use of noncompetition clauses. Concludes that physicians should carefully evaluate these clauses given their likely enforceability. Quotes Opinions 9.02, 9.06, 10.01, and 10.015. Loeser, *The Legal, Ethical, and Practical Implications of Noncompetition Clauses: What Physicians Should Know Before They Sign, 31 J. L. Med. & Ethics 283, 286, 287, 290 (2003).*

Journal 2000 Examines strikingly different approaches to enforcement of reasonable contractual restraints on competition in the medical and legal fields. Observes that most recent cases find the public harm caused by noncompetition agreements to be generally insufficient to deny enforcement. Quotes Opinion 9.02. Wilcox, *Enforcing Lawyer Non-Competition Agreements While Maintaining the Profession: The Role of Conflict of Interest Principles, 84 Minn. L. Rev. 915, 966 (2000).*

Journal 1999 Discusses the need for physicians to advocate on behalf of patients' rights in the context of health care delivery. Evaluates the nature and scope of the physician's role as advocate, noting that physicians cannot be expected to engage in attorney-like advocacy. Quotes Principles IV and VI, Fundamental Elements (2), (4), and (6) [now Opinion 10.01], Patient Responsibilities 5 [now Opinion 10.02], and Opinions 2.03, 2.07, 2.09, 2.16, 2.19, 3.06, 4.01, 4.04, 6.01, 7.02, 8.02, 8.03, 8.13, 8.132, 9.06, 9.07, and 9.131. Cites Opinions 5.05, 5.09, 7.01, 8.135, and 9.02. Sage, *Physicians as Advocates, 35 Hous. L. Rev. 1529, 1537, 1541, 1542, 1552-53, 1554, 1556, 1557, 1559, 1561-62, 1564, 1571, 1574, 1576, 1580 (1999).*

Journal 1998 Discusses the ramifications of physician license revocation for failing to pay child support. Points out that patients stand to lose access to trusted physicians and confidence in the health care system. Concludes that children need the most protection and that patients will have an easier time finding another physician than children will have finding another means for support. Quotes Opinion 5.05. Cites Opinions 9.02 and 9.06. Noyes, *Higher Penalties for Failing to Pay Child Support: A Look at Medical License Revocation, 19 J. Legal Med. 127, 138 (1998).*

Journal 1997 Examines noncompetition clauses in the medical field. Reviews policy concerns and historical and common-law analyses of agreements not to compete. Posits that the more commercialized the medical profession becomes, the more noncompetition clauses infringe upon the physician-patient relationship and patients' rights. Quotes Opinions 9.02 and 9.06. Cites Preamble and Opinion 6.11. Comment, *Noncompetition Clauses in Physician*

Employment Contracts in Oregon, 76 Or. L. Rev. 195, 204-06 (1997).

Journal 1997 Examines the judicial assessment of restrictive covenants within the legal and medical fields. Observes that courts tend to uphold physician, but not attorney, restrictive covenants. Concludes that covenants in medical practice should be treated in a manner similar to those in legal practice. Opinion 9.02. Levy, *Because Judges Went to Law School, Not Medical School: Restrictive Covenants in the Practices of Law and Medicine, 30 J. Health & Hosp. L. 89, 92, 101 (1997).*

Journal 1995 Analyzes South Carolina judicial treatment of covenants not to compete and liquidated damages provisions. Considers approaches in other jurisdictions and proposes guidelines for drafting contractual agreements. Quotes Opinion 9.06. Cites Opinion 9.01 (1982) [now Opinion 9.02]. Note, *Covenants Not to Compete and*

Liquidated Damages Clauses: Diagnosis and Treatment for Physicians, 46 S. C. L. Rev. 505, 514 (1995).

Journal 1991 Considers the question of whether physicians should provide medical treatment to those who come to them for second opinions. Concludes that each physician must individually decide whether to treat these patients. Quotes Opinions 6.11, 9.06, and 9.12. Cites Opinion 9.02. Ile, *Should Physicians Treat Patients Who Seek Second Opinions? 266 JAMA 273, 274 (1991).*

Journal 1982 Discusses the legal status of restrictive covenants in employment contracts against the background of the AMA's position discouraging such agreements as not serving the public interest. Observes that courts generally have upheld restrictive covenants if the limits are reasonable. Cites Opinion 9.01 (1982) [now Opinion 9.02]. Cooper, *Restrictive Covenants, 248 JAMA 3091, 3091 (1982).*

11.2.4 Transparency in Health Care

Journal 2003 Discusses conflicts of interest caused when managed care organizations provide financial incentives to physicians. Concludes that the focus of managed care is not well-suited for the doctor-patient relationship. Quotes Opinion 8.03. Cites Principle VII. References Opinion 8.051. Hall, *Bargaining With Hippocrates: Managed Care and the Doctor-Patient Relationship, 54 S. C. L. Rev. 689, 696, 735 (2003).*

Journal 2001 Discusses the prohibition on nonlawyer ownership of legal service providers. Considers how ethical rules and standards governing physicians have been directed toward preserving independent judgment. Concludes that ethical conflicts created by abandoning the prohibition on nonlawyer ownership of legal service providers may be managed by following the medical ethics model. Quotes Principle VI and Opinions 2.03, 2.09, 8.02, 8.021, 8.03, 8.05, 8.051, 8.054, and 8.13, and 8.132. Harris & Foran, *The Ethics of Middle-Class Access to Legal Services and What We Can Learn From the Medical Profession's Shift to a Corporate Paradigm, 70 Fordham L. Rev. 775, 817, 821, 822, 823, 824 (2001).*

Journal 1999 Discusses the push to mandate disclosure in managed care programs. Explains the dangers of disclosing too much information. Provides objectives and goals for disclosure. Quotes Opinion 8.051. References Opinions 8.032 and 8.13. Sage, *Regulating Through Information: Disclosure Laws and American Health Care, 99 Colum. L. Rev. 1701, 1753, 1758, 1760 (1999).*

Journal 1999 Explores the impact managed care organizations have had on health care. Explains that patients may not understand restrictions and incentives imposed by their managed care organizations when entering the program. Argues that such information should be disclosed at various times

during the period of plan coverage. Cites Opinions 2.03, 8.03, 8.032, 8.051, 8.13, and 8.132. Wolf, *Toward a Systemic Theory of Informed Consent in Managed Care, 35 Hous. L. Rev. 1631, 1641, 1658, 1661, 1662, 1679 (1999).*

S.D. Fla. 2001 Insured patients under health care plans sued managed care companies alleging improper nondisclosure of policies and procedures imposing restrictions on physicians' judgment as to appropriate medical treatment. The insureds sued under both the Racketeer Influenced and Corrupt Organizations Act (RICO) and the Employee Retirement Income Security Act (ERISA). The court, with one exception, dismissed without prejudice both the RICO and ERISA claims. Among the plaintiffs' arguments was that the defendants had included "gag clauses" in their physician contracts in violation of Opinion 8.053. *In Re Managed Care Litigation, 150 F.Supp.2d 1330, 1335.*

Journal 2006 Examines ethical dilemmas physicians may face as providers of pay-for-performance medical care. Concludes that this strategy offers a benefit to patients as long as physicians uphold stringent ethical standards and work together to ensure optimum patient care. Cites Principles I, V, VIII, and IX and Opinions 2.035, 2.095, 6.01, 8.021, 8.03, 8.0501, 8.053, 8.054, and 8.121. Bostick, Sade, & McMahon, *Report of the Council on Ethical and Judicial Affairs: Physician Pay-for-Performance Programs, 3 Ind. Health L. Rev. 429, 430, 431, 432-33, 434, 435, 436 (2006).*

Journal 2006 Discusses preemption of lawsuits against managed care organizations by the Employee Retirement Income Security Act of 1974 (ERISA). Proposes a "bifurcated legal regime" to decrease the protective scope of ERISA. Quotes Opinions 8.053 and 8.135. Madison, *ERISA and Liability for Provision of Medical Information, 84 N. C. L. Rev. 471, 540 (2006).*

Journal 2002 Examines how managed care has adversely affected information disclosure in the physician-patient relationship. Concludes that, unless courts expand applicability of principles of informed consent, patient self-determination and autonomy will continue to be undermined. Quotes Principle VIII and Opinions 8.03, 8.053, 8.054, and 8.08. Morris, *Dissing Disclosure: Just What the Doctor Ordered, 44 Ariz. L. Rev. 313, 344, 349, 362, 363, 366 (2002).*

Journal 2008 Explores the tension experienced by health care professionals who provide care and compete in a market economy. Concludes if health care professions continue commercializing, providers must strive to maintain ethical standards and appropriate professional-patient relationships. Quotes Opinion 8.054. Peltier & Guisti, *Commerce and Care: The Irreconcilable Tension Between Selling and Caring, 39 McGeorge L. Rev. 785, 794 (2008).*

Journal 2006 Discusses the evolution of health law in Virginia. Concludes that the area of health law continues to expand, develop, and be refined. Cites Opinions 3.03, 3.08, 5.01, 5.015, 5.02, 5.04, 5.055, 6.02, 6.021, 6.03, 6.04, 7.03, 7.04, 7.05, 8.054, 8.08, 8.081, 8.085, 8.115, 8.12, 8.14, 8.145, 8.19, and 9.045. Guanzon, *Health Care Law, 41 U. Rich. L. Rev. 179, 199 (2006).*

Journal 2005 Argues that in *Aetna v. Davila/Cigna v. Calad*, the Supreme Court missed an opportunity to overturn unjust ERISA policies. Concludes that the principle of complete ERISA preemption as articulated in these consolidated cases is unsatisfactory because it violates the separation of powers doctrine. Quotes Principle VIII. Cites Opinions 8.054, 8.13, 8.135, 9.123, 10.01, and 10.015. Nelson, *AETNA v. DAVILA/CIGNA v. CALAD: A Missed Opportunity, 31 Wm. Mitchell L. Rev. 843, 847, 849, 850, 880 (2005).*

Journal 2003 Reviews state laws designed to protect physicians acting as patient advocates in managed care organizations. Concludes that federal and state law must make it easier for physicians to challenge denials of or delays in patient care. Quotes Opinions 8.054, 8.13, and 10.01. Fentiman, *Patient Advocacy and Termination From Managed Care Organizations. Do State Laws Protecting Health Care Professional Advocacy Make Any Difference? 82 Neb. L. Rev. 508, 515-16, 517-18 (2003).*

Journal 1990 Discusses efforts of third-party payers to control health care expenditures for beneficiaries. Concludes that financial incentives to limit care and other cost-control techniques should be disclosed and that the rationale for such disclosure is compelling. Quotes Opinions 2.03, 2.09, and 8.03. Cites Opinions 2.19, 4.04, and 4.06. Hirshfeld, *Should Third Party Payors of Health Care Services Disclose Cost Control Mechanisms to Potential Beneficiaries? 14 Seton Hall Legis. J. 115, 130, 131, 144, 145, 146 (1990).*

D. N. J. 1999 Patient sued her managed care organization alleging that she suffered injuries due to failure to obtain timely approval for a nonmember physician to perform her back surgery. The plaintiff apparently relied on Opinion

8.13 to show that the defendant had a duty to advocate for her in seeking prompt approval for her surgery. The court, however, stated that the plaintiff's reference to the Opinion failed to establish such a duty because the Code of Medical Ethics does not have the force of law. *Pryzbowski v. US Health Care, Inc., 64 F. Supp. 2d 361, 370.*

S.D.N.Y. 1997 Employee brought suit against a health maintenance organization (HMO) under contract with her employer to provide health benefits. The suit alleged various theories of liability ranging from breach of implied contract to breach of fiduciary duties. Employee sought redress pursuant to the civil enforcement provisions of the Employee Retirement Income Security Act of 1974. The court granted HMO's motion to dismiss all claims except for the breach of fiduciary duty stemming from HMO's alleged policy of restricting the disclosure of noncovered treatments. The court quoted report of AMA Council on Ethical and Judicial Affairs [now Opinion 8.13] in holding that physicians have an ethical duty to fully disclose treatment options to patients regardless of whether treatment occurs in a managed care environment. *Weiss v. Cigna Healthcare, Inc., 972 F. Supp. 748, 751-52.*

Mass. Super. 2004 Defendants filed a motion for partial summary judgment in an action alleging they were liable for not disclosing their financial interests in an experimental program that the decedent participated in. The court denied the defendants' motion, referencing Opinion 8.13 in stating physicians should disclose financial incentives and restrictions placed on them by their HMO. *Darke v. Estate of Isner, 2004 WL 1325635, 3.*

Ohio Att'y Gen. 1999 State attorney general concluded that physicians who render opinions regarding the necessity of medical services for health insuring corporations are not engaged in the practice of medicine. Additionally, physicians who render opinions regarding medical necessity for appeals of adverse determinations do not fall under the regulatory, investigatory, or enforcement authority of the Ohio State Medical Board. Quoting Opinions 8.03, 8.11, and 8.13, the attorney general stated that physicians have an ethical duty to provide appropriate treatment for patients. *Ohio Att'y Gen. Op. No. 99-044, 1999 WL 692623.*

Journal 2006 Examines the process of physician deselection and the protections afforded to physicians. Concludes that physicians should be able to make a legal challenge to a dismissal made without cause. Quotes Opinion 8.13. Coppolo, *Not Just a Minimum Income Policy for Physicians: The Need for Good Faith and Fair Dealing in Physician Deselection Disputes, 48 Wm. and Mary L. Rev. 677, 686 (2006).*

Journal 2006 Examines external review systems used for adjudication of disputes between patients and managed care organizations. Concludes that external review systems do not satisfy constitutional due process requirements. Quotes Opinions and Reports of the Judicial Council Sec. 6, Para. 4 (1969) [now Opinion 8.05]. References Opinion 8.13. Hunter,

Managed Process, Due Care: Structures of Accountability in Health Care, 6 Yale J. Health Pol'y L. & Ethics 93, 107, 113 (2006).

Journal 2006 Argues for an alternative framework by which health ethics, policy, and law can address equitable distribution of health care. Concludes that a new paradigm would lead to a more efficient and compassionate system. References Opinions 2.22 and 8.13. Ruger, *Health, Capability, and Justice: Toward a New Paradigm of Health Ethics, Policy and Law, 15 Cornell J. L. & Pub. Pol'y 403, 425, 465 (2006).*

Journal 2006 Considers the role of informed consent and patient autonomy as a central tenet of bioethics. Concludes that the field should focus most strongly on serving the practical needs and desires of patients. References Opinion 8.13. Schneider, *After Autonomy, 41 Wake Forest L. Rev. 411, 429-30 (2006).*

Journal 2006 Critiques the Uniform Health-Care Decisions Act. Concludes that the Act poses dangers to disabled patients, and proposes safeguards against such dangers. References Opinion 8.13. Stith, *The Semblance of Autonomy: Treatment of Persons With Disabilities Under the Uniform Health-Care Decisions Act, 22 Issues L. & Med. 39, 63-64 (2006).*

Journal 2002 Observes that changes in the health professions challenge certain assumptions about professional ethics. Concludes that these long-standing assumptions must be re-examined. Cites Opinion 2.161. References Opinion 8.13. Kelley, *The Meanings of Professional Life: Teaching Across the Health Professions, 27 J. Med. & Phil. 475, 485, 490, 491 (2002).*

Journal 2002 Considers whether physicians should be required to disclose information regarding financial incentives received from patients' HMOs. Concludes that physicians should not be required to disclose these incentives. References Opinion 8.13. Reuland, *Health Maintenance Organizations and Physician Financial Incentive Plans: Should Physician Disclosure Be Mandatory? 27 Iowa J. Corp. L. 293, 312 (2002).*

Journal 2002 Examines whether managed care organizations should be obligated to disclose physician financial incentives that may limit patient care. Concludes that mandatory disclosure is in the best interest of patients and physicians. Quotes Opinions 2.03 and 8.13. Talesh, *Breaking the Learned Helplessness of Patients: Why MCOs Should Be Required to Disclose Financial Incentives, 26 Law & Psychol. Rev. 49, 60-61, 63 (2002).*

Journal 2001 Examines issues relating to health care cost containment. Concludes that, if physicians are to meet the goals assigned to them in a cost-constrained health care system, then professional standards must be reevaluated and modified to afford meaningful guidance for clinical decision-making in the face of health care spending controls. Quotes Opinions 2.03, 2.09, 2.095, 8.032, and 9.04. Cites Opinions 8.02, 8.021, 8.051, and 8.13. Agrawal, *Resuscitating Professionalism: Self-regulation in the Medical Marketplace, 66 Mo. L. Rev. 341, 354, 355, 360, 361, 378, 388 (2001).*

Journal 2001 Examines the doctrine of informed consent with respect to nontraditional issues, such as a physician's duty to disclose personal information. Concludes there must be a balance that will accommodate the needs of both the patient and the physician. References Opinion 8.13. Hanson, *Informed Consent and the Scope of a Physician's Duty of Disclosure, 77 N. D. L. Rev. 71, 89, 91 (2001).*

Journal 2000 Discusses and evaluates different systems for addressing consumer concerns about managed health care. Asserts that current legal systems for identifying and resolving consumer concerns are not understood by most consumers and are not accessible by many, especially the uninsured. Concludes that several immediate steps are realistic for moving toward reform. Cites Principle VI. References Opinions 8.13 and 9.065. Kinney, *Tapping and Resolving Consumer Concerns About Health Care, 26 Am. J. Law & Med. 335, 337, 375 (2000).*

Journal 2000 Reviews the case of *Corporate Health Insurance, Inc. v. Texas Dept. of Insurance* and discusses its impact on HMO liability in Texas. Considers the conflicts of interest managed care imposes upon physicians. Concludes that, without national amendments to the scope of ERISA, HMOs are not compelled to provide quality health care. References Opinion 8.13. Lockhart, *The Safest Care Is to Deny Care: Implications of Corporate Health Insurance, Inc. v. Texas Department of Insurance on HMO Liability in Texas, 41 S. Tex. L. Rev. 621, 628, 634 (2000).*

Journal 2000 Describes the fiduciary aspects of the physician-patient relationship. Explores the conflicts that may occur between physicians and pregnant women in the health care setting. Proposes legal strategies to address these conflicts. Quotes Opinions 8.08 and 10.01. References Opinion 8.13. Oberman, *Mothers and Doctors' Orders: Unmasking the Doctor's Fiduciary Role in Maternal-Fetal Conflicts, 94 Nw. U. L. Rev. 451, 456, 462, 493 (2000).*

Journal 1999 Describes the gag clause debate in managed care and analyzes the types of incentives that might limit physician-patient communication. Concludes that, to protect patient access to information about treatment options and their health plans, antigag legislation must be coupled with a thorough examination of the extent to which financial incentives will be permitted to impact managed health care delivery. Quotes Opinion 8.13. Krause, *The Brief Life of the Gag Clause: Why Antigag Clause Legislation Isn't Enough, 67 Tenn. L. Rev. 1, 4, 43 (1999).*

Journal 1999 Describes the development of managed care organizations. Examines professional associations' statements regarding managed care organizations. Argues that physicians and managed care organizations should be viewed as economically disciplined, moral cofiduciaries for patients. References Opinion 8.13. McCullough, *A Basic*

Concept in the Clinical Ethics of Managed Care: Physicians and Institutions as Economically Disciplined Moral Co-Fiduciaries of Populations of Patients, 24 J. Med. Phil. 77, 82-83, 87, 89, 91, 96 (1999).

Journal 1999 Explores the increased push toward mandatory disclosure laws regarding financial incentives imposed by managed care organizations. Discusses current laws and ethical guidelines. Emphasizes that efforts to mandate disclosure force physicians to focus on the effects of imposed incentives and the essence of the physician-patient relationship. References Opinions 8.032, 8.13, and 8.132. Miller & Sage, *Disclosing Physician Financial Incentives, 281 JAMA 1424, 1425 (1999).*

Journal 1999 Discusses the need for physicians to advocate on behalf of patients' rights in the context of health care delivery. Evaluates the nature and scope of the physician's role as advocate, noting that physicians cannot be expected to engage in attorney-like advocacy. Quotes Principles IV and VI, Fundamental Elements (2), (4), and (6) [now Opinion 10.01], Patient Responsibilities 5 [now Opinion 10.02], and Opinions 2.03, 2.07, 2.09, 2.16, 2.19, 3.06, 4.01, 4.04, 6.01, 7.02, 8.02, 8.03, 8.13, 8.132, 9.06, 9.07, and 9.131. Cites Opinions 5.05, 5.09, 7.01, 8.135, and 9.02. Sage, *Physicians as Advocates, 35 Hous. L. Rev. 1529, 1537, 1541, 1542, 1552-53, 1554, 1556, 1557, 1559, 1561-62, 1564, 1571, 1574, 1576, 1580 (1999).*

Journal 1999 Discusses financial incentives offered to physicians by managed care organizations. Argues that evidence of financial incentives should be admissible in medical malpractice cases. Quotes Opinion 8.13. References Opinion 8.132. Sugarman & Yarashus, *Admissibility of Managed Care Financial Incentives in Medical Malpractice Cases, 34 Tort & Ins. L. J. 735, 743, 746, 759 (1999).*

Journal 1998 Analyzes Hall's book *Making Medical Spending Decisions: The Law, Ethics and Economics of Rationing Mechanisms.* Discusses cost-based rationing for medical services and physician bedside rationing. Concludes that patients should be informed in advance when their physician may receive financial incentives for withholding care. Quotes Opinion 8.13. Agrawal, *Chicago Hope Meets the Chicago School, 96 Mich. L. Rev. 1793, 1804 (1998).*

Journal 1998 Discusses changes in the health care system. Explains why patients need more power in the managed care system. Suggests that patients should use class action suits as a method to assert power over managed care organizations. References Opinions 8.13 and 8.132. Cerminara, *The Class Action Suit as a Method of Patient Empowerment in the Managed Care Setting, 24 Am. J. Law & Med. 7, 16, 17, 23 (1998).*

Journal 1998 Discusses conflicts of interest in the physician-patient relationship arising out of use of financial incentives by managed care organizations. Considers how such conflicts are dealt with in the attorney-client relationship. Suggests that a financial incentive should be legally denounced if it unreasonably interferes with a physician's

duty to properly care for and treat patients. Quotes Preamble, Fundamental Elements (1) [now Opinion 10.01], and Opinions 4.04, 5.01, 8.03, 8.13, and 9.06. Cites Fundamental Elements (4) [now Opinion 10.01] and Opinions 2.07, 2.08, and 2.132. Hall, *Third-Party Payor Conflicts of Interest in Managed Care: A Proposal for Regulation Based on the Model Rules of Professional Conduct, 29 Seton Hall L. Rev. 95, 96, 107, 108, 109, 110, 111, 112, 134, 135, 136 (1998).*

Journal 1998 Asserts that managed care organizations assume fiduciary obligations by exercising discretionary control over the administration of an ERISA plan. Argues that ERISA requires managed care organizations and physicians to disclose financial incentives intended to influence physician decision-making. References Opinions 8.13 and 8.132. Johnson, *ERISA Doctor in the House? The Duty to Disclose Physician Incentives to Limit Health Care, 82 Minn. L. Rev. 1631, 1639, 1649, 1655 (1998).*

Journal 1998 Discusses changes in the health care system. Analyzes conflicts of interest arising from the practice of capitation. Argues that physicians should refuse to sign contracts with health care plans offering incentives that may present a temptation to undertreat patients. References Opinion 8.13. Kassirer, *Managing Care—Should We Adopt a New Ethic? 339 New Eng. J. Med. 397 (1998).*

Journal 1998 Expresses concern about the impact of managed care cost-containment practices on the physician-patient relationship. Advocates the need for disclosure of information about these practices to patients. Evaluates and recommends a Maryland law that requires such disclosure. Cites Opinion 8.13. Khanna, Silverman, & Schwartz, *Disclosure of Operating Practices by Managed-Care Organizations to Consumers of Healthcare: Obligations of Informed Consent, 9 J. Clinical Ethics 291, 293, 296 (1998).*

Journal 1998 Discusses quality and safety concerns arising under managed care systems. Explores benefits and detriments of the proposed patients' bill of rights. Advocates legislation to provide safeguards from cost-containment mechanisms utilized by managed care programs. Quotes Opinion 8.13. Misocky, *The Patients' Bill of Rights: Managed Care Under Siege, 15 J. Contemp. Health L. & Pol'y 57, 73 (1998).*

Journal 1998 Explores clinical freedom and the Hippocratic Oath. Discusses issues of patient trust and confidence. Suggests that a sense of confidence will not be present if managerial priorities are dominant factors in resource allocation. References Opinion 8.13. Newdick, *Public Health Ethics and Clinical Freedom, 14 J. Contemp. Health L. & Pol'y 335, 336, 339, 356, 359, 361 (1998).*

Journal 1998 Discusses communication conflicts between physicians and managed care organizations. Describes legal responses to gag provisions imposed by managed care organizations. Assesses the impact of gag practices on physician-patient communication. Quotes Opinion 8.13. Spielman, *After the Gag Episode: Physician*

Communication in Managed Care Organizations, 22 Seton Hall Legis. J. 437, 453, 461, 463 (1998).

Journal 1998 Argues that health maintenance organizations (HMOs) do not have an incentive to act reasonably because they are not held accountable under tort law. Points out that the duty to act reasonably is imposed on most of society in order to deter negligence. Advocates imposing the same duty on HMOs. References Opinion 8.13. Wertheimer, *Ockham's Scalpel: A Return to a Reasonableness Standard, 43 Vill. L. Rev. 321, 327 (1998).*

Journal 1997 Discusses the quality of neurological care and the ethical conflicts that are created by the drive to contain costs. Focuses on quality management and cost-containment programs and the conflicts created when neurologists attempt to reconcile the interests of patients and society. References Opinions 8.032 and 8.13. Bernat, *Quality of Neurological Care: Balancing Cost Control and Ethics, 54 Arch. Neurol. 1341, 1343, 1345 (1997).*

Journal 1997 Compares past ethical opinions to current opinions and notes the differences. Comments on the forces that have changed medical ethics through the years. Notes differing theories on the future course of medical ethics. Quotes Fundamental Elements (Preamble) and Opinions 5.05, 5.057, 7.01, 8.12, 9.12, and 9.131. Cites Fundamental Elements (5) and Opinions 8.115 and 8.13. Buchanan, *Medical Ethics at the Millennium: A Brief Retrospective, 26 Colo. Law. 141, 142, 143, 144, 145 (1997).*

Journal 1997 Examines the use of gag clauses in the managed care setting. Explores the conflict of interest between physicians' loyalty to HMOs and their duty to patients. Questions whether patients can give informed consent based on inadequate information. Emphasizes the need for more comprehensive regulation. Quotes Opinion 8.13. Comment, *Physician Gag Clauses—The Hypocrisy of the Hippocratic Oath, 21 So. Ill. U. L. J. 313, 318, 320 (1997).*

Journal 1997 Reviews the conflict between the economics of managed care and physicians' ethical obligations to patients. Questions whether a patient may give informed consent to treatment without knowledge of all available alternatives. Offers a proposal for disclosure of managed care cost-containment mechanisms and incentives to patients. Quotes Opinion 8.13. Hall, *A Theory of Economic Informed Consent, 31 Ga. L. Rev. 511, 521, 524-25 (1997).*

Journal 1997 Posits that cost-containment schemes in managed care systems have eroded the fiduciary duty physicians owe patients. Notes that managed care organizations (MCOs) are prohibiting patients from trusting and relying on physicians. Concludes that patients must seek quality assurance from sources other than their physicians. Quotes Opinions 2.03, 2.09, and 8.13. Jacobi, *Patients at a Loss: Protecting Health Care Consumers Through Data Driven Quality Assurance, 45 U. Kan. L. Rev. 705, 720, 721, 759 (1997).*

Journal 1997 Explores the responsibilities imposed on physicians by managed care and capitation. Notes that physicians are called on to act as gatekeepers, controlling access to specialty services and tests. Considers whether primary care physicians in capitated groups are satisfied with the quality of care they provide. References Opinion 8.13. Kerr, Hays, Mittman, Siu, Leake, & Brook, *Primary Care Physicians' Satisfaction With Quality of Care in California Capitated Medical Groups, 278 JAMA 308, 312 (1997).*

Journal 1997 Discusses the practice of physician deselection by managed care organizations. Suggests that deselection harms the physician-patient relationship and creates a conflict of interest. Argues that solutions to deselection should consider effects on the patient rather than on the physician. Quotes Principle III. Cites Principle I and Opinions 8.05 and 8.13. Liner, *Physician Deselection: The Dynamics of a New Threat to the physician-patient Relationship, 23 Am. J. Law & Med. 511, 513, 527 (1997).*

Journal 1997 Examines national health care reform and managed care. Notes that state regulatory policies in this context evidence common concerns. Suggests ways in which the government can promote patient and physician rights. References Opinion 8.13. Miller, *Managed Care Regulation: In the Laboratory of the States, 278 JAMA 1102, 1104, 1108-09 (1997).*

Journal 1997 Discusses physician frustration with managed care plans caused by gag clauses and cost-containment mechanisms. Reviews the development of managed care organizations and federal attempts at limiting the use of gag clauses. Concludes that gag clauses are inherently flawed and compromise quality health care. Quotes Principles II and V, Fundamental Elements (1), and Opinion 8.13. Note, *Physicians, Bound and Gagged: Federal Attempts to Combat Managed Care's Use of Gag Clauses, 21 Seton Hall Legis. J. 567, 601-02 (1997).*

Journal 1997 Describes gag provisions in managed care contracts. Explains the context in which gag provisions may undermine the physician-patient relationship, as well as the conflicts of interest they may create. Proposes legislation to address these problems. Quotes Opinion 8.13. Note, *Stop Gagging Physicians! 7 Health Matrix 187, 193, 200, 208-09 (1997).*

Journal 1997 Examines the need for change in interpretation of state laws under the saving clause of the Employment Retirement Income Security Act. Discusses any willing provider laws and concludes that they should receive saving clause protection. References Opinion 8.13. Pittman, *Any Willing Provider Laws and ERISA's Saving Clause: A New Solution for an Old Problem, 64 Tenn. L. Rev. 409, 416 (1997).*

Journal 1997 Discusses the need for balance between business ethics and medical ethics in the context of managed care. Explores two models for integrating ethics and managed care. Proposes the adoption of a collective responsibility model to improve quality of care. Quotes Principles

I, II, III, IV, and V. Cites Preamble. References Opinion 8.13. Regan, *Regulating the Business of Medicine: Models for Integrating Ethics and Managed Care, 30 Colum. J. L. & Soc. Probs. 635, 651, 656, 657 (1997).*

Journal 1997 Examines utilization review in the managed care context. Discusses a survey of third-party utilization review firms, noting practices that advance and undermine adherence to important professional norms. Quotes Opinion 9.031. References Opinion 8.13. Schlesinger, Gray, & Perreira, *Medical Professionalism Under Managed Care: The Pros and Cons of Utilization Review, 16 Health Affairs 106, 119, 120, 124 (1997).*

Journal 1996 Discusses the use of practice guidelines to improve medical care quality and to aid in decreasing health care costs. Evaluates pertinent ethical considerations. Concludes that, when used appropriately, guidelines have clinical value. References Opinion 8.13. Berger & Rosner, *The Ethics of Practice Guidelines, 156 Arch. Intern. Med. 2051, 2053, 2056 (1996).*

Journal 1996 Considers the economic implications for physicians brought about by the change from traditional fee-for-service care to capitation. Discusses capitation payments in the American health care system. Alludes to pertinent ethical issues. References Opinion 8.13. Bodenheimer & Grumbach, *Capitation or Decapitation: Keeping Your Head in Changing Times, 276 JAMA 1025, 1031 (1996).*

Journal 1996 Examines the business of health care and the ethical implications of managed care. Describes incentives that affect the delivery of health care. Suggests that a redistribution of excess revenues would help both patients and nonprofit hospitals coexist with managed care. Quotes Opinion 8.13. Bond, *Diverse and Perverse Incentives in Managed Care: Where Will the Pendulum Stop? 1 Widener L. Symp. J. 141, 151, 154 (1996).*

Journal 1996 Discusses the trend toward health care reform. Focuses on benefits and problems posed by managed mental health care. Posits that the moral problems of managed mental health care, including quality concerns, are curable. Concludes that managed mental health care may prove superior to fee-for-service care. References Opinion 8.13. Boyle, *Managed Care in Mental Health: A Cure, or a Cure Worse Than the Disease? 40 St. Louis U. L. J. 437, 448 (1996).*

Journal 1996 Discusses the threat managed health care poses to patients and physicians. Explores direct incentives given to physicians by managed care organizations and the impact these incentives have on physician behavior. Proposes possible methods for dealing with the problems that such incentives create. References Opinion 8.13. Greely, *Direct Financial Incentives in Managed Care: Unanswered Questions, 6 Health Matrix 53, 81 (1996).*

Journal 1996 Discusses the change from fee-for-service health care financing to managed care. Notes that cost-containment mechanisms modify physicians' behaviors and patients' access to health care. Emphasizes that physicians

must remain committed to following ethical guidelines. References Opinion 8.13. Hammes & Webster, *Professional Ethics and Managed Care in Dermatology, 132 Arch. Dermatol. 1070, 1072, 1073 (1996).*

Journal 1996 Discusses workers' compensation and the medical care provided to injured employees. Examines the effect of managed care on workers' compensation. Advocates focusing on prevention of injuries and quality of care. References Opinion 8.13. Hashimoto, *The Future Role of Managed Care and Capitation in Workers' Compensation, XXII Am. J. Law & Med. 233, 258, 259 (1996).*

Journal 1996 Considers challenges to the psychiatrist-patient relationship that are triggered by managed care cost-containment methodologies. Offers guidance to psychiatrists for addressing these challenges. References Opinions 2.095, 8.13, and 8.132. Hoge, *APA Resource Document: I. The Professional Responsibilities of Psychiatrists in Evolving Health Care Systems, 24 Bull. Am. Acad. Psychiatry Law 393, 405 (1996).*

Journal 1996 Discusses the problems managed care raises within the framework of the physician-patient relationship. Considers issues specific to psychiatry. Advocates legal regulation to improve upon and bring structural change to managed care systems. Cites Opinion 8.13. Hoge, *APA Resource Document: II. Regulatory Guidelines for Protecting the Interests of Psychiatric Patients in Emerging Health Care Systems, 24 Bull. Am. Acad. Psychiatry Law 407, 412, 418 (1996).*

Journal 1996 Considers procedural issues relative to patient protection in the context of capitated health care plans. Examines regulations governing capitated health plans and consumer protection issues. Offers suggestions regarding policy making, rate setting, dispute resolution, and judicial review. References Opinion 8.13. Kinney, *Procedural Protections for Patients in Capitated Health Plans, XXII Am. J. Law & Med. 301, 319-20 (1996).*

Journal 1996 Explains the conflict between managed care, which focuses on controlling costs, and traditional health care values, which focus on patient autonomy. Proposes a solution to this conflict requiring that patients incur certain economic consequences in obtaining health care and that managed care organizations disclose resource management techniques. References Opinion 8.13. Morreim, *Diverse and Perverse Incentives of Managed Care: Bringing Patients Into Alignment, 1 Widener L. Symp. J. 89, 129 (1996).*

Journal 1996 Discusses efforts to reduce health care costs. Considers whether personal financial incentives given to physicians decrease level of care given to patients. Suggests that, while financial incentives may create ethical concerns, they serve an important function by containing costs. Concludes that efforts to eliminate them completely are misguided. References Opinion 8.13. Orentlicher, *Paying Physicians More to Do Less: Financial Incentives to Limit Care, 30 U. Rich. L. Rev. 155, 167 (1996).*

Ill. App. 1999 Administrator of estate brought suit against physician and health maintenance organization (HMO). The suit alleged medical negligence and breach of a fiduciary duty to deceased for the physician's failure to disclose contract with the HMO that created incentives to minimize diagnostic tests and specialist referrals. The court quoted Opinion 8.132, stating that, while a violation of professional ethics does not in itself establish a breach of the legal standard of care, it is relevant in determining whether such a breach occurred. *Neade v. Portes, 303 Ill.App.3d 799, 710 N.E. 2d 418, 427.*

Journal 2002 Explores how courts have attempted to provide relief when managed care organizations cause harm. Concludes that the judiciary has evidenced respect for the legislative process in this context. Quotes Opinion 8.132. Spector, *Managed Healthcare Liability Issues, 32 Cumb. L. Rev. 311, 335-36 (2002).*

Journal 2001 Examines the changing duties of health care providers to disclose managed care financial incentives to patients. Concludes that managed care organizations, not physicians, should be obligated to make such disclosures. Quotes Opinion 8.132. Kurfirst, *The Duty to Disclose HMO Physician Incentives, 13 (3) Health Law 18, 18, 22 (2001).*

Journal 2001 Examines patient attitudes toward physician compensation models. Concludes that most wealthier, well-educated, Caucasian patients are the least satisfied with capitation. References Opinion 8.132. Pereira & Pearson, *Patient Attitudes Toward Physician Financial Incentives, 161 Arch. Intern. Med. 1313, 1316, 1317 (2001).*

Journal 2001 Examines the concept of fiduciary duty in the managed care context. Considers potential liability of health plans and providers for breach of this duty. Reviews the US Supreme Court decision in *Pegram v. Herdrich.* Concludes that *Pegram* left many unanswered questions concerning ERISA's fiduciary requirements for health plans and providers. Quotes Opinion 8.132. Rosoff, *Breach of Fiduciary Duty Lawsuits Against MCOs, 22 J. Legal Med. 55, 65 (2001).*

Journal 2000 Examines physician value neutrality (PVN). Defines PVN as providing a foundation to suggest physicians must keep their values—religious, political, or otherwise—out of the patient-physician relationship. Concludes it is not clear how values can be removed from the patient-physician relationship without removing the very thing PVN supporters are trying to protect, the intrinsic value of persons. References Opinions 2.01, 2.02, 8.032, 8.05, 8.08, and 8.132. Beckwith & Peppin, *Physician Value Neutrality: A Critique, 28 J. L. Med. & Ethics 67, 72-73 (2000).*

Journal 2000 Examines the fiduciary nature of the physician-patient relationship. Explores crucial policy implications of the *Neade v. Portes* decision. Concludes that policy makers, not courts, should address whether physician involvement in managed care plans fundamentally implies a profit motive. Quotes Opinion 8.132. Potter, *Failure to Disclose HMO Incentives and the Breach of Fiduciary*

Duty: Is a New Cause of Action Against Physicians the Best Solution? 34 USF. L. Rev. 733, 753 (2000).

Journal 1999 Considers the viability of a legal cause of action for negligent referral in the physician-patient relationship. Examines differences between the legal and medical professions and discusses variations in the applicable standards of care. Cites Opinion 8.132. Martin, *Legal Malpractice: Negligent Referral as a Cause of Action, 29 Cumb. L. Rev. 679, 686 (1999).*

Journal 1996 Considers challenges to the psychiatrist-patient relationship that are triggered by managed care cost-containment methodologies. Offers guidance to psychiatrists for addressing these challenges. References Opinions 2.095, 8.13, and 8.132. Hoge, *APA Resource Document: I. The Professional Responsibilities of Psychiatrists in Evolving Health Care Systems, 24 Bull. Am. Acad. Psychiatry Law 393, 405 (1996).*

Journal 1990 Examines various cost-control mechanisms utilized by prepaid health plans and other managed care programs and considers the impact of such mechanisms on clinical decision making. Emphasis is placed on the possible existence of conflicts of interest on the part of health care providers in this context. Quotes Opinions 8.03 and 8.13 [now Opinion 8.132]. Hirshfeld, *Defining Full and Fair Disclosure in Managed Care Contracts, 60 The Citation 67, 70 (1990).*

Journal 2006 Discusses preemption of lawsuits against managed care organizations by the Employee Retirement Income Security Act of 1974 (ERISA). Proposes a "bifurcated legal regime" to decrease the protective scope of ERISA. Quotes Opinions 8.053 and 8.135. Madison, *ERISA and Liability for Provision of Medical Information, 84 N. C. L. Rev. 471, 540 (2006).*

Cal. App. 2002 State agency appealed a writ of mandamus requiring it to approve managed care plan's proposed amendment to discontinue coverage of sexual dysfunction prescription drugs. Agency based its authority to disapprove on a statute empowering it to regulate health plan prescription drug coverage. California Court of Appeals affirmed. The court held that the agency exceeded its statutory authority. References Opinion 8.135 regarding managed care drug formulary systems. *Kaiser Foundation Health Plan, Inc. v. Zingale, 99 Cal. App. 4th 1018, 121 Cal. Rptr. 2d 741, 746.*

Journal 2000 Describes the American formulary system and the economic efficiencies that can be realized when physicians comply. Describes how the formulary system fits into and underlies health care electronic data interchange. Concludes that congressional action is needed to fully extend the formulary system to Medicaid programs in all 50 states. References Opinion 8.135. Buckles, *Electronic Formulary Management and Medicaid: Maximizing Economic Efficiency and Quality of Care in the Age of Electronic Prescribing, 11 U. Fla. J. L. & Pub. Pol'y 179, 182-83 (2000).*

11.2.5 Retainer Practices

Journal 2008 Explores the legal, ethical, and policy implications of concierge medicine. Argues physicians engaged in concierge care must strive to meet ethical and legal standards, and take care to communicate clearly with patients about services and fees. Quotes Opinion 8.055. Cites Principles II and VI and Opinion 8.055. Portman & Romanow, *Concierge Medicine: Legal Issues, Ethical Dilemmas, and Policy Challenges, 1 J. Health & Life Sci. L. 1, 4, 28-29 (2008).*

Journal 2007 Reviews the legal and ethical problems surrounding concierge medical practice. Concludes that concierge medicine should remain restricted to a small class of wealthy individuals. Cites Opinions 8.05, 8.055, 8.115, 9.06, and 9.065. Carnahan, *Concierge Medicine: Legal and Ethical Issues, 35 J. L. Med. & Ethics 211, 212-13 (2007).*

Journal 2007 Analyzes current retainer care practices. Concludes that retainer care offers some benefits, but should be regulated to prevent patients who pay a retainer from receiving quicker access to care. References Opinion 8.055. Pasquale, *The Three Faces of Retainer Care: Crafting a Tailored Regulatory Response, 7 Yale J. Health Pol'y L. & Ethics 39, 74 (2007).*

Journal 2006 Explores the legal and ethical issues surrounding concierge medicine. Concludes that concierge medicine is best restricted to a small class of wealthy individuals. Quotes Principle IX and Opinion 8.055. Cites Principle VI and Opinions 8.055, 8.11, 8.115, 9.065,

and 10.05. Carnahan, *Law, Medicine, and Wealth: Does Concierge Medicine Promote Health Care Choice, or Is It a Barrier to Access? 17 Stan. L. & Pol'y Rev. 121, 149-50, 151, 152, 153-54 (2006).*

Journal 2006 Discusses health care service fees and the Maryland "Hold Harmless" statute. Concludes that physicians may charge administrative fees for services not covered by insurance as long as they do not violate a statute or impede proper care. Quotes Opinions 4.01 and 8.055. Doherty & Freed, *User Fees in Health Care, 39 Md. B. J. 5, 9 (April 2006).*

Journal 2006 Evaluates legal implications of consumer-driven health care. Concludes that a system of consumer-driven health care is feasible and offers many benefits to patients. Quotes Opinions 8.055 and 9.065. Hall, *Paying for What You Get and Getting What You Pay For: Legal Responses to Consumer-Driven Health Care, 69 Law & Contemp. Prob. 159, 165 (2006).*

Journal 2005 Examines the practice of "boutique medicine" and considers legal and ethical implications. Concludes that boutique medical services would be ethical only if physicians used retainer money from their boutique clients to augment health care costs of the poor. Quotes Principles VII and IX and Opinion 8.055. Russano, *Is Boutique Medicine a New Threat to American Health Care or a Logical Way of Revitalizing the Doctor-Patient Relationship? 17 Wash. U. J. L. & Pol'y 313, 331, 332 (2005).*

11.3.1 Fees for Medical Services

Journal 2007 Highlights inconsistencies in applying judicial deference to medical ethics. Concludes that courts should afford greater deference to established medical ethics standards. Quotes Principle I and Opinions 2.06 and Ch. II, Art. I, Sec. 3 (May 1847) [now Opinion 5.02]. Cites Opinions 4.01 and 7.05. Lerman, *Second Opinion: Inconsistent Deference to Medical Ethics in Death Penalty Jurisprudence, 95 Geo. L. J. 1941, 1945, 1974-75, 1976, 1977 (2007).*

Journal 2006 Discusses health care service fees and the Maryland "Hold Harmless" statute. Concludes that physicians may charge administrative fees for services not covered by insurance as long as they do not violate a statute or impede proper care. Quotes Opinions 4.01 and 8.055. Doherty & Freed, *User Fees in Health Care, 39 Md. B.J. 5, 9 (April 2006).*

Journal 1999 Discusses the need for physicians to advocate on behalf of patients' rights in the context of health care delivery. Evaluates the nature and scope of the physician's role as advocate, noting that physicians cannot be expected to engage in attorney-like advocacy. Quotes Principles IV and VI, Fundamental Elements (2), (4), and (6) [now Opinion 10.01], Patient Responsibilities 5 [now Opinion 10.02], and

Opinions 2.03, 2.07, 2.09, 2.16, 2.19, 3.06, 4.01, 4.04, 6.01, 7.02, 8.02, 8.03, 8.13, 8.132, 9.06, 9.07, and 9.131. Cites Opinions 5.05, 5.09, 7.01, 8.135, and 9.02. Sage, *Physicians as Advocates, 35 Hous. L. Rev. 1529, 1537, 1541, 1542, 1552-53, 1554, 1556, 1557, 1559, 1561-62, 1564, 1571, 1574, 1576, 1580 (1999).*

Cal. App. 1992 Lower court held that a contingent fee agreement between plaintiff and a medical-legal consulting service violated public policy and was void. In reversing, appellate court referred to *Polo v. Gotchel* 225 N.J. Super. 492, 542 A.2d 947 (1987), and *Dupree v. Malpractice Research, Inc.*, 179 Mich. App. 254, 445 N.W.2d 498 (1989), which had relied on Opinion 8.04 (1984) [now Opinion 6.01] to hold that contingent fee consulting contracts were per se invalid. The court was unpersuaded by the reasoning of these decisions, stating that (1) the contingent fee agreement was with a company, not with a physician, and (2) the term "medical services" in the Opinion refers to patient treatment and not to consulting services provided in conjunction with the services of an attorney. *Ojeda v. Sharp Cabrillo Hosp., 8 Cal. App. 4th 1, 12, 13 n.11, 14, 10 Cal. Rptr. 2d 230, 237 n.11, 238.*

Mich. App. 1989 Plaintiffs, who settled an underlying medical malpractice suit, sought to invalidate contingent fee contract with expert witness service. Plaintiffs had paid witness and report fees, travel costs, and other expenses in advance according to a fee schedule but objected to a charge of 20% of their recovery. The court, citing Opinion 8.04 (1984) [now Opinion 6.01], held that the contingent fee contract for expert witnesses was repugnant to the public policy of preserving the plaintiff's recovery and preventing the exaggeration of favorable testimony and would not be enforced. Further, the court refused to consider defendant's quantum meruit claim, since some fees had been paid in advance, and any further attempt to collect fees would fail to deter such contracts. *Dupree v. Malpractice Research, Inc., 179 Mich. App. 254, 445 N.W.2d 498, 501.*

N.J. Super. 1987 Contingent fee agreement between plaintiff's attorney in a medical malpractice action and a medical-legal consulting service which linked plaintiff with potential expert witnesses violated public policy and was void. The court cited with approval Opinion 8.04 (1984) [now Opinion 6.01], which states that a physician's fees should not be based upon the outcome of litigation because of the risk that the physician may become more of an advocate than a healer. *Polo v. Gotchel, 225 N.J. Super. 429, 542 A.2d 947, 948.*

Tenn. 1998 Physician sued patient and patient's attorney for breach of contract after the patient settled a personal injury claim. Physician claimed that under contract, he was entitled to receive a contingency fee for services as the medical expert in the patient's case and contingency fees for medical services rendered. Alternatively, the physician claimed that he could recover under the theory of quantum meruit. The court held that the contingency fee both for the physician acting as a medical expert and for medical services violated public policy. The court quoted Opinions 6.01 and 9.07, stating that the Tennessee Board of Medical Examiners, which governs state medical licenses, had adopted the AMA's stance on contingency fees. The court also rejected the physician's argument that he should be allowed to recover under the theory of quantum meruit because the underlying contracts were void as against public policy. *Swafford v. Harris, 967 S.W.2d 319, 321-323.*

Journal 2011 Explains how to prepare for and take a physician's deposition for trial, including obtaining records and opinions and preserving answers. Cites Opinion 6.01. Radnor, *How to Prepare for and Take a Doctor's Deposition, 22 Prac. Litigator 40, 52 (May 2011).*

Journal 2009 Discusses financing assisted reproduction and adoption using specialty loans and the political and economic implications of such practices. Concludes parenthood loans could increase access to assisted reproduction and adoption for those otherwise unable to afford these services. Cites Opinion 6.01. Jacoby, *Show Me the Money: Making Markets in Forbidden Exchange: The Debt Financing of Parenthood, 72 Law & Contemp. Prob. 147, 156 (2009).*

Journal 2006 Examines ethical dilemmas physicians may face as providers of pay-for-performance medical care. Concludes that this strategy offers a benefit to patients as long as physicians uphold stringent ethical standards and work together to ensure optimum patient care. Cites Principles I, V, VIII, and IX and Opinions 2.035, 2.095, 6.01, 8.021, 8.03, 8.0501, 8.053, 8.054, and 8.121. Bostick, Sade, & McMahon, *Report of the Council on Ethical and Judicial Affairs: Physician Pay-for-Performance Programs, 3 Ind. Health L. Rev. 429, 430, 431, 432-33, 434, 435, 436 (2006).*

Journal 2006 Discusses health care reform in the interest of social justice. Concludes that such reform is feasible, but requires extensive planning and effort. References Opinion 6.01. Hyman, *Getting the Haves to Come Out Behind: Fixing the Distributive Injustices of American Health Care, 69 Law & Contemp. Probs. 265, 268-69 (2006).*

Journal 2006 Discusses the benefits and drawbacks to pay-for-performance medical care. Concludes that pay-for-performance may increase the quality of medical care if implemented correctly and with increased government support. Cites Opinion 6.01. Sage, *Pay For Performance: Will It Work in Theory? 3 Ind. Health L. Rev. 305, 308-09 (2006).*

Journal 2005 Argues that abolishing or weakening the tort liability system will not improve the quality of health care, but may diminish it. Concludes that a systems-based approach coupled with a liability system that encourages high-quality care may improve health care delivery in the US. Quotes Opinion 8.12. References Opinion 6.01. Hyman & Silver, *The Poor State of Health Care Quality in the U.S.: Is Malpractice Liability Part of the Problem or Part of the Solution? 90 Cornell L. Rev. 893, 926, 965 (2005).*

Journal 2001 Considers result-based compensation arrangements for medical services. Focuses on a 1994 AMA amendment to Opinion 6.01 that prohibits payment of physicians contingent upon outcome. Concludes that such arrangements may be appropriate in some circumstances. Quotes Opinion 6.01. Hyman & Silver, *Just What the Patient Ordered: The Case for Result-Based Compensation Arrangements, 29 J. L. Med. & Ethics 170, 170 (2001).*

Journal 2001 Explains the design and potential benefits of result-based compensation arrangements for health care. Concludes that a more reliable and efficient health care delivery system is fostered by such arrangements. Quotes Opinion 6.01. References Opinions 9.121 and 9.122. Hyman & Silver, *You Get What You Pay For: Result-Based Compensation for Health Care, 58 Wash. & Lee L. Rev. 1427, 1459, 1460, 1461, 1481-82 (2001).*

Journal 2000 Considers the rules governing expert testimony. Explores professional ethical standards affecting expert witnesses and concludes that codes of ethics have not succeeded in eliminating biased expert testimony. Recommends creation of an organization to assist courts in obtaining reliable expert witness testimony. Quotes Principle III and Opinion 6.01. Cites Principles I, II, and V and Opinions 1.02 and 9.07. Murphy, *Expert Witnesses at*

Trial: Where Are the Ethics? 14 Geo. J. Legal Ethics 217, 231-32 (2000).

Journal 1998 Examines mechanisms of oversight for expert witness testimony by medical, legal, legislative, and regulatory agencies. Points out that the amount of malpractice litigation will increase the need for medical expert witnesses. Concludes that improvements in this context must uphold principles of due process and be acceptable to the medical and legal communities. Cites Opinions 6.01, 8.04, and 9.07. McAbee, *Improper Expert Medical Testimony: Existing and Proposed Mechanisms of Oversight, 19 J. Legal Med. 257, 265 (1998).*

Journal 1991 Looks at the problem of high expert witness fees and lack of access to expert testimony by those who may need it. Proposes revamping the current system to allow certain types of contingent fee arrangements. Quotes Opinion 8.04 (1984) [now Opinion 6.01]. Note, *Contingent Expert Witness Fees: Access and Legitimacy, 64 So. Cal. L. Rev. 1363, 1374, 1382 (1991).*

Journal 1990 Examines conflicting court decisions that have addressed the appropriateness of medical-legal consulting services and their use of contingent fee arrangements. Concludes by discussing the need for a less troublesome solution to the problems plaintiffs face in malpractice and personal injury cases. Quotes Opinion 6.01. Cites Opinions 6.12 (1989) [now Opinion 6.05] and 9.07. Dillon, *Contingent Fees and Medical-Legal Consulting Services: Economical or Unethical? 11 J. Legal Med. 93, 101, 111 (1990).*

Wis. Sup. 2010 State petitioned for involuntary administration of psychotropic medication for defendant who was in custody after acquittal due to mental illness. Defendant argued that Wisconsin statute allowing for such treatment unconstitutionally violated his due process rights. The majority quotes Opinions 2.065 and 2.19 in finding the Wisconsin statute in question facially valid on procedural due process grounds. *State v. Wood, 323 Wis. 2d 321, 780 N.W.2d 63, 82-83.*

Journal 1994 Considers how greater patient autonomy has led to situations in which medical care may be viewed as futile. Suggests that the law has intruded too far into this area of medicine. Quotes Opinion 2.035. Cites Opinions 2.03, 2.095, 2.17, 2.19, 2.20, and 2.22. Cultice, *Medical Futility: When Is Enough, Enough? 27 J. Health & Hosp. Law 225, 230, 256 (1994).*

Journal 1991 Looks at the physician as a fiduciary and the law governing fiduciary relationships. Concludes that fiduciary concepts are a valuable basis for establishing ethical and legal guidelines for physician behavior. Quotes Opinions 2.19, 8.03 (1989) [now Opinion 8.032], and 8.06. Healey & Dowling, *Controlling Conflicts of Interest in the Doctor-Patient Relationship: Lessons From Moore v. Regents of the University of California, 42 Mercer L. Rev. 989, 997, 998 (1991).*

Journal 1991 Examines the issues surrounding judicial use of professional ethics codes in private litigation. Concludes

that judges should more extensively use professional ethics codes to define public policy, standards of care, and legal causes of action. Quotes Principle II and Opinion 2.19. Note, *Professional Ethics Codes in Court: Redefining the Social Contract Between the Public and the Professions, 25 Georgia L. Rev. 1327, 1335, 1351 (1991).*

Journal 1990 Discusses efforts of third-party payers to control health care expenditures for beneficiaries. Concludes that financial incentives to limit care and other cost-control techniques should be disclosed and that the rationale for such disclosure is compelling. Quotes Opinions 2.03, 2.09, and 8.03. Cites Opinions 2.19, 4.04, and 4.06. Hirshfeld, *Should Third Party Payors of Health Care Services Disclose Cost Control Mechanisms to Potential Beneficiaries? 14 Seton Hall Legis. J. 115, 130, 131, 144, 145, 146 (1990).*

Journal 1986 Discusses the Missouri living will statute and the Death-Prolonging Procedures Act. Examines the extent to which these laws ensure individuals the right to make choices regarding personal medical treatment in the event of terminal illness, even if they become incompetent. Quotes Opinion 2.12 (1981) [now Opinion 2.19]. Johnson, *The Death-Prolonging Procedures Act and Refusal of Treatment in Missouri, 30 St. Louis Univ. L. J. 805, 816 (1986).*

Journal 2008 Argues waiver of patient coinsurance costs creates unfair competition among physicians and has negative economic consequences for those paying providers. Suggests close monitoring of waivers will reduce inflation of health care charges, diminish interference with the health plan insurer–network provider relationship, and discourage overutilization of medical services. Quotes Opinion 6.12. Cites Opinion 6.13. Bernstein & Seybert, *Everyone Pays the Price When Healthcare Providers Waive Patients' Co-insurance Obligations, 21 Health Law. 20, 22 (Dec. 2008).*

Journal 2000 Examines civil and criminal liability in connection with the practice of professional courtesy fee waivers and discounts. Discusses conflicts between the long-standing traditional practice of professional courtesy and a prudent and ethical course under current law. Quotes Opinion 6.12. Cites Opinion 6.13. Schmidt, *Professional Courtesy Discounts Under Siege—Part II, 29 Colo. Law. 59, 62 (Jan. 2000).*

Journal 2011 Examines the Patient Protection and Affordable Care Act and its impact on patient access to physician services. Also considers the possibility that physicians might be required to provide services to all patients as a condition to practice. Concludes that regulations that try to conscript physician services would be practically ineffective, legally dubious, and unwise public policy. Quotes Opinion 9.06 and 10.015. Cites Opinion 2.09. Kapp, *Conscripted Physician Services and the Public's Health, 39 J. L. Med. & Ethics 414, 414, 418 (2011).*

Journal 2009 Discusses methods of allocation and rationing of health care resources in an effort to curb health care costs and how these methods impact the elderly. Concludes that in order to make the greatest use of the available resources, an equitable policy regarding elder health care must be adopted and adhered to. Quotes Opinion 2.09. Smith, *The Elderly and Health Care Rationing, 7 Pierce L. Rev. 171, 181 (2009).*

Journal 2008 Argues that as a matter of public health, physicians must control antibiotic administration to combat antibiotic resistance. Concludes that despite limited incentives for antibiotic conservation, physicians must acknowledge their important role in mitigating the public health threat of antibiotic resistance. Quotes Principles VII and VIII and Opinions 2.09 and 10.015. Cites Opinion 2.03. Saver, *In Tepid Defense of Population Health: Physicians and Antibiotic Resistance, 34 Am. J. L. & Med. 431, 457 (2008).*

Journal 2003 Discusses the practice of gainsharing and argues that providing physicians and hospitals with certain financial incentives to reduce health costs may be of value in health care reform. Concludes with suggestions for how best to proceed in this difficult context. Quotes Opinions 2.03, 2.09, 4.04, and 8.03. References Opinion 8.13. Saver, *Squandering the Gain: Gainsharing and the Continuing Dilemma of Physician Financial Incentives, 98 Nw. U. L. Rev. 145, 219, 221, 222 (2003).*

Journal 2001 Examines issues relating to health care cost containment. Concludes that, if physicians are to meet the goals assigned to them in a cost-constrained health care system, then professional standards must be reevaluated and modified to afford meaningful guidance for clinical decision-making in the face of health care spending controls. Quotes Opinions 2.03, 2.09, 2.095, 8.032, and 9.04. Cites Opinions 8.02, 8.021, 8.051, and 8.13. Agrawal, *Resuscitating Professionalism: Self-regulation in the Medical Marketplace, 66 Mo. L. Rev. 341, 354, 355, 360, 361, 378, 388 (2001).*

Journal 2001 Discusses the prohibition on nonlawyer ownership of legal service providers. Considers how ethical rules and standards governing physicians have been directed toward preserving independent judgment. Concludes that ethical conflicts created by abandoning the prohibition on nonlawyer ownership of legal service providers may be managed by following the medical ethics model. Quotes Principle VI and Opinions 2.03, 2.09, 8.02, 8.021, 8.03, 8.05, 8.051, 8.054, 8.13, and 8.132. Harris & Foran, *The Ethics of Middle-Class Access to Legal Services and What We Can Learn From the Medical Profession's Shift to a Corporate Paradigm, 70 Fordham L. Rev. 775, 817, 821, 822, 823, 824 (2001).*

Journal 1997 Posits that cost-containment schemes in managed care systems have eroded the fiduciary duty physicians owe patients. Notes that managed care organizations (MCOs) are prohibiting patients from trusting and relying on physicians. Concludes that patients must seek quality assurance from sources other than their physicians. Quotes Opinions 2.03, 2.09, and 8.13. Jacobi, *Patients at a Loss: Protecting Health Care Consumers Through Data Driven Quality Assurance, 45 U. Kan. L. Rev. 705, 720, 721, 759 (1997).*

Journal 1996 Explores changing health care delivery environment and proposes a new approach to medical ethics. Suggests ways to improve the roles of care managers in capitated systems. Advocates disclosure of information to patients regarding coverage limitations and cost-containment policies. Quotes Opinion 2.09. Malinowski, *Capitation, Advances in Medical Technology, and the Advent of a New Era in Medical Ethics, XXII Am. J. Law & Med. 331, 337 (1996).*

Journal 1996 Discusses the health care system as it pertains to the elderly. Observes that age-based rationing decisions create significant value conflicts. Suggests that, in developing national health policy, decisions regarding resource allocation for the elderly must incorporate principles of ethical and moral reasoning. Quotes Opinion 2.09. Smith, *Our Hearts Were Once Young and Gay: Health Care Rationing and the Elderly, 8 U. Fla. J. L. & Pub. Pol'y 1, 21 (1996).*

Journal 1994 Considers how patients with insufficient financial resources place physicians in a conflict-of-interest situation with respect to patient needs and the financial interests of the physician, other patients, and society. Suggests that rules of contract and malpractice law do not provide satisfactory guidelines to resolve these conflicts. Cites Opinions 2.09 and 2.095. Mehlman & Massey, *The Patient-Physician Relationship and the Allocation of Scarce Resources: A Law and Economics Approach, 4 Kennedy Inst. Ethics J. 291, 292 (1994).*

Journal 1994 Observes that health care reform proposals present significant challenges to the role and ethics of attending physicians. Emphasizes that reform proposals must set forth the role envisioned for physicians and must articulate an acceptable ethical framework within which physicians may fulfill that role. Quotes Opinions 4.04, 9.121, and 9.122. Cites Opinions 2.03, 2.09, 5.01, and 8.03. Wolf, *Health Care Reform and the Future of Physician Ethics, 24 Hastings Center Rep. 28, 32, 40 (March/April 1994).*

Journal 1993 Discusses the problem of physicians withholding needed medical treatment from HIV-infected infants. Concludes that current law should be expanded to eliminate this discrimination. Quotes Opinions 2.09, 2.17, 2.20, 2.22, 4.04, and 8.03. Crossley, *Of Diagnoses and Discrimination: Discriminatory Nontreatment of Infants With HIV Infection, 93 Columbia L. Rev. 1581, 1620, 1621 (1993).*

Journal 1993 Defines the physician-patient relationship within the framework of contract, tort, and fiduciary law. Concludes that the law does not require a physician to provide care for the nonpaying patient. Quotes Opinion 2.09. Mehlman, *The Patient-Physician Relationship in an Era of Scarce Resources: Is There a Duty to Treat? 25 Conn. L. Rev. 349 (1993).*

Journal 1992 Examines the major health care rationing issues facing the US including increasing costs and decreasing access. Concludes that the standard of care should not be changed and that rationing should be a separate enterprise undertaken pursuant to explicit criteria. Quotes Opinions 2.03, 2.09, and 4.04. Hirshfeld, *Should Ethical and Legal*

Standards for Physicians Be Changed to Accommodate New Models for Rationing Health Care? 140 Univ. Pa. L. Rev. 1809, 1816 (1992).

Journal 1991 Focuses on the denial of insurance benefits for experimental medical procedures. Explains the de novo review process under ERISA. Concludes that there is need for a structure that will permit greater objectivity in the context of data collection as well as judicial determination. Cites Opinions 2.03 and 2.09. Note, *Denial of Coverage for "Experimental" Medical Procedures: The Problem of De Novo Review Under ERISA, 79 Kentucky L. J. 801, 824 (1990-1991).*

Journal 1990 Discusses economic considerations in clinical decision-making, with emphasis on the standard of care. Concludes that organized medicine has made valuable contributions through development of practice parameters that offer guidance in the exercise of clinical judgment. Cites Opinions 2.03 and 2.09. Hirshfeld, *Economic Considerations in Treatment Decisions and the Standard of Care in Medical Malpractice Litigation, 264 JAMA 2004, 2007 (1990).*

Journal 2001 Explores the extent to which pediatricians should rely on their expertise when prescribing therapies and durable medical equipment for children with special health care needs. Emphasizes the importance of the pediatrician's role in this context and urges pediatricians to comply with pertinent AMA guidelines and relevant state and federal laws. Quotes Opinion 8.06. References Opinion 9.132. Sneed, May, & Stencel, *Physicians' Reliance on Specialists, Therapists, and Vendors When Prescribing Therapies and Durable Medical Equipment for Children With Special Health Care Needs, 107 Pediatrics 1283, 1287, 1288, 1289 (2001).*

11.3.2 Fees for Nonclinical and Administrative Services

Journal 1992 Discusses the ethical and legal boundaries of medical treatment. Concludes that minor boundary violations occur frequently, but warns that if they become too frequent or serious, physicians risk substantial liability. Quotes Opinion 6.07 (incorrectly cited as 6.06). Simon, *Treatment Boundary Violations: Clinical, Ethical, and Legal Considerations, 20 Bull. Am. Acad. Psychiatry Law 269, 282 (1992).*

Journal 2007 Examines the ethical obligations of a corporate health lawyer. Concludes that the ethical health lawyer must balance obligations to the client with obligations to patients and the public. Quotes Opinion 8.09. Weeks, *Loopholes: Opportunity, Responsibility, or Liability? 35 J. L. Med. & Ethics 320, 322 (2007).*

11.3.3 Interest and Finance Charges

Cal. App. 1968 Plaintiff-physician sought dissolution of a medical partnership with defendant's decedent, and also sought a larger percentage of the partnership receipts based upon an alleged oral agreement. Defendant cross-claimed to enjoin plaintiff from taking physical control of the partnership offices and patient records. The trial court enjoined plaintiff from treating previous patients, requiring that he return all medical records and pay defendant all fees received from patients he had treated during the time of dispute. The appellate court reversed insofar as the injunction prohibited the plaintiff from treating the patient who desired to continue to receive his services or prevented access to medical records essential for this purpose, citing Opinions and Reports of the Judicial Council Sec. 7, Para. 16, Sec. 5, Para. 21, and Sec. 9 (1966) [now Opinions 6.08, 5.02, and 5.05] to support view that patients may not be regarded as the subject of ownership. *Jones v. Fakehany, 261 Cal. App. 2d 298, 67 Cal. Rptr. 810, 815, 816 n.1.*

Journal 2010 Describes how physicians act as bankers in financing fertility treatments for patients and how this significantly contributes to medical debt and bankruptcies. Proposes regulations which would address these issues within fertility markets. Quotes Opinion 6.08. Cites Opinion 2.055. Hawkins, *Doctors as Bankers: Evidence From Fertility Markets, 84 Tul. L. Rev. 841, 848, 874 (2010).*

Journal 2010 Examines competing methods of measuring the role of medical debt in bankruptcies. Concludes that court records alone reveal very little about the burden of medical bills on financially distressed families and ultimately diminish bankruptcy cases in which medical bills were particularly significant. References Opinion 6.08. Holman & Jacoby, *Managing Medical Bills on the Brink of Bankruptcy, 10 Yale J. Health Pol'y, L. & Ethics 239, 255 (2010).*

Journal 2008 Reviews current physician practices of collecting money from indebted patients. Concludes that physicians should continue to refrain from aggressive debt collection. Quotes Opinions 6.08 and 6.12. Hall & Schneider, *The Professional Ethics of Billing and Collections, 300 JAMA 1806, 1807 (2008).*

11.3.4 Fee Splitting

Ill. App. 2004 Appellant physicians moved for a declaration that flat and percentage-based fees assessed by respondents for inclusion on a list of health care providers constituted fee-splitting and was a violation of state law. The trial court found that the percentage-based fee, but not the flat fee, violated the Illinois Medical Practice Act, but denied appellants recovery for past fees paid. The appellate court, quoting Opinion 6.02, found that both flat and percentage-based fees constituted fee-splitting and violated the Medical Practice Act, but still denied recovery for past fees paid. *Vine Street Clinic v. Healthlink, Inc., 353 Ill. App. 3d 929, 819 N.E.2d 363, 367.*

Kan. App. 1985 Members of a medical partnership sought an injunction to enforce a covenant not to compete against defendant-physician, a former partner. Defendant asserted that the covenant was void as against public policy relying on Opinion 9.02 (1984). The court, however, ruled that the covenant was reasonable as defined by precedent and that it was bound to follow this precedent as opposed to the AMA's position regarding such covenants. Defendant further argued enforcement of the covenant was precluded because the partnership had violated ethical norms, apparently referring to Opinions 6.03 and 6.04 (1984) [now Opinions 6.02 and 6.03], which were part of partnership contract. The court held that defendant was estopped from complaining about the partnership's actions due to his own conduct. *Axtell Clinic v. Cranston, No. 56,745 (Kan. Ct. App. June 20, 1985) (LEXIS, States Library, Kan. file).*

Mass. 1955 Plaintiff-physician was charged under state licensing statute by defendant-board with conspiracy and fee-splitting. Both parties sought a declaratory judgment as to whether the defendant-board had jurisdiction to determine plaintiff's guilt or innocence. In holding that the board was qualified to determine if plaintiff's actions constituted gross misconduct under the statute, the court referred to Principles Ch. I, Secs. 1 and 6 (1947) [now Principle II and Opinion 6.02] delineating, in part, limitations on payment for medical services. These provisions, the court said, reflected the medical profession's understanding of its peculiar obligations. *Forziati v. Board of Registration in Medicine, 333 Mass. 125, 128 N.E.2d 789, 791.*

Mass. Super. 1998 Plaintiff-surgeon filed suit against a medical group practice claiming that the defendants reduced referrals to him because he declined to join the group. Plaintiff claimed that the decline harmed his surgical practice. He alleged that the group's practice of taking 10% of members' income constituted unethical and illegal kickbacks. The court held that the decline in referrals was not connected to plaintiff not being a member of the group. The court also found that the plaintiff had not presented evidence that the decline in referrals harmed his practice. Finally, the court found that the fees paid by members of the group practice were gatekeeper fees rather than referral fees. The court quoted Opinion 6.02, in support of its decision that

the defendants' fees did not constitute fee splitting. Further, the court referenced Opinion 8.032 concluding that a self-referral was not necessarily unethical if disclosed to the patient. *Boman v. Southeast Medical Services Group, 1998 WL 1182063, 11-12.*

Journal 2010 Examines medical tourism and the referral-type fees foreign providers pay to brokers to bring patients from the United States. Concludes that while medical tourism is a viable option for uninsured or underinsured patients, disclosure of broker's fees would enhance competition and patient trust. Quotes Opinion 6.021, References Opinions 6.02 and 6.021. Spece, *Medical Tourism: Protecting Patients From Conflicts of Interest in Broker's Fees Paid by Foreign Providers, 6 J. Health & Biomedical L. 1, 3, 19 (2010).*

Journal 2007 Examines the effectiveness of banning conflicts of interest in order to promote ethical medical research. Concludes that regulation of research practice should be based on the overall nature of relationships rather than on purely financial issues. Cites Opinion 6.02. Sage, *Some Principles Require Principals: Why Banning "Conflicts Of Interest" Won't Solve Incentive Problems in Biomedical Research, 85 Tex. L. Rev. 1413, 1458 (2007).*

Journal 2006 Discusses the evolution of health law in Virginia. Concludes that the area of health law continues to expand, develop, and be refined. Cites Opinions 3.03, 3.08, 5.01, 5.015, 5.02, 5.04, 5.055, 6.02, 6.021, 6.03, 6.04, 7.03, 7.04, 7.05, 8.054, 8.08, 8.081, 8.085, 8.115, 8.12, 8.14, 8.145, 8.19, and 9.045. Guanzon, *Health Care Law, 41 U. Rich. L. Rev. 179, 199 (2006).*

Journal 2002 Suggests a reconceptualization for bioethics that integrates an analysis of the history of moral change. Concludes that bioethical textbooks should include discussion about the history of bioethics and medical ethics. Quotes Opinion 2.20. References Opinions 6.02, 6.03, 6.04 [now Opinion 8.06], and 8.032. Baker, *Bioethics and History, 27 J. Med. & Phil. 447, 455, 469 (2002).*

Journal 2001 Evaluates current forms of cybermedicine and Internet resources that support it. Explores patient and regulatory concerns, including privacy issues, insurance reimbursement problems, licensure, and liability, which may thwart the growth of cybermedicine. Concludes that cybermedicine may facilitate delivery of cost-effective, quality medical care. Quotes Opinions 5.05, 6.02, and 6.03. Scott, *Cybermedicine and Virtual Pharmacies, 103 W. Va. L. Rev. 407, 441, 451 (2001).*

Journal 1999 Provides a historical account of fee splitting and the corporate practice of medicine doctrine. Suggests that legislation on kickbacks should allow an exception for goods and services supplied at fair market value. Concludes that the legislature's approach to fee splitting should be revised to fit contemporary circumstances. References Opinion 6.02. Jacobs & Goodman, *Splitting Fees or*

Splitting Hairs? Fee Splitting and Health Care—The Florida Experience, 8 Annals Health L. 239, 244 (1999).

Journal 1998 Explores aspects of trust in physician-patient relations. Discusses the transformation of the health care system and the need for regulation. Points out that too much involvement by politicians and legislators will put the health care system at risk. References Opinions 6.02 and 8.03. Mechanic, *The Functions and Limitations of Trust in the Provision of Medical Care,* 23 J. Health Pol. Pol'y & Law 661, 667 (1998).

Journal 1985 Initially describes how existing doctrines protect the value of autonomy in the context of the physician-patient relationship, then examines various problems in the current protective scheme. Concludes by recommending the creation of an independent articulable protected interest in patient autonomy. Quotes Principles II and IV. Cites Opinions 4.04 (1984) [now Opinions 8.03 and 8.032] and 6.03 (1984) [now Opinion 6.02]. Shultz, *From Informed Consent to Patient Choice: A New Protected Interest,* 95 Yale L. J. 219, 275 (1985).

Journal 2003 Discusses financial incentive programs for physicians who enroll patients in clinical trials. Concludes that more regulatory oversight is needed to protect research subjects and the integrity of the medical research process. Quotes Opinions 6.03 and 8.031. Lemmens & Miller, *The Human Subjects Trade: Ethical and Legal Issues Surrounding Recruitment Incentives,* 31 J. L. Med. & Ethics 398, 407 (2003).

Concordance

To aid readers in navigating the updated *Code of Medical Ethics*, the Concordance below maps previous Opinion numbers and titles of the 2014-2015 edition to their new, updated numbers and titles in this 2016 edition.

OPINION NUMBER (2014-2015)	OPINION TITLE (2014-2015)	OPINION NUMBER (2016)	OPINION TITLE (2016)
2.01	Abortion	4.2.7	Abortion
2.015	Mandatory Parental Consent to Abortion	2.2.3	Mandatory Parental Consent to Abortion
2.02	Physicians' Obligations in Preventing, Identifying and Treating Violence and Abuse	8.10	Preventing, Identifying, and Treating Violence and Abuse
2.03	Allocation of Limited Medical Resources	11.1.3	Allocating Limited Health Care Resources
2.035	Futile Care	5.5	Medically Ineffective Interventions
2.037	Medical Futility in End-of-Life Care	5.5	Medically Ineffective Interventions
2.04	Artificial Insemination by Known Donor	4.2.2	Gamete Donation
		4.2.3	Therapeutic Donor Insemination
2.05	Artificial Insemination by Anonymous Donor	4.2.2	Gamete Donation
		4.2.3	Therapeutic Donor Insemination
2.055	Ethical Conduct in Assisted Reproductive Technology	4.2.1	Assisted Reproductive Technology
2.06	Capital Punishment	9.7.3	Capital Punishment
2.065	Court-Initiated Medical Treatments in Clinical Cases	9.7.2	Court-Initiated Medical Treatment in Criminal Cases
2.067	Torture	9.7.5	Torture
2.068	Physician Participation in Interrogation	9.7.4	Physician Participation in Interrogation
2.07	Clinical Investigation	7.1.1	Physician Involvement in Research
		7.1.2	Informed Consent in Research
		7.1.3	Study Design and Sampling
		7.1.5	Misconduct in Research
		7.2.1	Principles for Disseminating Research Results
2.071	Subject Selection for Clinical Trials	7.1.3	Study Design and Sampling
2.075	The Use of Placebo Controls in Clinical Trials	7.1.1	Physician Involvement in Research
		7.3.1	Ethical Use of Placebo Controls in Research

OPINION NUMBER (2014-2015)	OPINION TITLE (2014-2015)	OPINION NUMBER (2016)	OPINION TITLE (2016)
2.076	Surgical "Placebo" Controls	7.3.1	Ethical Use of Placebo Controls in Research
2.077	Ethical Considerations in International Research	7.3.3	International Research
2.078	Guidelines to Prevent Malevolent Use of Biomedical Research	7.1.3	Study Design and Sampling
		7.2.1	Principles for Disseminating Research Results
2.079	Safeguards in the Use of DNA Databanks in Genomic Research	7.3.7	Safeguards in the Use of DNA Databanks
2.08	Commercial Use of Human Tissue	7.3.9	Commercial Use of Human Biological Materials
2.09	Costs	11.3.1	Fees for Medical Services
2.095	The Provision of Adequate Health Care	11.1.1	Defining Basic Health Care
2.10	Fetal Research Guidelines	7.3.4	Maternal-Fetal Research
		7.3.5	Research Using Human Fetal Tissue
2.105	Patenting Human Genes	7.2.3	Patents and Dissemination of Research Products
2.11	Gene Therapy	7.3.6	Research in Gene Therapy and Genetic Engineering
2.12	Genetic Counseling	4.1.1	Genetic Testing and Counseling
		4.1.2	Genetic Testing for Reproductive Decision Making
2.13	Genetic Engineering	7.3.6	Research in Gene Therapy and Genetic Engineering
2.131	Disclosure of Familial Risk in Genetic Testing	4.1.1	Genetic Testing and Counseling
2.132	Genetic Testing by Employers	4.1.3	Third-Party Access to Genetic Information
2.135	Insurance Companies and Genetic Information	4.1.3	Third-Party Access to Genetic Information
2.136	Genetic Information and the Criminal Justice System	4.1.4	Forensic Genetics
2.137	Ethical Issues in Carrier Screening of Genetic Disorders	4.1.3	Third-Party Access to Genetic Information
2.138	Genetic Testing of Children	2.2.5	Genetic Testing of Children
2.139	Multiplex Genetic Testing	4.1.1	Genetic Testing and Counseling
2.14	In Vitro Fertilization	4.2.1	Assisted Reproductive Technology
2.141	Frozen Pre-Embryos	4.2.5	Storage and Use of Human Embryos
2.145	Pre-Embryo Splitting	—	*Withdrawn*
2.146	Research with Stem Cells	7.3.8	Research with Stem Cells
2.147	Cloning to Produce Children	4.2.6	Cloning for Reproduction
2.15	Transplantation of Organs from Living Donors	6.1.1	Transplantation of Organs from Living Donors
2.151	Cadaveric Organ Donation: Encouraging the Study of Motivation	6.1.3	Studying Financial Incentives for Cadaveric Organ Donation
2.152	Solicitation of the Public for Directed Donation of Organs for Transplantation	6.2.2	Directed Donation of Organs for Transplantation

OPINION NUMBER (2014-2015)	OPINION TITLE (2014-2015)	OPINION NUMBER (2016)	OPINION TITLE (2016)
2.155	Presumed Consent and Mandated Choice for Organs from Deceased Donors	6.1.4	Presumed Consent and Mandated Choice for Organs from Deceased Donors
2.157	Organ Donation After Cardiac Death	6.1.2	Organ Donation After Cardiac Death
2.16	Organ Transplantation Guidelines	6.2.1	Guidance for Organ Transplantation from Deceased Donors
2.161	Medical Applications of Fetal Tissue Transplantation	7.3.5	Research Using Human Fetal Tissue
2.162	Anencephalic Neonates as Organ Donors	6.1.6	Anencephalic Newborns as Organ Donors
2.165	Umbilical Cord Blood Banking	6.1.5	Umbilical Cord Blood Banking
2.169	The Ethical Implications of Xenotransplantation	6.3.1	Xenotransplantation
2.17	*Quality of Life*	—	*Withdrawn*
2.18	Surrogate Mothers	4.2.4	Third-Party Reproduction
2.19	Unnecessary Medical Services	11.3.1	Fees for Medical Services
2.191	Advance Care Planning	5.1	Advance Care Planning
2.20	Withholding or Withdrawing Life-Sustaining Medical Treatment	5.3	Withholding or Withdrawing Life-Sustaining Treatment
2.201	Sedation to Unconsciousness in End-of-Life Care	5.6	Sedation to Unconsciousness in End-of-Life Care
2.21	Euthanasia	5.8	Euthanasia
2.211	Physician-Assisted Suicide	5.7	Physician-Assisted Suicide
2.215	Treatment Decisions for Seriously Ill Newborns	2.2.4	Treatment Decisions for Seriously Ill Newborns
2.22	Do-Not-Resuscitate Orders	5.4	Orders Not to Attempt Resuscitation (DNAR)
2.225	Optimal Use of Orders Not-to-Intervene and Advance Directives	5.2	Advance Directives
2.23	HIV Testing	8.1	Routine Universal Screening for HIV
2.24	Impaired Drivers and Their Physicians	8.2	Impaired Drivers and Their Physicians
2.25	The Use of Quarantine and Isolation as Public Health Interventions	8.4	Ethical Use of Quarantine and Isolation
2.30	Information from Unethical Experiments	7.2.2	Release of Data from Unethical Experiments
2.40	Radio Frequency ID Devices in Humans	1.2.9	Use of Remote Sensing and Monitoring Devices
3.01	*Nonscientific Practitioners*	—	*Withdrawn*
3.02	Nurses	10.4	Nurses
3.03	Allied Health Professionals	10.5	Allied Health Professionals
3.04	Referral of Patients	1.2.3	Consultation, Referral and Second Opinions
3.041	*Chiropractic*	-	*Proposed to withdraw*
3.05	Physician Employment by a Nonphysician Supervisee	10.2	Physician Employment by a Nonphysician Supervisee
3.06	Sports Medicine	1.2.5	Sports Medicine

OPINION NUMBER (2014-2015)	OPINION TITLE (2014-2015)	OPINION NUMBER (2016)	OPINION TITLE (2016)
3.08	Sexual Harassment and Exploitation Between Medical Supervisors and Trainees	9.1.3	Sexual Harassment in the Practice of Medicine
3.09	Medical Students Performing Procedures on Fellow Students	9.2.5	Medical Students Practicing Clinical Skills on Fellow Students
4.01	Admission Fee	11.3.1	Fees for Medical Services
4.02	*Assessment, Compulsory*	—	*Withdrawn*
4.03	Billing for Housestaff and Student Services	11.3.1	Fees for Medical Services
4.04	Economic Incentives and Levels of Care	11.2.2	Conflicts of Interest in Patient Care
4.05	Organized Medical Staff	9.5.1	Organized Medical Staff
4.06	Physician-Hospital Contractual Relations	11.2.3	Contracts to Deliver Health Care Services
4.07	Staff Privileges	9.5.2	Staff Privileges
5.01	*Advertising and Managed Care*	—	*Withdrawn*
5.015	Direct-to-Consumer Advertisements of Prescription Drugs	9.6.7	Direct-to-Consumer Advertisement of Prescription Drugs
5.02	Advertising and Publicity	9.6.1	Advertising and Publicity
5.025	Physician Advisory or Referral Services by Telecommunication	2.3.1	Health Information Sites and Services Outside of Patient-Physician Relationships
5.026	The Use of Electronic Mail	2.3.2	Electronic Communication with Patients
5.027	Use of Health-Related Online Sites	1.2.12	Ethical Practice in Technology
5.04	Communications Media: Standards of Professional Responsibility	3.1.5	Professionalism in Relationships with Media
5.045	Filming Patients in Health Care Settings for Public Education	3.1.4	Audio or Visual Recording Patients for Public Education
5.046	Filming Patients for the Education of Health Care Professionals	3.1.3	Audio or Visual Recording Patients for Education in Health Care
5.05	Confidentiality	3.2.1	Confidentiality
5.051	Confidentiality of Medical Information Postmortem	3.2.2	Confidentiality Postmortem
5.055	Confidential Care for Minors	2.2.2	Confidential Health Care for Minors
5.059	Privacy in the Context of Health Care	3.1.1	Privacy in Health Care
5.0591	Patient Privacy and Outside Observers to the Clinical Encounter	3.1.2	Patient Privacy and Outside Observers of the Clinical Encounter
5.06	*Confidentiality: Attorney-Physician Relation*	—	*Withdrawn*
5.07	Confidentiality: Computers	3.3.2	Confidentiality and Electronic Medical Records
5.075	Confidentiality: Disclosure of Records to Data Collection Companies	3.2.4	Access to Medical Records by Data Collection Companies
5.08	*Confidentiality: Release of Information to Insurance Company Representatives*	—	*Withdrawn*
5.09	Confidentiality: Industry-Employed Physicians and Independent Medical Examiners	3.2.3	Industry-Employed Physicians and Independent Medical Examiners

OPINION NUMBER (2014-2015)	OPINION TITLE (2014-2015)	OPINION NUMBER (2016)	OPINION TITLE (2016)
5.10	A Physician's Role Following a Breach of Electronic Health Information	3.3.3	Breach of Security in Electronic Medical Records
6.01	Contingent Fees	11.3.1	Fees for Medical Services
6.02	Fee Splitting	11.3.4	Fee Splitting
6.021	Financial Incentives to Patients for Referral	9.6.3	Incentives to Patients for Referrals
6.03	Fee Splitting: Referrals	11.3.4	Fee Splitting
6.05	Fees for Medical Services	11.3.1	Fees for Medical Services
6.07	Insurance Form Completion Charges	11.3.2	Fees for Nonclinical and Administrative Services
6.08	Interest Charges and Finance Charges	11.3.3	Interest and Finance Charges
6.09	Laboratory Services	11.3.1	Fees for Medical Services
6.10	Services by Multiple Physicians	11.3.1	Fees for Medical Services
6.12	Forgiveness or Waiver of Insurance Copayment	11.1.4	Financial Barriers to Health Care Access
6.13	Professional Courtesy	11.3.1	Fees for Medical Services
7.01	Records of Physicians: Availability of Information to Other Physicians	3.3.1	Management of Medical Records
7.02	Records of Physicians: Information and Patients	3.3.1	Management of Medical Records
7.025	Records of Physicians: Access by Non-Treating Medical Staff	3.3.1	Management of Medical Records
7.03	Records of a Physician Upon Retirement or Departure from a Group	3.3.1	Management of Medical Records
7.04	Sale of a Medical Practice	3.3.1	Management of Medical Records
7.05	Retention of Medical Records	3.3.1	Management of Medical Records
8.01	Missed Appointment Charges	11.3.2	Fees for Nonclinical and Administrative Services
8.02	Ethical Guidelines for Physicians in Administrative or Other Non-Clinical Roles	10.1	Ethics Guidance for Physicians in Nonclinical Roles
8.021	Ethical Obligations of Medical Directors	10.1.1	Ethical Obligations of Medical Directors
8.03	Conflicts of Interest: Guidelines	11.2.2	Conflicts of Interest in Patient Care
8.031	Conflicts of Interest: Biomedical Research	7.1.1	Physician Involvement in Research
		7.1.4	Conflicts of Interest in Research
8.0315	Managing Conflicts of Interest in the Conduct of Clinical Trials	7.1.1	Physician Involvement in Research
		7.1.2	Informed Consent in Research
		7.1.4	Conflicts of Interest in Research
8.0321	Physician Self-Referral	9.6.9	Physician Self-referral
8.04	Consultation	1.2.3	Consultation, Referral, and Second Opinions
8.041	Second Opinions	1.2.3	Consultation, Referral, and Second Opinions
8.043	Ethical Implications of Surgical Co-Management	2.3.7	Surgical Co-management

OPINION NUMBER (2014-2015)	OPINION TITLE (2014-2015)	OPINION NUMBER (2016)	OPINION TITLE (2016)
8.045	Direct-to-Consumer Diagnostic Imaging Tests	9.6.8	Direct-to-Consumer Diagnostic Imaging Tests
8.047	Industry Representatives in Clinical Settings	10.6	Industry Representatives in Clinical Settings
8.05	Contractual Relations	11.2.1	Professionalism in Health Care Systems
		11.2.3	Contracts to Deliver Health Care Services
8.0501	Professionalism and Contractual Relations	11.2.1	Professionalism in Health Care Systems
		11.2.3	Contracts to Deliver Health Care Services
8.051	Conflicts of Interest Under Capitation	11.2.1	Professionalism in Health Care Systems
		11.2.4	Transparency in Health Care
8.052	Negotiating Discounts for Specialty Care	1.2.3	Consultation, Referral, and Second Opinions
		11.3.4	Fee Splitting
8.053	Restrictions on Disclosure in Health Care Plan Contracts	11.2.3	Contracts to Deliver Health Care Services
		11.2.4	Transparency in Health Care
8.054	Financial Incentives and the Practice of Medicine	11.2.1	Professionalism in Health Care Systems
		11.2.3	Contracts to Deliver Health Care Services
		11.2.4	Transparency in Health Care
8.055	Retainer Practices	11.2.5	Retainer Practices
8.056	Physician Pay-for-Performance Programs	11.2.1	Professionalism in Health Care Systems
		11.2.3	Contracts to Deliver Health Care Services
8.06	Prescribing and Dispensing Drugs and Devices	9.6.6	Prescribing and Dispensing Drugs and Devices
8.061	Gifts to Physicians from Industry	9.6.2	Gifts to Physicians from Industry
8.062	Sale of Non-Health-Related Goods from Physicians' Offices	9.6.5	Sale of Non-Health-Related Goods
8.063	Sale of Health-Related Products from Physicians' Offices	9.6.4	Sale of Health-Related Products
8.07	Expedited Partner Therapy	8.9	Expedited Partner Therapy
8.08	Informed Consent	2.1.1	Informed Consent
8.081	Surrogate Decision Making	2.1.2	Decisions for Adult Patients Who Lack Capacity
8.082	Withholding Clinical Information from Patients	2.1.3	Withholding Information from Patients
8.083	Placebo Use in Clinical Practice	2.1.4	Use of Placebo in Clinical Practice
8.085	Waiver of Informed Consent for Research in Emergency Situations	7.1.2	Informed Consent in Research
		7.3.2	Research on Emergency Medical Interventions
8.087	Medical Student Involvement in Patient Care	9.2.1	Medical Student Involvement in Patient Care
8.088	Resident Physicians' Involvement in Patient Care	9.2.2	Resident and Fellow Physicians' Involvement in Patient Care

OPINION NUMBER (2014-2015)	OPINION TITLE (2014-2015)	OPINION NUMBER (2016)	OPINION TITLE (2016)
8.09	Laboratory Services	1.2.3	Consultation, Referral, and Second Opinions
		11.3.1	Fees for Medical Services
		11.3.2	Fees for Nonclinical and Administrative Services
8.095	Reporting Test Results: General Guidelines	2.1.5	Reporting Clinical Test Results
8.1	*Lien Laws*	—	*Withdrawn*
8.11	*Neglect of Patient*	—	*Withdrawn*
8.115	Termination of the Physician-Patient Relationship	1.1.5	Terminating a Patient-Physician Relationship
8.12	Patient Information	8.6	Promoting Patient Safety
8.121	Ethical Responsibility to Study and Prevent Error and Harm	8.6	Promoting Patient Safety
8.13	Managed Care	11.2.1	Professionalism in Health Care Systems
		11.2.3	Contracts to Deliver Health Care Services
		11.2.4	Transparency in Health Care
8.132	Referral of Patients	11.2.2	Conflicts of Interest in Patient Care
		11.2.4	Transparency in Health Care
8.135	Cost Containment Involving Prescription Drugs in Health Care Plans	11.2.1	Professionalism in Health Care Systems
		11.2.4	Transparency in Health Care
8.14	Sexual Misconduct in the Practice of Medicine	9.1.1	Romantic or Sexual Relationships with Patients
8.145	Sexual or Romantic Relations Between Physicians and Key Third Parties	9.1.2	Romantic or Sexual Relationships with Key Third Parties
8.15	Substance Abuse	9.3.1	Physician Health and Wellness
8.16	Substitution of Surgeon without Patient's Knowledge or Consent	2.1.6	Substitution of Surgeon
8.17	Use of Restraints	1.2.7	Use of Restraints
8.18	Informing Families of a Patient's Death	2.3.4	Informing Families of a Patient's Death
8.181	Performing Procedures on the Newly Deceased for Training Purposes	9.2.3	Performing Procedures on the Newly Deceased
8.19	Self-Treatment or Treatment of Immediate Family Members	1.2.1	Treating Self or Family
8.191	Peers as Patients	10.3	Peers as Patients
8.21	Use of Chaperones During Physical Exams	1.2.4	Use of Chaperones
9.01	Accreditation	9.5.3	Accreditation
9.011	Continuing Medical Education	9.2.6	Continuing Medical Education
9.0115	Financial Relationships with Industry in Continuing Medical Education	9.2.7	Financial Relationships with Industry in Continuing Medical Education
9.012	Physicians' Political Communications with Patients and Their Families	2.3.5	Political Communications
9.02	Restrictive Covenants	11.2.3.1	Restrictive Covenants

OPINION NUMBER (2014-2015)	OPINION TITLE (2014-2015)	OPINION NUMBER (2016)	OPINION TITLE (2016)
9.021	Covenants-Not-to-Compete for Physicians-in-Training	11.2.3.1	Restrictive Covenants
9.025	Advocacy for Change in Law and Policy	1.2.10	Political Action by Physicians
9.03	Civil Rights and Professional Responsibility	9.5.4	Civil Rights and Medical Professionals
9.0305	Physician Health and Wellness	9.3.1	Physician Health and Wellness
		9.3.2	Physician Responsibilities to Impaired Colleagues
9.031	Reporting Impaired, Incompetent or Unethical Colleagues	9.3.2	Physician Responsibilities to Impaired Colleagues
		9.4.2	Reporting Incompetent or Unethical Behavior by Colleagues
9.032	Reporting Adverse Drug or Device Events	8.8	Required Reporting of Adverse Events
9.035	Gender Discrimination in the Medical Profession	9.5.5	Gender Discrimination in Medicine
9.037	*Signing Bonuses*	—	*Withdrawn*
9.04	Discipline and Medicine	9.4.2	Reporting Incompetent or Unethical Behavior by Colleagues
		9.4.3	Discipline and Medicine
9.045	Physicians with Disruptive Behavior	9.4.4	Physicians with Disruptive Behavior
9.05	Due Process	9.4.1	Peer Review and Due Process
9.055	Disputes Between Medical Supervisors and Trainees	9.2.4	Disputes Between Medical Supervisors and Trainees
9.06	*Free Choice*	—	*Withdrawn*
9.065	Caring for the Poor	11.1.4	Financial Barriers to Health Care Access
9.0651	Financial Barriers to Health Care Access	11.1.4	Financial Barriers to Health Care Access
9.0652	Physician Stewardship of Health Care Resources	11.1.2	Physician Stewardship of Health Care Resources
9.067	Physician Obligation in Disaster Preparedness and Response	8.3	Physicians' Responsibilities in Disaster Response and Preparedness
9.07	Medical Testimony	9.7.1	Medical Testimony
9.08	New Medical Procedures	7.2.1	Principles for Disseminating Research Results
9.09	Patent for Surgical or Diagnostic Instrument	7.2.3	Patents and Dissemination of Research Products
9.095	The Use of Patents and Others Means to Limit Availability of Medical Procedures	7.2.1	Principles for Disseminating Research Results
		7.2.3	Patents and Dissemination of Research Products
9.10	Peer Review	9.4.1	Peer Review and Due Process
9.11	Ethics Committees in Health Care Institutions	10.7	Ethics Committees in Health Care Institutions
9.115	Ethics Consultations	10.7.1	Ethics Consultations
9.12	*Patient-Physician Relationship: Respect for Law and Human Rights*	—	*Withdrawn*

OPINION NUMBER (2014-2015)	OPINION TITLE (2014-2015)	OPINION NUMBER (2016)	OPINION TITLE (2016)
9.121	Racial and Ethnic Health Care Disparities	8.5	Disparities in Health Care
9.122	Gender Disparities in Health Care	8.5	Disparities in Health Care
9.123	Disrespect and Derogatory Conduct in the Patient-Physician Relationship	1.2.2	Disruptive Behavior by Patients
9.124	Professionalism in the Use of Social Media	2.3.3	Professionalism in the Use of Social Media
9.13	Physicians and Infectious Diseases	9.3.1	Physician Health and Wellness
9.131	*HIV-Infected Patients*	—	*Withdrawn*
9.132	Health Care Fraud and Abuse	11.3.1	Fees for Medical Services
9.133	Routine Universal Immunization of Physicians for Vaccine-Preventable Disease	8.7	Routine Universal Immunization of Physicians
9.14	Quality	1.1.6	Quality
10.01	Fundamental Elements of the Patient-Physician Relationship	1.1.3	Patient Rights
10.015	The Patient-Physician Relationship	1.1.1	Patient-Physician Relationships
10.016	Pediatric Decision-Making	2.2.1	Pediatric Decision Making
10.017	Gifts from Patients	1.2.8	Gifts from Patients
10.018	Physician Participation in Soliciting Contributions from Patients	2.3.6	Soliciting Charitable Contributions from Patients
10.02	Patient Responsibilities	1.1.4	Patient Responsibilities
10.03	Patient-Physician Relationship in the Context of Work-Related and Independent Medical Examinations	1.2.6	Work-Related and Independent Medical Examinations
10.05	Potential Patients	1.1.2	Prospective Patients
10.06	Physician Exercise of Conscience	1.1.7	Physician Exercise of Conscience

Index of Cases

The cases below cross-reference the relevant provision(s) of the version of the Principles and Opinions as they appeared in the 2014-2015 edition of the *Code of Medical Ethics (Code)*. The Concordance maps the updated Opinions in the present volume to their predecessors in the 2014-2015 edition of the *Code*.

Index of Articles

The articles below cross-reference the relevant provision(s) of the version of the Principles and Opinions as they appeared in the 2014-2015 edition of the *Code of Medical Ethics (Code)*. The Concordance maps the updated Opinions in the present volume to their predecessors in the 2014-2015 edition of the *Code*.

American Bar Association Task Force on Mental Disability and the Death Penalty (Igasaki et al), *Recommendation and Report on the Death Penalty and Persons With Mental Disabilities*, 30 Mental & Physical Disability L. Rep. 668, 676 (2006) [2.06].

Anderson, *A Medical-Legal Dilemma: When Can "Inappropriate" Nutrition and Hydration Be Removed in Indiana?* 67 Ind. L. J. 479, 480 (1992) [2.20].

Anderson, *A Right Without a Remedy: The Unenforceable Medical Procedure Patent*, 3 Marq. Intell. Prop. L. Rev. 117, 132, 140 (1999) [9.08, 9.09].

Anderson, *Distinguishing Patentable Process Claims From Unpatentable Laws of Nature in the Medical Technology Field*, 59 Ala. L. Rev. 1203 (2008) [9.08].

Andrews, *Harnessing the Benefits of Biobanks*, 33 J. L. Med. & Ethics 22, 25 (2005) [2.08].

Andrews, *The Gene Patent Dilemma: Balancing Commercial Incentives With Health Needs*, 2 Hous. J. Health L. & Pol'y 65, 74, 104 (2002) [2.08, 9.095].

Andrews, *Two Perspectives: Rights of Donors: Who Owns Your Body? A Patient's Perspective on Washington University v. Catalona*, 34 J. L. Med. & Ethics 398, 404 (2006) [2.08].

Andrews & Jaeger, *Confidentiality of Genetic Information in the Workplace*, XVII Am. J. Law & Med. 75, 78 (1991) [5.05].

Annas, *Toxic Tinkering—Lethal-Injection Execution and the Constitution*, 359 New Engl. J. Med. 1512 (2009) [2.06].

Annas, Glantz, & Mariner, *The Right of Privacy Protects the Doctor-Patient Relationship*, 263 JAMA 858, 861 (1990) [2.20].

Antommaria, *Conscientious Objection in Clinical Practice: Notice, Informed Consent, Referral, and Emergency Treatment*, 9 Ave Maria L. Rev. 81, 98 (2010) [8.115].

Antommaria, *How Can I Give Her IV Antibiotics at Home When I Have Three Other Children to Care For? Using Dispute System Design to Address Patient Provider Conflicts in Health Care*, 29 Hamline J. Pub. L. & Pol'y 273 (2008) [8.115].

Appelbaum, Jorgenson, & Sutherland, *Sexual Relationships Between Physicians and Patients*, 154 Arch. Intern. Med. 2561, 2561 (1994) [8.14].

Aral, Mosher, & Cates, *Self-reported Pelvic Inflammatory Disease in the United States, 1988*, 266 JAMA 2570, 2573 (1991) [9.121].

Ares, *An Uncommon Skin Condition Illustrates the Need for Caution When Prescribing for Friends*, 20 J. Am. Acad. of Nurse Prac. 389, 390 (2008) [8.115, 8.19].

Ariens, *"Playing Chicken": An Instant History of the Battle Over Exceptions to Client Confidences*, 33 J. Legal Prof. 239 (2009) [IV].

Ashburn, Wilson, & Eisenstein, *Human Tissue Research in the Genomic Era of Medicine*, 160 Arch. Intern. Med. 3377, 3378 (2000) [2.132].

Avraham, *Private Regulation*, 34 Harv. J. L. & Pub. Pol'y 543, 614-15 (2011) [III].

Awad, *Attorney-Client Sexual Relations*, 22 J. Legal. Prof. 131, 190 (1998) [8.14].

Bagley, *Patent First, Ask Questions Later: Morality and Biotechnology in Patent Law*, 45 Wm. & Mary L. Rev. 469, 500 (2003) [9.095].

Bahnassi, *Keeping Doctors Out of the Interrogation Room: A New Ethical Obligation That Requires the Backing of the Law*, 19 Health Matrix 447 (2009) [Preamble; 2.06, 2.067, 2.068].

Bailey, *The Legal, Financial, and Ethical Implications of Online Medical Consultations*, 16 J. Tech. L. & Pol'y 53, 95 (2011) [10.015].

Baker, *Bioethics and History*, 27 J. Med. & Phil. 447, 455, 469 (2002) [2.20, 6.02, 6.03, 8.032, 8.06].

Baker, *In Defense of Bioethics*, 37 J. of Law, Med. and Ethics 83, 87 (2009) [3.01].

Baker & Emanuel, *The Efficacy of Professional Ethics: The AMA Code of Ethics in Historical and Current Perspective*, 30 Hastings Center Rep. S13, S14 (July/Aug. 2000) [I].

Balint, *Issues of Privacy and Confidentiality in the New Genetics*, 9 Alb. L. J. Sci. & Tech. 27, 32 (1998) [IV].

Banks, *Legal and Ethical Safeguards: Protection of Society's Most Vulnerable Participants in a Commercialized Organ Transplantation System*, XXI Am. J. Law & Med. 45, 77, 79, 95-96, 103-04 (1995) [2.15, 2.167].

199 Am. J. Obstet. Gynecol. 232.e1, 232.e1 (2008) [10.01].

Cherry, *Polymorphic Medical Ontologies: Fashioning Concepts of Disease, 25 J. Med. & Phil. 519, 532 (2000)* [2.03].

Childress, *Ethics, Public Policy, and Human Fetal Tissue Transplantation Research, 1 Kennedy Inst. Ethics J. 93, 116 (June 1991)* [2.10].

Childress, *The Failure to Give: Reducing Barriers to Organ Donation, 11 Kennedy Inst. Ethics J. 1, 13, 14 (2001)* [2.155].

Chopko, *Responsible Public Policy at the End of Life, 75 U. Det. Mercy L. Rev. 557, 573 (1998)* [2.211].

Chouhan & Draper, *Modified Mandated Choice for Organ Procurement, 29 J. Med. Ethics 157, 162 (2003)* [2.155].

Chow, *Health Courts: An Extreme Makeover of Medical Malpractice With Potentially Fatal Complications, 7 Yale J. Health Pol'y L. & Ethics 387, 399 (2007)* [9.07].

Christensen & Orlowski, *Iatrogenic Cardiopulmonary Arrests in DNR Patients, 11 J. Clinical Ethics 14, 15, 20 (2000)* [2.22].

Chudoba, *Conscience in America: The Slippery Slope of Mixing Morality With Medicine, 36 Sw. U. L. Rev. 85, 86, 103, 104, 105 (2007)* [Preamble; V, VI, VIII].

Cibas, Alexander, Benson, Patricio de Agustín, Doherty, Faquin, Middleton, Miller, Raab, White, & Mandel, *Indications for Thyroid FNA and Pre-FNA Requirements: A Synopsis of the National Cancer Institute Thyroid Fine-Needle Aspiration State of the Science Conference, 36 Diagnostic Cytopathology 390, 394 (2008)* [8.08].

Clark, *Autonomy and Death, 71 Tul. L. Rev. 45, 89 (1996)* [2.21, 2.211].

Clark, *Confidential Communications in a Professional Context: Attorney, Physician, and Social Worker, 24 J. Legal Prof. 79, 92 (2000)* [5.05].

Clark, *Medical Ethics at Guantanamo Bay and Abu Ghraib: The Problem of Dual Loyalty, 34 J. L. Med. & Ethics 570, 573 (2006)* [2.067].

Clark, *Medication Errors in Family Practice, in Hospitals and After Discharge From the Hospital: An Ethical Analysis, 32 J. L. Med & Ethics 349, 354 (2004)* [10.01].

Clark, *Oregon's Death with Dignity Act and Alleged Patient Euthanasia After Hurricane Katrina—The Government's Role, 18 Health Lawyer 1, 8 (2006)* [2.211].

Clayton, *The Web of Relations: Thinking About Physicians and Patients, 6 Yale J. Health Pol'y, L. & Ethics 465, 473 (2006)* [8.061].

Clemmens, *Creating Human Embryos for Research: A Scientist's Perspective on Managing the Legal and Ethical Issues, 2 Ind. Health L. Rev. 95, 99 (2005)* [2.14].

Closen, *HIV-AIDS, Infected Surgeons and Dentists, and the Medical Profession's Betrayal of Its Responsibility to Patients, 41 N. Y. L. Sch. L. Rev. 57, 65, 71-72, 129 (1996)* [9.131].

Cohen, *An Examination of the Right of Hospitals to Engage in Economic Credentialing, 77 Temp. L. Rev. 705, 741 (2004)* [8.032].

Cohen, *Holistic Health Care: Including Alternative and Complementary Medicine in Insurance and Regulatory Schemes, 38 Ariz. L. Rev. 83, 92 (1996)* [3.01].

Cohen, *The Open Door: Will the Right to Die Survive Washington v. Glucksberg and Vacco v. Quill? 16 In Pub. Interest 79, 94 (1998)* [2.20, 2.211].

Cohen, *Toward a Bioethics of Compassion, 28 Ind. L. Rev. 667, 673, 681-82, 683 (1995)* [2.01, 2.211, 8.18].

Cohen & Cohen, *Required Reconsideration of "Do-Not-Resuscitate" Orders in the Operating Room and Certain Other Treatment Settings, 20 Law Med. & Health Care 354, 356 (1992)* [2.22].

Cohen, Dicecco, & Levin, *Failure to Communicate: When It Comes to Hospital Patient Care, Communication Between Doctor and Nurse Should Be Seamless. If It's Not, Patients Suffer. Here's How to Find Out if a Miscommunication Is at the Core of Your Client's Case, 46 Trial 38, 40-41 (May 2010)* [3.02, 9.045].

Cohen-Almagor, *A Critique of Callahan's Utilitarian Approach to Resource Allocation in Health Care, 17 Issues L. & Med. 247, 261 (2002)* [2.037].

Cohn, Berger, Holzman, Lockhart, Reuben, Robertson, & Selbst, *Guidelines for Expert Witness Testimony in Medical Liability Cases, 94 Pediatrics 755, 756 (1994)* [9.07].

Index

This edition of the *Code of Medical Ethics* has been revised and modernized, and the index reflects this. Subject headings follow natural phrases more frequently than in the past. For example, previous editions used inverted headings, such as "Education, medical." In this edition, the term, "Medical education" is used instead. Also, because of Opinion updates, previous topics/subject headings have been consolidated. Two prime examples of this are the current headings "Minors" and "Violence." Earlier indexes listed "Adolescence," "Children," etc. But these are now all consolidated under "Minors." Similarly, specific types of violence and abuse were listed in such headings as "Child abuse," "Intimate partner violence," etc. These are all consolidated under "Violence."

Pages in this index that appear in italics refer to Annotations of Opinions, which are found on pages *249-453*.

E

Q